IMMUNOLOGIC AND INFECTIOUS REACTIONS IN THE LUNG

Edited by

Charles H. Kirkpatrick
Herbert Y. Reynolds

National Institute of Allergy
and Infectious Disease
National Institutes of Health
Bethesda, Maryland

MARCEL DEKKER, INC.   New York and Basel

CONTRIBUTORS

Malcolm S. Artenstein, M.D.   Chief, Department of Bacterial Diseases, Walter Reed Army Institute of Research, Washington, D.C.

John R. Benfield, M.D.   Professor of Surgery, University of California at Los Angeles School of Medicine, and Chief of Pulmonary Surgery, Harbor General Hospital, Torrance, California

John Bienenstock, M.D.   Professor of Medicine and Associate Professor of Pathology, McMaster University Medical Center, Hamilton, Ontario, Canada

Rebecca H. Buckley, M.D.   Associate Professor of Pediatrics and Immunology, Duke University School of Medicine, Durham, North Carolina

Antonino Catanzaro, M.D.   Assistant Professor of Medicine, University of California at San Diego School of Medicine, San Diego, California

Robert M. Chanock, M.D.   Chief, Laboratory of Infectious Diseases, National Institute of Allergy and Infectious Diseases, National Institutes of Health, Bethesda, Maryland

Robert L. Clancy, M.D.   Assistant Professor of Medicine, McMaster University Medical Center, Hamilton, Ontario, Canada

Wallace A. Clyde, Jr., M.D.   Professor of Pediatrics and Bacteriology, University of North Carolina School of Medicine, Chapel Hill, North Carolina

Davis C. Dale, M.D.*   Senior Investigator, Clinical Physiology Section, Laboratory of Clinical Investigation, National Institute of Allergy and Infectious Diseases, National Institutes of Health, Bethesda, Maryland

Anthony S. Fauci, M.D.   Senior Investigator and Head, Clinical Physiology Section, Laboratory of Clinical Investigation, National Institute of Allergy and Infectious Diseases, National Institutes of Health, Bethesda, Maryland

---

Present Affiliation
*Associate Professor of Medicine, University of Washington School of Medicine, Seattle, Washington

Gerald W. Fernald, M.D.   Associate Professor of Pediatrics, The University of North Carolina School of Medicine, Chapel Hill, North Carolina

Jordan N. Fink, M.D.   Professor of Medicine, The Medical College of Wisconsin, Milwaukee, Wisconsin

John I. Gallin, M.D.   Senior Investigator, Clinical Physiology Section, Laboratory of Clinical Investigation, National Institute of Allergy and Infectious Diseases, National Institutes of Health, Bethesda, Maryland

Christopher S. Henney, Ph.D.   Associate Professor of Medicine, Division of Immunology, The Johns Hopkins University School of Medicine, Baltimore, Maryland

H. Benfer Kaltreider, M.D.   Assistant Professor of Medicine and Co-Chief, Respiratory Care, San Francisco Veterans Administration Hospital, University of California School of Medicine, San Francisco, California

Allen P. Kaplan, M.D.   Senior Investigator and Head, Allergic Diseases Section, Laboratory of Clinical Investigation, National Institute of Allergy and Infectious Diseases, National Institutes of Health, Bethesda, Maryland

Charles H. Kirkpatrick, M.D.   Senior Investigator and Head, Clinical Allergy and Hypersensitivity Section, Laboratory of Clinical Investigation, National Institute of Allergy and Infectious Diseases, National Institutes of Health, Bethesda, Maryland

Bernard B. Levine, M.D.   Professor of Medicine, New York University School of Medicine, New York, New York

Harold H. Newball, M.D.*   Staff Associate, Pulmonary Branch, National Heart and Lung Institute, The Johns Hopkins University School of Medicine, Baltimore, Maryland

Philip S. Norman, M.D.†   Professor of Medicine, The Johns Hopkins University School of Medicine, Baltimore, Maryland

Eric A. Ottesen, M.D.‡   Senior Staff Associate, Laboratory of Clinical Investigation, National Institute of Allergy and Infectious Diseases, National Institutes of Health, Bethesda, Maryland

Robert M. Parrott, M.D.   Director, Children's Hospital National Medical Center, and Chairman, Department of Child Health and Development, George Washington University School of Health Sciences, Washington, D.C.

Present Affiliation
*Assistant Professor, Department of Respiratory Diseases, The Johns Hopkins University School of Medicine, Baltimore, Maryland
†Professor of Medicine, Good Samaritan Hospital, Baltimore, Maryland
‡Laboratory of Parasitic Diseases, National Institute of Allergy and Infectious Diseases, National Institutes of Health, Baltimore, Maryland

James E. Pennington, M.D.* Senior Staff Associate, Laboratory of Clinical Investigation, National Institute of Allergy and Infectious Diseases, National Institutes of Health, Bethesda, Maryland

Daniel Y. E. Perey, M.D. Associate Professor of Pathology, Host Resistance Programme, McMaster University Medical Center, Hamilton, Ontario, Canada

Stephen H. Polmar, Ph.D., M.D. Assistant Professor of Pediatrics, Case Western Reserve University School of Medicine, Cleveland, Ohio

Herbert Y. Reynolds, M.D. Senior Investigator and Head, Bacterial Diseases Section, Laboratory of Clinical Investigation, National Institute of Allergy and Infectious Diseases, National Institutes of Health, Bethesda, Maryland

Edward C. Rosenow III, M.D. Consultant, Division of Thoracic Diseases and Internal Medicine, Mayo Clinic and Mayo Foundation, and Assistant Professor of Medicine, Mayo Medical School, Rochester, Minnesota

Lynn Spitler, M.D. Assistant Professor of Medicine, University of California School of Medicine, San Francisco, California

Present Affiliation
*Peter Bent Brigham Hospital and Harvard Medical School, Boston, Massachusetts

FOREWORD

Many techniques for updating and assimilating new information in medicine have been proposed. As scientific reports proliferate, we hear shrill complaints about the amount of material that must be covered by the scientist and the physician in order to "keep up" with the latest and best information. There is no substitute for review by an expert to help others interpret the significance of new data and concepts.

This series of monographs is both expert and timely. There has been an expansion of research on respiratory and pulmonary problems. This expansion reflects a renewed public awareness of the importance of lung disease and a new awareness by researchers of opportunity to apply modern biological techniques to the study of the lung in health and disease.

It is my view that this series makes a comprehensive contribution to the science and practice of medicine and to the hopes we have for more effective concepts of preventive medicine.

Theodore Cooper, M. D.
Assistant Secretary for Health
Department of Health, Education,
and Welfare

PREFACE

One of the principal contacts the human organism has with his environment is the 10,000 or so liters of ambient air that enters and leaves the respiratory tract during normal daily activities, Inspired air, which has so many essential ingredients for survival, also contains noxious gases and a variety of particulate materials which must be cleared or excluded from the lungs to maintain good health. To accomplish this the respiratory tract is equipped with a variety of physical and cellular mechanisms for defense against the hostile elements in air. Green has described this complex system as an umbrella of defense.*

Deposition of large particles in the lungs is prevented by anatomic filtration in the nose and the turbidity imparted to the air stream in the pharynx and tracheobronchial passages. Particles larger than 2-$3\mu m$ in diameter are deposited on the mucus and cleared from the airways by ciliary action and coughing.

The smaller inhaled particles (0.5-$3\mu m$) include many infectious agents, and may be deposited distal to the ciliated epithelial portions of the respiratory tract in the alveolar spaces. Here a different clearance apparatus is present in which fluid components in the alveoli—a mixture of lipids, immunoglobulins and enzymes, and phagocytic cells interact to inactivate and remove particles either by way of the respiratory tract or through lymphatic channels to the hilar and mediastinal lymph nodes. When the local defenses fail, components of the inflammatory response recruit polymorphonuclear cells and other cellular and humoral factors from the intravascular compartment and systemic mobilization of the hosts' immune defenses is accomplished.

The purpose of this monograph, "Immunologic and Infectious Reactions in the Lung" is to explore the various immunologic components of host-defense that operate in the lungs. The presentation is divided into three parts. First, the anatomic and functional components of the lungs defenses are reviewed and the responses to challenges with antigens and certain infectious

---

*G. M. Green, The J. Burns Amberson Lecture—In defense of the lung, *Am. Rev. Respir. Dis.*, **102**:691-703 (1970).

agents are considered. Part II concerns the disease states that occur as a consequence of deficiencies in the defense mechanisms or aberrant responses to drugs and environmental or unidentified antigens.

The third section dwells on techniques and phenomena, both conventional and projected, that enhance or reconstitute the hosts' defenses and thereby either prevent disease or have direct therapeutic effects. These therapies were reviewed from the rationale of their specific interactions with the immunologic processes.

Charles H. Kirkpatrick, M.D.
Herbert Y. Reynolds, M.D.
Bethesda, Maryland

INTRODUCTION

This monograph, *Immunologic and Infectious Reactions in the Lung,* marks the initiation of a series that will cover various aspects of modern *Lung Biology in Health and Disease.* Conceived late in 1972, the series has been made possible through the enthusiastic support of the many scientists who were approached. Until now, nearly 200 researchers from several countries have been involved in the twelve titles that are already in production or planned.

This series clearly reflects the remarkable blossoming of pulmonary investigation during the last decade, a decade during which investigators have become aware that nonrespiratory metabolic and "defense" functions of the lung are as important as the respiratory functions. There is now abundant evidence that all of these functions are closely related and interdependent. Alterations in the processes of gas exchange will be followed by impairment of the other functions; and conversely, disorders of the nonrespiratory functions will eventually lead to disturbances in the respiratory functions. While numerous research efforts are directed toward defining this interdependence more precisely, others are uncovering the fundamental processes that underlie all aspects of lung function. New approaches and new disciplines are being brought to bear on explorations of the lung as a whole, its cells and even its cellular components. The enormous body of new knowledge that has emerged from these new approaches to lung biology is addressed by the editors and authors of this series of monographs.

Special tribute should be paid to the editors to, and contributors of, this monograph, the first to appear. Through their unrelenting effort, Drs. C. H. Kirkpatrick and H. Y. Reynolds managed to complete the manuscript for this volume in about one year.

The volumes that soon will follow will cover topics in basic molecular biology applied to the lung, various aspects of lung development, the evolution of the respiratory system as it is reflected in different species, and various facets of pulmonary medicine, from early detection and pathogenesis to treatment.

Claude Lenfant, M.D.
Bethesda, Maryland

ix

CONTENTS

Contributors   iii
Foreword   Theodore Cooper   vi
Preface   vii
Introduction   ix

PART ONE   **Contributions of Immunologic Process to Defense**
                  of the Lung   1

1/   FLUID AND CELLULAR MILIEU OF THE HUMAN
         RESPIRATORY TRACT   3

Herbert Y. Reynolds and Harold H. Newball

   I   Introduction   3
   II   Types of Respiratory Cells Analyzed   5
   III   Protein Identified in the Lower Respiratory Tract   10
          Acknowledgment   23
          References   23

2/   BRONCHUS ASSOCIATED LYMPHOID TISSUE (BALT):
         ITS RELATIONSHIP TO MUCOCAL IMMUNITY   29

John Bienenstock, Robert L. Clancy, and Daniel Y. E. Perey

   I   Introduction   29
   II   Historic   31
   III   Anatomy of Balt   31
   IV   Function of Balt   38
   V   Discussion and Speculation   44
          References   52

3/   CELL-MEDIATED IMMUNE REACTIONS IN THE LUNG   59

Christopher S. Henney

   I   Introduction   59

                                                                             xi

  II   T-cell Effector Functions and Methods for Assaying
            Cell-mediated Immunity   60
  III   Demonstrations of Cell-mediated Immunity in the
            Respiratory Tract   61
  IV   The Role of Cell-mediated Immunity in Lung Defenses   63
  V   Unanswered Questions   66
        Acknowledgments   69
        References   69

4/   INITIATION OF IMMUNE RESPONSES IN THE LOWER
     RESPIRATORY TRACT WITH RED CELL ANTIGENS   73

     H. Benfer Kaltreider

  I   Introduction   73
  II   The Biology of the Immune Response of Systemic
            Lymphoid Tissue to Red Cell Antigens   74
  III   Normal Structure—Function Relationships of the
            Upper and Lower Respiratory Tracts   78
  IV   Biology of the Immune Response of the Respiratory
            Tract to Red Cell Antigens   85
  V   Future Directions   95
        Addendum   96
        Acknowledgments   97
        References   97

5/   PULMONARY IMMUNE MECHANISMS IN *MYCOPLASMA
     PNEUMONIAE* DISEASE   101

     Gerald W. Fernald and Wallace A. Clyde, Jr.

  I   Introduction   101
  II   Nature of the Organism   102
  III   Natural *M. Pneumoniae* Disease   102
  IV   Studies in Volunteers   107
  V   Experimental Models of *M. pneumoniae* Disease   108
  VI   Pathogenesis of *M. pneumoniae* Disease   121
  VII   Conclusion   125
        References   126

6/   RESPIRATORY SYNCYTIAL VIRUS   131

     Robert H. Parrot

  I   Introduction   131
  II   Pathogenesis   136
  III   Unresolved Questions   140
        References   140

7/ INTERACTION OF *PSEUDOMONAS* BACTERIA WITH
ANTIBODIES AND CELLS IN THE LUNG   143

Herbert Y. Reynolds

   I   Introduction   143
   II   Materials and Methods   145
   III   Results   146
   IV Discussion   155
   V   Summary   156
       References   157

8/ THE ROLE OF CHEMOTAXIS IN THE INFLAMMATORY-
IMMUNE RESPONSE OF THE LUNG   161

John I. Gallin

   I   Introduction   161
   II   Methods   161
   III   Chemotactic Factors-Fluid Phase Components   162
   IV Cellular Derived Chemotactic Stimuli   166
   V   Eosinophil Chemotaxis   169
   VI Chemotactic Activity of Products of Bacterial
         Growth and Virus-Infected Tissues   169
   VII Mechanism of the Leucocyte Response to
         Chemotactic Factors   170
   VIII Clinical Disorders of Chemotaxis and Their
         Association with Pulmonary Pathology   170
   IX Conclusions and Speculations   171
       References   172

PART TWO   Diseases that are Consequences of Aberrant or
              Deficient Immunologic Reactions in the Lung   179

9/ EXPERIMENTAL INFECTIONS OF THE LUNG   181

David C. Dale

   I   Introduction   181
   II   Methods   182
   III   Basic Concepts from Experimental Studies   183
   IV Current and Proposed Research   186
       References   186

10/ IMMUNODEFICIENCY AND PULMONARY DISEASE   191

Stephen H. Polmar

   I   Introduction   191
   II   Antibody Deficiency Syndromes   192

III	Cell–mediated Immunodeficiency Syndromes	198
IV	Phagocyte Dysfunction Syndromes	202
V	Concluding Remarks	205
	References	205

11/ ASTHMA AND ATOPIC HYPERSENSITIVITY 211

Charles H. Kirkpatrick

I	Introduction	211
II	The Atopic Patient	212
III	Immunopathology of Asthmatic Patients	218
IV	Concluding Comments	221
	References	222

12/ HYPERSENSITIVITY PNEUMONITIS 229

Jordan N. Fink

I	Introduction	229
II	Etiology of Hypersensitivity Pneumonitis	230
III	Clinical Features	232
IV	Laboratory Findings	234
V	Diagnosis	239
VI	Therapy	240
	References	240

13/ PULMONARY VASCULITIS 243

Anthony S. Fauci

I	Introduction	243
II	Mechanisms of Pulmonary Vasculitis	244
III	Diseases with Pulmonary Vasculitis	245
IV	Treatment	252
V	Summary	256
	References	256

14/ DRUG-INDUCED HYPERSENSITIVITY DISEASE OF THE LUNG 261

Edward C. Rosenow III

I	Introduction	261
II	Types of Adverse Reactions	262
III	Diagnosis of Allergic Drug Reactions	263
	References	282

15/ EOSINOPHILIA AND THE LUNG 289

Eric A. Ottesen

I   Introduction 289
II Clinical States 290
III The Eosinophil 295
IV Mechanisms of Eosinophilia 302
V   Pulmonary Eosinophilia Reconsidered 316
VI Summary 322
    Acknowledgment 322
    References 324

PART III **Treatment and Prophylaxis of Lung Diseases** 333

16/ REPLACEMENT THERAPY FOR PREVENTION AND
TREATMENT OF PULMONARY INFECTIONS 335

Rebecca H. Buckley

I   Introduction 335
II Indications and Contraindications 336
III Types of Therapy 339
    References 350

17/ KINETICS OF PENETRATION AND CLEARANCE OF
ANTIBIOTICS IN RESPIRATORY SECRETIONS 355

James E. Pennington

I   Introduction 355
II Pharmacokinetics of Antibodies in Bronchial Secretions 356
III Clinical Studies 358
IV Animal Model 362
V   Antibiotic Aerosols and Tracheobronchial Instillations 368
VI Summary 371
    References 371

18/ VACCINES FOR NONBACTERIAL DISEASE OF THE
LOWER RESPIRATORY TRACT 375

Robert M. Chanock

I   Viruses and Mycoplasmas of Sufficient Importance in
    Lower Respiratory Tract Disease to Warrant
    Attempts at Immunoprophylaxis 375
II Obstacles to Successful Immunoprophylaxis 377

III Nature of Resistance to Respiratory Tract
     Viruses and Mycoplasmas   379
IV   Vaccines Licensed for Prevention of Viral
     Respiratory Disease   383
V   Experimental Inactivated Vaccines   386
VI   Experimental Live Vaccines   388
     References   398

19/ ANTIBACTERIAL VACCINES FOR LOWER LUNG
     INFECTIONS   407
     Malcolm S. Artenstein

I   Introduction   407
II   Pertussis   408
III Tuberculosis   410
IV   Vaccination Against Pneumococcal Pneumonia   412
     References   416

20/ GENETIC FACTORS IN ATOPIC ALLERGIC DISEASE   419
     Bernard B. Levine

I   Introduction   419
II   Clustering of Asthma, Eczema, and Hay Fever   421
III Genetic Factors in Atopy   425
IV   Genetic Studies on Reagin Production in Mice   426
V   Genetic Studies in Allergic Man   433
VI   Clinical Application of Genetic Studies   439
     References   441

21/ THE PHARMACOLOGIC MODULATION OF MEDIATOR
     RELEASE FROM HUMAN BASOPHILS AND MAST CELLS   445
     Allen P. Kaplan

I   Introduction   445
     References   454

22/ IMMUNOTHERAPY (DESENSITIZATION) IN ALLERGIC
     CONDITIONS OF THE RESPIRATORY TRACT   461
     Philip S. Norman

I   Introduction   461
II   Controlled Efficacy Studies in Pollen Allergy   463
III Blocking Antibodies   471
IV   Untoward Reactions   475
V   Standardization   478
     References   478

23/ TRANSPLANTATION OF THE LUNG   485

John R. Benfield

I   Introduction   485
II   The Reimplantation Response   487
III   The Allograft Response   492
IV   Human Lung Transplantation   503
V   The Future   508
   References   512

24/ TRANSFER FACTOR IN DISEASES OF THE LUNG   519

Antonio Catanzaro and Lynn Spitler

I   Cell-mediated Immunity in Lung Disease   519
II   Transfer Factor   528
III   The Role of Potential Role of Transfer Factor
      in Treatment of Lung Diseases   536
   References   542

AUTHOR INDEX   549
SUBJECT INDEX   591

Part I

TREATMENT AND
PROPHYLAXIS OF LUNG DISEASES

1

Fluid and Cellular Milieu of the Human Respiratory Tract

HERBERT Y. REYNOLDS

National Institute of Allergy and Infectious Diseases
National Institutes of Health
Bethesda, Maryland

HAROLD H. NEWBALL

The Johns Hopkins University School of Medicine
Baltimore, Maryland

I. Introduction

Transnasal fiberoptic bronchoscopy [1,2] permits easy and nontraumatic access to the lower respiratory tract. In addition to a direct view and biopsy of endobronchial lesions, bronchial lavage of segmental portions of the lung is routine to obtain cytopathologic material and bacteriologic specimens. With the increasing use of diagnostic fiberoptic bronchoscopy [3], analysis of protein components and functional assessment of respiratory cells recovered from bronchial fluid will most likely become more important in the evaluation of pulmonary disease. Recently, bronchial washings obtained with the bronchofiberscope from smokers and nonsmokers were analyzed for immunoglobulins and alveolar macrophage enzymes [4-6].

In this initial chapter, we would like to define, so far as is possible, the milieu of the normal human respiratory tract which can serve as a basis for alterations in disease states discussed in later chapters. Several components of the bronchoalveolar environment will be analyzed: (a) recoverable respiratory cells; (b) proteins, including immunoglobulins and enzymes; (c) complement activity; and (d) lipids (surfactant). Results from bronchial lavage of 42 subjects [6] will be used as a basis for comparison with and discussion of other relevant observations about these components of the human respiratory tract.

Because cigarette smoking is so prevalent, it is impossible to exclude the healthy smoker from the ranks of normal adults. Therefore, in attempting to describe the protein and cellular environment of the lower human respiratory tract, cigarette smokers have been classified as normal. However, frequent comparisons between smokers and nonsmokers will point out some obvious differences, which, in the future, could change the "normal" category by eliminating smokers.

A. Subject Selection and Bronchial Lavage Procedure

Patients were hospitalized at the clinical center of the National Institutes of Health and scheduled for diagnostic fiberoptic bronchoscopy as part of an initial evaluation for a variety of intrathoracic lesions. Patients selected for bronchial lavage had minimal parenchymal lesions in an upper lobe, such as coin lesions, residual infiltrates, or asymmetric mediastinal enlargements. Lower-lung fields were free of detectable disease, both roentgenographically and by physical examination. Patients were not receiving drugs, specifically no antineoplastic medications, and all had peripheral blood counts within normal values. Normal young adult volunteers, participating in clinical projects at the National Institutes of Health, underwent limited bronchoscopy for selective lavage of the lingula lobe.

Bronchoscopies were performed with a fiberoptic bronchoscope (model BF-T 5B2, Olympus Corporation of America, New Hyde Park, NY). Patients were premedicated intramuscularly with atropine (0.6 mg) and merperidine (50 mg) and volunteers with diazepam (10 mg). Local anesthesia of the respiratory tract was obtained with topical 2% lidocaine spray. Following the usual bronchoscopic examination in patients, the bronchoscope was positioned in a segmental lobe orifice of the lower lobe, contralateral to the involved upper lobe. Sterile saline (0.9% sodium chloride), in a volume of 50 ml, was infused through the bronchoscope, into the lung segment, and aspirated into a sterile container. The wash was repeated once (total 100 ml of saline). Voluntary coughing was encouraged to aspirate the lavage fluid completely. For normal volunteers, the lavage procedure varied only in that three 50-ml saline washings were done. A complete blood count and a 5-ml clotted blood specimen were obtained from each participant within 2 hr after the procedure. All subjects were examined regularly during the 24–hr interval after bronchoscopy. Inspiratory rales were usually audible for 2 to 6 hr in the area of the lung lavaged. All subjects tolerated bronchoscopy well and had no subsequent effects from the procedure.

B. Methods

The lavage fluid was strained through several layers of very loose cotton gauze to remove mucus and then centrifuged for 5 min at 1800 rpm at 25°C. The supernatant fluid was decanted and concentrated 30 to 50-fold to a 2-ml volume in a Amicon Diaflo chamber containing an UM-10 filter at 4°C. The volume was finally adjusted to 1 ml by negative pressure dialysis in a collodion bag. A 0.2-ml aliquot of this concentrated fluid was analyzed immediately for hemolytic complement activity, and a 0.3-ml portion was separated into size components in a sucrose density gradient. To the remaining fluid, gentamicin sulfate (5 μg/ml), and penicillin G, (1000 U/ml) were added to retard bacterial growth. The specimen was stored at 4°C. Serum from clotted blood was also stored at 4°C. Various qualitative and quantitative protein and lipid analyses, to be described later, were done on bronchial fluids and sera.

Respiratory cells were suspended at a density of $2-3 \times 10^6$ cells per milliliter in modified Hank's balanced salt solution.* Cell viability by eosin dye exclusion [7], a cell count, and differential cell counts on a wet mount and a Wright-Giemsa stained smear were done. In sizing the various respiratory cells distributed in an unstained wet mount, the diameter of a cell was measured in two planes with an eye micrometer, under oil emersion (960X), and the average diameter expressed in microns; a differential count was made from 500 cells. Because it is difficult to distinguish between small lymphocytes (diameter 7-8 μm) and small alveolar macrophages (diameter about 10μm), the phagocytic properties of macrophages were used for further identification. Staining macrophages with neutral red [8] and the ingestion of polystyrene latex balls (mean diameter 1.1μm) helped to separate these cells. Phase-contrast microscopy also helped this differentiation. Respiratory macrophages seemed to segregate into three general groups and have been arbitrarily so classified (Table 1). Large macrophages (diameter 20-40μm) are giant cells with multiple nuclei, but most macrophages are intermediate in size (14-19μm). Cells in the third group are about the size of peripheral blood monocytes (9-11μm) and are difficult to differentiate from lymphocytes even in stained cell preparations.

II. Types of Respiratory Cells Analyzed

A. Respiratory Cell and Bronchial Lavage Fluid Recovery in Groups of Smokers and Nonsmokers

In Table 1, a composite of the groups of subjects is given with additional details about the number, viability, and types of respiratory cells obtained by endo-

---

*Prepared without Ca++ and Mg++ ions and phenol red.

TABLE 1 Composition of Subject Groups and Recovery in Bronchial Fluid of Total Protein, Respiratory Cells and Cell Types

Age (yr)	Lavage fluid recovery %	Protein recovery Mg/ml	Number respiratory cells ($\times 10^6$)	Cell viability %	Lymphocytes %	Macrophages (%) by size[a]		
						(L)	(I)	(S)
Nonsmokers, Normal Volunteers (n = 5)[b]								
20±0.5[b] (19–22)	66.4±9.4 (50–93)	4.2±0.6 (2.7–6.1)	12.8±2.7 (6.0–21.0)	94.2±1.1 (90–96)	15.2±2.6 (11–20)	7.6±1.6 (5–14)	70.2±3.2 (63–79)	18.6±3.0 (15–30)
Smokers, Normal Volunteers (n = 5)[b]								
21±0.8 (19–23)	74.0±7.6 (58–95)	5.6±0.8 (2.8–7.6)	39.8±5.3 (25.0–54.0)	94.0±1.4 (90–98)	6.0±2.3 (1–12)	8.4±2.5 (5–18)	72.2±8.4 (40–85)	19.6±9.4 (9–47)
Nonsmokers, Patients (n = 11)[c]								
52.1±3.0 (30–63)	48.3±6.3 (30–80)	3.8±0.8 (1.3–7.6)	6.3±2.0 (1.0–10.9)	87.7±3.0 (75–99)	18.0±3.2 (9–37)	6.2±2.2 (2–25)	63.4±6.2 (48–86)	24.3±3.4 (13–35)
Smokers, Patients (n = 21)[c]								
48.0±2.4 (22–62)	43.0±4.0 (10–77)	2.5±0.3 (0.7–5.2)	14.4±4.5 (1.6–77.0)	82.2±3.5 (40–95)	7.9±1.2 (4–21)	8.5±2.2 (2–23)	62.4±4.0 (55–82)	25.7±4.4 (12–37)

[a]Cell diameter was determined in wet mount and average cell diameter expressed in microns; large macrophages $>20\mu$; intermediate size, 14–19μm; small size, 9–13μm.

[b]Normal volunteers had three 50-ml lavages of lingula lobe.

[c]Patients, smokers, and nonsmokers had two 50-ml lavages.

[d]Mean ±SE and the range observed for each group are given.

bronchial lavage. The ages of the volunteers ranged from 19 to 23 yr and they were generally about 30 yr younger than most of the patients. Patients in the smoking category had a mean cigarette pack-year (pk-yr) history of 35 ±6.0 yr (range 3-70 pk-yr); volunteers in the smoking group had a much briefer smoking history of about 2 pk-yr (range 1-3). The fractional recovery of infused lavage from the lower lobes of patients was not as great as that in volunteers. This was particularly evident in patients who smoked. Ventilatory pulmonary function tests had shown that about 40% (8 of 21) of the smokers had clinically unsuspected mild-to-moderate obstructive lung disease, and smaller fluid recoveries and protein values were obtained in these subjects (34.6% fluid recovery, mean Lowry protein 1.25 mg/ml). It was noted previously that lavage fluid-return is poor in subjects with structural lung changes, such as emphysema [9].

The yield of cells obtained from the lungs of patients who smoked was greater than that from nonsmokers, but variability was such that the difference was not statistically significant. In contrast, the mean recovery of cells from volunteers who were smokers was three times greater than that from nonsmoking volunteers (Student's *t* test, P<0.005). The viability of respiratory cells was less in both groups of patients. Finally, the mean percentages of lymphocytes detected in the two groups of smokers were less than those found in respective groups of nonsmokers (P<0.005). This suggested that the greater number of cells recovered from smokers' lungs was due to increased numbers of macrophages. However, the distribution of macrophages of various sizes was virtually the same for all groups (Table 1). Differential cell counts also included 1% to 2% polymorphonuclear cells, and 3% to 6% ciliated epithelial cells, which invariably were nonviable. Although the lavage fluid appeared clear, cell pellets usually contained 2% to 8% red blood cells. In contrast to nonsmokers, respiratory cell pellets obtained from smokers appeared gray and dirty and the cytoplasm of alveolar macrophages was filled with yellowish-brown granules.

Our findings support previous studies [4,5,10,11] in which the recovery of respiratory cells from bronchial lavage of cigarette smokers was increased but the respiratory cell mixture from smokers contained fewer lymphocytes. This would suggest that smoking caused selective hyperplasia of the alveolar macrophage population and enlargement of the lymphoreticular system of the lung. The net result would be an increase in the number of phagocytic cells. Surprisingly, in young volunteers only a brief history of cigarette smoking appeared to be sufficient to induce these greater numbers of respiratory cells.

B. Alveolar Macrophages

Alveolar macrophages attach well to plastic or glass surfaces. They can be established in tissue culture and maintained for periods of 3 to 6 wk [12]. These in vitro cultures have been used to study macrophage phagocytosis and metabolism [12] and to identify macrophage surface receptors. Alveolar macrophages have membrane receptors for IgG [13,14] and for the third component (C3) of complement [14]. Specifically, macrophages bind two fragments of C3, C3b, and the enzymatic cleavage fragment (C3 inactivator) C3d [15]. Alveolar macrophages do not bind immune complexes formed with IgM antibody (i.e., erythrocytes sensitized with IgM antibody-EA [15]). This result is not surprising because IgM immunoglobulin usually is not found in secretions from the lower respiratory tract and is not part of the normal respiratory milieu [6].

The identity of alveolar macrophage membrane receptors is important in understanding the response of these cells to foreign particulate materials (0.5 to 3μm size), which are inhaled into the lungs and deposited in terminal airways (alveoli) [16]. In the alveoli, macrophages are the principal means of clearing particulate matter and are the phagocytic cells which initially attempt to inactivate infectious microorganisms.

Although animal studies indicate that pulmonary macrophages originate from the bone marrow [17], little is known of the origin or fate of these cells in man. Because the lungs of cigarette smokers have substantially increased numbers of macrophages, the possibility of proliferative capacity of human alveolar macrophages is important. If these cells can proliferate, then the population of macrophages in the lung may be locally self-sustaining. Recently [18,19], pulmonary cells from normal human subjects were shown to incorporate [3H] thymidine label for scheduled DNA synthesis. The percentage of macrophages incorporating label, presumably for nuclear DNA, varied between 0.35 and 1.25; this low labeling index was interpreted as representative of a small growth fraction. Thus, some human pulmonary macrophages are probably capable of replication, and the macrophage compartment could be sustained in part by local cell proliferation as well as by an influx of cells from peripheral blood and from bone marrow [18]. In certain circumstances, the lung macrophages appear to be a sheltered or self-sufficient population of cells, little affected by irradiation or chemotherapeutic agents, which regularly supress peripheral blood and bone-marrow cellular elements. In a recent report [13], alveolar macrophages lavaged from three patients with acute leukemia were functionally and morphologically normal despite intensive antineoplastic treatment of these patients, which caused prolonged leukopenia. Peripheral blood monocytes were virtually absent in these patients for 40 to 60 days prior to bronchial lavage. The incorporation of [3H] thymidine by the alveolar macrophages suggested that these cells have the capacity to replicate and hence maintain their numbers in the lungs. We have observed that respiratory cells recovered from bronchial lavage from dogs (10 kg body weight) given 350 R of total body irradiation to produce predictable peripheral blood leukopenia in 6 days and bone marrow arrest [20] do not begin to diminish in number for at least 3 wk following irradiation (H. Reynolds, unpublished preliminary observation). Similarly, in humans receiving daily therapeutic doses of prednisone or a dose of cyclophosphamide sufficient to create leukopenia (WBC 1000/mm^3), for intervals of months to years, neither drug caused qualitative changes in the types of respiratory cells recovered at bronchoscopy (H. Reynolds, unpublished observations).

These kinds of observations raise several questions: (a) What stimuli are necessary to maintain or replete the lymphoreticular cell population in the lungs? (b) What subtle metabolic effects do cytotoxic drugs induce in macrophages, which could impair their phagocytic and bactericidal capacities, since immunosuppressed people are more susceptible to infections, including respiratory infections? (c) What is the effective life-span of lung macrophages and what portion of this time is necessary for differentiation from monocyte to macrophage?

C. Lymphocytes in the Respiratory Tract

The other cell type readily recovered by bronchial lavage is the lymphocyte. Morphologically, these lymphocytes are about 7μm in diameter, contain very few cytoplasmic granules, and stain deeply with Wright-Giemsa. Lymphocytes accounted for 11% to 17% of the respiratory cells recovered by lavage from normal nonsmoking subjects [21,22]; in both groups of nonsmokers (Table 1), the average was approximately 17%. As already mentioned, fewer lymphocytes were identified in respiratory cell differential counts from smokers. Two relevant questions can be raised: (a) What is the anatomic origin of these cells? (b) What lymphocyte subpopulations can be identified (T or B cells)?

First, the lymphocytes in alveoli could originate from multiple sites. Circulating blood lymphocytes could escape through the pulmonary capillary endothelium; however, pulmonary endothelium is a continuous type, with cells linked by tight junctions [23,24] that create only small intracellular clefts approximately 40 Å wide. The egress of essentially nonmotile cells, such as lymphocytes, could be slow and difficult because they must pass through the capillary endothelium, the interstitial space, and the alveolar epithelium before reaching the alveolar lumen. Alternatively, lymphocytes located in the submucosa of the lower respiratory tract [25], or in lymphoid aggregates associated with the trachea and major bronchi (BALT) [26], might be redistributed to the alveoli. Finally, one must consider that the situation is an artificial one in that the vigor of bronchial lavage may wash lymphocytes to distal portions of the lung and cause an artifactual mixture of cell types.

Second, as to the identity of the lymphocytes in bronchial lavage fluids, more information is available. Daniele et al. [22] have found that from 15% to 19% of the lymphocytes recovered by bronchial lavage were B cells, and 47% were T cells on the basis of spontaneous rosette formation with unsensitized sheep erythrocytes. Although a high proportion of lung lymphocytes were not identified as either T or B (34%) and classified as "null" cells, the T:B ratio of lung lymphocytes may be comparable to that found for normal peripheral blood lymphocytes. In the dog, Kaltreider and Salmon [27] observed that most respiratory lymphocytes were B cells because they had the ability to produce antibody to sheep erythrocytes after intrabronchial immunization. Reynolds et al. [28] reported that about 38% of rabbit respiratory lymphocytes were nonadherent to glass bead–wool columns [29]; Rosenthal and coworkers [29] reported that similar nonadherent cells from guinea pig lymph nodes were enriched for T cells. Certainly, ample evidence has accumulated from animal studies that immune respiratory lymphocytes can be stimulated to produce lymphokines, such as migration inhibition factor, by appropriate antigen stimulation [30–37]. This function has been considered an in vitro correlate of delayed hypersensitivity or cellular immunity [38], and a function of T lymphocytes. With some justification, it appears that respiratory lymphocytes comprise a mixed population of T and B cells.

III. Proteins Identified in the Lower Respiratory Tract

Tracheobronchial fluids [39–42] obtained by limited lavage (a single 10-ml saline wash of major bronchi at the approximate level of the carina and with recovery of about 1-ml fluid) have contained principally: albumin; immunoglobulins A and G; and in trace amounts, a variety of proteins [41], such as amylase, lysozyme, lactoferrin, a_1-antitrypsin, haptoglobin, transferrin, and so forth. Following lavage (250 ml) by fiberoptic bronchoscopy [4], specimens from normal smokers, when compared with those from nonsmokers, contained increased amounts of IgG but comparable amounts of IgA.

Immunoelectrophoreses on all concentrated bronchial specimens and sera were developed with antisera to human serum and saliva. A precipitin pattern of only six to eight arcs was found consistently for bronchial specimens, suggesting that relatively few proteins were present in adequate concentration to be easily detected. Oüchterlony analysis identified 14 protein constituents (Table 2). Matching bronchial and serum specimens were placed in adjacent antigen wells in the agar so that precipitin lines of identity could be seen in both specimens. The origins of the specific antisera used in these precipitation reactions were given in detail previously [6]. Bronchial and serum specimens from smoking and nonsmoking subjects had no significant qualitative differences. Serum

TABLE 2 Identification of Major Proteins in Bronchial Secretions

Component	Positive (N)	
	Nonsmokers ($n = 16$)	Smokers ($n = 26$)
Albumin	A[a]	A
Transferrin	A	A
a_1-antitrypsin	15(94)[b]	24(92)
a_2-macroglobulin	2(13)	3(12)
Immunoglobulin		
M	1(6)	1(4)
A	A	A
G	A	A
D	N[c]	N
E	N	N
"Free" secretory component	10(63)	18(70)
Bound secretory component	A	A
Complement		
Clq	N	N
C3	2(13)	5(20)
C4	1(6)	3(12)

[a]A = detected in all specimens.
[b]Number in parentheses is percent positive.
[c]N = not detected in any specimen.

specimens were reactive for all components, except IgE and bound and free secretory piece. Apparently, bronchial fluid is much less complex than serum in its protein composition and is not just an ultrafiltration of intravascular plasma proteins.

The components found consistently in concentrated bronchial fluids were: albumin; transferrin; a_1-antitrypsin; IgA with secretory component reactivity; IgG; and in about 67% of specimens, detectable "free" or unbound secretory component. Only C3 was detected in about 17% of bronchial specimens. However, Table 6 shows that low levels of complement activity were present. IgG_1 was detected in all bronchial specimens but other gamma-chain subclasses were not regularly present. IgM was detected in 2 of 42 (5%) bronchial specimens. Our Oüchterlony system would detect IgM at a concentration of 0.01 mg/ml. IgM was not present in human bronchial lavage in previous reports [4,39,40,42] and was only detected in about 5% of bronchial secretions obtained from rabbits [43]. The evidence would indicate that IgM is not a prominent constituent of normal respiratory fluids.

Each freshly concentrated bronchial lavage specimen and paired serum were separated into size components in sucrose density gradients; a representative separation is shown in Figure 1. Protein components were identified in various gradient fractions, and the sedimenting position of the catalase and IgG

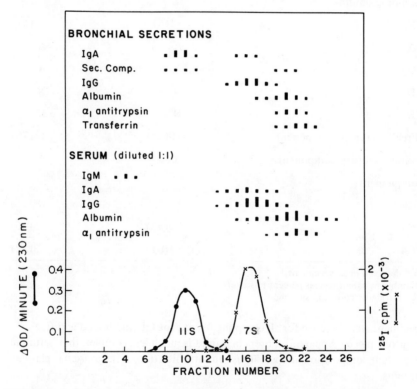

FIGURE 1 Bronchial secretions and serum were simultaneously separated in 10% to 40% linear sucrose density gradients by ultracentrifugation. Fractions from each gradient were comparable and the positions of the 11 S and 7S markers were the same in each gradient. The position of the 11 S catalase marker (●) was determined enzymatically and is plotted as optical density per minute (OD/min); the radiodinated 7 S marker position (X) is shown as counts per minute (cpm). The relative concentrations of immunoglobulins and other proteins in each gradient fraction are denoted by vertical bars. (Reprinted by permission of the C. V. Mosby Co., from Ref. [6]).

marker proteins are shown. IgA was detected in two regions of the gradient: in those fractions which contained the 11 S catalase material and in fractions which contained human IgG and ^{125}I-labeled rabbit IgG. IgA identified in the 11 S region showed reactivity for secretory component, whereas 7 S IgA did not. Of 40 gradient separations of bronchial fluid, 31 contained 7 S IgA. Polymeric forms (between 7 S and 11 S) were not detected in bronchial secretions. As shown in Table 2, free secretory component was present in about 67% of the bronchial specimens, and was also present in gradient fractions sedimenting with albumin. a_1-Antitrypsin and transferrin were found in fractions partially overlapping with albumin, but a_1-antitrypsin was not found in any gradient fraction containing IgA.

Sucrose density gradient fractions which contained 11 S IgA, 7 S IgA, and IgG, and free secretory component were collected and pooled from each gradient, dialyzed against borate–saline buffer to remove sucrose and concentrated to 0.1 ml with negative pressure dialysis. The IgA concentration was measured by radial immunodiffusion in pooled fractions. To measure 11 S IgA, a colostral or bronchial secretory IgA standard was used; to quantitate 7 S IgA, a serum standard was used. The relative amount of 7 S IgA to total IgA was found. About 9.4% ±3.6 ($n = 20$) of IgA in bronchial fluids was present as 7 S IgA; a significant difference between smokers and nonsmokers was not found. Again, concentrated fractions of 7 S IgA did not show reactivity for secretory component.

It was of interest to find that IgA in bronchial fluid was not exclusively 11 S secretory IgA, but approximately 9% of the IgA was monomeric 7 S IgA, which was indistinguishable from serum IgA. Also, unbound secretory component, which is synthesized by epithelial cells [44], was detected free in bronchial fluid and not in association with IgA. This finding reemphasizes the independent origin of secretory component. The predominant specie of serum IgA in humans is the monomeric form [45], in contrast to the dog and mouse, for example, where circulating IgA is almost exclusively in dimeric form [46,47] and IgA is rarely found in secretory fluids as a monomer. In humans, about 20% of IgA in nasal fluids [48] and colostrum [49] is 7 S IgA, which is similar to serum IgA. Uncertainty persists, however, as to the origin of this material. Is it derived directly from serum or does it represent the secretory molecule which has undergone dissociation or failed to complex with secretory component [45]? We feel that this IgA is probably derived from the intravascular space. Of practical significance is the fact that separation and purification of IgG by gel filtration chromatography from bronchial fluids is complicated by monomeric IgA, which elutes in the IgG fractions because of its similar size.

A. Quantitation of Major Proteins in Bronchial Fluids

The major proteins in concentrated bronchial fluids were quantitated by radial immunodiffusion (Table 3) so that ratios of these components in bronchial

TABLE 3 Quantitation of Selected Proteins and Immunoglobulins in Concentrated Bronchial Fluid (mg/ml)

Groups	Albumin	IgA[a]	IgG	IgE[b]	Total protein (mg/ml)
Nonsmokers Volunteers (n = 5)	1.42±0.22[c] (0.9–1.9)	0.91±0.11 (0.5–1.1)	0.17±0.05 (0.1–0.4)	77.2±8.2 (52.0–100.0)	4.2±0.6 (2.7–6.1)
Smokers Volunteers (n = 5)	1.53±0.15 (0.9–1.8)	0.80±0.14 (0.4–1.1)	0.52±0.19 (0.2–1.0)	32.0±6.2 (20.0–52.0)	5.6±0.8 (2.8–7.6)
Nonsmokers Patients (n = 8)	1.84±0.52 (0.5–3.0)	1.07±0.36 (0.4–2.9)	0.55±0.15 (0.1–1.2)	ND[d]	3.8±0.8 (1.3–7.6)
Smokers Patients (n = 17)	1.0±0.13 (0.3–1.9)	0.60±0.10 (0.1–1.5)	0.41±0.08 (0.15–1.2)	95.3±25.1 (20.0–300.0)	2.5±0.3 (0.7–5.2)

[a]An 11 S IgA standard and a purified serum IgG standard were used to calculate bronchial values.
[b]Nanograms per milliliter.
[c]Mean ± SE and range for group given.
[d]Not done.

specimens could be found and compared for individual subjects (Table 4). For these quantitative measurements, 11 S secretory IgA standards were prepared from human bronchial secretions and colostrum, and 7 S IgG was purified from human serum [6]. Serum values were not included in Table 4, but serum protein and immunoglobulin values were within accepted normal ranges for all subjects, and mean determinations for the four subject groups were comparable. In bronchial fluids from smoker patients, albumin quantitative values were uniformly lower, which probably reflected the smaller amount of protein recovered in some of these lavages (Table 1). The mean IgG concentration in nonsmoker volunteers was significantly lower (P <0.05) than the mean value obtained for the volunteers who smoked; a similar result was not found between the two patient-groups. IgA values were not significantly different between any of the subject-groups. Although IgE was not detected in bronchial fluid or serum by double diffusion immunoprecipitation, we attempted to quantitate it with a more sensitive method [6]. However, normal bronchial fluids had small amounts of IgE, which is in contrast to nasal washings and sputum from patients with extrinsic asthma where its concentration is considerably greater [50,51].

For each bronchial specimen and its paired serum, individual ratios of IgG: albumin, IgA:albumin, and IgG:IgA concentrations were calculated [39,42] and then a resultant mean ratio was determined for each group of subjects (Table 4). Such a presentation provides a pattern, or a profile, of the protein composition and circumvents variations in total protein concentration among individual specimens that make the mean quantitative values less informative (Table 3). In bronchial secretions the mean IgG:albumin ratio of 0.12 calculated for nonsmoker volunteers was less than that for the other groups and reflects the lower IgG concentrations in bronchial fluids given in Table 3. Of particular interest was the comparison of mean IgG:IgA ratios because of a previous report [4] that the lavage fluid from smokers contained increased amounts of IgG but not IgA when compared with nonsmoker controls. The mean IgG:IgA ratios for the groups of volunteers differed significantly (P <0.05); although there is an apparent difference between patient groups of smokers and nonsmokers, the difference is not quite significant statistically (Student's t test, value $t = 1.80$ P~0.08). However, these overall results substantiate a conclusion that IgG is increased, relative to IgA, in bronchial fluids obtained from smokers. However, when the degree of smoking (pk-yr history) was compared with the individual IgG:IgA ratio for each smoker, no association was found (Spearman's rank correlation). When the comparison was repeated using the smoker's age and IgG:IgA ratio, a negative correlation was found between increasing age and higher IgG levels (rank correlation coefficient $r = -0.61$, P <0.01). Smoking may still be the single determinant in elevating IgG values in bronchial fluid but it is surprising that the

TABLE 4 Comparison of Combined Protein Ratios Obtained From Quantitative Values of Individual Bronchial Specimens and Serum by Subject Groups

Groups	Bronchial fluid			Serum		
	IgG/Alb[a]	IgA/Alb	IgG/IgA	IgG/Alb	IgA/Alb	IgG/IgA
Nonsmokers Volunteers ($n = 5$)	0.12±0.02[b] (0.07–0.22)	0.72±0.12 (0.54–0.96)	0.19±0.04 (0.10–0.33)	0.23±0.02 (0.17–0.26)	0.05±0.01 (0.03–0.08)	6.04±0.60 (4.0–8.4)
Smokers Volunteers ($n = 5$)	0.32±0.10 (0.20–0.60)	0.51±0.06 (0.30–0.60)	0.70±0.20 (0.2–1.3)	0.21±0.01 (0.20–0.23)	0.04±0.01 (0.02–0.06)	6.08±0.78 (3.7–7.6)
Nonsmokers Patients ($n = 8$)	0.33±0.05 (0.20–0.58)	0.71±0.16 (0.33–2.80)	0.54±0.15 (0.10–0.95)	0.40±0.04 (0.32–0.61)	0.07±0.01 (0.05–0.10)	6.0±0.41 (4.0–7.6)
Smokers Patients ($n = 17$)	0.36±0.04 (0.20–0.60)	0.63±0.12 (0.20–1.5)	1.04±0.19 (0.3–2.6)	0.39±0.04 (0.24–0.60)	0.08±0.01 (0.03–0.12)	6.04±0.82 (3.2–9.0)

[a]IgG value (mg/ml)/albumin value (mg/ml).
[b]Mean±SE of combined ratios, and ratio range observed for the group.

degree of smoking had no influence and that the younger age smokers might well have higher IgG levels. Certainly, other determinants need to be investigated.

In contrast, mean ratios in bronchial specimens, compared with similar ratios in paired sera for the groups, show several expected differences. The IgA: albumin ratio in bronchial secretions is about 0.64, but it is about 0.06 in serum, which emphasizes the relative increase of IgA in bronchial fluid specimens. Likewise, bronchial and serum ratios of IgG:IgA are much different, reflecting the preponderance of IgG in intravascular globulin fractions.

B. a_1 -Antitrypsin

The glycoprotein a_1 -antitrypsin is present in human serum and in various exocrine fluids, such as colostrum and gastrointestinal secretions [52] and bronchial alveolar fluid (Table 2). This glycoprotein, capable of inhibiting the proteolytic activity of trypsin and other proteinases, has become important because of the association of a_1 -antitrypsin deficiency with the early development of chronic obstructive pulmonary disease (emphysema).

a_1 -Antitrypsin concentrations in serum and respiratory secretions obtained from groups of nonsmokers and smokers are given in Table 5. For comparison, values for a_1 -antitrypsin have been measured in subjects with cystic fibrosis. From these patients with cystic fibrosis, 24-hr sputum specimens were obtained and then bronchial lavage performed as part of other studies in which tracheobronchial clearance was measured.* People with cystic fibrosis usually have a chronic infection of the respiratory tract and produce secretions that contain thick mucus as well as many polymorphonuclear leukocytes (PMN). Cellular components in the lavage fluid from these subjects contained about 85% PMNs, and cell viability was only 30%. The protein concentration of lavage fluid concentrates from subjects with cystic fibrosis was greater than that in the lavage fluid from nonsmokers and smokers, so that values for a_1 -antitrypsin should not be compared. Concentrations of a_1 -antitrypsin did not differ significantly between groups of nonsmokers and smokers. Serum levels of a_1 -antitrypsin were somewhat higher for the group with cystic fibrosis, but still within the normal range for serum, from 2 to 4 mg/ml [53]. Appreciable amounts of a_1 - antitrypsin were detected in both lavage and sputum specimens from the group with cystic fibrosis.

These a_1 -antitrypsin levels are best interpreted within the context of several recent and provocative observations made by Cohen [54]. With

---

*Lavage specimens kindly provided by Dr. Robert E. Wood, Pediatric Metabolism Branch, National Institute of Arthritis, Metabolism and Digestive Diseases, Bethesda, Md.

TABLE 5 a_1-Antitrypsin in Serum and Respiratory Fluids (mg/ml)

	Serum	Bronchial lavage concentrate[a]	Sputum[b]
Nonsmokers (n = 12)	2.63±0.17[c]	0.04±0.02	ND[d]
Smokers (n = 16)	3.11±0.13	0.05±0.02	ND
Cystic Fibrosis (n = 7)	3.93±0.17	0.15±0.04	0.17±0.06

[a]Bronchial lavage fluid concentrated to final volume 1 ml.
[b]Sputum from patients with cystic fibrosis was centrifuged at 12,000 rpm for 30 min. and supernatant fluid used.
[c]Mean concentration ± SE.
[d]Not determined.

fluorescent techniques, he observed that a_1-antitrypsin was present intracellularly in human alveolar macrophages but was present to a lesser degree in a subject deficient in serum a_1-antitrypsin (ZZ phenotype). Alveolar macrophages were able to assimilate a_1-antitrypsin from serum, and presumably they would be able to do it from alveolar fluid by an endocytotic mechanism. Furthermore, he identified an alveolar macrophage protease (cathepsin), which might be an emphysema–producing enzyme, that is inhibited by a_1-antitrypsin [54]. The implications are that an autoregulatory mechanism may exist in macrophages, or within the alveoli, which can neutralize proteolytic activity possibly deleterious to lung structures.

Many more macrophages can be lavaged from the lungs of cigarette smokers than from the lungs of nonsmokers [4–6,10]. The compensatory increase of these cells, however, may constitute an additional burden of macrophage enzymes for the smoker, which must be neutralized by appropriate inhibitors, such as a_1-antitrypsin, to prevent insidious destruction of lung tissue. Therefore, we anticipated finding increased amounts of a_1-antitrypsin in lavage fluid concentrates from smokers but did not, as shown in Table 5. Subjects with cystic fibrosis, who have vast numbers of degenerating PMNs in their lavage fluid and sputum, potentially have large amounts of lysozomal enzymes in respiratory secretions, which could, in part, perpetuate chronic irritation of the respiratory tree or contribute to mucus secretion and ultimately degenerative lung changes. It appears that patients with cystic fibrosis may attempt some compensation by having higher serum levels of a_1-antitrypsin and perhaps increased respiratory levels of this material. In conclusion, enzymatic digestion of lung tissues could occur as a consequence of increased amounts of macrophage enzymes in cigarette smokers [54], which are not adequately inactivated by a concomitant increase in specific inhibitors in alveolar fluids. More obvious are the results of a decreased level of enzyme-inhibitor in people deficient in a_1-antitrypsin.

Because an adequate concentration of a_1-antitrypsin in respiratory fluids seems critical, the method of its transport into these secretions becomes important. Recently, Tomasi and Hauptman [52] found that a_1-antitrypsin binds to serum-derived IgA and can be released from this IgA complex when the complex is incubated in such exocrine secretions as colostrum or intestinal contents. They suggest that a_1-antitrypsin could be transported into body lumens attached to IgA and then released. The ingredients are present in bronchial alveolar fluid, supporting such an hypothesis of transport into the respiratory tract. Small amounts of apparently serum-derived 7 S IgA are present, yet a_1-antitrypsin is present in a noncomplexed form. These interactions are of considerable interest, and further investigation is deserved.

C. Complement Activity in Bronchial Fluids

As shown in Table 2, few concentrated bronchial lavage specimens had detectable complement components by qualitative analysis; however, with more sensitive measurement of hemolytic complement activity, complement was identified.

Complement activity was measured in concentrated bronchial specimens and in fresh serum within 3 to 4 hr after lavage (Table 6). C4 and C6 titers [55, 56] were obtained for nine patients who smoked and for the two groups of normal volunteers. Except for the titer of C4 in patients who smoked, C4 complement activity in the bronchi was about 3% of that in concomitant serum specimens and C6 titers were about 1%; the concentration of albumin in bronchial fluids was about 3.5% of that in serum. Complement activity is known to be labile and activity undoubtedly was lost in the lavage and concentrating procedures. Nevertheless, the complement activity found in normal bronchial secretions, compared with that in serum was roughly proportional to the albumin ratio found between bronchial secretions and serum.

The functional presence of small amounts of complement in the overall, coordinated host-defense system of the normal lower respiratory tract is unclear. Two examples can be given. First, fixation of complement by IgA still seems to be unsettled [57-61]. The interaction of complement components and secretory IgA antibody obtained from the respiratory tract has not been investigated to our knowledge. Second, the presence of complement per se as part of an immune complex is an insufficient stimulus in itself to promote particle ingestion by alveolar macrophages. We found that erythrocytes coated with only IgG antibodies (EA) are avidly ingested by macrophages, particularly as the duration of the in vitro culture of macrophages increases [15]. In contrast, erythrocytes sensitized with IgM antibody to which complement (C3) is attached (EAC) bind to about 90% of in vitro macrophages to form rosettes. Yet these immune erythrocyte complexes (EAC), which attach to the macrophage membrane only by a presumed C3 receptor, are never phagocytosed [15]. It should be added

TABLE 6 Complement Titers in Concentrated Bronchial Lavage Fluid and Serum[a]

	Albumin content (mg/ml)	Complement Components	
		C4[b] (X 10^3)	C6[c]
Smoker normals (n = 5)			
Bronchial fluid	1.53±0.15	4.1±0.6[d]	4.6±1.7
Serum	43.0±3.4	145.1±22.1	412.5±55.7
Ratio[e]	0.036	0.028	0.011
Nonsmoker normals (n = 5)			
Bronchial fluid	1.42±0.20	4.3±0.8	4.7±1.0
Serum	38.8±2.0	167.0±24.5	518.8±52.0
Ratio[e]	0.037	0.026	0.009
Smoker patients (n = 9)			
Bronchial fluid	1.13±0.39	1.4±0.2	2.9±1.1
Serum	34.4±3.4	172.1±26.1	398.9±67.6
Ratio[e]	0.033	0.008	0.007

[a]Fifty- to 100-fold concentration to 1 ml at 4°C immediately after lung lavage and separation of cells.
[b]Serum C4 titer for normal controls, 141,005±5,300.
[c]Serum C6 titer for normal controls, 443.8±28.0.
[d]Mean±SE and range for group given.
[e]Bronchial fluid/serum ratio of means.

that erythrocytes coated with IgM antibody (EA) do not form rosettes and are not ingested by macrophages because macrophages lack an IgM surface receptor.

D. Lipid Components (Pulmonary Surfactant) in Bronchial Lavage Fluids

Following centrifugation of bronchial lavage fluid, the pelleted sediment is separated visibly into a bottom layer of brown cellular material, which contains respiratory cells, and above it a layer of white flocculent foamy acellular material which upon further analysis was surface-active and is designated pulmonary surfactant. Lipids, both polar and nonpolar (neutral), are present in both layers of the sediment and have been thoroughly analyzed in smoking (cigarette) and nonsmoking volunteers by Finley and Ladman [11]. The white acellular layer is considered to contain the surfactant. Of the neutral lipids analyzed in surfactant, free cholesterol and cholesterol esters accounted for 70% and free fatty acids and trigylcerides accounted for the rest. Of the phospholipids (polar lipids), phosphatidyl choline was predominent (64%). Although no qualitative differences were found among the lipid patterns of smokers and nonsmokers, quantitatively, lavage fluid from smokers contained about one–seventh of the white acellular material (surfactant) and phosphatidyl choline as did surfactant obtained from nonsmokers [11]. A conservative interpretation of these find-ings has been suggested [62], because of possible inefficient sampling of the lavaged lung area. Nevertheless, interesting information has been obtained which apparently distinguishes between two groups of normal subjects on the basis of their smoking history.

In our subjects, qualitative lipid analyses were done. Both neutral and polar lipids (phospholipids) were separated by thin–layer chromatography with the methods and appropriate solvents previously described [11,43]. We, too, were unable to detect any qualitative differences in the lipid patterns of smokers and nonsmokers, although total lipid content was found to be less in endobron-chial fluid obtained from smokers, as previously reported [11]. For neutral lipids, cholesterol and its esters were readily identified in bronchial specimens. The phospholipids separated into five major components of which phosphatidyl choline was predominant; in semiquantitative order, phosphatidyl ethanolamine was followed by phosphatidyl inositol and serine.

The significance of the lower levels of surfactant in smokers is not yet determined; however, is this deficit of surfactant due to its increased removal from the lungs of smokers or due to decreased production by Type II granular pneumocytes in alveoli? The implication has been raised that less surfactant in smokers could lower surface tension in the alveoli, thus promoting alveolar hyperinflation, which could be involved in the pathogenesis of emphysema [63]. Furthermore, it has been suggested that surfactant and alveolar lipid production is diverted toward synthetic processes of alveolar macrophages, which are found in increased numbers in smokers [11]. The high percentage of neutral lipids present as free or esterfied cholesterol in surfactant is of interest. Because the numbers of alveolar macrophages are increased, presumably to enhance phago-cytosis and clearance of noxious alveolar material, one wonders if the reduced percentage of free cholesterol found in the white layer of bronchial lavage from smokers (n = 7) 14.9 ±7.2 as compared with nonsmokers (n = 6) 31.3 ±16.3 [11] could reflect the increased utilization of cholesterol to repair macrophage cell membranes ingested during macrophage endocytosis [64]? Such questions are speculative but do point to an area of potentially useful investigation con-cerning the supply of alveolar nutrients for respiratory cell metabolism. These interactions have been approached with various animal models reviewed [62,65 66], but human data are still sparse.

E. Summary

As an aid to the diagnosis of pulmonary diseases, the analysis of bronchial-alveolar fluid components would be helpful, if results could be compared with normal findings. In an attempt to establish normal values, selective bronchial lavage by transnasal fiberoptic bronchoscopy was done in 42 subjects who were separated into groups of cigarette smokers and nonsmokers, because smoking is so prevalent in the normal population.

Because some of the patients who were heavy cigarette smokers had obstructive lung disease as disclosed by abnormal ventilatory pulmonary function tests, the fractional recovery of lavage fluid from the lower lobe was not as great as that in nonsmokers. Lingula lobe lavage, done in the 10 normal volunteers, was a more satisfactory procedure because the recovery of lavage fluid was greater. The bronchoscope can be positioned easily in the lingula and with gravity aiding the return of lavage fluid, this site seemed to be preferable for lavage. We were impressed that limited lavage, as a part of diagnostic bronchoscopy, was without hazard and apparently innocuous.

In smokers, the recovery of respiratory cells was greater, reflecting an increase in the number of alveolar macrophages, whereas nonsmokers had fewer macrophages but more lymphocytes. The milieu of the lower respiratory tract is quite different from that of the intravascular space, assuming that bronchoalveolar lavage is a representative sampling of the lung airways. The protein composition of concentrated bronchial fluid was seemingly less complex than that of plasma or serum. Only a few major proteins and enzymes were consistently identified in concentrated bronchial fluids: albumin, transferrin, a_1-antitrypsin, IgG, IgA, and free secretory component. IgA was found principally as 11 S secretory IgA, but 9% of IgA was in monomeric form and possibly of intravascular origin. Complement activity (C4 and C6 components) and IgE were in minimal quantities, and IgM was not present. Also, in smokers versus nonsmokers, the ratio of IgG:IgA in bronchial secretions was greater, indicating a relative increase of IgG; otherwise there were no significant qualitative or quantitative differences between the groups. It is not known whether this increase in IgG is the product of local immunoglobulin synthesis in the submucosa of the respiratory tract, or whether local irritation from smoking has increased transudation of IgG from the intravascular space. It was surprising that in young volunteers a brief history of cigarette smoking was sufficient to induce changes that might be associated with chronic smoking—greater numbers of respiratory cells and higher levels of IgG in bronchial fluids.

Acknowledgment

We appreciate the courtesy of the *Journal of Laboratory and Clinical Medicine* and the C. V. Mosby Co. in allowing us to reproduce portions of this manuscript, which have been previously published.

References

1. J. F. Smiddy, G. R. Kerby, and W. E. Ruth, The flexible fiberoptic bronchoscope in pulmonary diagnosis and therapy. Transcript 30th VA–Armed Forces Pulmonary Disease Research Conference, 1971, pp. 30.

2. M. A. Sackner, A. Wanner, and J. Landa, Applications of bronchofiberoscopy, *Chest,* Suppl. **62**:70–78S (1972).

3. W. F. Credle, Jr., J. F. Smiddy, and R. C. Elliott, Complications of fiberoptic bronchoscopy, *Am. Rev. Respir. Dis.,* **109**:67–72 (1974).

4. P. M. Sharp, G. A. Warr, and R. R. Martin, Effects of smoking on bronchial immunoglobulins, *Clin. Res.,* 21:672 (1973), (abstr.).

5. E. T. Cantrell, G. A. Warr, D. L. Busbee, and R. R. Martin, Induction of aryl hydrocarbon hydroxylase in human pulmonary alveolar macrophages by cigarette smoking, *J. Clin. Invest.,* **52**:1881–1884 (1973).

6. H. Y. Reynolds and H. H. Newball, Analysis of proteins and respiratory cells obtained from human lungs by bronchial lavage, *J. Lab. Clin. Med.,* **84**:559–573 (1974).

7. J. H. Hanks and J. H. Wallace, Determination of cell viability, *Proc. Soc. Exp. Biol. Med.,* **98**:188–192 (1958).

8. Z. A. Cohn and E. Weiner, The particulate hydrolases of macrophages. II. Biochemical and morphological responses to particle ingestion, *J. Exp. Med.,* **118**:1009–1019 (1963).

9. T. N. Finley, E. W. Swenson, W. S. Curran, G. L. Huber, and A. J. Ladman, Bronchopulmonary lavage in normal subjects and patients with obstructive lung disease, *Ann. Intern. Med.,* **66**:651–658 (1967).

10. J. O. Harris, E. W. Swenson, and J. E. Johnson, III, Human alveolar macrophages: Comparison of phagocytic ability, glucose utilization, and ultrastructure in smokers and nonsmokers, *J. Clin. Invest.,* **49**:2086–2096 (1970).

11. T. N. Finley and A. J. Ladman, Low yield of pulmonary surfactant in cigarette smokers, *N. Engl. J. Med.,* **286**:223–227 (1972).

12. A. B. Cohen and M. J. Cline, The human alveolar macrophage: Isolation, cultivation *in vitro,* and studies of morphologic and functional characteristics, *J. Clin. Invest.,* **50**:1390–1398 (1971).

13. D. W. Golde, T. N. Finley, and M. J. Cline, The pulmonary macrophage in acute leukemia, *N. Engl. J. Med.,* **290**:875–878 (1974).

14. H. Y. Reynolds, J. P. Atkinson, H. H. Newball, and M. M. Frank, Receptors for immunoglobulins and complement on human and rabbit alveolar macrophages, *Clin. Res.*, **22**:427 (1974) (abstr.).

15. H. Y. Reynolds, J. P. Atkinson, H. H. Newball, and M. M. Frank, Receptors for immunoglobulin and complement on human alveolar macrophages, *J. Immunol.*, **114**:1813–1819 (1975).

16. G. M. Green, The J. Burns Amberson Lecture–In defense of the lung, *Am. Rev. Respir. Dis.*, **102**:691–703 (1970).

17. J. J. Godleski and J. D. Brain, The origin of alveolar macrophages in mouse radiation chimeras, *J. Exp. Med.*, **136**:630–643 (1972).

18. D. W. Golde, L. A. Byers, and T. N. Finley, Proliferative capacity of human alveolar macrophage, *Nature* (London), **247**:373–375 (1974).

19. D. W. Golde, T. N. Finley, and M. J. Cline, Proliferative characteristics of the human alveolar macrophage, *Clin. Res.*, **22**:503 (1974) (abstr.).

20. D. C. Dale, H. Y. Reynolds, J. E. Pennington, R. J. Elin, T. W. Pitts, and R. G. Graw, Granulocyte transfusion therapy of experimental Pseudomonas pneumonia, *J. Clin. Invest.*, **54**:664–671 (1974).

21. P. E. G. Mann, A. B. Cohen, T. N. Finley, and A. J. Ladman, Alveolar macrophages: Structural and functional differences between non–smokers and smokers of marijuana and tobacco, *Lab. Invest.*, **25**:111–120 (1971).

22. R. P. Daniele, M. D. Altose, B. G. Salisbury, and D. T. Rowlands, Jr., Characterization of lymphocyte subpopulations in normal lungs, *Chest*, suppl., **67**:52–535 (1975).

23. U. Smith and J. W. Ryan, Electron microscopy of endothelial and epithelial components of the lungs: Correlations of structure and function, *Fed. Proc.*, **23**:1957–1966 (1973).

24. J. P. Szidon, G. G. Pietra, and A. P. Fishman, The alveolar–capillary membrane and pulmonary edema, *N. Engl. J. Med.*, **286**:1200–1204 (1972).

25. R. VanFurth and F. Aiuti, Immunoglobulin synthesis by tissue of the gastro–intestinal and respiratory tracts. In *Protides of Biological Fluids.* Proceedings of the Sixteenth Colloquium. Vol. 1969. London, Pergamon Press, 1969, pp. 479–484.

26. J. Bienenstock, N. Johnston, and D. Y. E. Perey, Bronchial lymphoid tissue I. Morphologic characteristics, *Lab. Invest.*, **28**:686–692 (1973).

27. H. B. Kaltreider and S. E. Salmon, Immunology of the lower respiratory tract: Functional properties of bronchoalveolar lymphocytes obtained from the normal canine lung, *J. Clin. Invest.*, **52**:2211–2217 (1973).

28. H. Y. Reynolds, R. E. Thompson, and H. B. Devlin, Development of cellular and humoral immunity in the respiratory tract of rabbits to *Pseudomonas* lipopolysaccharide, *J. Clin. Invest.*, **53**:1351–1358 (1974).

29. A. S. Rosenthal, J. M. Davie, D. L. Rosenstreich, and J. T. Blake, Depletion of antibody–forming cells and their precursors from complex cell populations, *J. Immunol.*, **108**:279–281 (1972).

30. B. Galindo and Q. N. Myrvik, Migratory response of granulomatous alveolar cells from BCG–sensitized rabbits, *J. Immunol.*, **105**:227–237 (1970).

31. C. S. Henney and R. H. Waldman, Cell–mediated immunity shown by lymphocytes from the respiratory tract, *Science* (Wash. D.C.), **169**:696–697 (1970).
32. R. H. Waldman and C. S. Henney, Cell–mediated immunity and antibody responses in the respiratory tract after local and systemic immunization, *J. Exp. Med.*, **134**:482–494 (1971).
33. G. L. Truitt and G. B. Mackaness, Cell–mediated resistance to aerogenic infection of the lung, *Am. Rev. Respir. Dis.*, **104**:829–843 (1971).
34. G. W. Fernald, W. A. Clyde, Jr., and J. Bienenstock, Immunoglobulin-containing cells in lungs of hamsters infected with Mycoplasma pneumoniae, *J. Immunol.*, **108**:1400–1408 (1972).
35. G. Biberfeld, Macrophage migration inhibition in response to experimental *Mycoplasma pneumoniae* infection in the hamsters, *J. Immunol.*, **110**:1146–1150 (1973).
36. E. Seravalli and A. Taranta, Release of macrophage migration inhibitory factor(s) from lymphocytes stimulated by streptococcal preparations, *Cell. Immunol.*, **8**:40–54 (1973).
37. J. C. Spencer, R. H. Waldman, and J. E. Johnson, III, Local and systemic cell–mediated immunity after immunization of guinea–pigs with live or killed M. tuberculosis by various routes, *J. Immunol.*, **112**:1322–1328 (1974).
38. B. R. Bloom, In vitro approaches to the mechanism of cell–mediated immune reactions, *Adv. Immunol.*, **13**:101–208 (1971).
39. R. I. Keimowitz, Immunoglobulins in normal human tracheobronchial washings, *J. Lab. Clin. Med.*, **63**:54–59 (1964).
40. P. L. Masson, J. F. Heremans, and J. Prignot, Studies on the proteins of human bronchial secretions, *Biochim. Biophys. Acta,* **111**:466–478 (1965).
41. The proteins of respiratory secretions. In *Molecular Biology of Human Proteins.* Vol. I. Edited by H. E. Schultze and J. F. Heremans. Amsterdam, Elsevier Publishing Co., 1966, pp. 816–831.
42. G. A. Falk, A. J. Okinaka, and G. W. Siskind, Immunoglobulins in the bronchial washings of patients with chronic obstructive pulmonary disease, *Am. Rev. Respir. Dis.*, **105**:14–21 (1972).
43. H. Y. Reynolds and R. E. Thompson, Pulmonary host defenses I. Analysis of protein and lipids in bronchial secretions and antibody responses after vaccination with Pseudomonas aeruginosa, *J. Immunol.*, **111**:358–368 (1973).
44. T. B. Tomasi, Jr. and J. Bienenstock, Secretory immunoglobulins, *Adv. Immunol.*, **9**:1–97 (1968).
45. T. B. Tomasi, Jr., Secretory immunoglobulins, *N. Engl. J. Med.*, **287**:500–506 (1972).
46. J. P. Vaerman and J. F. Heremans, Origin and molecular size of immunoglobulin A in the mesenteric lymph of the dog, *Immunology,* **18**:27–38 (1970).

47.   H. Y. Reynolds and J. S. Johnson, Structural units of canine serum and secretory immunoglobulin A, *Biochemistry,* **10**:2821–2827 (1971).

48.   R. D. Rossen, R. H. Alford, W. T. Butler, and W. E. Vannier, The separation and characterization of proteins intrinsic to nasal secretions, *J. Immunol.,* **97**:369–378 (1966).

49.   T. B. Tomasi, Jr., E. M. Tan, A. Solomon, and R. A. Prendergast, Characteristics of an immune system common to certain external secretions, *J. Exp. Med.,* **121**:101–123 (1965).

50.   K. Ishizaka and R. W. Newcomb, Presence of IgE in nasal washings and sputum from asthma patients, *J. Allergy,* **46**:97 (1970).

51.   R. H. Waldman, C. Virchow, and D. S. Rowe, IgE levels in external secretions, *Int. Arch. Allergy,* **44**:242–248 (1973).

52.   T. B. Tomasi, Jr. and S. P. Hauptman, The binding of alpha₁ antitrypsin to human IgA, *J. Immunol.,* **112**:2274–2277 (1974).

53.   R. G. Townley, F. Ryning, H. Lynch, and A. W. Brody, Obstructive lung disease in hereditary alpha 1 antitrypsin deficiency, *J.A.M.A.,* **214**:325–331 (1970).

54.   A. B. Cohen, Interrelationships between the human alveolar macrophage alpha-1-antitrypsin, *J. Clin. Invest.,* **52**:2793–2799 (1973).

55.   T. A. Gaither, D. W. Alling, and M. M. Frank, A new one step method for the functional assay of the fourth component (C₄) of human and guinea pig complement, *J. Immunol.,* **113**:574–583 (1974).

56.   J. E. May and M. M. Frank, Complement–mediated tissue damage: Contribution of the classical and alternate complement pathways in the Forssman reaction, *J. Immunol.,* **108**:1517–1525 (1972).

57.   M. Adinolfi, A. A. Glynn, M. Lindsay, and C. M. Milne, Serological properties of IgA antibodies to *Escherichia coli* present in human colostrum, *Immunology,* **10**:517–526 (1966).

58.   M. E. Kaplan, A. P. Dalmasso, and M. Woodson, Complement–dependent opsonization of incompatible erythrocytes by human secretory IgA, *J. Immunol.,* **108**:275–278 (1972).

59.   D. S. Eddie, M. L. Schulkind, and J. B. Robbins, The isolation and biologic activities of purified secretory IgA and IgG anti–*Salmonella typhimurium* "O" antibodies from rabbit intestinal fluid and colostrum, *J. Immunol.,* **106**:181–190 (1971).

60.   I. D. Wilson, Studies of the opsonic activity of human secretory IgA using an in vitro phagocytosis system, *J. Immunol.,* **108**:726–730 (1972).

61.   A. Zipursky, E. J. Brown, and J. Bienenstock, Lack of opsonization potential of 11S human Secretory IgA, *Proc. Soc. Exp. Biol. Med.,* **142**:181–184 (1973).

62.   J. A. Clements, Smoking and pulmonary surfactant (Editorial), *N. Engl. J. Med.,* **286**:261–262 (1972).

63.   T. E. Morgan, Pulmonary surfactant, *N. Engl. J. Med.,* **284**:1185–1193 (1971).
64.   Z. Werb and Z. A. Cohn, Plasma membrane synthesis in the macrophage following phagocytosis of polystyrene latex particles, *J. Biol. Chem.,* **247**: 2439–2446 (1972).
65.   T. E. Morgan, Biosynthesis of pulmonary surface–active lipid, *Arch. Intern. Med.,* **127**:401–407 (1971).
66.   A. Naimark, Cellular dynamics and lipid metabolism in the lung, *Fed. Proc.,* **32**:1967–1976 (1973).

2

Bronchus Associated Lymphoid Tissue (BALT): Its Relationship to Mucocal Immunity

JOHN BIENENSTOCK, ROBERT L. CLANCY, and
DANIEL Y. E. PEREY

McMaster Medical Center
Hamilton, Ontario, Canada

I. Introduction

The average adult, at rest, breathes in more than 500 ft^3 of air every day. Despite the efficiency of the upper respiratory tract in clearing the respired air of particulate matter, a substantial amount of fine particles, including potential pathogens, must constantly reach the lower respiratory tract. What immune resistance mechanisms does the lung possess to deal with these potential invaders?

Since the lungs are not generally regarded as lymphoid organs, it is of interest to note that Humphrey and coworkers [1,2], in 1958, showed that following intravenous hyperimmunization with particulate antigens, lung tissue was the most important tissue source of antibody, surpassing bone marrow, spleen, and lymph glands. Clearly the implication of this work is that there exists in lung tissue a substantial population of immunocompetent cells, which it might be presumed to be particularly well placed from the point of view of initiating

Supported by the Canadian Thoracic Society, the Medical Research Council of Canada and the Ontario Provincial Research Council, Canada.

host responses against pathogens. Yet, in a recent authoritative monograph on the lung, Spencer [3] devoted only half a page to the lymphoid tissue of the lung.

It would appear that the lung, as an organ, is an important component of the immune response, even when antigen is introduced parenterally. It is reasonable to speculate that this contribution might be enhanced after antigen is introduced locally through the tracheobronchial tract.

We first became interested in pulmonary lymphoid tissue during a series of experiments designed to investigate the effect of local passive instillation of immune complexes into the rabbit bronchial tract [4]. Despite an extensive acute inflammatory response in bronchial and alveolar tissue, clearly defined follicular lymphoid aggregates, closely related to the bronchial mucosa, did not appear to participate directly in this acute host response. Moreover, the number, size, distribution, and appearance of these lymphoid aggregates did not differ from those of normal animals, which had not received immune complexes. As a result of these observations, we extended our investigations into other animal species, including man. We noted subepithelial follicular lymphoid aggregates in most species studied and termed them bronchus-associated lymphoid tissue (BALT) [5,6]. Since the mucosa of the normal lung possesses relatively few immunoglobulin-containing cells in the lamina propria, several questions about the function of BALT, in terms of host-resistance, in general, and local immunity in particular, can be raised.

1. What is the derivation of cells comprising BALT follicles?

2. What is the destination of these cells?

3. Is the formation of BALT dependent on antigenic stimulation?

4. Is there a relationship between BALT lymphocytes and IgA production?

5. Is there a relationship between BALT, mast cells, basophils, and IgE production?

6. Does the BALT contain actual or potential effector cells of cell-mediated immunity?

7. How does BALT differ from other mucosa-associated lymphoid tissue?

8. Is there an immunologic system common to mucosal surfaces?

We shall restrict ourselves, in this review, to the description of BALT, our attempts to ascertain its functional nature, and speculation as to its significance and relationships to other lymphoid tissue.

II. Historic

Burdon-Sanderson [7], in 1868, may have been the first person to have mentioned lymphoid tissue within the bronchial walls, and he appears to have concluded that this lymphoid tissue was the first site of disease in experimental tuberculosis of the guinea pig. Klein [8], in 1875, wrote: "these lymphoid follicles in the bronchial walls are therefore in every respect analogous to the lymph follicles found in other mucous membranes, e.g., tonsils and in the intestine...." Detailed illustrations (Fig. 1) and extensive and careful investigation of this lymphoid tissue is available in this reference. The most complete review of the function and morphology of this lymphoid tissue is to be found in the book by Miller [9], published in 1937, in which there is a detailed account of the studies of a large number of investigators who had worked in this general area between 1868 and the 1930s. Simson and Strachan [10], in 1931, published an account of this lymphoid tissue in bronchial tissue obtained from children. This report contains some excellent early photomicrographs of the BALT and some interesting references, particularly relating to tuberculosis and silicosis. It is not our intention here to provide a complete historic account and, to this end, we would refer the reader to Klein [8], Miller [9], Brundelet [11] and von Seebach and Schoeler [12].

III. Anatomy of BALT

A. Macroscopic

Lymphoid tissue could be detected in situ by the acetic acid fixation procedure of Carlens [13]. The lymphoid tissue appeared as white opacities (Fig. 2). These lymphoid areas can, with practice, be discerned under the dissecting microscope, since at high magnification the areas of epithelium overlying the lymphoid follicles have a different appearance. The BALT follicles in chicken consist of mucosal projections into the lumen of large bronchi expecially and can be detected easily at low magnification under the dissecting microscope. The distribution of lymphoid tissue is random, down the length of the bronchial tract as far as the small bronchioles. In addition, it is concentrated around bifurcations (Fig. 2). In the chicken, large amounts of tissue can be seen in the trachea as well [14], and this lymphoid tissue has been shown in situ, using the staining technique of Moe [15].

B. Microscopic

The BALT in the rabbit [5,6], in which most studies have been performed, tends to consist of isolated aggregates of one or two follicles lying at some point

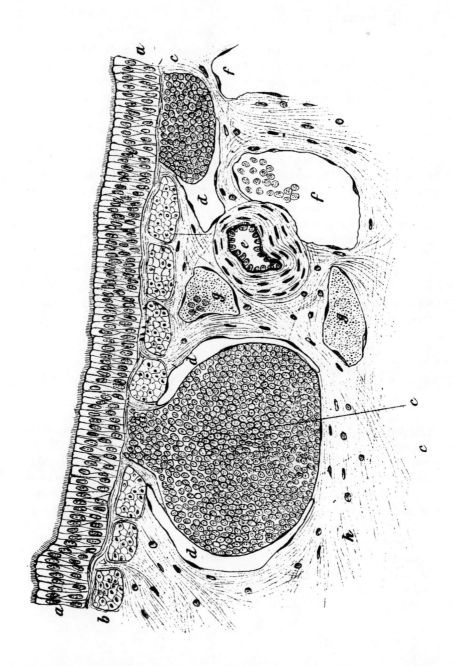

FIGURE 1 From Klein (1875) [8]. "Longitudinal section through a small bronchus of a guinea pig's lung. (a) Ciliated epithelium; (b) Circular coat of unstriped muscles transversely cut; (c) Lymphatic follicles belonging to the wall of lymphatic vessels, (d); (e) Branch of pulmonary artery; (f) Lymphatic vessels; (g) The same filled with granular material (coagulated plasm). In some of the lymphatic vessels clusters of lymph-corpuscles are to be found." Note the absence of epithelial change over the follicle, and the absence of lymphocytes in epithelium.

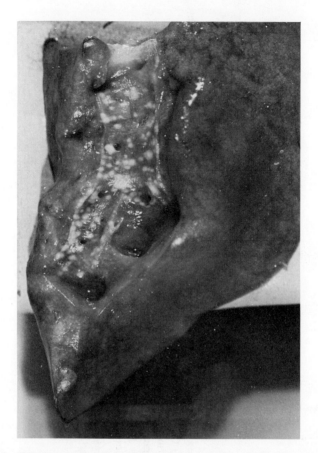

FIGURE 2   Rabbit lung treated with acetic acid. White opacities are **BALT** and
are found around bifurcations. Reprinted from *Lab. Invest.*, 28:686, 1973, by
courtesy of the Williams and Wilkins Company.

immediately below the epithelium (Fig. 3). The overlying epithelium often ex-
hibits a change in histologic appearance from columnar and cuboidal to a flattened irregular shape. The epithelium is heavily infiltrated with lymphocytes
from underlying follicles (Fig. 4). This epithelium is reminiscent of the lymphoepithelium found overlying Peyer's patches in the gut. The epithelium over the
central point of the follicle tends to be deficient in glandular tissue and goblet
cells. The cilia, which appear to be regularly distributed over the surrounding
columnar epithelium, are less numerous and may be totally absent over the
lymphoepithelium. Special histologic techniques have confirmed the absence of
glandular tissue and goblet cells in the lymphoepithelium. The basement membrane under the lymphoepithelium is frequently interrupted, and the transverse
collagenous and muscle bundles are often fragmented and heavily infiltrated with
lymphocytes.

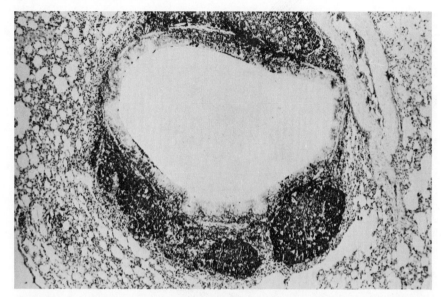

FIGURE 3 Transverse section of rabbit bronchus stained with hematoxylin and eosin showing BALT (40X). Reprinted from *Lab. Invest.*, 28:686, 1973, by courtesy of the Williams and Wilkins Company.

Most cells of the BALT follicles are mononuclear and consist mainly of lymphocytes with scattered reticulum cells and occasional macrophage–like cells. Using hematoxylin and eosin staining, we noticed circular or, more frequently, crescent–shaped areas of cells with nuclei that stain lighter than the surrounding sheets of lymphocytes. Rare plasma cells, judged either on classic appearance or by staining with methyl–green pyronine, have been seen within the lymphoid follicles. Occasional plasma cells were found in the lamina propria, adjacent to the follicles, particularly close to the lymphoepithelium. No true classic germinal center, as seen in the cortex of stimulated peripheral lymph nodes, have been found in BALT. Eosinophils are occasionally seen in overlying epithelium, especially when this is several layers thick.

In the cartilaginous bronchi, BALT often undertakes a 'collar stud' appearance, in which the major mass of lymphoid tissue lies below the cartilage and is connected by a narrow neck of lymphocytes that passes between two cartilaginous plates to an expanded lymphocytic collection immediately under the epithelium. The overlying epithelium in these cases is usually columnar in type, but always heavily infiltrated with lymphocytes. This may either reflect the greater distance between the epithelium and the follicle, or the planes of section.

In the chicken, unlike the mammalian species examined, the BALT contains clear–cut avian germinal centers, as seen commonly in spleen and cecal tonsils. In the mammalian species, the antiluminal portion of the follicles often

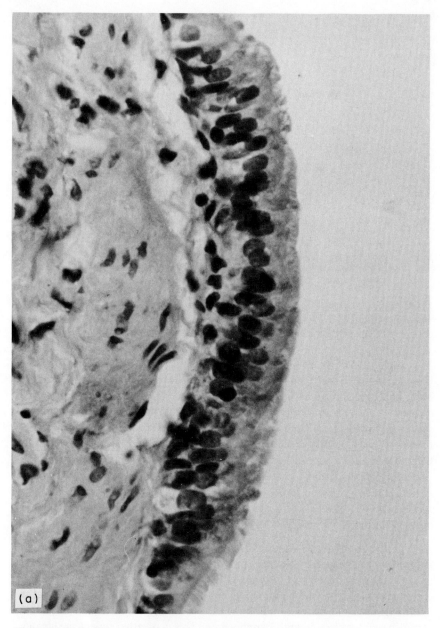

FIGURE 4(a)   Tissue sections stained with hematoxylin and eosin of normal
bronchial epithelium (380X).

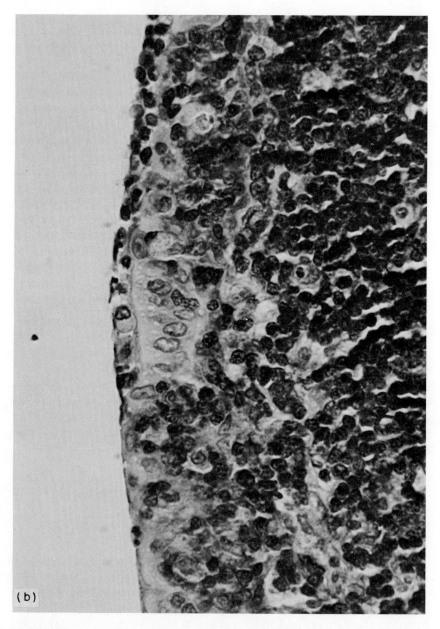

(b)

FIGURE 4(b) Lymphoepithelium overlying BALT (380X).

contains thin-walled vessels (presumed lymphatics). These have also been reported in the original descriptions of BALT by Klein [8].

C. Ultrastructural

The epithelium overlying the BALT often lacks cilia but possesses short microvilli [16]. Some of the characteristics of gut lymphoepithelium, described by Bockman [17], were also seen in BALT lymphoepithelium. Electron microscopy has documented the presence of lymphocytes with well-developed or developing endoplasmic reticulum, particularly toward the outside of the BALT follicles. It appears that these cells have been termed plasma cells by Chamberlain et al. [16] who also noted, in their ultrastructural studies of rat BALT, postcapillary venules with high cuboidal endothelium, typical of sites of lymphocyte emigration. In the BALT and bronchial epithelium, we have seen cells with numbers of dark homogeneous cytoplasmic granules. These have not been distinguished from macrophage or granulocyte granules, but the appearance is often of partially degranulated mast cells and is somewhat reminiscent of the granular lymphocytes we and others have described in the gut [18].

All these morphologic studies indicate that mammalian BALT differs significantly from peripheral lymphoid tissues, since it lacks classic germinal centers and is devoid of plasma cells. Frequently, BALT can be seen to relate closely to the bronchial epithelium, where it forms a characteristic lymphoepithelium. Although lymphocytes form the major constituents of BALT follicles, one can also observe, particularly with electron microscopy, the presence of granular cells reminiscent of basophils and mast cells. In the chicken, however, BALT is seen to protrude into the bronchial lumen and is made up of densely packed sheets of lymphocytes as well as classic avian germinal centers.

IV. Function of BALT

A. Derivation

To gain insight into the origin of BALT cells, we performed cytokinetic studies in rabbits, using intravenous injections of tritiated thymidine [6], and studied the fate of intravenously injected autologous thoracic-duct lymphocytes labeled in vitro with either tritiated uridine or thymidine [19]. We compared the labeling patterns and indices of BALT follicles as well as other lymphoid tissues (Fig. 5). The results of in vivo labeling studies indicate that a few isolated and scattered BALT lymphocytes become heavily labeled within 1 hr after the injection of thymidine. Superimposed upon this pattern, one occasionally sees small, defined

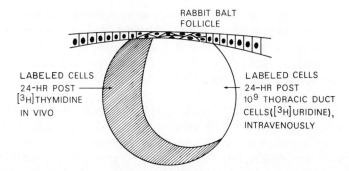

FIGURE 5 Schematic summary of autoradiographic findings in the rabbit BALT after in vivo [^{3}H] thymidine and intravenous transfer of 10^9 thoracic duct cells labeled invitro with [^{3}H] uridine.

areas of heavily labeled cells usually near the periphery of the BALT follicle. Labeled cells were rarely seen in the lymphoepithelium at this time, but 24 hr after the injection of thymidine, there still remained scattered, heavily labeled cells throughout the lymphoid sheet of BALT follicles. A substantial number of labeled cells within the lymphoepithelium were now seen. We interpreted these data to represent cells labeled at the time thymidine was injected and subsequently migrated to the epithelium without further proliferation. Lightly labeled cells were now evident in the crescent-shaped areas at the periphery of follicles, and this pattern may reflect the proliferation of the well-defined, heavily labeled cells seen at 1 hr.

To assess whether BALT follicles contain lymphocytes from the recirculating pool, thoracic–duct lymphocytes, obtained after short–term thoracic–duct drainage, were labeled in vitro with tritiated uridine (Fig. 5). This technique led to the labeling of most thoracic–duct lymphocytes, which were then washed and reinjected intravenously into the respective original donors. Autoradiographs of tissue sections, 24 hr later, revealed a distinct labeling pattern within BALT follicles. Lightly labeled cells were seen scattered throughout the sheets of lymphocytes, whereas areas we interpreted as labeled after the in vivo injection of thymidine were completely devoid of labeled cells. In the other lymphoid tissues, we could clearly identify thymus–dependent areas, as classically described. Incubation of thoracic–duct lymphocytes with tritiated thymidine in vitro, labeled less than 10% of the cells. When these were reinjected into autologous recipients, only rare, heavily labeled cells could be found in BALT follicles.

In summary, therefore, cytokinetic studies indicate that BALT is made up of both locally derived and replicating cells, as well as recirculating cells which form the pool of thymus–derived lymphocytes. The appearance of heavily labeled cells within the lymphoepithelium 24 hr after in vivo labeling would suggest that these cells represent an outward migration through the bronchial epithelium. This interpretation of a thymus–derived cellular component of BALT is supported by our observation [20] of the killing of 18% of cells in suspensions derived from BALT follicles (Table 1) with a specific goat antirabbit thymus-lymphocyte antigen antiserum (RTLA [21]). Moreover, neonatal thymectomy of chicks combined with sublethal total body x-irradiation also leads to partial depletion of the sheets of lymphocytes in the BALT of this species. However, surgical neonatal thymectomy, in both chickens and rats, in the absence of subsequent x-irradiation has failed to demonstrate a cell deficit in BALT. All of these studies, therefore, indicate that at least part of the BALT lymphocytes belongs to thymus–derived cell lines. However, this cell population would seem to represent, at best, one-quarter of the total BALT lymphocytes and one must, therefore, consider the possibility that the remaining BALT lymphocytes represent B cells or other lymphocytes not bearing T- or B-cell markers.

The direct immunofluorescent technique was used on cell suspensions to determine the heavy–chain class of receptors on B lymphocytes. We have made single–cell suspensions from rabbit bronchial mucosa by stripping the mucosal membrane from the parenchyma of the lung, washing the mucosa in Hank's balanced salt solution with 3% bovine serum albumin (HBSS-BSA), and grinding the tissue in a loose-fitting teflon homogenizer. Clumps and tissue debris were allowed to settle briefly at room temperature, and the dissociated cells were obtained from the supernatant by centrifugation at 300 g and washed once in HBSS-BSA. These cells were then subjected to a discontinuous BSA gradient and the interface between 10% and 28% was removed, washed, and resuspended in HBSS-BSA. Better than 90% of these cells were lymphocytes, with a viability greater than 95%, according to the trypan blue exclusion technique. These cell suspensions are considered to represent mainly BALT because of the predominance of this lymphoid tissue relative to the few lymphocytes scattered through the rest of the lamina propria, although no direct evidence exists to support this at present.

Results of direct immunofluorescence [20] on living cells with specific antisera to α, μ, and γ heavy chains [22] were compared to those obtained with splenic lymphocytes prepared by Ficoll-Hypaque buoyant–density separation techniques (Table 1). It can be seen that only 50% of the BALT cells possess membrane immunoglobulins, assuming that only a single class is represented on any individual cell membrane. Since another 20% of BALT cells bear the RTLA marker, this leaves approximately one-third of the BALT cells not possessing either a T- or B-cell marker. When the same BALT suspensions were fixed and stained for cytoplasmic fluorescence with the same reagents, less than 1% of the total stained with any anti–immunoglobulin antiserum. This result corroborated

TABLE 1 Surface Markers of Lymphocytes from
Various Rabbit Tissue Sources

Tissue source	RTLA[a] (Percent cytotoxicity)	Membrane immunoglobulins[b] (No. positive per 10^3 cells)		
		IgA	IgM	IgG
Thoracic duct	72.4±4.9[c]	108±13	108±13	61±8
BALT	18.4±3.9	172±24	168±31	75±10
Peyer's patches	16.6±4.0	299±39	320±42	168±15
Gut mucosa	11.1±3.4	73±6	62±8	32±4
Spleen	19.7±5.7	30±4	98±10	47±4

[a]Fradelizi et al. [21].
[b]Direct immunofluorescence.
[c]± standard error (SE).

our earlier findings, with the same reagents, on tissue sections of bronchial wall containing BALT, in which we did not find immunoglobulin-containing cells within the BALT follicles. This could be interpreted as providing further supportive evidence that the cell suspensions are representative of BALT tissue. In tissue sections, very few immunoglobulin-containing cells were seen at any time in normal bronchial lamina propria. Those cells that were seen were predominantly IgA-containing. Personal experience with immunofluorescence from normal mice, hamsters, rabbits, and man confirmed the relative scarcity of immunoglobulin-containing cells in the bronchial lamina propria, especially when compared to other lymphoid tissues and to gut.

In further experiments designed to characterize the nature of BALT cells, suspension culture in the presence of phytohemagglutinin and pokeweed mitogens at optimal concentrations, determined from dose-response curves of spleen-lymphocyte cultures, revealed little or no stimulation [23].

The experimental evidence to date suggests that both B and T cells comprise at least part of the cell constituents of BALT. To test the influence of the thymus and bursa on the ontogeny of BALT, we performed extirpative experiments in newly hatched chicks. As stated earlier, neonatal surgical thymectomy had, by itself, little effect upon the morphology of BALT. Similarly, surgical bursectomy at hatching did not influence the structure of BALT significantly. Agammaglobulinemic birds, which had been bursectomized and x-irradiated at hatching, lacked germinal centers throughout their lymphoid tissues, including the BALT. The combination of surgical thymectomy plus bursectomy at hatching, in the absence of further treatment, led to marked disorganization of BALT with partial depletion of lymphocytes and total absence of germinal centers at 5 months of age [19]. On the other hand, the spleen and cecal tonsils of these same birds were grossly normal, and both possessed germinal centers. We conclude, on the basis of our studies in chickens, that both an intact thymus and bursa are necessary for the normal ontogenetic development of BALT and that the germinal centers, evident in avian BALT, may differ from those seen in other peripheral lymphoid tissues.

Failure to demonstrate plasma cells within BALT, despite the presence of B cells therein, strongly suggests that BALT differs from other peripheral lymphoid tissues and may indeed serve as a site of differentiation for both B and T cells, which may complete their full differentiation outside BALT. With this thesis in mind, cell-transfer experiments were carried out, as discussed in the following section.

B. Destination

The eventual destination of cells present at a given time in BALT could be either the lumen of the bronchial tract, the tissue of the bronchial tract itself, or migration to other sites in the body. We must first consider the possibility that these cells migrate to the lumen. Most of the BALT follicles are separated at some point by a single layer of epithelium, which in most cases is heavily infiltrated with lymphocytes. That many of these lymphocytes may be derived from the BALT itself, is suggested by our cytokinetic data referred to earlier. Older morphologic studies described openings or "mouths" in the epithelium overlying what we have termed BALT. These authors described breaks in the epithelium through which lymphocytes and macrophages can come into contact with the contents of the lumen [11,12]. These were present in normal rat lung, but were exaggerated following inhalation of quartz dust [12]. Evidence that lymphocytes derived from Peyer's patches may find their way to the lumen of the gut has been brought forward by Faulk and coworkers [24], so that this phenomenon may not be unique to BALT. It is unlikely that lymphocytes from the upper respiratory tract would be found in bronchial washings because of the ciliary action of tracheobronchial epithelia. Thus, most of these cells may emanate from the lower respiratory tract. As discussed elsewhere in this review, functional studies of lymphocytes found in bronchial washings of both guinea pigs and mice have demonstrated the production of migration-inhibition factor (MIF) upon challenge with the relevant antigen after specific local antigenic immunization [25, 26]. Further, lymphocytes obtained from dog bronchial washings have been shown to synthesize immunoglobulins when cultured in vitro and were thought to be primarily B lymphocytes [27]. Similarly, plaque-forming cells have been detected in rabbit bronchial washings after local immunization with sheep red cells [28]. We obtained evidence [29], from comparative studies between BALT and lymphocytes from bronchial washings in the same animals, that spontaneous proliferation rates, as judged by in vitro incorporation of $[^3H]$ thymidine, always corresponded, i.e., whenever one was high so was the other, and vice versa. Further, introduction of antigen through the bronchial tract invariably caused an increase in turnover of cells from both sources, a phenomenon not found with parenteral immunization. All of these studies suggest that one potential fate of BALT lymphocytes is the lumen of the respiratory tract, either by direct migration or after recirculation.

We obtained evidence with cell-transfer studies into lethally irradiated allogeneic rabbit recipients that at least some BALT cells may go on to differentiate into IgA-producing cells [30]. Fifty million cells from the BALT of several rabbits were prepared separately and injected together into single recipients, which had received lethal (1000 R) irradiation on the same day. Parallel studies were done with allogeneic Peyer's patch cells. The recipients were killed 6 days later, and spleen cell-suspensions were made, fixed, and treated with antiheavy chain reagents in order to determine the number of immunoglobulin–containing cells in the spleen suspensions. At the same time, sections were taken from spleen, lung, and gut and subjected to direct immunofluorescence to obtain a qualitative estimate of the numbers of cells of a given immunoglobulin class in repopulated tissues.

In the spleen cell-suspensions following BALT transfer, there were 10 times as many IgA-producing cells as either IgG or IgM cells. BALT transfer resulted in repopulation of both gut and lung lamina propria with IgA-producing cells. Very few IgG- or IgM-producing cells were seen in either tissue. The numbers of IgA-producing cells in the lamina propria of the gut were similar for Peyer's patch and BALT cell-transfers. Relatively few IgA-producing cells were seen in the lamina propria of the bronchi, an observation that corresponded to the few IgA-producing cells normally found in this tissue. There was a greater concentration of IgA-producing cells close to Peyer's patches and BALT than in the rest of the tissue, and occasional BALT and Peyer's patch follicles were seen in tissue sections that possess membrane fluorescence positive for IgA but not for other classes of immunoglobulins. At no time were cytoplasmic fluorescent cells seen in either BALT or Peyer's patches.

The transfer of homologous lymph node cells resulted in the repopulation of spleen, predominantly by IgG-containing cells, whereas the lamina propria of both gut and lung was almost devoid of immunoglobulin–containing cells of any class.

It is significant that in these transfer experiments, cells from the BALT repopulated the lamina propria of both the lung and gut with IgA-producing cells, as did Peyer's patch cells. It is unlikely that the stimulus for the differentiation of cells going on to IgA production and the repopulation of the gut and lung lamina propria is somehow related to an allogeneic effect [31], since in parallel experiments we have shown that autologous Peyer's patch cell-transfer resulted in the same repopulation of IgA-producing cells in the gut and lung, although in this instance relatively few IgA-producing cells were seen in the spleens of recipients [32]. This quantitative difference does, however, suggest that stimuli other than antigen (perhaps T lymphocytes) can provide a proliferative drive that would amplify the IgA cell-producing population.

V. Discussion and Speculation

A. Does the Development of BALT Depend on Antigenic Stimulation?

A potential stimulus for the formation of BALT is inhaled antigens. Newborn rabbits do not possess BALT [5], which only differentiates later. Germ-free rats have been shown, by several groups [5,33,34], to possess BALT. However, Jericho [35] was unable to find intrapulmonary lymphoid tissue in pigs even at 39 days of age. In the human, BALT also appears after birth [36].

Since germ-free animals are clearly not antigen-free, these observations do not necessarily exclude the role of antigen in the development of this tissue. To overcome this problem, we transplanted mouse fetal lung and gut subcutaneously into syngeneic male adult recipients [6] and observed the development, both in lungs and gut, of subepithelial lymphoid aggregates. As in germ-free animals, these aggregates were smaller than those seen in conventional animals. Similar observations have been made by Andrews [37] on the lung following transplantation of fetal tissue into mammary fat pads of mice, and previously by Laws and Flaks [38]. Giddens et al. [39] observed the development of BALT in germ-free rats maintained on an antigen-free diet. Notwithstanding the conclusions of Jericho et al. [35,40,41] and Emery and Dinsdale [36], these findings suggest to us that the BALT, like Peyer's patches, do not necessarily require exposure to antigen for their development, although antigen may be required for the expansion and proliferation of this tissue as, for example, occurs with Peyer's patches in conventionalization of germ-free animals [42].

B. Does BALT Have a Reticuloendothelial Function?

Ultrastructural examination of BALT has shown that components of the reticuloendothelial system are present [16]. Many authors have proposed that BALT may function as a mechanism for disposing of dust and particulate matter [11, 43]. Macklin [44] suggested that these lymphoid aggregates were found in the lower respiratory tract and constituted "sumps" in which dust collected, trapped, and remained indefinitely. In this respect, Burdon–Sanderson [7] suggested, over 100 years ago, that the BALT in guinea pigs was the first site of disease in experimental tuberculosis. Emery and Dinsdale [36] have not found carbon particles in BALT (lymphoreticular aggregates) in human lungs. Another approach to the removal of dust and particulate matter has been taken by Brundelet [11] and Akazaki [43], who postulated that the BALT is in direct communication with the lumen through openings in the bronchial epithelium and provides an exit for macrophages, which track along peribronchial connective tissue and are eventually removed from the lung by ciliary action. This view has, however, not been supported by the more recent observations of von Seebach and Schoeler [12] who, despite their concurrence with the break in epithelium and lymphobronchial openings, think that it is a route for migration of lymphocytes rather than of macrophages.

Our own attempts to find more direct evidence for a reticuloendothelial function with BALT of rabbits by both the intravenous and intrabronchial instillation of india ink have failed to demonstrate any localization of carbon particles within BALT [6]. Since it is difficult to refute the ultrastructural findings of macrophage–like cells within BALT, one must assume that these cells are either destined to leave the lymphoid aggregates or, if they do remain within BALT, that they do not phagocytose particulate matter, although they may be involved in antigen processing. In that respect, we have failed to demonstrate significant antigen–binding in sections of BALT obtained from animals, which were either parenterally or locally immunized with specific antigens, despite the clear demonstration of specific antigen–binding within the spleen of parenterally immunized animals [45]. Since the site of antigen localization in both gut and bronchial lamina propria may be influenced by the nature of the antigen and the previous experience of the host [46], further studies along these lines in regard to BALT must be performed.

Of the 20 to 40 million cells which can be recovered in the tracheobronchial washings from a normal rabbit, most are alveolar macrophages [42]; only 5% to 10% are lymphocytes. Aerosol immunization increases both the yield of cells and the proportion of lymphocytes [28]. Much has been written on the phagocytic and scavenger function of these macrophages, but little is known of the role of this cell type in the local immune response. Recent studies of mouse irradiation chimeras have shown that essentially all alveolar macrophages are of bone marrow origin, although some local cell division probably occurs [48]. These cells may well play a major role in modifying the local immune response to inhaled antigen, since all particulate antigen entering their vicinity is rapidly and efficiently phagocytosed [49]. It is clear that adherent cells (presumably macrophages) collaborate with T and B lymphocytes during the immune response. Further, lymphokines released from T lymphocytes in vitro can arm alveolar macrophages, with a subsequent nonspecific increase in their capacity to kill certain injected organisms [50]. Lymphokines also inhibit the migration of rabbit alveolar macrophages from capillary tubes [51], however controversy exists regarding this response in different species [52]. Further, it is not so clear that such activation occurs as readily in vivo [53]. The relative inability of immune spleen lymphocytes to adoptively immunize mice against an aerogenic infection with *Listeria monocytogenes* [53] suggests that alveolar macrophages may not come into appropriate contact with circulating T cells, at least in the initial stage of infection. However, rechallenge of mice convalescent from an aerogenic infection with the same organisms, stimulated a prompt and massive recruitment of circulating monocytes [53], suggesting a readily available macrophage reserve, presumably from a precursor bone marrow pool.

Although it has been stated that the chief immunoglobulin synthesized by lymphocytes in the lower respiratory tract is IgG in the dog [27], washings of the bronchial tract and secretions from most mammalian species clearly show the predominance of IgA [54]. Biggar and coworkers [55] suggested that the alveolar macrophage may possess different surface receptors than its peripheral blood counterpart and thus could potentially be enhanced by the opsonic effect of locally produced IgA antibody. However, Reynolds and coworkers [56] recently showed that in respiratory tract secretions, IgG may be the most important opsonizing antibody. Further investigation of all classes of locally produced antibodies and their relationship to the local alveolar macrophage is of great importance; more so since there is controversy about the role of IgA in opsonization [57].

Alveolar macrophages have been identified as plaque–forming cells in direct assays of local primary immune responses [28]. Whether this occurs directly through a nonimmune mechanism, or through locally derived or circulating antibody, has not been established.

It can be concluded that the alveolar macrophage probably plays a complex and important role in both afferent and efferent limbs of the local immune response in the lung. Before this role can be clearly defined, much more needs to be learned with respect to the normal physiology of this cell; the normal mechanisms of handling of antigen by the respiratory tract; and the identification of the function, source, and circulation characteristics of lymphocytes and immunoglobulins contained within the bronchoalveolar space.

C. Is There any Relationship Between BALT and Basophils or Mast Cells?

Examination of preparations of BALT cells in suspension stained supravitally with toluidine blue has led to the observation that there are appreciable numbers of cells with metachromatic granules in the cytoplasm, which have the appearance of primitive mast cells [58]. Since mast cells are known to be present in the bronchial lamina propria [59] a systematic attempt was initiated to look for them in BALT tissue. Our preliminary results with electron microscopy and light microscopy, with special stains, revealed basophil-like cells, particularly in the peripheral zone of the BALT follicles. These cells are also seen in the epithelium above the basement membrane adjacent to the BALT follicles.

We recently described granular lymphocytes [18] in preparations of rabbit gut mucosa. These cells have single round nuclei and contain in their cytoplasm an average of five metachromatic granules (range 1-20). Similar cells are found in the gut epithelium on tissue section, as was recently described by Collan [60] in the rat. As yet, we do not know whether they also exist in the lung. Considerable discussion has appeared in literature regarding this cell type and it is well known that "globule leukocytes" and epithelial leukocytes are present in mucosal epithelia throughout the body [61,62,63]. Murray et al. [63] suggested that globule leukocytes and mast cells, and presumably granular lymphocytes, are one and the same cell, whereas Whur [64] thinks they are different. Collan [60] also thinks of them as being more related to the leukocyte series than to mast cells. We obtained evidence that granular lymphocytes obtained from the gut can be degranulated with phytohemagglutinin and concanavalin A but not with pokeweed mitogen [65]. In this regard, they possess properties similar to human, hamster, and rabbit peripheral blood basophils [66,67] as well as T cells. We have also shown that these cells release histamine, concomitant with degranulation. The origin of the mast cell and basophil is not well understood, but it has been suggested [68] that in the rat embryo the mast cell arises from loose connective tissue and not bone marrow. Most recently, we have shown that the rabbit basophil bears the thymus (RTLA) marker [69], and it is interesting to note that Burnet [70] suggested, in 1965, that thymic lymphocytes could transform into mast cells. The relationship between mast cells, basophils, granular lymphocytes, "globule leukocytes" [63], "theliolymphocytes" [62], and the aggregated lymphoid tissue either of lung or gut is completely unclear at present. The presence of these cells in bronchial epithelium, regardless of source, could play an important role in triggering the immune release of bronchoconstrictors. Indeed this possibility is suggested by the recent observation that inhalation of specific antigen by parenterally sensitized guinea pigs led to bronchoconstriction, even though the antigen did not penetrate the epithelial basement membrane [71].

D. What is the Relationship Between BALT Cells and Cell-mediated Immunity?

Lymphocytes comprise some 5% to 10% of the normal bronchoalveolar cell population. Plasma cells are not common in bronchial washings but may be found

after several days of in vitro culture [27]. B lymphocytes from bronchial washings can form plaques [48] and synthesize immunoglobulins [27]. Although
IgM and IgG production has been demonstrated by these techniques, it remains
to be shown whether IgA is also synthesized. The presence of T lymphocytes in
normal bronchial secretions is less well established. Phytohemagglutinin responsive lymphocytes could not be found following bronchial lavage of normal dogs
[27]. Our own preliminary data in rabbits support this observation and further
suggest that only 6% of lymphocytes washed from the normal rabbit bronchus
may have a thymic marker [72]. Local immunization with either a hapten-
protein antigen or a virus vaccine [25,73] has induced local cell-mediated immunity in lymphocytes from bronchial washings from guinea pigs as detected by
the specific release of MIF [25]. Instillation of high doses of antigen into the
respiratory tract led to systemic cell-mediated immunity [74], but it was not
established whether this resulted from the documented systemic distribution of
the antigen [74] or from emigration of locally sensitized cells. Similar findings
have been obtained in relation to plaque-forming cells in the mouse [26]. However, specifically sensitized cells in bronchial washings may belong to the recirculating pool and appear as a result of a local nonspecific stimulus [74]. Demonstration of memory for local cell-mediated immunity, as was shown for bronchial IgA antibody [75], may be of considerable biologic importance in view of
the limited time course of the primary immune response in bronchial washings as
detected by MIF [26]. Our own studies with cells from bronchial washings and
BALT have shown a similar time course for antigen-specific lymphocyte stimulation. Since it has been suggested that MIF can be released equally by both B
and T lymphocytes [76], the observation of local MIF release may well relate to
B-cell migration from the BALT.

The role of BALT cells, if any, in direct lymphocytotoxicity still has not
been demonstrated and no evidence exists on the possibility that antibody-
mediated lymphocytotoxicity can occur with BALT cells. In this regard, the
role of secretory IgA might well be worth pursuing.

E. What is the Relationship of BALT to IgA Production?

We have shown that in BALT, IgA and IgM are the predominant immunoglobulin
cell-surface receptors [20]. This appears to be true also for cells in the thoracic
duct as well as in Peyer's patches, but is not the case for cells in peripheral
lymphoid tissue, such as the spleen. When BALT cells are transferred into lethally irradiated allogeneic rabbits, the predominant immunoglobulin synthesized in
the repopulated spleens in IgA. This observation, similar to that obtained by
Craig and Cebra [77] with Peyer's patch cell transfer, suggests that a population
or subpopulation of BALT cells has the potential to develop into IgA-producing
cells. Nevertheless, in the spleen this observation may be irrelevant to the normal

physiologic processes, as suggested by our recent experiments [32] in which the injection of Peyer's patch cells into autologous lethally x-irradiated rabbits gave rise to a very reduced number of IgA-producing cells in the spleen when compared to that of allogeneic recipients. The same numbers of IgA-containing cells were seen in the lung and gut mucosae of both types of recipients. We have taken these data to indicate that an allogeneic effect was capable of inducing greater proliferation of IgA-containing cells in the spleen. In the absence of an allogeneic effect, both BALT and gut-associated lymphoid tissue (GALT) normally contains precursors of IgA-producing cells, which can repopulate the lamina propria of both the gut and lung. The nature of the stimulus for this differentiation is not known but could possibly be due to local exposure to antigens or to the specific microenvironmental influence of mucosal lymphoid aggregates.

F. Are T Cells Necessary for IgA Production?

Several lines of indirect evidence suggest that the thymus may be involved in the differentiation of IgA-producing cells. Serum IgA levels in nude mice are extremely low [78], and neonatal thymectomy in rabbits leads to low levels of serum IgA and markedly reduced serum IgA antibody responses to a hapten-albumin reagent [79]. Similarly, adult thymectomy combined with lethal total-body x-irradiation and reconstitution with allogeneic rabbit fetal liver cells decreased serum IgA [80]. We produced a model of IgA deficiency in the chicken in which bursectomy and thymectomy at hatching, without further treatment, resulted in the complete absence of both serum and secretory IgA up to 5 months of age [81]. These animals were markedly deficient in IgG but had normal levels of IgM. Their BALT follicles, which normally contain germinal centers, were completely disorganized and totally deficient in germinal centers, whereas the cecal tonsils, which are classic peripheral lymphoid tissue [82], were grossly normal and possessed germinal centers. The interaction of thymus- and bursa-derived cells, necessary for the phenotypic expression of IgA synthesis, may conceivably occur in the mucosal aggregates themselves.

Helper T cells have been demonstrated in Peyer's patches [83], and the 20% or so of RTLA positive cells in young adult rabbit BALT [20] may provide this function. In the repopulation experiments quoted above, it is conceivable that the T- and B-cell populations necessary for this interaction may have been supplied directly in the donor-cell population.

G. What is the Relationship of BALT to
IgM and IgG Production?

The role of BALT in this regard is unknown. Direct immunization of Peyer's patches appears to be the best-known method of priming the rat for IgM antibody production [84], and it is also known that most B cells have, at one time or another, probably expressed IgM on their cell surface [85]. Cooper and coworkers [85] postulate that a cell must go through an IgG phase from IgM before arriving at an IgA-synthesizing stage. No direct evidence exists to support this hypothesis. All available indirect evidence can so far be taken either to support this hypothesis or to support the suggestion that the initial B cell can bypass the IgG stage and go on to IgA production. It is true that in IgA deficiency in both chicken [86,81] and man [87], IgM-producing cells predominate in the mucosae. It is possible that this defect represents a subtle thymic–bursal imbalance which, although allowing lymphocytes to express IgA on their cell surface [88], does not permit the cell to go on to IgA synthesis and may divert the cell to IgM production for export. In this view, the capacity of BALT cells for IgM synthesis would be compatible with priming for IgM production after Peyer's patch immunization. It is interesting that the solution to this problem may also lie in the nature of the antigen presented. We have previously shown that *Mycoplasma* infection of the respiratory tract in hamsters resulted in a local IgM and not an IgA immune response [89]. Other antigens may well give rise to different responses, as would be evidenced by the immunofluorescent studies of Martinez–Tello et al. [90] and Callerame et al. [91] who found that both IgG- and IgA-producing cells predominated in the human bronchial lamina propria after a variety of respiratory tract infections. How many of these cells were, in fact, locally derived from mucosal aggregates as opposed to other sites is an important question yet to be resolved.

H. What is the Relationship of BALT to IgE Synthesis?

That the respiratory and gastrointestinal tracts are characterized by a predominance of IgA- as well as IgE-producing cells relative to other lymphoid organs [92], has been established. Further, IgE-producing cells often predominate in biopsies of the lamina propria from bronchi of patients with chronic respiratory tract disease [93], and evidence for local synthesis of IgE has been obtained in secretions from the respiratory tract in various diseases by Waldman et al. [94] and by Ishizaka and Newcombe [95]. Tada and Ishizaka [92], using antihuman IgE reagents in the monkey, reported IgE in Peyer's patch follicles. Thus the possibility exists that mucosal aggregates of both lung and gut may supply cells committed to the production of IgE destined for other mucosal surfaces. No evidence currently exists for this, but the possibility must be seriously entertained.

I. What Evidence is There for an Immunologic System Common to Mucosal Surfaces?

We described mucosal aggregates with morphologic characteristics similar to those of mucosal aggregates of the gut in the respiratory tract of a number of

TABLE 2 Comparison of Various Parameters and Properties of BALT, Peyer's Patch, and Lymph Node Lymphocytes

Properties	BALT	Peyer's patch	Lymph node
Lymphoepithelium	+	+	—
T–cell content (RTLA) (%)	18	20	70
B–cell content (membrane Ig) (%)	40[a]	78[a]	b
Plasma cells (cytoplasmic Ig)	–	–	+
Germinal centers			
(chickens)	+	+	+
(mammals)	–	–	+
(IgA deficiency [chickens])	–	?	+
Particulate clearance	? (–)	±	+
Repopulation with Peyer's patch cells	+	+	–
with BALT cells	+	+	–
with lymph node cells	–	–	+
Potential for predominant repopulation with IgA cells	+	+	–
Proliferative response to PHA	–	(+)	+
PWM	–	(+)	+

For explanation of abbreviations see text.
Range of reactions from –, ±, (+) to +.
[a]IgM = IgA > IgG.
[b]IgM = IgG > IgA.

mammalian species, including man. (For a summary and comparison of many of these characteristics see Table 2). These lymphoid aggregates are generally subepithelial and covered by a lymphoepithelium consisting, at some point, of flattened epithelial cells often heavily infiltrated with lymphocytes. The aggregates themselves do not possess immunoglobulin-containing cells and are made up, in part, of B cells, a subpopulation of which appears to be committed to eventual IgA production, and is capable of repopulating the lamina propria of the respiratory tract and gut.

Both the lung and gut are subjected to bombardment by potential pathogens, both are characterized by a secretory IgA local immunoglobulin system, and both are derived from endoderm. That these mucosal aggregates lie in sentinel positions, for example at bifurcations of main and stem bronchi, would clearly be an efficient way of priming other mucosal sites with cells specifically proliferating under the influence of antigen. The number of cells from BALT or Peyer's patches which go back to the lamina propria of the bronchi is compatible with the number of IgA-producing cells normally found in the absence of infection. This does not negate the findings of local IgA-antibody immune responses following local instillation of antigen either into the respiratory tract or gut, since the levels of sensitivity of antibody detection in secretions, particularly against viruses, is low and extremely small amounts of antibody synthesized after such a primary immunization would not be detected. To find out whether this occurs, much better techniques with higher sensitivity would have to be developed. Tissues would have to be examined to demonstrate specific antibody synthesis to the relevant antigen. However, the implications of this finding for the practice of immunization are considerable. Thus, it might be possible to obtain effective protection of mucosal surfaces by feeding the antigen orally in a practical and effective form. This would avoid the emerging concept that to achieve local immunization it is necessary to administer the antigen locally.

It is our feeling that these mucosal lymphoid aggregates may not be found just in the lung and gut but might be part of a wider mucosal immunologic system. Bang and Bang [14] have shown similar lymphoid aggregates in the lateral nasal gland and Harderian gland ducts of germ free-chickens. Ham [96], in his classic treatise on histology, refers to such mucosal lymphoid aggregates as lymphatic nodules "to provide a line of defense behind such wet epithelial membranes ... beneath the epithelial membranes lining the upper respiratory passes, the intestine and the urinary tract." Whether all of these mucosal aggregates as well as lymphoid tissue in other sites, such as mammary gland, salivary gland, and so forth, have any common function is, at this point, unknown, but remains an attractive hypothesis quite easily open either to refutation or verification.

References

1. J. H. Humphrey and B. D. Sulitzeanu, The use of (^{14}C) amino acids to study sites and rates of antibody synthesis in living hyperimmune rabbits, *Biochem. J.,* **68**:146–161 (1958).
2. B. A. Askonas and J. H. Humphrey, Formation of specific antibodies and gamma globulin in vitro. A study of the synthetic ability of various tissues from rabbits immunized by different methods, *Biochem. J.,* **68**:252–261 (1958).
3. H. Spencer. In *Pathology of the Lung.* New York, Pergamon Press, 1968, p. 58.
4. J. Bienenstock and N. Johnston. Immune complex disease: Effect of introduction of immune complexes into the tracheobronchial tree. In *Immune Reactions and Experimental Models in Rheumatic Diseases.*

Proceedings of the Fourth Canadian Conference on Research in the Rheumatic Diseases. Edited by D. A. Gordon. Toronto, University of Toronto Press, 1971, p. 145.

5. J. Bienenstock, N. Johnston, and D. Y. E. Perey, Bronchial lymphoid tissue. I. Morphologic characteristics, *Lab. Invest.*, **28**:686–692 (1973).

6. J. Bienenstock, N. Johnston, and D. Y. E. Perey, Bronchial lymphoid tissue. II. Functional characteristics, *Lab. Invest.*, **28**:693–698 (1973).

7. Burdon–Sanderson in Eleventh Report of the Medical Officer of the Privy Council, 1868. Quoted in *The Lung.* Edited by W. S. Miller. Springfield, Ill., Charles C. Thomas, 1937, pp. 101–102.

8. E. Klein. In *The Anatomy of the Lymphatic System. II. The Lung.* London, Smith, Elder and Co., 1875.

9. W. S. Miller. In *The Lung.* Springfield, Ill., Charles C. Thomas, 1937.

10. F. W. Simson and A. S. Strachan, *Publ. S. Afr. Inst. Med. Res.*, **26**:231 (1931).

11. P. J. Brundelet, Experimental study of the dust–clearance mechanism of the lung, *Acta Pathol. Microbiol. Scand.*, 175 (1965) (Suppl.).

12. H. B. von Seebach and K. Schoeler, Das lymphoepitheliale system der rattenlunge bei experimenteller quarzstaub–belastung. The pulmonary lymphatic system of the rat following experimental exposure to quartz dust, *Virchows Arch. A.*, **350**:205–215 (1970).

13. O. Carlens, Studien über das lymphatische Gewebe des Darmkanals bei einigen Haustieren, mit besonderer Berücksichtigung der embryonalen Entwicklung, der Mengenverhältnisse und der Alterinvolution dieses Gewebes in Dünndarm des Rindes. *Z. Anat. Entwicklungsgesch*, **86**:393–493 (1928).

14. B. G. Bang and F. B. Bang, Localized lymphoid tissues and plasma cells in paraocular and paranasal organ systems in chickens, *Am. J. Pathol.*, **53**: 735–751 (1968).

15. H. Moe, Mapping goblet cells in mucous membranes, *Stain Technol.*, **27**: 141–146 (1952).

16. D. W. Chamberlain, C. Nopjaroonsri, and G. T. Simon, Ultrastructure of the pulmonary lymphoid tissue, *Am. Rev. Respir. Dis.*, **108**:621–631 (1973).

17. D. E. Bockman and M. D. Cooper, Pinocytosis by epithelium associated with lymphoid follicles in the bursa of Fabricius, appendix, and Peyer's patches. An electron microscopic study, *Am. J. Anat.*, **136**:455–477 (1973).

18. O. Rudzik and J. Bienenstock, Isolation and characteristics of gut mucosal lymphocytes, *Lab. Invest.*, **30**:260–266 (1974).

19. J. Bienenstock, O. Ruzdik, R. L. Clancy, and D. Y. E. Perey. In *Proceedings of the International Symposium on the Immunoglobulin A System*, Birmingham, Alabama, October 1973. Edited by F. W. Kraus, et al. New York, Plenum Publishing Corp., 1974.

20. O. Rudzik, R. Clancy, D. Perey, J. Bienenstock, and D. Singal, The distribution of a rabbit thymic antigen and membrane immunoglobulins in

lymphoid tissue, with special reference to mucosal lymphocytes, *J. Immunol.,* **114**:1–4 (1975).

21.   D. P. Fradelizi, C. T. Chou, B. Cinader, and S. Dubiski, A membrane antigen of rabbit thymus cells, *Cell. Immunol.,* **7**:484–501 (1973).

22.   D. Y. E. Perey, D. Frommel, R. Hong, and R. A. Good, The mammalian homologue of the avian bursa of Fabricius. II. Extirpation, lethal x–irradiation, and reconstitution in rabbits. Effects on humoral immune responses, immunoglobulins, and lymphoid tissues, *Lab. Invest.,* **22**:212–227 (1970).

23.   R. Clancy and J. Bienenstock, The proliferative response of lymphocytes from mucosa–associated lymphoid tissues to phytohaemagglutinin and pokeweed mitogen. Unpublished data.

24.   W. P. Faulk, J. N. McCormick, J. R. Goodman, J. M. Yoffey, and H. H. Fudenberg. Peyer's patches: Morphologic studies, *Cell. Immunol.,* **1**: 500–520 (1970).

25.   C. S. Henney and R. H. Waldman, Cell–mediated immunity shown by lymphocytes from the respiratory tract, *Science,* **169**:696–697 (1970).

26.   D. R. Nash, Direct and indirect plaque forming cells in extrapulmonary lymphoid tissue following local vs systemic injection of soluble antigen, *Cell. Immunol.,* **9**:234–241 (1973).

27.   H. B. Kaltreider and S. E. Salmon, Immunology of the respiratory tract. Functional properties of bronchoalveolar lymphocytes obtained from the normal canine lung, *J. Clin. Invest.,* **52**:2211–2217 (1973).

28.   M. Holub and R. E. Hauser, Lung alveolar histiocytes engaged in antibody production, *Immunology,* **17**:207–226 (1969).

29.   R. Clancy and J. Bienenstock, *J. Immunol.,* in press, (1975).

30.   O. Rudzik, R. Clancy, D. Perey, R. Day, and J. Bienenstock, Repopulation with IgA containing cells of bronchial and intestinal lamina propria after transfer of homologous Peyer's patch and bronchial lymphocytes, *J. Immunol.,* in press, (1975).

31.   D. H. Katz and B. Benacerraf, The regulatory influence of activated T cells on B cell responses to antigen, *Adv. Immunol.,* **15**:1–94 (1972).

32.   O. Rudzik, D. Y. E. Perey and J. Bienenstock. Unpublished data.

33.   W. E. Giddens and C. K. Whitehair. In *Germ–Free Biology.* Edited by E. A. Mirand and N. Black. New York, Plenum Publishing Corp., 1969, p. 75.

34.   W. E. Giddens, C. K. Whithair, and G. R. Carter, Morphologic and microbiologic features of trachea and lungs in germfree, define–flora, conventional, and chronic respiratory disease–affected rats, *Am. J. Vet. Res.,* **32**: 115–129 (1971).

35.   K. W. F. Jericho, Intrapulmonary lymphoid tissue of healthy pigs, *Res. Vet. Sci.,* **11**:548–552 (1970).

36.   J. L. Emery and F. Dinsdale, The postnatal development of lymphoreticular aggregates and lymph nodes in infants' lungs, *J. Clin. Pathol.,* **26**:539–545 (1973).

37. E. J. Andrews, The survival and differentiation of embryonic lung tissues in diffusion chambers and in mammary fat pads of mice, *Anat. Rec.,* **172**: 89–96 (1972).

38. J. O. Laws and A. Flaks, Pulmonary adenomata induced by carcinogen treatment in organ culture, *Br. J. Cancer,* **20**:550–554 (1966).

39. W. E. Giddens, Morphologic and microbiologic features of trachea and lungs in germfree, defined–flora, conventional, and chronic respiratory disease–affected rats. Quoted in *Am. J. Vet. Res.,* **32**:115–129 (1971).

40. K. W. F. Jericho, P. K. C. Austwick, R. T. Hodges, and J. Dixon, Intra-pulmonary lymphoid tissue of pigs exposed to aerosols of carbon particles, of Salmonella oranienburg, of *Mycoplasma granularum,* and to an oral inoculum of larvae of *Metastrongylus apri, J. Comp. Pathol.,* **81**:13–21 (1971).

41. K. W. F. Jericho, J. B. Derbyshire, and J. E. T. Jones, Intrapulmonary lymphoid tissue of pigs exposed to aerosols of haemolytic streptococcus group L and porcine adenovirus, *J. Comp. Pathol.,* **81**:1–11 (1971).

42. M. Pollard, M. Sharon, and N. Sharon, Responses of the Peyer's patches in germ–free mice to antigenic stimulation, *Infect. Immun.,* **2**:96–100 (1970).

43. K. Akazaki, Über das Fruhstadium der Reaktion des Lungengewebes bei Einführung der verschiedenen Staubarten, *Beitr. Pathol. Anat. Allg. Pathol.* **97**:439–480 (1936).

44. C. C. Macklin, Pulmonary sumps, dust accumulations, alveolar fluid, and lymph vessels, *Acta Anat.,* **23**:1–33 (1955).

45. R. Clancy and J. Bienenstock, The Proliferative response of bronchus-associated lymphoid tissue after local and systemic immunization, *J. Immunol.,* **112**:1997–2001 (1974).

46. R. L. Hunter, Antigen trapping in the lamina propria and production of IgA antibody, *J. Reticuloendothel. Soc.,* **11**:245–252 (1972).

47. Q. N. Myrvik, E. S. Leake, and B. Fariss, Studies on pulmonary alveolar macrophages from the normal rabbit: A technique to procure them in a high state of purity, *J. Immunol.,* **86**:128–132 (1961).

48. J. J. Godleski and J. D. Brain, The origin of alveolar macrophages in mouse radiation chimeras, *J. Exp. Med.,* **136**:630–643 (1972).

49. G. M. Green and E. H. Kass, The role of the alveolar macrophage in the clearance of bacteria from the lung, *J. Exp. Med.,* **119**:167–176 (1964).

50. F. T. Valentine and H. S. Lawrence, Cell–mediated immunity, *Adv. Intern. Med.,* **17**:51–93 (1971).

51. T. Kawai, S. Salvaggio, J. O. Harris, and P. Arquembourg, Alveolar macro-phage migration inhibition in animals immunized with thermophilic actino-mycete antigen, *Clin. Exp. Immunol.,* **15**:123–130 (1973).

52. R. W. Leu, A. L. Eddleston, J. W. Hadden, and R. A. Good, Mechanism of action of migration inhibitory factor (MIF). I. Evidence for a receptor for MIF present on the peritoneal macrophage but not on the alveolar macro-phage, *J. Exp. Med.,* **136**:589–603 (1972).

53. G. B. Mackaness, The J. Burns Amberson lecture–The induction and

expression of cell–mediated hypersensitivity in the lung, *Am. Rev. Respir. Dis.,* **104**:813–828 (1971).

54.   T. B. Tomasi and J. Bienenstock, Secretory Immunoglobulins, *Adv. Immunol.,* **9**:1 (1968).
55.   W. D. Biggar, B. Holmes, and R. A. Good, Opsonic defect in patients with cystic fibrosis of the pancreas, *Proc. Natl. Acad. Sci.,* **69**:1716–1719 (1971).
56.   H. Y. Reynolds and R. E. Thompson, Pulmonary host defenses. II. Interaction of respiratory antibodies with Pseudomonas aeruginosa and alveolar macrophages, *J. Immunol.,* **111**:369–380 (1973).
57.   A. Zipursky, E. Brown and J. Bienenstock, Lack of opsonization potential of 11S human secretory γA, *Proc. Soc. Exp. Biol. Med.,* **142**:181–184 (1973).
58.   O. Rudzik, R. Clancy and J. Bienenstock. Unpublished data.
59.   G. L. Brinkman, N. Brooks, and V. Bryant, The ultrastructure of the lamina propria of the human bronchus, *Am. Rev. Respir. Dis.,* **99**:219–228 (1969).
60.   Y. Collan, Characteristics of nonepithelial cells in the epithelium of normal rat ileum, *Scand. J. Gastroenterol.,* Suppl. 7:1–66 (1972).
61.   D. Darlington and A. W. Rogers, Epithelial lymphocytes in the small intestine of the mouse, *J. Anat.,* **100**:813–830 (1966).
62.   K. E. Fichtelius, The gut epithelium—A first level lymphoid organ? *Exp. Cell Res.,* **49**:87–104 (1968).
63.   M. Murray, H. R. P. Miller, and W. F. H. Jarrett, The globule leukocyte and its derivation from the subepithelial mast cell, *Lab. Invest.,* **19**:222–234 (1968).
64.   P. Whur and H. S. Johnston, Ultrastructure of globule leucocytes in immune rats infected with *Nippostrongylus brasiliensis* and their possible relationship to the Russell body cell, *J. Pathol. Bacteriol.,* **93**:81–85 (1967).
65.   R. P. Day, O. Rudzik, and J. Bienenstock. Unpublished data.
66.   W. A. Hook, S. F. Dougherty, and J. J. Oppenheim, Histamine release from hamster mast cells and human basophils by nonspecific mitogens, *Fed. Prod.,* **32**:1000 (1973)
67.   R. P. Day, J. Dolovich, and J. Bienenstock, Characteristics of tritiated histamine uptake and release by human basophils, *Fed. Proc.,* 752 (1973).
68.   J. W. Combs, D. Lagunoff, and E. P. Benditt, Differentiation and proliferation of embryonic mast cells of the rat, *J. Cell Biol.,* **25**:577–592 (1965).
69.   R. P. Day, D. Singal, and J. Bienenstock, Presence of thymic antigen on rabbit basophils, *J. Immunol.,* **114**:1333–1336 (1975).
70.   F. M. Burnet, Mast cells in the thymus of NZB mice, *J. Pathol. Bacteriol.,* **89**:271–284 (1965).
71.   J. B. Richardson, J. C. Hogg, R. Bouchard, and D. L. Hall, Localization of antigen in experimental bronchoconstriction in guinea pigs, *J. Allergy Clin. Immunol.,* **52**:172–181 (1973).
72.   R. Clancy, D. Singal, and J. Bienenstock. Unpublished data.
73.   R. H. Waldman, C. S. Spencer, and J. E. Johnson, Respiratory and systemic cellular and humoral immune responses to influenza virus vaccine administered parenterally or by nose drops, *Cell. Immunol.,* **3**:294–300 (1972).

74. D. Nash and B. Holle, Local and systemic cellular immune responses in guinea pigs given antigen parenterally or directly into the lower respiratory tract, *Clin. Exp. Immunol.,* **13**:573–583 (1973).

75. J. L. F. Gerbrandy and E. A. Van Dura, Anamnestic secretory antibody response in respiratory secretions of intranasally immunized mice, *J. Immunol.,* **109**:1146–1148 (1972).

76. T. Yoshida, H. Sonosaki, and S. Cohen, The production of migration inhibition factor by B and T cells of the guinea pig, *J. Exp. Med.,* **138**: 784–797 (1973).

77. S. W. Craig and J. J. Cebra, Peyer's patches: An enriched source of precursors for IgA–producing immunocytes in the rabbit, *J. Exp. Med.,* **134**: 188–200 (1971).

78. A. L. Luzzati and E. B. Jacobson, Serum immunoglobulin levels in nude mice, *Eur. J. Immunol.,* **2**:473–474 (1972).

79. J. D. Clough, L. H. Mims, and W. Strober, Deficient IgA antibody responses to arsanilic acid bovine serum albumin (BSA) in neonatally thymectomized rabbits, *J. Immunol.,* **106**:1624–1629 (1971).

80. D. Y. E. Perey, D. Frommel, R. Hong, and R. A. Good, The mammalian homologue of the avian bursa of Fabricius. II. Extirpation, lethal x–irradiation, and reconstitution in rabbits. Effects on humoral immune responses, immunoglobulins, and lymphoid tissues, *Lab. Invest.,* **22**:212–227 (1970).

81. D. Y. E. Perey and J. Bienenstock, Effects of bursectomy and thymectomy on ontogeny of fowl IgA, IgG and IgM, *J. Immunol.,* **111**:633–637 (1973).

82. J. Bienenstock, J. Gauldie, and D. Y. E. Perey, Synthesis of IgG, IgA, IgM by chicken tissues: Immunofluorescent and ^{14}C amino acid incorporation studies, *J. Immunol.,* **111**:1112–1118 (1973).

83. D. H. Katz and D. Y. E. Perey, Lymphocytes in Peyer's patches of the mouse: Analysis of the constituent cells in terms of their capacities to mediate functions of mature T and B lymphocytes, *J. Immunol.,* **111**: 1507–1513 (1973).

84. G. N. Cooper and K. Turner, Immunological responses in rats following antigenic stimulation of Peyer's patches. 3. Local and general sequelae, *Aust. J. Exp. Biol. Med. Sci.,* **46**:415–424 (1968).

85. M. D. Cooper, A. R. Lawton, and P. W. Kincade, A two–stage model for development of antibody–producing cells, *Clin. Exp. Immunol.,* **11**:143–149 (1972).

86. P. W. Kincade and M. D. Cooper, Immunoglobulin A: Site and sequence of expression in developing chicks, *Science,* **179**:398–400 (1973).

87. S. Eidelman and S. D. Davis, Immunoglobulin content of intestinal mucosal plasma–cells in ataxia telangiectasia, *Lancet,* **1**:884–886 (1968).

88. A. R. Lawton, A. S. Royal, K. S. Self, and M. D. Cooper, IgA determinants on B–lymphocytes in patients with deficiency of circulating IgA, *J. Lab. Clin. Med.,* **80**:26–33 (1972).

89. G. W. Fernald, W. A. Clyde, and J. Bienenstock, Immunoglobulin–containing cells in lungs of hamsters infected with *Mycoplasma Pneumoniae,* *J. Immunol.,* **108**:1400–1408 (1972).

90. F. J. Martinez–Tello, D. G. Braun, and W. A. Blanc, Immunoglobulin pro-
     duction in bronchial mucosa and bronchial lymph nodes, particularly in
     cystic fibrosis of the pancreas, *J. Immunol.*, **101**:989–1003 (1968).

91. M. L. Callerame, J. J. Condemi, K. Ishizaka, S. G. O. Johansson, and
     J. Vaughan, Immunoglobulins in bronchial tissues from patients with
     asthma, with special reference to immunoglobulin E, *J. Allergy*, **47**:187–
     197 (1971).

92. T. Tada and K. Ishizaka, Distribution of gamma E–forming cells in lymph-
     oid tissues of the human and monkey, *J. Immunol.*, **104**:377–387 (1970).

93. M. A. Gerber, F. Paronetto, and S. Kochwa, Immunohistochemical
     localization of IgE in asthmatic lungs, *Am. J. Pathol.*, **62**:339–352 (1971).

94. R. H. Waldman, C. Virchow, and D. S. Rowe, IgE levels in external secre-
     tions, *Int. Arch. Allergy Appl. Immunol.*, **44**:242–248 (1973).

95. K. Ishizaka and R. W. Newcomb, Presence of gamma E in nasal washings
     and sputum from asthmatic patients, *J. Allergy*, **46**:197–204 (1970).

96. A. W. Ham. In *Histology*. New York, Lippincott Co., 1969, p. 313.

3

Cell-mediated Immune Reactions in the Lung

CHRISTOPHER S. HENNEY

The Johns Hopkins University School of Medicine
Baltimore, Maryland

I. Introduction

Immune phenomena depend on cells of the lymphocyte series for their expression. Currently two major subpopulations of immunocompetent lymphoid cells are recognized; (a) that which depends on the thymus for differentiation (such cells are consequently termed thymus-derived lymphocytes or T cells), and (b) that which differentiates independently of the thymus. In birds, the latter cells require the Bursa of Fabricius for development, and although the mammalian analogue of this organ is unknown, these lymphocytes are termed B cells. This subdivision of lymphoid-cell elements, based on their mode of differentiation, corresponds broadly with their immune functions: T cells are the effectors of cell-mediated immune reactions, whereas B cells are precursors of antibody-forming plasma cells which mediate humoral immunity.

Cell-mediated and humoral immune mechanisms are often complementary in the protective sense, and antigenic challenge almost invariably leads to both cell-mediated and humoral immune responses. In protective terms, there seems to be some degree of specialization in the two arms of the immune response: humoral immunity is often viewed as the dominant protective mechanism against pyogenic infection and against toxin-producing infections, whereas cell-mediated immunity is commonly thought to be primarily involved in immune surveillance, in protection against the development of neoplastic growth, and in rejection of allografted tissue. These functional designations are, of course, crude ones. Recently, antibody-independent immune protection against bacterial and viral antigens has been demonstrated in an increasing number of studies. Such studies have aroused much interest in cell-mediated immunity and its possible role in defense against microbial infection. Nowhere has this resurgence of interest been more apparent than in investigations of the lung, where a number of conditions, generally accepted to have an immune etiology, have always been difficult to explain solely in terms of antibody involvement.

It has been known for a long time that the respiratory tract has associated lymphoid tissue [1,2], and about 7 to 8 yr ago it was demonstrated that immune responses could be elicited at lymphoepithelial surfaces (e.g., the gut) in a manner independent of systemic immunity [3]. Therefore, studies of immune responses in the respiratory tract were a natural development. Initial attempts to provoke immune responses in the air spaces of the lung were soon rewarded [4,5]. Antibody production in the respiratory tract was found to reflect immune responses at other mucosal surfaces, being characterized by increased amounts of antibody of the IgA isotype in a structural form not generally found in serum (secretory IgA) [6,7]. Humoral immune responses alone were the subject of early study, principally because the assay procedures available to measure antibody production were much more sensitive and remain more quantifiable than comparable assays for cell-mediated immunity.

II. T-cell Effector Functions and Methods for Assaying Cell-mediated Immunity

The delayed hypersensitivity skin test has been the reaction classically used to define the presence of cell-mediated immunity. This assay, while still used widely, suffers principally from difficulties associated with quantitation. Additionally, in studies of local (lung-associated) cell-mediated responses, measurements of systemic immunity by skin testing may not be relevant. In recent years, studies on the mechanisms of T-cell effector functions suggested that various in vitro correlates of the delayed hypersensitivity skin reaction might be of use in measuring cell-mediated immune responses. While the mechanism(s) of cell-mediated immune phenomena remain the subject of debate, two basic effector processes have been identified: (a) T cells from immune animals can by cytotoxic, lysing, in an immunologically specific manner, cells that carry membrane antigens against which the host is immune (reviewed in [8]); and (b) T cells from immune animals, in the presence of homologous antigen, synthesize and subsequently secrete, a number of biologically active soluble factors, often collectively referred to as "lymphokines" (reviewed in [9]).

The cytolytic activity of T-effector cells is thought to be the basis of allograft rejection and to represent an important pathway for the destruction of neoplasms [10]. Lymphokines are currently defined only in terms of their myriad biologic activities, which include cell-migration inhibitory factors(s), chemotactic factor(s), and cytotoxic factor(s) [9]. These soluble products of effector T cells probably play a salient role in most cell-mediated immune phenomena, specifically and characteristically in the delayed hypersensitivity skin-test reaction, in which they are thought to be responsible for the mononuclear cell-infiltration routinely observed.

The relationship between the cytolytically active T cell and cells that produce "lymphokines" in the presence of antigen, is at present unknown, although recent evidence suggests that they may be distinct T-cell types [11]. While still awaiting characterization, lymphokines have nevertheless presented the immunologist with useful tools for assessing cell-mediated immunity in vitro (reviewed in [12]). One of the most widely used in vitro assay for lymphokine activity is the macrophage migration-inhibition (MIF) assay [12,13]. This assay depends on the antigen-induced synthesis of a lymphocyte-derived factor which prevents the migratory movement of a number of cell types, including macrophages [12]. Release of this factor in cultures containing lymphocytes and homologous antigen, is taken as direct evidence of "lymphokine"-producing T cells (and thus of cell-mediated immunity) in the lymphocyte population under study. This system has proven particularly useful for assaying cell-mediated immune functions of bronchoalveolar lymphocytes [7,14,15].

III. Demonstrations of Cell-mediated Immunity in the Respiratory Tract

Cell-mediated immune responses in the respiratory tract remained, until recently, a matter of speculation, although circumstantial evidence of its presence was readily forthcoming. Guinea pigs sensitized to ovalbumin by intramuscular administration of antigen in complete Freund's adjuvant were shown to be rendered exquisitely sensitive to subsequent antigen administration by aerosol [16]. Such antigenic challenge led to an inflammatory response in alveoli and peribronchial tissues, showing a strong histologic resemblance to classic delayed hypersensitivity (DHS) skin-test reactions [16].

More conclusive observations were made by Miyamoto et al., who transferred tuberculin skin-test positivity to normal guinea pigs with immune spleen cells and then subjected the recipient animals to aerosolized PPD [17]. A pneumonitis developed in which the inflammatory exudate was not only pre-dominantly mononuclear (as is the DHS skin test), but reached its peak with a characteristic time lag (48 hr) after antigen administration. These experiments established that delayed type hypersensitivity reactions (presumably mediated by immune T cells) could be elicited in the lung.

Definitive indications of a "local" cell-mediated immune response fol-lowed a developing awareness of the mechanisms of T-cell effector functions and the associated introduction of suitable in vitro assay systems. By assessing the MIF-producing capacity of alveolar lymphocytes, Henney and Waldman [7,14] were able to demonstrate directly the stimulation of cell-mediated immunity in the air spaces of the lung. Guinea pigs were immunized either parenterally or locally (nose drops) with dinitrophenylated human IgG (DNP-HGG), and the cell-mediated immune response of the secretory surface of the lower respiratory tract was investigated and compared to the systemic (spleen) cell-mediated immune response. Cellular immunity was assayed, employing peritoneal exudate cells from normal guinea pigs as migratory indicator cells in an MIF assay [12]. Splenic lymphocytes from animals immunized subcuta-neously strongly inhibited the migration of normal guinea pig macrophages in the presence of antigen; but lymphoid cells obtained from bronchial washings from these animals exhibited little or no inhibition of macrophage migration (Fig. 1a). In animals immunized intranasally with nose drops, on the other hand, splenic lymphocytes showed virtually no inhibition of macrophage migration; but, bronchial lymphocytes strongly inhibited macrophage migration in the presence of antigen (Fig. 1b). Thus, nose-drop immunization gave rise to a significantly greater local cellular immune response than did parenteral immuni-zation [7,14].

Although the antigen employed in such studies (DNP-HGG) can be con-sidered esoteric, in terms of relating physiologic significance to these demonstra-tions, two important facts emerge: (a) cell-mediated immune responses can be elicited in the respiratory tract, and (b) such responses can occur independently of systemic immunity.

In more recent studies, employing a variety of microbial organisms known to invade the respiratory tract primarily, the generality of these findings have been confirmed in man [18]. Localized stimulation of the respiratory tract with aerosolized antigen has been shown to give rise to cell-mediated immune re-sponses to *Mycobacterium tuberculosis,* to influenza virus and to mumps virus. In all cases, following aerosolized antigen, lymphocytes from alveolar aspirates demonstrated an ability to secrete MIF in the presence of homologous antigen; peripheral blood leukocytes from the same individuals showed minimal evidence

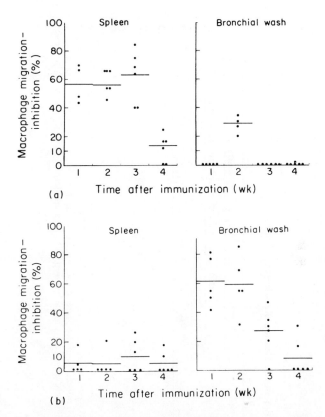

FIGURE 1 Percent inhibition of macrophage migration at various times after immunization of guinea pigs with dinitrophenylated human IgG: (a) in the foot pads (b) as nose drops. Each point represents one determination of migration inhibition. The horizontal lines represent the mean inhibition. Cells were obtained from the spleen and bronchial washings of the same animals. Reproduced from *J. Exp. Med.*, 134:482, 1971, by permission of the publishers.

of cell-mediated immunity. On the other hand, antigen administered subcutaneously was associated with systemic cell-mediated immunity, whereas bronchoalveolar lymphocytes demonstrated little ability to produce MIF [18]. Typical data are shown in Table 1.

IV. The Role of Cell-mediated Immunity in Lung Defenses

Current evidence suggests an important role for cell-mediated immunity in host defenses against microbial infection [19,20]. Such demonstrations do not, of

TABLE 1 Demonstration of Cell-Mediated Immunity in the Human Respiratory Tract: Correlations with Systemic Immunity

Antigen	Mode of administration	Lymphocyte source			
		Inhibition (%) of macrophage migration[a]			
		Before immunization		After immunization	
		Blood	Lung	Blood	Lung
Mumps	Subcutaneous	<10	<10	42	<20
	Aerosol	<10	<10	<20	42
Influenza	Subcutaneous	<10	<10	30	<20
	Aerosol	<10	<10	<20	33

[a]Lymphoid cells 3×10^6, were incubated with 10^7 guinea pig peritoneal macrophages for 48 hr at 37°C in the presence and in the absence of homologous antigen. In such assays, >20% inhibition of cell migration in the presence of antigen is considered evidence of MIF production. The above data are mean values gleaned from studies of approximately 25 patients in each group. The data are derived from the study of Jurgenson et al.: J. Infect. Dis., 128:730 (1973).

course, allow the conclusion that cell-mediated immunity plays a salient role in the lung's defense against infection, although clearly the fact that such responses can be mounted in the air spaces of the lung supports the feasibility of such a protective mechanism. If local cell-mediated immune responses are important to the lung's protection, how are such defense reactions likely to be effected?

Cytolytically active T cells are probably of little consequence in lung defenses, although potentially they could be of protective importance. Lytically active T cells, directed against viral antigens, have been widely shown to destroy virus-bearing cells in vitro [21,22], so that such activity could severely limit the replication of viruses superficially expressed in cell membranes. To date, however, there has been no demonstration of lytically active cells in the air spaces of the lung, although there is no reason why, following appropriate antigenic stimulation, they should not be elicited there. Lymphokines are much more likely mediators of lung-defense processes. In a series of elegant studies by Mackaness and his collaborators [23-26], direct evidence was produced for the involvement of T cell-derived soluble factors in combatting bacterial infection. These investigators have shown that in the presence of antigen and "sensitized" T cells, macrophages are endowed with the ability to destroy intracellular facultative parasites (e.g., *Listeria monocytogenes, Mycobacterium tuberculosis, Salmonella typhimurium, Brucella*) following phagocytosis; a destructive capacity these phagocytic cells normally do not possess. Incubation of homologous antigen with immune lymphoid-cell populations gave rise to a cell-free supernate, which could activate or "arm" macrophages in the same manner. One interpretation of this phenomenon is that a lymphokine, produced as a result of antigen T-cell interactions, increases lysosomal enzyme production in the macrophage and consequently enhances the phagocytic cell's bacteriolytic capacity. Clearly this is a potentially important defense mechanism, involving cooperation between lymphocytes and mononuclear phagocytic cells, the major cellular elements found in the air spaces of the respiratory tract. Protection in vivo by this mechanism has indeed been shown: the cell-mediated immune response elicited in mice by *L. monocytogenes* provides a strikingly effective defense against subsequent inhalation challenge with antigen [25]. Similarly, Yamamoto et al. [15] established that following aerosol vaccination of mice with BCG, lung cells produced lymphokines (e.g., MIF) in the presence of antigen. This lymphokine-producing capacity of alveolar cells correlated excellently with the acquired resistance of the host to airborne infection with *Mycobacterium tuberculosis* H_{37}Rv. Interestingly, there was no correlation between delayed hypersensitivity skin tests and resistance to airborne infections in these animals [15].

It should be pointed out that in their original observations, Mackaness and Truitt [25,26] commented on the "deficient" ability of the lung to mount a cell-mediated immune response. This conclusion was based on two observations: (a) Following a primary systemic immunization with *L. monocytogenes,* animals resisted a secondary challenge in aerosol form, but alveolar macrophages handled the administration of secondary infection much less readily than did hepatocytes after an intravenous challenge with *Listeria*. Indeed, kinetic studies implied that the destruction of *Listeria* in the lung was mediated by macrophages derived from the peripheral circulation [25]. (b) Following adoptive intravenous transfer of spleen cells from animals exhibiting immunity against *L. monocytogenes* to normal animals, there was only a modest protective effect against subsequent aerosol challenge with *Listeria* [26].

There are several problems in ascribing these observations to the deficiency of the lung as an organ for mounting cell-mediated immune responses. The system employed in the above studies requires two cell types: (a) the lymphocyte, which "triggers" the reaction, and (b) the macrophage, which is the effector cell. Clearly, if the alveolar macrophage has an impaired phagocytic capacity relative to cells from the peripheral circulation, then there could be defective clearance of microorganisms irrespective of the number of immune T cells present in the lung compartment. The experiments in which immune spleen cells were transferred intravenously to normal animals, and the capacity of these animals to resist aerosolized antigen was assayed, depend on the degree to which T cells from the peripheral circulation penetrate into the air spaces of the lung. Truitt's experiments [26] suggest that this penetration may be poor; they do not address the issue of the lung's capacity to mount cell-mediated immune responses. The direct confrontation of this issue, transferring alveolar cells from a locally stimulated animal, has apparently not yet been carried out.

At this time there seems to be no reason to suppose that the lung has an impaired capacity to mount cell-mediated immune responses, although there is some indication that when the effector cell is a macrophage (as in the experiments of Mackaness and Truitt) alveolar cells may not perform as efficiently as do cells from the peripheral circulation.

It can easily be schematized, in a teleologic way, that other products of "activated" lymphocytes (lymphokines) could cooperate with "macrophage-arming" factors in contributing to host defenses. Chemotactic factors, by increasing cellular infiltration, and migration inhibitory factors, by preventing cellular traffic from leaving sites of antigenic stimulation, could clearly contribute to focusing host cells to sites of microbial infiltration. Further studies will undoubtedly evaluate these postulated contributions more definitively.

V. Unanswered Questions

It is thus apparent that cell-mediated responses can occur in the respiratory tract, and that such responses can apparently be expressed autonomously of systemic immunity. Several important questions remain, perhaps the most intriguing of which is the source of the precursor cells whose progeny mount the immune responses expressed in the lung. This question is pertinent to discussions of humoral as well as cell-mediated immune responses.

The dichotomy of local immunity from systemic responses would suggest, if not demand, the local existence of precursors of both B- and T-lymphocyte effector cells. The absence of erythrocytes from the bronchoalveolar cell populations would, furthermore, indicate that the cells are derived from the airside of the pulmonary capillary bed [27]. Clearly, the bronchial epithelium, with its well-developed lymphoid cell infiltrate, is the obvious candidate tissue for such precursor cells. Several observations suggest, however, that this is not the source. Bienenstock et al. [28] observed no changes in bronchial-associated lymphoid tissue following thymectomy. More specifically, Kaltreider and Salmon [27], in studies of the cell types present in bronchopulmonary washings of unimmunized dogs, were unable to demonstrate cells reacting to the plant mitogen phyto-hemagglutinin (PHA). In most species so far studied, it is the thymus-derived lymphocyte that primarily, if not exclusively, undergoes increased nucleic acid synthesis (blastogenesis) in the presence of PHA. Kaltreider and Salmon, arguing by analogy, concluded, not unreasonably, that the PHA-responsive cell is also a T cell in the dog, and that there are consequently no T cells in the unstimulated bronchial lumen. It may be, however, that unresponsiveness to the T-cell mitogen reflected not the total absence of T cells from the lung but the relative immaturity of the T-cell compartment, for in several species immature T cells are not responsive to PHA. Although Kaltreider [27] found no PHA-responsive cells in the resting lung, following the instillation of sheep erythrocytes into the air spaces cells that could be stimulated by PHA were readily demonstrable. At this time, it is unclear whether this represents a T-cell recruitment caused by the inflammation of local irritation or a differentiation of T cells under antigen "drive." Clearly, this is a central and important issue, affecting the entire concept of "local" cell-mediated immune responses. The same arguments clearly apply to the induction of local humoral responses, for although precursors of antibody-forming cells can be shown normally to inhabit the air spaces of the respiratory tract [27], it is uncertain, as Kaltreider et al. pointed out [29], whether these are static residents capable of in situ proliferation following antigenic stimulation or whether they represent the normal traffic of immunologically competent cells through the alveolar compartment.

In a careful study of the number of antibody-forming cells (AFC) in lymphoid tissue following the instillation of sheep erythrocytes into the air spaces of the lung, Kaltreider et al. [29] found maximal activity in hilar lymph nodes. Although at high doses of antigen AFC were also present in broncho-alveolar washings, at lower doses, AFC were demonstrable in draining lymph nodes at a time when no AFC were found in alveolar aspirates. These findings appear to cast serious doubts on our current concepts of local immunity, for clearly the implications are that antibody–forming cells in lung air spaces were derived from the peripheral circulation.

This hypothesis makes at least two demands: (a) that lymphocytes from the peripheral circulation can enter the air spaces of the lung, and (b) that intact macromolecules (or, at least, an immunogenic degradation product) can escape from the lung into the systemic circulation. Evidence for both of these tenets can be found. Chamberlain et al. [30] recently observed the infiltration of peripheral lymphocytes into peribronchial tissue through postcapillary venules and the passage of lymphocytes into bronchoalveolar air spaces between epithelial cells. Nash and Holle [31] found that considerable quantities of high molecular weight (>150,000) antigens escape from the lung intact into the systemic circulation.

The relative contribution of systemic immunity to the lung's immune defenses is, at present, unclear; the presence of secretory IgA molecules, with antibody activity, in bronchial air spaces remains, however, very substantial evidence that true "local" responses can, and do, occur.

The question of "local" cell–mediated immunity is a much more open issue. The observation of lymphoid cells trafficking from the circulation to the bronchoalveolar air spaces raises doubts as to the origin of cell–mediated immune responses demonstrated, to date, in the lung. The strongest argument for "local" cell–mediated immune responses are demonstrations of lymphokine (MIF) production by bronchoalveolar lymphocytes at a time when populations of splenic (and peripheral blood) lymphoid cells fail to synthesize MIF [7,14,18]. If effector cells were not produced locally, they would need either to "home" or to concentrate in the lung to give the observed effects; neither of these phenomena has been demonstrated.

The role of the bronchial lymphoepithelium in the lung's immune response remains unknown. If it does not provide B- and T-effector lymphocyte precursors (as Kaltreider's studies seem to suggest), what is its function, and what is its relationship to the lymphoid system in general and to mucosal immunity in particular? These questions clearly await, and demand, further study. The greatest barriers to resolution of these issues so far have been technical ones: the lack of sensitive quantitative techniques to assess cell–mediated immunity. Hopefully, with the development of such techniques, the answers to some of these crucial questions will be forthcoming.

Acknowledgments

I wish to thank Dr. R. H. Waldman, University of Florida and Dr. M. Plaut, Johns Hopkins University, for most helpful discussions.

The original work presented here was supported by grants from the National Institute of Allergy and Infectious Disease and the National Science Foundation and was carried out while in receipt of a Research Career Development Award from the National Institute of Allergy and Infectious Disease.

This is communication No. 120 from the O'Neill Memorial Laboratories.

References

1. E. Klein. *The Anatomy of the Lymphatic System*. Vol. 2. London, Smith, Elder and Co., 1875.
2. J. Bienenstock, N. Johnston, and D. Y. E. Perey, Bronchial lymphoid tissue. I. Morphologic characteristics, *Lab. Invest.*, **28**:686–692 (1973).
3. T. B. Tomasi and J. Bienenstock, Secretory immunoglobulins, *Adv. Immunol.*, **9**:1–96 (1968).
4. J. S. Remington, K. L. Vosti, A. Lietze, and A. L. Zimmerman, Serum proteins and antibody activity in human nasal secretions, *J. Clin. Invest,.* **43**:1613–1624 (1964).
5. R. H. Waldman, S. H. Wood, E. J. Torres, and P. A. Small, Influenza antibody response following aerosol administration of inactivated virus, *Am. J. Epidemiol.*, **91**:575–584 (1970).
6. T. B. Tomasi, E. M. Tam, A. Solomon, and R. A. Prendergast, Characteristics of an immune system common to certain external secretions, *J. Exp. Med.*, **121**:101–124 (1965).
7. R. H. Waldman and C. S. Henney, Cell mediated immunity and antibody responses in the respiratory tract following local and systemic immunization, *J. Exp. Med.*, **134**:482–494 (1971).
8. C. S. Henney, On the mechanism of T–cell mediated cytolysis, *Transplant Rev.*, **17**:37–70 (1973).
9. B. R. Bloom, In Vitro approaches to the mechanism of cell mediated immune reactions, *Adv. Immunol.*, **13**:101–208 (1971).
10. J. C. Cerottini and K. T. Brunner, Cell mediated cytotoxicity, allograft rejection and tumor immunity, *Adv. Immunol.*, **18**:67–132 (1974).
11. C. S. Henney, J. Gaffney, and B. R. Bloom, On the role of soluble mediators in T–cell mediated cytolysis, *J. Exp. Med.*, **140**:837 (1974).

12. B. R. Bloom and P. R. Glade. In *In Vitro Methods in Cell Mediated Immunity*. Edited by R. R. Bloom and P. R. Glade. New York, Academic Press, 1971.

13. J. R. David, Cellular hypersensitivity and immunity, *Prog. Allergy*, **16**:300–449 (1972).

14. C. S. Henney and R. H. Waldman, Cell–mediated immunity shown by lymphocytes from the respiratory tract, *Science*, **169**:696–697 (1970).

15. K. Yamomoto, R. L. Anacker, and E. Ribi, Macrophage migration inhibition studies with cells from mice vaccinated with cell walls of *Mycobacterium bovis:* Relationship between inhibitory activity of lung cells and resistance to airborne challenge with *Mycobacterium tuberculosis* H37Rv, *Infect. Immunol.*, **1**:595–599 (1970).

16. B. Pernis, Role of lymphocytes in infiltrative lung disease, *Arch. Environ. Health*, **10**:289–294 (1965).

17. J. Miyamoto, J. Kabe, M. Noda, N. Kobayashi, and K. Miura, Physiologic and pathologic respiratory changes in delayed type hypersensitivity reaction in guinea pigs, *Am. Rev. Respir. Dis.*, **103**:509–515 (1971).

18. P. F. Jurgenson, G. N. Olsen, J. E. Johnson, E. W. Swenson, E. M. Ayoub, C. S. Henney, and R. H. Waldman, Cell–mediated immunity in the lower respiratory tract to tuberculin, mumps, and influenza virus, *J. Infect. Dis.*, **128**:730–735 (1973).

19. L. A. Glasgow, Cellular immunity in host resistance to viral infections, *Arch. Intern. Med.*, **126**:125–134 (1970).

20. R. J. North, The relative importance of blood monocytes and fixed macrophages to the expression of cell–mediated immunity to infection, *J. Exp. Med.*, **132**:521–545 (1970).

21. C. Lundstedt, Interaction between antigenically different cells. Virus–induced cytotoxicity by immune lymphoid cells in vitro, *Acta. Pathol. Microbiol. Scand.*, **75**:139–152 (1969).

22. G. A. Cole, R. A. Prendergast, and C. S. Henney. In Vitro correlates of lymphocytic choriomeningitis (LCM) virus–induced immune response. In *Lymphocytic Choriomeningitis Virus and Other Adanoviruses*, Monograph. Edited by F. Lehmann–Grube. Wein–New York, Springer–Verlag, 1973, pp. 61–71.

23. G. B. Mackaness, The influence of immunologically committed lymphoid cells on macrophage activity In Vitro, *J. Exp. Med.*, **129**:973–992 (1969).

24. D. D. McGregor, F. T. Koster, and G. B. Mackaness, The mediator of cellular immunity. I. The life span and circulation dynamics of the immunologically committed lymphocyte, *J. Exp. Med.*, **133**:389–399 (1970).

25. G. L. Truitt and G. B. Mackaness, Cell mediated resistance to aerogenic infection of the lung, *Am. Rev. Respir. Dis.*, **104**:829–843 (1971).

26. G. B. Mackaness, The induction and expression of cell mediated hypersensitivity in the lung, *Am. Rev. Respir. Dis.*, **104**:813–828 (1971).

27. H. B. Kaltreider and S. E. Salmon, Immunology of the lower respiratory tract. Functional properties of bronchoalveolar lymphocytes obtained from the normal canine lung, *J. Clin. Invest.,* **52**:2211–2217 (1973).
28. J. Bienenstock, N. Johnston, and D. Y. E. Perey, Bronchial lymphoid tissue. II. Functional characteristics, *Lab. Invest.,* **28**:693–698 (1973).
29. H. B. Kaltreider, L. Kyselka, and S. E. Salmon, Immunology of the lower respiratory tract. II. The plaque–forming response of canine lymphoid tissue to sheep red blood cells following intrapulmonary or intravenous immunization, *J. Clin. Invest.,* **54**:263–270 (1974).
30. D. W. Chamberlain, C. Nopajaroonsri, and G. T. Simon, Ultrastructure of the pulmonary lymphoid tissue, *Am. Rev. Respir. Dis.,* **108**:621–631 (1973).
31. D. R. Nash and B. Holle, Local and systemic cellular immune responses in guinea pigs given antigen parenterally or directly into the lower respiratory tract, *Clin. Exp. Immunol.,* **13**:573–583 (1973).

4

Initiation of Immune Responses in the Lower Respiratory Tract with Red Cell Antigens

H. BENFER KALTREIDER

University of California School of Medicine
San Francisco, California

I. Introduction

The immune response to heterologous erythrocytes, administered by a variety of routes, has been studied extensively both in vivo and in vitro. The results of these studies have contributed enormously to our understanding of the cellular mechanisms involved in the generation of immune responses to antigenic stimulation. In much of this research, sheep red blood cells (SRBC) were used as the antigenic stimulus and were administered to mice or rats either intravenously, subcutaneously, or intraperitoneally. The SRBC is frequently used because of its high degree of immunogenicity (ability to evoke an immune response), and because exquisitely sensitive assays are available to detect and quantitate the specific antibody-forming cell response in a variety of tissues.

This work was supported in part by grants AT–12296 from the U. S. Public Health Service, research funds from the San Francisco Veterans Administration Hospital and was aided by grants from the California Lung Association, the School of Medicine Committee on Research Evaluation and Allocation (Ackerman Fund), and the Academic Senate Committee on Research (Ethyl Fine Fund and Cook Fund). Part of this work was performed while Dr. Kaltreider was a U.S. Public Health Service Postdoctoral Fellow (HL–05705), and part while he was a recipient of an NIH Special Fellowship (1 F03 HL–53181–01).

In contrast to systemic modes of immunization, the intrapulmonary route for administering SRBC has not been thoroughly studied. The rationale for immunizing the respiratory tract with SRBC is that (a) it is a particulate antigen with a size comparable to that of airborne substances capable of reaching distal air spaces of the lung; (b) as a particulate antigen, its mode of clearance from distal air spaces should resemble that of naturally occurring particles and differ from that of soluble antigens; (c) it is a complex natural antigen, as are bacteria and viruses, and might be expected to evoke immune responses at least analogous to those elicited by naturally occurring infectious agents; and (d) the cells responsible for antibody-mediated immune responses to the SRBC among various lymphoid populations derived from the respiratory tract can be detected with a high degree of sensitivity.

The instillation of SRBC into the respiratory tract is not intended as a "physiologic" probe but rather as a deliberate experimental perturbation of the local environment in order to characterize the inherent capabilities and limitations of immune functions as they exist in the distal air spaces of the lung. This approach basically represents the application of an experimental system, proven to be productive of knowledge in systemic lymphoid organs, to the lung, which is not generally considered a formal component of the systemic immune apparatus. By this means, the unique features of respiratory tract immunity may be defined and separated from those which are similar to systemic lymphoid tissue.

The purpose of this chapter is to (a) review briefly current concepts of cellular events involved in the generation of immune responses to SRBC in rodent lymph nodes and spleen; (b) correlate structural and functional relationships between airways of the lung and their associated lymphatic tissue; and (c) review in detail experimental work pertinent to the response of respiratory tract lymphoid tissue to local immunization with sheep erythrocytes.

II. The Biology of the Immune Response of Systemic Lymphoid Tissue to Red Cell Antigens

A. The Antigen

Antigens or immunogens are substances which, when introduced into a recipient, evoke a specific antibody response, or specifically sensitize lymphocytes involved in cell-mediated immunity, or both. Antigenic determinants are those small portions of antigen molecules toward which specific antibody activity is directed. Erythrocytes, particularly the SRBC, are classified as complex natural immunogens and are characterized by multiple antigenic determinates on their surface membranes [1]. The surface components of the SRBC responsible for its immunogenicity have not been well characterized chemically, but appear to reside in or on the external plasma membrane [1]. The protein components of the cell surface can be labeled with ^{125}I [2] and the fate of administered antigen traced either by tissue counting (gamma emission) or by autoradiography (beta emission). It is assumed that the ^{125}I and the antigenic determinates are closely linked, such that the tissue content of radioactivity accurately reflects the amount of antigen present.

B. Fate of Antigens Administered by Various Routes

The most extensively studied routes of antigen administration are the intravenous, subcutaneous, intramuscular, and intraperitoneal. Antigens, both soluble and particulate, given by these routes, in the absence of adjuvant, disappear from the site of injection and are disseminate rapidly throughout the body. Either blood, or lymphatic vessels, or both may participate in the systemic distribution of antigen. The factors regulating the drainage system that participates predominately have not been clearly defined and vary with the route of immunization.

Antigens (soluble and particulate) delivered by the intravenous route are clearly distributed by the vascular system and concentrate predominately in the liver and, to a lesser extent, in the spleen, bone marrow, lymph nodes, and lung [3]. Ingraham [4] injected SRBC stromata intravenously into rabbits and mice and found that after 100 min 4% of the antigen was trapped in the lung as opposed to 87% in the liver and 2% in the spleen. Rather large amounts of incompatable red cells given intravenously also localize in the lungs of sheep [5]. However, until recently, these observations have not been further investigated [6] (See Section IV, B).

The mechanism by which antigen is trapped in organs with a rich network of sinusoids (i.e., liver, spleen, and bone marrow) is explained by the ready availability of mononuclear phagocytes in sinusoidal walls [7]. By contrast, the exact mechanism by which intravenous antigen is trapped in the lung is not clear. Heinemann and Fishman [8] recently reviewed the blood–filtering mechanism of the lung and suggested that mechanical sieving of the blood by the pulmonary capillary bed is the major mechanism. Once trapped in the pulmonary vascular bed, some particulates clearly gain access to pulmonary lymphatic tissue [6,8,9].

Antigen administered subcutaneously (e.g., footpad) tends to drain through regional lymph nodes where it is partially trapped by sinusoidal phagocytes; the remainder reaches the blood circulation through the thoracic duct. Nossal and Ada [10] summarized data relevant to the distribution of a variety of antigens after injection into the footpad. Except for the high concentration in regional lymph nodes, the organ–distribution of antigen resembles that following intravenous immunization.

The most important natural route of antigen entry is probably through the respiratory and gastrointestinal tracts, yet the fate of antigen applied directly to mucosal or bronchoalveolar surfaces has been least well studied. A great deal of investigation has been directed toward elucidating mechanisms responsible for the clearance of particles deposited on respiratory surfaces [11-13] (See Section III, B.), but little of this work has attempted to correlate particle deposition with subsequent immune responses in the lung.

The fate of antigens in contact with respiratory surfaces appears to depend on the ability of the antigen to resist enzymatic degradation and to penetrate cellular, physical, and chemical barriers provided by respiratory epithelium [14]. Some soluble molecules can escape degradation, penetrate mucosal surfaces, and reach the submucosa. Particulate materials are generally excluded unless they are infective (eg., virus) and destroy the integrity of the mucosal epithelium or are administered in high doses [12]. Although collections of organized lymphoid tissue exist in the lamina propia and submucosa of the entire respiratory tract, it is nòt known how much of the absorbed antigens are trapped locally and whether or not systemic dissemination, resembling that after parenteral immunization, occurs. This is an area in which much more experimental investigation is required.

C. Interaction of Antigen and Phagocytic Cells

Once antigen gains access to the body, the efficiency of antigen-trapping by mononuclear phagocytes of the reticuloendothelial system in an unprimed host depends on the physicochemical properties of the antigen. Particulate antigens, such as SRBC, are trapped and retained far more efficiently than are soluble antigens [10]. Only a small percentage of the original dose is retained in organized lymphatic tissue 48 hr after injection. Preformed circulating antibody enhances the uptake of antigens by the reticuloendothelial system [3,10]. The enhancement phenomenon by specific antibody results in a marked increase in the uptake of intravenously administered antigens by the lung [3]. The mechanism has not been fully elucidated.

Uptake of particulate antigen by macrophages is by phagocytosis, a process that requires energy and results in an intracellular phagocytic vacuole [15,16]. These vacuoles fuse with lysosomes and hydrolytic enzymes are activated, resulting in the rapid degradation and excretion of most of the antigen [17]. A minority of the ingested antigen appears to be retained for long periods of time within the phagocytes. The antigenic material which remains associated with phagocytes is probably partially degraded, but retains its immunogenic properties and appears to be responsible for the highly efficient initiation of immune responses [18]. It has been demonstrated in vitro that macrophages must be present in order to initiate an immune response by mouse spleen cells to SRBC [19].

All of the above work was performed using peritoneal exudate cells, spleen macrophages, or monocyte–derived macrophages. Virtually nothing is known about the role of the alveolar macrophage in the induction of immune responses (See Section III, F).

D. Cellular Basis of Immune Responses to Red Cell Antigens

The immune response to SRBC has been studied extensively both in vivo and in vitro. The results of these studies constitute the basis for modern concepts of antibody–mediated immune responses in general. The pioneering in vivo work of Miller and Mitchell [20,21] and the in vitro studies of Mishell and Dutton [22] have been expanded by many investigators, and these studies were reviewed in detail [23-25].

Two types of experimental systems have been used. The in vivo model consists of either neonatally thymectomized or lethally irradiated mice, reconstituted with suspensions of various syngeneic (genetically compatable) cell types (eg., spleen, thymus, bone marrow). These animals are then challenged intravenously with SRBC and after an appropriate period of time the recipient's spleen cells are assayed for antibody–forming cells, using a hemolytic plaque technique [26]. The in vitro system involves short–term tissue culture of various combinations of murine lymphoid cells, together with SRBC (antigen). The cultured cells are then assayed for hemolytic plaque activity at various times. Correlation between the in vivo and in vitro response to SRBC has been good, so that the availability of a reliable in vitro system has provided the opportunity to perform a wide variety of experimental manipulations not technically possible in the intact animal model.

From these studies, it has become apparent that the interaction of at least three distinct cell types is required for maximal expression of immunity against SRBC. Antigen–specific cells are lymphocytes which are thought to be precommitted to recognize a specific antigenic determinant. These cells make up two distinct classes of lymphocytes: (a) bone marrow–derived lymphocytes (B cells) and (b) thymus–derived lymphocytes (T cells). The third type of cell required for optimal expression of immunity against the SRBC is the glass–adherent, mononuclear phagocyte (macrophage, A cell). These three cell types are believed to reside in close approximation within organized lymphatic tissues (e.g., spleen and lymph nodes).

The successful initiation of an immune response to SRBC requires the presentation of antigen (either intact or modified by macrophages) to both antigen–specific T and B cells. The interaction of these three cells with antigen leads to massive proliferation of lymphoid cells accompanied by differentiation of T and B cells. This results in the products of the immune response: B cells differentiate into specific antibody-producing plasma cells; T cells become "sensitized" T cells (effectors of cell-mediated immune reactions). "Memory cells" are also generated and these may be derived from T cells, B cells, or both and are important in the anamnestic response to a second exposure to antigen.

While the SRBC system has been studied most thoroughly, the above outlined series of events appears to be directly applicable to other complex antigens. During the remainder of this chapter, it is important to bear in mind (a) the cellular events constituting the immune response when interpreting data obtained from immunization of the respiratory tract and (b) that it is very likely that this complex series of events required a high degree of lymphatic tissue organization to efficiently effect an immune response.

III. Normal Structure—Function Relationships of the Upper and the Lower Respiratory Tracts

A. Definition of the Upper and the Lower Respiratory Tracts

The entire air-tissue interface of the respiratory tract is lined with epithelial cells [9]. From the trachea proximally to the terminal bronchioles distally, this lining consists of tightly-packed ciliated epithelial cells of progressively diminishing thickness. At the point where terminal bronchioles bifurcate into respiratory bronchioles (bronchoalveolar junction), the ciliated epithelium becomes a single layer of low cuboidal cells, and these become progressively thinner over alveolar ducts and alveoli [9]. As the respiratory epithelium becomes thinner, the peribronchial lymphoid tissue located in the lamina propria becomes more closely approximated to the air-tissue interface and, hence, more accessible to airborne antigens.

Because a number of structural and functional differences exist between airways above and below the bronchoalveolar junction, it is convenient to arbitrarily use this point to demarcate the upper from the lower respiratory tract. In considering immune functions of the respiratory tract, it is operationally useful to consider "mucosal immunity" (upper respiratory tract) separately from immunologic events occurring distal to the bronchoalveolar junction (lower respiratory tract). In the remainder of this chapter, this operational definition will be employed.

B. Clearance of Particulates From the Respiratory Tract

The clearance of inhaled particulate materials from both the upper and the lower respiratory tract is currently under intensive investigation and the present state

of knowledge regarding this subject has recently been summarized [11-13,27].
It is not the purpose of this chapter to review respiratory tract clearance in detail
but only to summarize the major mechanisms operative in the upper and the
lower respiratory tracts as the basis for a rational discussion of the fate of antigens applied to respiratory surfaces.

The major clearance mechanism for particles deposited in the upper respiratory tract is the mucociliary transport system. Approximately 90% of
particles with diameters greater that 2 to 3μm are deposited on the mucous layer
overlying ciliated epithelium. Deposition occurs by direct impaction of particles
against the walls of the airway walls caused by the aerodynamic properties of
bulk airflow and the geometric configuration of upper airways. These particles
are carried from the terminal bronchioles to the trachea by the flow of visco-
elastic fluid consisting of a sol and a gel phase of complex physicochemical
structure which is propelled along the surface of upper airways by the wave like
motion of beating cilia. The mucociliary transport mechanism is rapid; 90% of
the particles are cleared in the first hour. Under normal circumstances, this
clearance mechanism helps maintain bacteriologic sterility of the bronchial
mucosa [28].

In contrast to the mucociliary transport mechanism of the upper respiratory tract, the clearance of particles from those portions of lung distal to the
ciliated epithelium (lower respiratory tract) is poorly understood and requires a
long period of time to accomplish (days to years). Approximately 90% of the
particles with diameters of 0.5 to 3.0μm will penetrate to the lower respiratory
tract. Since bulk air–flow virtually ceases in the distal air spaces, particle deposition occurs by sedimentation and by diffusion.

The fate of particles deposited in the distal air spaces depends on the dose
of exposure and the physicochemical properties of the material. If the exposure
is light, nontoxic, and avirulent, the vast majority of particles are ingested by
alveolar macrophages and these are eliminated by several mechanisms: (a) Some
macrophages reach the mucociliary blanket through air passages by mechanisms
as yet undefined. (b) Some travel by interstitial "short cuts," using either free
tissue spaces or lymphatic channels and pass through the "lymphoepithelial
organ" (See Section III, C.) at the bronchoalveolar junction and there re-enter
air spaces to gain access to the mucociliary blanket [11]. (c) Some particle-
laden phagocytes enter long-term storage sites in subpleural regions and in perivascular and in peribronchial lymphoid tissue. The ultimate fate of this material
is unknown, but most authors agree that at low doses, very little if any reaches
the hilar lymph nodes or vascular spaces. Whether or not immune responses
occur in these lymphoid storage areas is not known.

By contrast, after massive exposure to noxious particles, virulent organisms,
or liquid suspensions of particulates, the phagocytic capacity of alveolar macrophages is apparently overwhelmed and an acute inflammatory reaction, with

consolidation, occurs. Under these conditions, particulate materials, either alone or within phagocytes, may gain access to lymphatic channels, or blood vessels, or both, and reach regional lymph nodes (hilar) or systemic lymphoid tissue. In general, particulates absorbed from the lower respiratory tract are cleared by lymphatic channels rather than by blood vessels [9]. Whether such particulate antigens are retained completely in the hilar lymph nodes or whether they become disseminated systemically, as with parenteral modes of immunization, is a question that must be answered.

C. Lymphoid Apparatus of the Respiratory Tract

A description of bronchial lymphoid tissue has been presented elsewhere in this monograph (Chapter 2). A brief discussion of pulmonary lymphoid tissue will be presented here as it relates to the immune response of the lung to red cell antigens.

Nagaishi [9] recently reviewed the lymphatic system of the lung. From his discussion, several general statements appear warranted. (a) lymphoid tissue (collection of lymphocytes and reticulum cells) occurs throughout the entire respiratory tract, from nasopharynx to respiratory bronchiole. (b) The degree to which lymphoid tissue is organized decreases as one proceeds anatomically from proximal airways to distal or peripheral air spaces. (c) while lymphoid tissue is predominately related to the walls of the airway, it is also associated with pulmonary vessels, both arteries and veins. (d) all lymphoid tissue, so far examined, is intimately related to lymphatic channels.

According to Nagaishi [9], at least three levels of lymphoid tissue organization exist in the lung: (a) lymph nodes, (b) lymphoid nodules, and (c) lymphoid infiltrations. True lymph nodes with follicular organization and a well-defined capsule exist proximally, being confined to regions of the trachea, the carina, and the mainstem bronchi. The latter are collectively known as the hilar lymph node complex.

Lymphoid nodules resemble a primary lymph follicle but do not have a capsule. They are closely related to bronchial walls and may extend from the subepithelial region, throughout the submucosa, and infiltrate and surround the adventitia. Chamberlain and coworkers [29] recently studied the ultrastructure of the bronchial lymphoid nodule of the rat. These studies confirmed the follicular structure demonstrated by light microscopy. They noted an abundance of lymphatic and blood vessels within the lymphoid nodule. In addition, lymphocytes appeared to be passing through the endothelial cells of postcapillary venules, suggesting a lymphocyte recirculation mechanism analogous to that described in systemic lymph nodes [30]. These investigators noted that lymphocytes were present between respiratory epithelial cells and postulated a transit route between lymphoid nodules and airways.

In the lower respiratory tract, aggregates of lymphoid infiltrations are scattered throughout the lamina propria of terminal and respiratory bronchioles. Near the junction of ciliated epithelial cells of terminal bronchioles and the alveolar epithelial lining cells (bronchoalveolar junction), there exist particularly prominent collections of lymphocytes, which may even protrude into the air spaces. This structure brings into close approximation the bronchoalveolar epithelium, lymphocytes, phagocytes, blood vessel, and the blind pocket origin of lymphatic vessels. They have been called, by von Hayek [31], the "lympho-epithelial organ" of the bronchoalveolar junction. The anatomic location of this structure suggests that it plays an important role in immune functions of the lower respiratory tract.

The lung is richly endowed with lymphatic vessels closely related to lym-phatic tissue of the bronchial tree and the pulmonary arteries and veins. Inter-alveolar septa are devoid of lymphatic channels. Lymphatic capillaries appear to originate as blind pouches at or about the junction of the terminal and respira-tory bronchioles, in close proximity to the "lymphoepithelial organ." While the details of the route of lymph flow are not entirely clear, it is evident that most pulmonary lymphatic channels drain ultimately into the hilar lymph node complex [9].

D. Methods for Sampling Lymphoid Tissue From the Respiratory Tract

Peribronchial lymphoid tissue in the lower respiratory tract is difficult to study because lymphoid collections are small and diffusely dispersed along airways [9]. One approach to the study of immunocytes derived from the lower respiratory tract is bronchopulmonary lavage. This technique has been widely used to obtain alveolar macrophages for metabolic and functional study [32]. In several species, particularly the guinea pig, dog, and man, there are in addition to macrophages, substantial numbers of lymphocytes which can be recovered from broncho-pulmonary-lavage fluids. Several investigators have employed this technique to study both cell-mediated [33-35] (See Chapter 6) and antibody-mediated im-mune reactions [36-38] (See Section IV, B.) in peripheral air spaces of the lung. Kaltreider and Salmon [39] performed bronchopulmonary lavage on normal living dogs and found, by light microscopy, that approximately 25% of the sampled cell population consisted of lymphocytes. Ultrastructural studies showed that these cells were lymphocytes of various sizes and typical plasma cells.

The validity of bronchopulmonary lavage as a method of sampling lymphoid tissue from the lower respiratory tract rests on at least two assumptions: (a) that the cell population obtained is a representative sample of lymphoid tissue as it exists in situ in the lower respiratory tract, and (b) that these cells are, in fact, derived from the lower respiratory tract (terminal bronchioles and distal air spaces) and not from large upper airways. The actual anatomic derivation of lymphocytes obtained by bronchopulmonary lavage is not certain. They may represent cells normally free in bronchoalveolar air spaces, although lymphocytes have not been described in this location by ultrastructure analyses. More likely, bronchoalveolar lymphocytes are derived from the lamina propria of respiratory bronchioles (lymphoepithelial organ), the delicate surface epithelium of which has been mechanically disrupted by the lavage procedure. Erythrocytes are absent from the lavage-cell population when the procedure is performed on intact lungs, demonstrating that bronchoalveolar lymphocytes are derived from the air side of pulmonary capillaries [39]. Obviously, direct evidence with respect to the origin of these lymphocytes would be valuable for the interpretation of their biologic function.

The organized lymph nodes (hilar nodes), which ultimately drain the periphery of the lung, are clustered around the trachea and mainstem bronchi [9]. These are readily obtained, fully intact, by dissection after the experimental animal has been sacrificed. Thus, without undue difficulty, it is possible to obtain two anatomically separated populations of immunocytes from the lung in order to study their response to antigenic stimulation. One population (bronchoalveolar lymphocytes) is probably closely related to the air-tissue interface and might be expected to make direct contact with airborne antigens. The hilar lymph node population is anatomically well defined and probably comes in contact with most materials carried by lymphatic drainage from all parts of the lung [9]. In addition, both lymphoid populations are closely related to blood vessels and both may be accessible to blood-borne antigens.

E. Functional Properties of Lymphoid Tissue Obtained From the Respiratory Tract

Although the morphologic description of peribronchial lymphoid tissue by light microscopy is relatively complete, there is very little information with respect to the functional capabilities of these immunocytes. Bronchial lymphoid tissue of the respiratory tract has been examined histologically with fluorescent antisera to immunoglobulins. Plasma cells staining positively for immunoglobulin have been demonstrated in the submucosal collections of lymphoid tissue [40,41]. IgA containing plasma cells have been particularly prominent. These observations demonstrate that immunoglobulin producing plasma cells and probably their B-cell precursors are present in peribronchial lymphoid tissue of the upper respiratory tract. Whether or not T cells are also present in these cell populations is an unanswered question. It is obviously important to know whether the full complement of immunocompetent cells (B cells, T cells, and phagocytes) are present in bronchial lymphoid tissue of the upper airways. This knowledge would help settle the question of whether a de novo immune response is limited to the respiratory mucosa, or whether participation of immunocytes from the systemic immune apparatus is also required, and it would increase our understanding of mucosal immune mechanisms.

The functional properties of bronchoalveolar lymphocytes obtained by lavage of normal dog lungs have been characterized by Kaltreider and Salmon [39]. The lymphocyte B and T cells were identified, using functional rather than morphologic criteria. The presence of B cells was established by demonstrating de novo synthesis of IgG in vitro by the bronchoalveolar-cell population (Fig. 1a). The blastogenic response to phytohemagglutinin (PHA) was used as a measure of the presence or absence of T cells. By this criterion, T cells were not detected in populations derived from normal dog lungs (Fig. 1b). Thus, it appears that the lymphoid cell population sampled by bronchopulmonary lavage of the normal

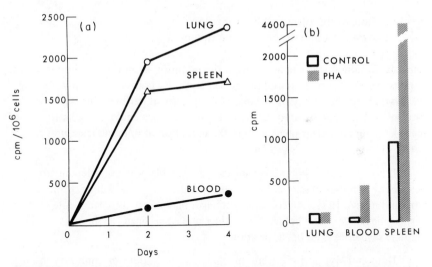

FIGURE 1 Comparison of IgG synthetic capacities of lung, blood, and spleen leukocytes (a) with blastogenic response to PHA of aliquots of the same cell populations (b). The differences in lymphocyte types among the three tissues are clear. Immunoglobulin synthesis was measured by radioimmunoassay. Endogenously labeled IgG ($[^3H]$ leucine) was detected in supernates by the immunologically specific binding of labeled immunoglobulin to plastic tubes coated with antiserum to canine IgG. The response to PHA measured by the incorporation of $[^{14}C]$ thymidine into DNA. Reproduced by permission from *J. Clin. Invest.*, 52:2211–2217 (1973).

dog lung is composed predominately of B cells and that T cells are either absent, present in very small numbers, or are too undifferentiated to respond to PHA. Although absent normally, PHA-responsive T cells can be recruited into broncho-alveolar-cell populations by intrapulmonary immunization [39].

The distributions of lymphocyte types in bronchoalveolar cells differs markedly from that of blood and spleen leukocytes (Fig. 1a and b). The spleen is composed of both T and B cells, the blood contains predominately T cells, while the bronchoalveolar population contains immunoglobulin-producing B cells. The lymphocyte-type composition of canine lymph nodes resembles that of spleen leukocytes, and no detectable differences in this regard were found between hilar and peripheral lymph nodes [42].

Thus, bronchoalveolar lymphocytes appear to differ markedly from both systemic lymphoid populations and organized lymphatic tissue from the lung (hilar lymph nodes). Since bronchoalveolar cells do not reflect simply the lymphoid population of peripheral blood, the argument that they are derived from peribronchiolar lymphoid tissue is strengthened.

F. Role of the Alveolar Macrophage in the Afferent Limb of the Immune Response

The role of mononuclear phagocytes in the initiation of an optimal immune response to SRBC was reviewed in Section II, C. By contrast, virtually nothing is known about the ability of alveolar macrophages to perform this function. Dutton [43] has commented that the lung macrophage could not substitute for the splenic mononuclear phagocyte in the induction of immune responses in vitro.

It is clear that alveolar macrophages are capable of energy-dependent phagocytosis and of myeloperoxidase-independent bacterial killing, both in vitro and in vivo [27]. Alveolar macrophages play a very important role in particle clearance, but whether or not they process antigen for the induction of immune responses is an open question.

Hunt and Myrvik [45] were unable to passively transfer immunity in rabbits with alveolar macrophages containing intracellular immunoglobulin. Mackaness [46] suggested that the role of some alveolar macrophages, especially in immunized animals, may be to prevent antigen from entering into the afferent limb of the immune response. If this is true, then the functional role of the alveolar macrophage (with respect to initiation of immunity) is clearly different from that of phagocytic cells in the in-vitro and in-vivo mouse-spleen system. If the function of the normal alveolar macrophage is to "keep antigen out," then immune responses to antigens delivered to the lower respiratory tract must either depend on free or naked antigen gaining access to phagocytes within the lung parenchyma itself or on the recruitment into air spaces of mononuclear phagocytes of tissue or blood origin.

Our total lack of understanding about the role of the alveolar macrophage in the initiation of an immune response to particulate antigen is a glaring deficiency in our knowledge and renders the task of interpreting relevant experimental data very difficult. This is an area badly in need of more research

IV. Biology of the Immune Response of the Respiratory Tract to Red Cell Antigens

A. Response of Respiratory Mucosa to Red Cell Antigens

The vast majority of the work on the respiratory mucosal immune response to particulate antigens applied locally (nasopharynx or aerosol) has been carried out using live or killed viral vaccines. Recently these studies were extensively reviewed [14]. The investigations leave little doubt that application of soluble or particulate antigens to respiratory mucosal surfaces results in humoral and cell-mediated immune responses. Both the qualitative and quantitative nature of this response depends on the properties of the antigen and the magnitude of the dose. In general, the greater the dose, or the more soluble or more virulent the antigen (the greater the ability to penetrate the mucosa), the quantitatively greater and more widespread is the specific immune response. For example, locally applied killed virus may evoke only a secretory IgA specific-antibody response, whereas a virulent virus may result in detectable systemically circulating antibody titers of other classes of immunoglobulin as well.

Whatever the antigen or nature of the immune response, it must be emphasized that little is known about the details of the mechanisms of the cell-cell interactions which initiate and perpetuate the immune response to locally applied antigen. It is not known, for example, whether genetically appropriate T and B cells reside in the respiratory submucosa in such a way as to initiate a primary immune response in situ to a new antigen or whether immunocompetent cells from the systemic immune apparatus must somehow cooperate with, or migrate into, the collections of submucosal lymphoid cells. It is certainly likely, but not demonstrated, that during the secondary response, or in the case of crossreacting antigens, memory cells, which are in and of themselves capable of mounting a secondary immune response, reside in the submucosa. A resolution of these uncertainties is fundamental to any understanding or definition of "local immunity" in the strictest sense.

The serious problems in studying respiratory immune reactions are (a) inherent uncertainties involved in antigen delivery by aerosol, both in terms of the amount of antigen delivered and its distribution; and (b) difficulties in collecting and processing bronchial secretions and peribronchial lymphocytes. In addition, the anatomic relationships between respiratory mucosa and subjacent lymphoid tissue varies with the level of the bronchial tree, and it is reasonable to suppose that mechanisms of immune responses vary as well.

Lieberman and coworkers [47], used the canine tracheal pouch (a surgically separated segment of trachea which appears anatomically and physiologically normal) to study the response of this segment of respiratory mucosa to the local application of SRBC. They observed a prompt and parallel rise in hemagglutinating antibody activity in both serum and tracheal secretions. The latter contained IgA antibody activity, which was not detectable in serum. Although the tracheal pouch model is somewhat nonphysiologic, these experiments do demonstrate that antigens derived from SRBC are capable of penetrating a defined segment of upper respiratory mocosa and can elicit an antibody–mediated immune response expressed both locally and systemically. In this system, the mucociliary transport system is interrupted and the SRBC remain in prolonged contact with the tracheal mucosa.

To the author's knowledge, the studies by Lieberman et al. represent the only attempt to achieve segmental immunization of upper respiratory mucosa using SRBC antigens. It would be of significance to devise experimental models in which various segmental levels of the upper respiratory tract could be reliably immunized with a variety of antigens, and the specific secretory and serum antibody responses compared and contrasted to define similarities or differences at various levels of the tracheobronchial tree. It would be of fundamental importance to work out the mechanisms of interaction of immunocompetent cells derived from the submucosa with those in regional lymph node tissue, such as has been done in gastrointestinal mucosa [48].

B. Response of the Lower Respiratory Tract to Red Cell Antigens

During the past five years, several investigators have studied the effect of immunizing the lower respiratory tract of rabbits and of dogs with SRBC [36-39]. For these studies saline suspensions of SRBC were instilled into the lungs through a catheter inserted into the airways. At some later time, bronchoalveolar cells or alveolar exudates were collected by bronchopulmonary lavage, and other tissues were obtained by dissection. Specific antibody-forming cells (AFC) against SRBC were detected in suspensions of nucleated cells by the Jerne plaque technique [26]. The effect of administering SRBC intravenously, on pulmonary lymphoid tissue has been studied as well [36,38].

Studies in Rabbits

Holub and Hauser [36] first demonstrated that local immunization of the rabbit respiratory tract with SRBC caused specific AFC to appear in alveolar exudates. Their observations established the practicability of applying the SRBC system to the lung, and laid the groundwork for subsequent studies that have enhanced our understanding of the immune response to particulate antigens of the lower respiratory tract.

These investigators immunized rabbits with saline suspensions of SRBC (4×10^9 cells per 4ml) by three routes: (a) directly into upper airways through an intratracheal catheter placed at the level of the carina (intratracheal route); (b) directly into the pulmonary parenchyma by injecting through a needle passed through the chest wall (intrapulmonary route); and (c) intravenously. All three routes of immunization caused similar levels of hemolytic and hemagglutinating antibodies in serum, although a rise in titer after intratracheal instillation was delayed [36].

Instillation of SRBC by the intratracheal route (solid bars) resulted in the greatest number of AFC in alveolar exudates, while there were remarkably few in the mediastinal lymph nodes and in the spleen (Fig. 2). These results indicate that even when fairly large doses of SRBC in liquid suspension are instilled into the upper airways of the respiratory tree, efficient mechanisms are operative which exclude antigen from regional lymph nodes and from systemic lymphoid tissue (spleen). Since this particular mode of immunization does not permit one to accurately delineate the anatomic site at which the antigen is deposited, the efficient clearance mechanism might either be mucociliary, or alveolar, or both. Nevertheless, it is clear from these data that AFC appeared and were concentrated in cell populations sampled by bronchopulmonary lavage (bronchoalveolar cells). The site of origin and the anatomic derivation of these AFC are unknown, but one might speculate that they were generated in peribronchial lymphoid tissue (e.g., the "lymphoepithelial organ") independently of regional lymph nodes. This interpretation is consistent with Holub and Hauser's data [36].

After equivalent numbers of SRBC were injected directly into the pulmonary parenchyma (horizontal crosshatch bars) percutaneously (intrapulmonary route), Holub and Hauser [36] observed an entirely different pattern of AFC response (Fig. 2). Very high concentrations of AFC were found in regional lymph nodes, whereas lower but substantial concentrations appeared in alveolar exudates and in the spleen. The authors concluded that this mode of immuniza-

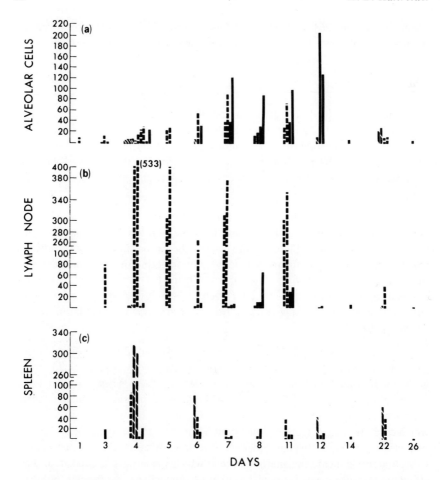

FIGURE 2 Number of specific antibody–forming cells from rabbits after intratracheal (solid bars), intrapulmonary (horizontal crosshatch bars) and intravenous
(diagonal crosshatch bars) immunization with 4.0 ml of 20% SRBC. Bars represent the number of AFC found in the direct assay of cells from individual rabbits.
(a) AFC among alveolar exudate cells, (b) AFC among mediastinal lymph node
cells, and (c) AFC among spleen cells. Reprinted by permission from *Immunology*,
17:207–226 (1969).

tion effectively disrupts normal anatomic structures of the pulmonary parenchyma
and allows SRBC to enter lymphatic channels and blood vessels, in addition to the
air spaces. From relative concentrations of AFC in lymph nodes and spleen, one
would suggest that most of the SRBC were drained by the lymphatic channels and
that relatively few entered vascular spaces in immunogenic form. This hypothesis

would be consistent with the concept that normally efficient antigen–clearance mechanisms had been bypassed by physical disruption of these functional barriers to particle entry. Mechanics of this particular method of immunization would suggest that SRBC are also deposited in distal air spaces (alveoli and terminal bronchioles), and it may be that this is required for the generation of AFC in alveolar exudates observed after both intratracheal and intrapulmonary immunization.

As might be expected after intravenous administration (diagonal crosshatch bars), AFC were concentrated mainly in the spleen; none was found in the lung.

Ford and Kuhn [37] recently confirmed and extended some of the observations made by Holub and Hauser [36], using intratracheal administration of SRBC [37]. They found that AFC obtained from alveolar exudates were (a) predominately IgM-secreting during the primary immune response and IgG-secreting during the secondary response; (b) sensitive to metabolic inhibitors, such as puromycin and actinomycin D; and (c) three times as concentrated as those contained in spleen-cell suspensions from the same animal. Both groups of investigators noted that approximately 20% of alveolar AFC resembled alveolar macrophages morphologically. While this observation is of interest, it is beyond the scope of this review to evaluate the controversy regarding whether or not macrophages synthesized antibody, though it is generally accepted that they do not. Ford and Kuhn [37] used the more sensitive Cunningham modification [49] of the Jerne plaque assay and found higher numbers of AFC in alveolar exudates than did Holub and Hauser [36]. However, their background plaques in unimmunized controls were high, accounting for almost 50% of AFC found in alveolar exudates from immunized animals [50].

Studies in Dogs

Experiments described in the previous section all suffer from the drawback that the exact anatomic site of antigen deposition is not precisely known. As pointed out previously, immune responses to particulate antigens may differ at various levels of the respiratory tract. In an attempt to circumvent this uncertainty, Kaltreider and Salmon [39] developed a method for instilling SRBC directly into the air spaces of the lower respiratory tract of intact living dogs. A double-lumen balloon catheter was passed, under fluoroscopic control, into a lower lobe bronchus and "wedged" in a bronchus about 4 mm in diameter. The balloon is inflated and a 20% to 50% (v/v) suspension of SRBC in saline is instilled into the pulmonary lobule. The inflated balloon was kept in position for 45 min to allow absorption of the saline into lymphatics and the vascular system. It was then assumed that the SRBC were confined to, and retained in, distal air spaces.

Using $[^{125}I]$-labeled SRBC, Turner and Kaltreider [6] have shown that this procedure results in a very localized consolidation of pulmonary parenchyma, which is limited to the region of lung into which the SRBC were placed. Radioactivity was confined exclusively to the pulmonary consolidation and was not detectable in other portions of the lung or tracheobronchial tree at 24 to 96 hr postimmunization. It appears that this method of immunization results in the reliable application of SRBC to the lower respiratory tract.

The fate of the intrapulmonary administered antigen is currently under study [6]. It appears from early data that (a) massive numbers of mononuclear and polymorphonuclear phagocytes, containing both radioactivity and fragmented SRBC membranes, can be retrieved from the consolidated lobule during the first 48 hr by bronchopulmonary lavage; (b) the SRBC are apparently phagocytosed rapidly and degraded in the lung, with only 3.5% of the administered dose remaining at 96 hr and; (c) despite the enormous amount of radioactive antigen administered into bronchoalveolar spaces, only the hilar lymph nodes consistently contained tissue-bound radioactivity, which accounted for only 10^{-6} of the dose administered. These preliminary data suggest that even massive, inflammatory-producing doses of SRBC are handled effectively by alveolar clearance mechanisms, which prevent generalized dissemination of antigen.

The studies of Holub and Hauser [36] and of Ford and Kuhn [37] showed that immunization of the respiratory tract elicits an immune response and that specific AFC accumulate in bronchoalveolar spaces, but they do not suggest the origin or the fate of immunologically committed cells. In an attempt to clarify the mechanisms involved in the initiation of immune responses to intrapulmonary immunization and in the accumulation of specific AFC in bronchoalveolar spaces, Kaltreider, and colleagues [38] studied the distribution in various canine lymphoid tissues of specific AFC as a function of the route of immunization (intravenous versus intrapulmonary) and as a function of the dose of SRBC.

The kinetics of appearance, the concentration, and the tissue distribution of AFC in dog lymphoid tissues after intrapulmonary and after intravenous immunization with 5×10^{10} SRBC are shown in Figure 3a and 3b. Both immunization routes resulted in a typical IgM-mediated primary immune response, the kinetics of which were mutually identical and similar to those of other animal species. The tissue distribution of AFC, however, were distinctively different for each of the two routes of immunization. After intrapulmonary administration of SRBC, specific AFC were concentrated in bronchoalveolar cells (lung), the hilar lymph nodes, and in peripheral blood leukocytes, but not in peripheral lymph nodes or spleen. By contrast, intravenous immunization produced AFC predominately in the spleen, in the bronchoalveolar cells, and in the blood; relatively few were produced in hilar and peripheral lymph nodes. It is evident that the distribution

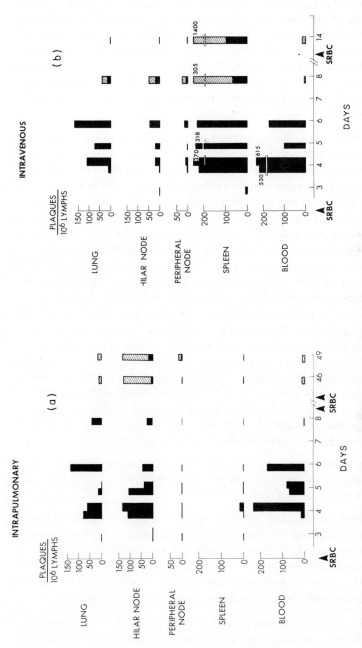

FIGURE 3 Plaque–forming response to **SRBC** of lymphocytes derived from various canine tissues as a function of time after immunization by the intrapulmonary route (a) and after immunization by the intravenous route (b). Each vertical column of bars represents the results of a single experiment on one dog. Solid bars, direct (IgM) plaques; hatched bars, indirect (IgG) plaques. IgA plaques were not detected in any tissue. Reproduced by permission from *J. Clin. Invest.*, 54:263–270 (1974).

of AFC is distinctly nonrandom, despite the free circulation of AFC in blood. It
is likely that the tissue distribution of AFC, occurring with both immunization
routes, reflects the distribution of administered SRBC antigens [6]. The absence
of AFC in spleen and peripheral lymph nodes after intrapulmonary immunization
constitutes functional evidence that SRBC did not enter vascular spaces in immunogenic amounts; in this sense the immune response was "local." However, the
free circulation of AFC in blood argues that the effect of local immunization is
indeed generalized.

At equivalent doses, both immunization routes are about equally effective
in populating bronchoalveolar spaces with AFC. (Recently obtained data suggest
that the intravenous route is actually superior to the intrapulmonary in this respect). Yet, the intrapulmonary route is clearly superior to the intravenous route
in generating AFC in the regional (hilar) lymph nodes. This constitutes clear
evidence for a dissociation between the two pulmonary-derived lymphoid populations (bronchoalveolar versus hilar nodes). The reasons for these phenomena
are unclear. One could speculate that the generation of an immune response
after intrapulmonary immunization depends on the penetration of alveolar clearance mechanisms by SRBC, and by this process, antigenic material gains access
both to lymphatic channels draining to hilar nodes and to peribronchial lymphatic tissue. On the other hand, after the intravenous administration of SRBC,
particulate antigen must enter lymphoid tissue through the blood vessels. By
virtue of the huge pulmonary capillary blood flow and the rich vascularity of
peribronchial lymphoid tissue, large amounts of antigen could be trapped in these
tissues, while relatively little might reach hilar lymph nodes, resulting in fewer
AFC. This formulation is supported by [^{125}I] SRBC studies of Turner and
Kaltreider [6], who have shown that at appropriate intravenous doses, large
amounts of antigen are trapped by lung tissue and are recoverable, in part, by
bronchopulmonary lavage; little reaches the hilar lymph nodes.

During the secondary response, after both routes of immunization, the AFC
were predominately IgG and IgM antibody-producing cells; IgA-producing cells
were not found in any of the tissues studied.

These observations are in agreement with those of Ford and Kuhn [37] and
suggest that hilar nodes and peribronchial lymphoid tissue of the lower respiratory tract are qualitatively different from the rich IgA-producing lymphatic
tissue of the upper respiratory tract. The findings of Fernald and coworkers
[41] that IgM and IgG antibody predominated in the lower respiratory tract of
hamsters challenged with Mycoplasma basically agrees with this concept.

The AFC response of canine lymphoid tissues to SRBC after both intrapulmonary and intravenous immunization is dose-dependent (Fig. 4a and b); as
the administered dose is reduced, the tissue concentration of AFC diminshes.
After intrapulmonary immunization with log-fold reductions in the number of

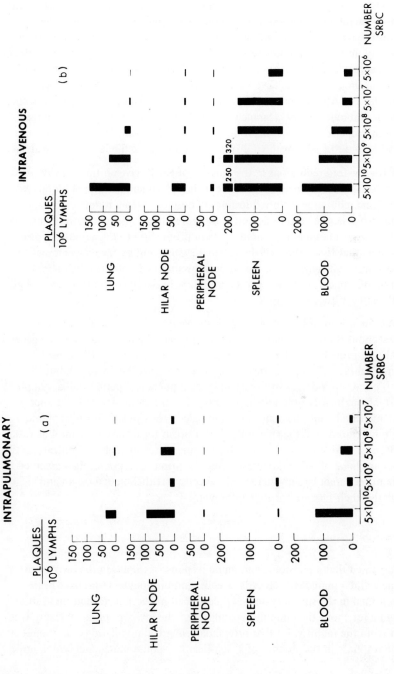

FIGURE 4 Effect on the plaque-forming response of various canine lymphoid tissues of three log-fold reductions in the number of SRBC administered by the intrapulmonary route (a) and of four log-fold reductions in the number of IV administered SRBC (b). Jerne plaque assays were performed either 4 or 5 days after immunization. Reproduced by permission from *J. Clin. Invest.,* 54:263–270 (1974).

SRBC, AFC become undetectable in bronchoalveolar spaces, but are consistently present in the hilar lymph nodes and blood. This suggests that in the canine model, as opposed to the rabbit, SRBC instilled into the lower respiratory tract consistently initiate an immune response in the regional lymph nodes rather than in peribronchial lymphoid tissue. This may reflect the mechanics of alveolar clearance in the canine lung. Even at the lowest dose (5×10^7 SRBC), significant numbers of AFC appeared in hilar lymph nodes. Thus, despite the efficiency of alveolar and mucociliary clearance mechanisms, the bronchopulmonary tree serves as an imperfect barrier, allowing immunogenic quantities of SRBC antigens, over a wide range of administered doses, to enter organized hilar lymphoid tissue.

With log-fold reductions in the number of SRBC given intravenously, AFC gradually disappears from all tissues except the spleen and peripheral blood. Assuming the requirement for a "threshold" dose of antigen to initiate an immune response, the pattern depicted in Figure 4b is consistent with the notion that AFC are generated in lymphoid tissue in proportion to the amount of antigen reaching that tissue through the vascular system and by the efficiency of the particle-trapping mechanism in the tissue's vascular bed. Studies with [^{125}I] - labeled SRBC appear to show a good correlation between concentrations of AFC and radioactivity [6].

A comparison of Figures 4a and 4b shows that, in fact, at equivalent doses the intravenous route is actually more efficient than the intrapulmonary in generating AFC in bronchoalveolar cells, whereas the reverse is true with respect to hilar lymph nodes. This phenomenon has been commented on above, but it serves to point out a degree of functional independence of peribronchial lymphatic tissue from hilar lymph node structures. From Figures 4a and 4b it appears that the hilar nodes are the major immunologic "target organ" for intrapulmonary administration and the spleen the target organ for intravenous administration of SRBC over a wide range of doses. Both routes result in high concentrations of AFC in peripheral blood leukocytes during the primary response. It is assumed that the major target organ generates these cells, but their actual origin and, particularly, their fate are entirely unknown.

Formulation

If it is assumed that a physiologic immune response to SRBC in the lung requires the same cellular ingredients (B cells, T cells, and phagocytes) that have been found optimal in the spleen system and described in Section II, then these studies have told a lot about the immune capabilities of the lower respiratory tract. It is evident from the rabbit work that bronchoalveolar cell populations can mount an immune response in the absence of a significant response in regional lymph nodes.

This implies that if antigen gets to the proper place, the peribronchial and peribronchiolar lymphoid tissue contains or recruits locally, T cells, B cells, and phagocytes, which are fully immunocompetent with respect to the SRBC. Data derived from the dog suggests that in this animal the predominate immune response occurs in regional lymph nodes, where the full complement of immunocytes is to be expected. The difference between the species may represent differences in alveolar clearance mechanisms rather than in immunocompetence of peribronchial lymphoid tissue.

Indeed after intravenous immunization of the dog, a brisk AFC response *is* observed in bronchoalveolar cells, suggesting simply that this route affords a better presentation of antigen to peribronchial lymphoid tissue. While the mode of transfer of antigen from the vascular to the bronchoalveolar cell compartment is not understood, it is clear that it occurs and results in an immune response in the lower respiratory tract. The rabbit does not appear to exhibit this phenomenon, but it has been inadequately studied to date.

The apparently distinctive distribution of AFC as a function of the immunization route is dose-dependent and most likely reflects the distribution of antigen. The compartmentalization model of a "local immune" response is therefore a relative phenomenon and reflects functional parameters, rather than strict anatomic boundaries, and is clearly dose dependent [14,34,35,38].

V. Future Directions

It is clear, from a review of these few studies, that the SRBC antigen is a useful probe in exploring the nature of antibody-mediated immune mechanisms in response to particulate antigens delivered to the respiratory tract. The data presented need to be confirmed in other species and extended to other antigens and to mechanisms of cell-mediated immunity.

Systems for delivery of antigens into various levels of the respiratory tree, with precise localization of their deposition, need to be developed. Advances in understanding pulmonary clearance mechanisms need to be applied to antigenic materials, correlating mode and efficiency of clearance with the nature and location of immune responses. Differences and similarities between immune responses of the upper versus the lower respiratory tract need to be defined more extensively.

A great deal more needs to be known about the characteristics of the alveolar macrophage with respect to its role in the afferent limb of the immune response. Do these cells function predominately to "keep antigen out"? If so, what is the nature of this difference between alveolar macrophages and other body phagocytes, which appear to facilitate immune responses to some antigens? Does antigen penetrate the respiratory tract as naked particles, or are phagocytes required?

The nature and derivation of the bronchoalveolar cell population needs to be characterized further. What lymphoid population is actually being sampled by bronchopulmonary lavage? Is it a representative or a physiologically meaningful sample?

How complete, functionally, is the submucosal peribronchial and peribronchiolar lymphoid apparatus? Are all necessary cellular elements present to initiate de novo antibody and cell-mediated immune responses, or is interaction with the central immune apparatus required?

The techniques of electron microscopy coupled with electron-dense tracers, autoradiography, and fluorescent microscopy ought to provide a great deal of badly needed structure-function correlation with respect to pulmonary lymphoid tissue and its relationship to immunizing antigens and resultant antibody formation.

The observation that intravenous particulates are extremely effective in evoking a pulmonary antibody-mediated immune response should be explored further to define the details of the mechanisms involved. Does the same hold true for soluble antigenic substances? What are the implications for parenteral versus respiratory immunization against infection?

Finally, the data obtained with particulates, such as the SRBC or with defined protein antigens, should be translated into physiologic terms in an attempt to dissect the immune mechanisms involved in defense against pathogenic materials inhaled into the lungs and those involved in the pathogenesis of lung tissue injury.

Addendum

Since final preparation of this manuscript, a study relevant to this chapter appeared in the published literature [51]. Nash examined both the direct and indirect AFC response in hilar lymph nodes and in the spleens of mice immunized with solubilized SRBC as a function of the route of immunization. After intratracheal immunization, [35,36,51], IgM-, IgG-, and IgA-producing AFC were demonstrated in the hilar nodes, but not in the spleen; after intravenous immunization, many AFC (predominately IgM and IgG) appeared in the spleen, while a small but significant number were detected in the hilar nodes. After a second intratracheal instillation of antigen, a brisk AFC response occurred in the spleen as well as in the hilar nodes. This observation suggests that subthreshold amounts of solubilized antigen had reached the spleen during primary immunization, rendering an anamnestic response possible upon a second exposure to antigen. These studies agree in general with those in the rabbit and dog [36-38]. They also serve to point out that the physicochemical form of the antigen may well affect its distribution after respiratory administration. The solubilized membranes of SRBC may efficiently penetrate mucosal and alveolar barriers, thereby gaining access to pulmonary lymphatics and blood vessels. The bronchoalveolar cells were not assayed for AFC in this study.

Acknowledgments

This work was supported by research funds from the Veterans Administration and by NIH Grant AI-12296 and was aided by grants from the California Lung Association, the Academic Senate Committee on Research (Ethyl Fine Fund and Cook Fund) and a US Public Health Service Training Grant in pulmonary diseases (HL-05705).

References

1. G. J. V. Nossal and G. L. Ada, Antigens and the afferent limb of the immune response. In *Antigens, Lymphoid Cells, and the Immune Response.* Chapter 2. New York, Academic Press, 1971, pp. 5-37.
2. J. J. Marchalonis, An enzymatic method for the trace iodination of immunoglobulins and other proteins, *Biochem. J.,* **118**:229-305 (1969).
3. D. H. Campbell and J. S. Garvey, Nature of retained antigen and its role in immune mechanisms, *Adv. Immunol.,* **3**:261-313 (1963).
4. J. S. Ingraham, Artificial radioactive antigens, *J. Infect. Dis.,* **96**:105-117 (1955).
5. D. F. J. Halmagyi, B. Starzecki, J. McRae, and G. J. Horner, The lung as the main target organ in the acute phase of transfusion reaction in sheep. *J. Surg. Res.,* **3**:418-429 (1963).
6. F. N. Turner and H. B. Kaltreider. Unpublished data. 1973-74.
7. F. J. Fenner, The biology of animal viruses. In *The Pathogenesis and Ecology of Viral Infections.* New York, Academic Press, 1965.
8. H. O. Heinemann and A. P. Fishman, Nonrespiratory functions of mammalian lung, *Physiol. Rev.,* **49**:1-47 (1969).
9. C. Nagaishi, Lymphatic system, Chapter 3. In *Functional Anatomy and Histology of the Lung.* Baltimore, Md., University Park Press, 1972, pp. 102-179.
10. G. J. V. Nossal and G. L. Ada, Organ distribution of antigens. In *Antigens*

Lymphoid Cells, and the Immune Response. Chapter 4. New York, Academic Press, 1971, pp. 38–59.

11. R. V. Lourenco, Inhaled Aerosol symposium, *Arch. Intern. Med.,* **131**:21–166 (1973).

12. G. M. Green, Pulmonary clearance of infectious agents, *Annu. Rev. Med.,* **19**:315–336 (1968).

13. A. D. Tucker, J. H. Wyatt, and D. Undery, Clearance of inhaled particles from alveoli by normal interstitial drainage pathways. *J. Appl. Physiol.,* **35**:719–732 (1973).

14. R. D. Rossen and W. T. Butler, Immunologic responses to infection at mucosal surfaces. In *Viral and Mycoplasmal Infections of the Respiratory Tract.* Edited by V. Knight. Chapter 3. Philadelphia, Lea and Febiger, 1973, pp. 23–52.

15. J. M. Rhodes and I. Ling, Antigen uptake in vivo by peritoneal macrophages from normal mice and those undergoing primary or secondary responses, *Immunology,* **14**:511–515 (1967).

16. B. Vernon–Roberts. *The Macrophage.* Edited by R. J. Harrison and R. M. H. McMinn. London, Cambridge University Press, 1972.

17. B. Ehrenreich and Z. A. Cohn, Pinocytosis by macrophages, *J. Reticuloendothel. Soc.,* **5**:230–242 (1968).

18. E. R. Unanue, The regulatory role of macrophages in antigenic stimulation, *Adv. Immunol.,* **15**:95–165 (1972).

19. K. D. Shortman, E. Diener, P. Russell, and W. D. Armstrong, The role of non–lymphoid accessory cells in the immune response to different antigens, *J. Exp. Med.,* **131**:461–482 (1970).

20. A. F. A. Miller and G. F. Mitchell, Cell to cell interaction in the immune response. I. Hemolysin–forming cells in neonatally thymectomized mice reconstituted with thymus or thoracic duct lymphocytes, *J. Exp. Med.,* **128**:801–820 (1968).

21. G. F. Mitchell and J. F. A. P. Miller, Cell to cell interaction in the immune response II. The source of hemolysin–forming cells in irradiated mice given bone marrow and thymus or thoracic duct lymphocytes, *J. Exp. Med.,* **128**:821–837 (1968).

22. R. I. Mishell and R. W. Dutton, Immunization of dissociated spleen cell cultures from normal mice, *J. Exp. Med.,* **126**:423–442 (1967).

23. D. H. Katz and B. Benacerraf, The regulatory influence of activated T cells on B cell responses to antigen, *Adv. Immunol.,* **15**:1–94 (1972).

24. G. J. V. Nossal and G. L. Ada. In *Antigens, Lymphoid Cells, and the Immune Response.* Chapters 8, 9, and 11. New York, Academic Press, 1971.

25. N. A. Mitchison, K. Rajewsky, and R. B. Taylor, Cooperation of autogenic determinants and of cells in the induction of antibodies. In *Developmental Aspects of Antibody Formation and Structure.* Edited by J. Stenzel and I. Riha. Vol. 2. New York, Academic Press, 1971, p. 547.

26. N. K. Jerne, A. A. Nordin, and C. Henry, The agar plaque technique for

recognizing antibody-producing cells. In *Cell Bound Antibodies.* Edited by B. Amos and H. Koprowski. Philadelphia, Wistar Institute Press, 1963, pp. 109–125.

27. G. M. Green, The J. Burns Amberson Lecture–In defense of the Lung, *Am. Rev. Respir. Dis.,* **102**:691–703 (1970).

28. K. H. Kilburn, Cilia and mucus transport as determinants of the response of lung to air pollutants, *Arch. Environ. Health,* **14**:77–91 (1967).

29. D. W. Chamberlain, C. Nopajaroonsri, and G. T. Simon, Ultrastructure of the pulmonary lymphoid tissue, *Am. Rev. Respir. Dis.,* **108**:621–631 (1973).

30. J. L. Gowans and E. J. Knight, The route of re-circulation of lymphocytes in the rat, *Proc. R. Soc. London, Ser. B.,* **159**:257–282 (1964).

31. H. von Hayek, Lymph vessels, lymph nodes, and lymphoid tissue. In *The Human Lung.* New York, Hafner Publishing Co., Inc., 1960, pp. 298–314.

32. W. Myrvik, E. Leake, and F. Fariss, Studies on pulmonary alveolar macrophages from the normal rabbit: A technique to procure them in a high state of purity, *J. Immunol.,* **86**:128–132 (1961).

33. R. H. Waldman and C. S. Henney, Cell–mediated immunity and antibody responses in the respiratory tract after local and systemic immunization, *J. Exp. Med.,* **143**:482–494 (1971).

34. R. H. Waldman, C. S. Spencer, and J. E. Johnson, III, Respiratory and systemic cellular and humoral immune responses to influenza virus vaccine administered parenterally or by nose drops, *Cell. Immunol.,* **3**:294–300 (1972).

35. D. R. Nash and B. Holle, Local and systemic cellular immune responses in guinea–pigs given antigen parenterally or directly into the lower respiratory tract, *Clin. Exp. Immunol.,* **13**:573–583 (1973).

36. M. Holub and R. E. Hauser, Lung alveolar histiocytes engaged in antibody production, *Immunology,* **17**:207–226 (1969).

37. R. J. Ford and C. Kuhn, Immunologic competence of alveolar cells: I. The plaque–forming response to particulate and soluble entigens and II. Modification of the plaque–forming response by inhibitors, tolerance, and chronic stimulation, *Am. Rev. Respir. Dis.,* **107**:763–770 and 771–775 (1973).

38. H. B. Kaltreider, L. Kyselka, and S. E. Salmon, Immunology of the lower respiratory tract: II. The plaque–forming response of canine lymphoid tissues to sheep erythrocytes after intrapulmonary or intravenous immunization, *J. Clin. Invest.,* **54**:263–270 (1974).

39. H. B. Kaltreider and S. E. Salmon, Immunology of the lower respiratory tract: I. Functional properties of bronchoalveolar lymphocytes obtained from the normal canine lung, *J. Clin. Invest.,* **52**:2211–2217 (1973).

40. T. B. Tomasi, Jr., Secretory Immunoglobulins, *New Engl. J. Med.,* **287**: 500–506 (1972).

41. G. W. Fernald, W. A. Clyde, Jr., and J. Bienenstock, Immunoglobulin-containing cells in lungs of Hamsters infected with *Mycoplasma pneumoniae, J. Immunol.,* **108**:1400–1408 (1972).

42. H. B. Kaltreider and S. E. Salmon. Unpublished data.

43. R. W. Dutton, Personal communication. In *Mediators of Cellular Immunity*. Edited by L. H. Lawrence and M. Lundy. New York, Academic Press, 1974.

44. A. B. Cohen and M. J. Cline, The human alveolar macrophage: Isolation, cultivation in vitro, and studies of morphologic and functional characteristics, *J. Clin. Invest.*, **50**:1390–1398 (1971).

45. W. B. Hunt and Q. N. Myrvik, Demonstration of antibody in rabbit alveolar macrophages with failure to transfer antibody production, *J. Immunol.*, **93**: 677–681 (1964).

46. G. B. Mackaness, The J. Burns Amberson Lecture—The induction and expression of cell mediated hypersensitivity in the lung, *Am. Rev. Respir. Dis.*, **104**:813–828 (1971).

47. P. Lieberman, H. Patterson, V. Petersen, L. Chakrin, J. Wardell, Jr., and J. Ricks, Effect of antigen variation on production of antibody in canine tracheal secretions, *J. Immunol.*, **107**:1349–1356 (1971).

48. J. F. Heremans and H. Brazin, Antibodies induced by local antigenic stimulation of mucosal surfaces, *Ann. N. Y. Acad. Sci.*, **190**:268–275 (1971).

49. A. J. Cunningham, A method of increased sensitivity for detecting single antibody–forming cells, *Nature* (London), **207**:1106–1107 (1965).

50. R. J. Ford, Jr. and C. Kuhn, Immunologic competence of alveolar cells. II. Modification of the plaque–forming response by inhibitors, tolerance, and chronic stimulation, *Am. Rev. Respir. Dis.*, **107**:771–774 (1973).

51. D. R. Nash, Direct and indirect plaque–forming cells in extrapulmonary lymphoid tissue following local vs. systemic injection of soluble antigen, *Cell. Immunol.*, **9**:234–241 (1973).

5

Pulmonary Immune Mechanisms in *Mycoplasma Pneumoniae* Disease

GERALD W. FERNALD and WALLACE A. CLYDE, JR.

The University of North Carolina School of Medicine
Chapel Hill, North Carolina

I. Introduction

Mycoplasma pneumoniae disease is one of the most common acute respiratory problems of man. The organism has certain unique properties among species of pathogenic mycoplasmas, and mediates its effects through extracellular parasitism of the respiratory mucosal surface. Observations of the natural human disease and studies in experimental animals have demonstrated a wide variety of immunologic phenomena related to *M. pneumoniae* infections. These effects coupled with the nature of the host–parasite relationship make the disease a good model for studying immune mechanisms of the respiratory tract. Evidence is accumulating indicating that there is a significant role of host factors as determinants of disease expression in this instance.

The author's investigations cited were supported by contracts DA-49-193-MD-2189 and DADA-17-71-C-1095 from the U.S. Army Medical Research and Development Command, Department of the Army. G.W.F. is recipient of Research Career Development Award 1-K04-AI-42544, and W.A.C., Jr. of Award 1-K03-AI-9676, from the National Institute of Allergy and Infectious Diseases, U.S. Public Health Service.

The following discussion will review our current understanding of the pathogenesis of *M. pneumoniae* disease. This has been gained through insights concerning the biology of the organism, certain observations of natural and experimental infections in man, and particularly through development of a variety of model systems.

II. Nature of the Organism

Despite the widespread occurrence of mycoplasmas as disease agents in animals, birds, plants, and insects, among the species indigenous to man, only the pathogenicity of *M. pneumoniae* has been proved [1]. The morphology of the organism is filamentous; it measures approximately 0.1 to 2μm [2] and is motile [3]. One end of the minute rod is differentiated into a specialized device which enables the organism to attach itself to host membranes and to the surfaces of culture vessels. Biologic properties of the organism, which determine virulence, have not been established, although it has been postulated that its possession of neuraminic acid receptors and its ability to generate peroxide are important features [4]. A major antigenic determinant, reactive in many serologic tests, is a glycolipid hapten in the mycoplasma membrane [5-7]. This substance is similar or identical to moieties found in spinach and some bacteria [8]. Recently, it was shown that a crude lipopolysaccharide extract of the organism resembles the I antigen of human erythrocyte membranes [9].

III. Natural *M. pneumoniae* Disease

Many studies of *M. pneumoniae* disease have dealt with its epidemiology, clinical features, diagnosis, treatment, and prevention. Despite the frequency of this disease, its benign nature has obviated intensive clinical investigation of pathogenetic mechanisms in the natural host. No attempt will be made to review all of these studies in this section; rather, selected points that relate to experimental disease and current concepts of the pathogenesis of the disease will be emphasized.

A. Microbiology of the Disease

Studies conducted in family units indicate an incubation period of approximately 3 wk [10]; shorter periods have been reported in studies in volunteers [11], possibly relating to the more direct route of inoculation. As symptoms and signs of the disease appear, *M. pneumoniae* can be recovered from the nasal mucosa, nasopharynx, throat, trachea, and sputum, indicating extensive colonization of the respiratory tract. Surface parasitism of respiratory epithelial cells from sputum has been demonstrated with immunofluorescence [12] and electron microscopic means [13]. The organism does not appear to be invasive, although there are sporadic reports of its isolation from the middle ear, tympanic membrane, pleural space, and cutaneous bullae [14]. Carriage of the organism in the upper respiratory tract may persist for several weeks during the convalescent phase of the illness, even if appropriate antibiotic therapy was applied.

B. Host-Response to Infection

Prominent constitutional symptoms and signs are the earliest manifestations of *M. pneumoniae* disease, often preceding by several days the onset of overt respiratory illness. Malaise, headache, and fever may be evidence of reaction to toxic products of the organism initially, or to byproducts of immune processes that occur later during the course of the illness. Injury to the respiratory mucosa is evidenced by protracted coughing, sore throat, increased secretions, and slight hemoptysis. Generally the disease is mild and self-limited. The rare fatalities that have occurred provide limited insight into the response of host tissues to infection.

Pathology

The lungs are increased in weight, usually showing patchy areas of consolidation, congestion, hemorrhage, atelectasis, or emphysema. Features of bronchitis, bronchiolitis, and interstitial pneumonitis can be seen microscopically (Fig. 1). The air passages may contain mucoid or purulent exudates consisting of desquamated epithelium, macrophages, polymorphonuclear leukocytes, and fibrin. The epithelial layers appear thickened due to the presence of edema, congestion, and infiltration by lymphocytes and plasma cells [15]. Opportunities to visualize mycoplasmas in the tissues have been rare since the advent of contemporary methodology, and no successes have been reported [16].

Immunopathology

Certain aspects of *M. pneumoniae* disease, seen occasionally, may have an immunologic basis; since evidence of extrapulmonary spread of the mycoplasma is lacking, involvement of the other organ systems may be related to antigenic similarities between parasite and host. These include hemolytic anemia, thromboembolic phenomena, skin rashes, central nervous system syndromes, and arthritis [14]. The pathogenesis of these manifestations has not been established, but detection of several peculiar serologic reactions suggests mediating pathways.

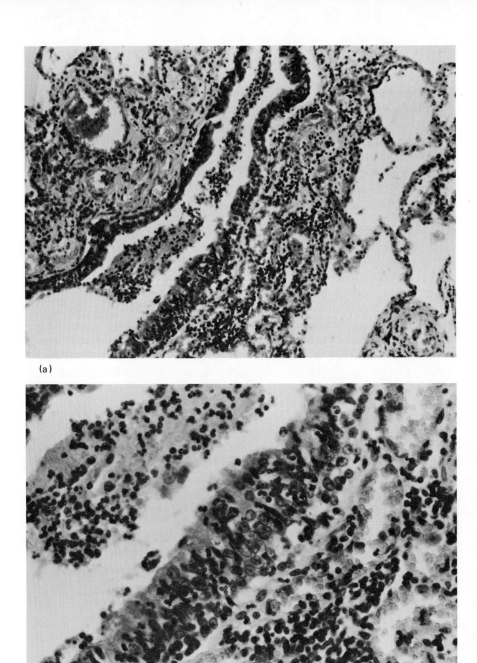

FIGURE 1 Histopathology of *M. pneumoniae* disease in man. Hematoxylin-eosin stained section from autopsied lung. (a) 40×; (b) 100×.

The cold–hemagglutinin response has been associated with *M. pneumoniae* pneumonia for many years, serving as a simple but useful diagnostic tool in many cases. The IgM antibodies involved appear early during the course of the disease [17]. It has been assumed that this is a nonspecific antibody response, from the point of view that a similar response occurs in a diverse group of disease entities and that absorption of positive sera with erythrocytes does not remove *M. pneumoniae* antibodies measurable by other serologic methods [18]. However, it is now apparent that cold agglutinins are directed against the I antigen of human erythrocyte membranes [19]. The significance of this response is supported by the finding that a lipopolysaccharide extract of *M. pneumoniae,* but not whole organisms, will inhibit the cold agglutination process [9]. Thus, in certain patients, what appears to be an autoimmune response may be an early reaction to organism products that resemble the I antigen. The pathologic role of this in vitro phenomenon is not clear. It is inferred that attachment of the antibody to erythrocyte membranes is the basis for hemolysis or thrombosis; although gross hemagglutination does not occur at body temperature, the possibility for more subtle reactions exists in vivo.

Antibodies reactive with other tissues have been reported in some patients with *M. pneumoniae* disease [20]. Like cold hemagglutinins, these antibodies are of the IgM class and can be detected by a complement–fixation method utilizing normal brain, liver, heart, or lung as antigen. This may be the basis for the development of heterophile antibodies and positive Wasserman reactions in some patients. It is uncertain whether these antibodies have pathologic significance in vivo. In one series, patients with *M. pneumoniae* infections with central nervous system complications all had antibrain IgM, but similar antibodies were found in patients who did not have nervous system problems [20].

Agglutinins for streptococcus–strain MG in some patients with *M. pneumoniae* infections appear to be explained by the sharing of a glycosyl diglyceride by both organisms [7]. Similarities between lipids of the mycoplasma and those found in host tissues may explain some of the other curious serologic reactions indicated above.

Immunology

Since *M. pneumoniae* is not an invasive organism, stimuli for host immune responses must be initiated at the respiratory mucosal surface, by means of organism–product absorption, or through interactions of organisms and phagocytes, or both. The lung and its regional nodes would therefore serve as the primary responding immune organ, providing those evidences of immune reactivity which can be detected in respiratory secretions and peripheral blood. Support for this concept is circumstantial, based on the occurrence of mature plasmacytes in the bronchial lamina propria in addition to macrophages and polymorphonuclear leukocytes in the endobronchial exudate (Fig. 1). In one fatal case, *M. pneumoniae* was recovered from the lungs, and mediastinal lymph nodes [16].

A plethora of techniques has been developed to measure serum antibodies in *M. pneumoniae* disease, including immunofluorescence, complement fixation, growth or metabolic inhibition of organisms, direct and indirect hemagglutination, complement-mediated killing, and radioimmunoprecipitation. It will not serve the purpose of this chapter to review all of these tests, which have various diagnostic and seroepidemiologic applications. These reactions—measured in vitro—reflect host experience and immunity, but it is not known whether the antibodies involved are direct mediators of resistance to reinfection. The serologic methods measure antibodies of the IgM, IgA, and IgG classes, with variable sensitivity dependent upon the type of reaction involved [17,21,22]. The classes of globulins follow the usual sequential pattern in their appearance, aiding differentiation of primary and secondary immune responses.

Respiratory tract secretions of patients with *M. pneumoniae* disease contain antibodies directed against the organism, as detected recently by more sensitive methods than previously used serologic techniques. In a study of sputa by immunofluorescence, IgA, IgG, and IgM antibodies were found in the order of frequency stated [23]. It is not clear whether these globulins represented transudation of serum through the injured mucosa, whether they were locally produced by plasmacytes in lesions, or whether the IgA was of the secretory (11 S) type. More recent studies using radioimmunoprecipitation have demonstrated *M. pneumoniae*-specific secretory IgA in nasal washings [24] (See Section IV). The biologic significance of surface antibodies can only be inferred from present data, augmented with information from studies in experimental models, to be considered later. The globulins could function to immobolize organisms, to prevent attachment to host cells, to inhibit replication and vital metabolic processes, or to enhance phagocytosis.

The significance of cell-mediated immunity in *M. pneumoniae* infections has received less attention. This parameter of the immune response has been examined in several ways. Peripheral blood lymphocytes from patients can be shown to undergo blastogenesis in the presence of the mycoplasma antigens in vitro [25]. This effect lasts several years after infection, and correlates well with the serum growth-inhibiting antibody for the organism [26]. Another measure of cell-mediated immunity has concerned the inhibition of peripheral leukocyte migration by *M. pneumoniae* antigens [27]. The cell system in this case is less pure, since it contains polymorphonuclear leukocytes in addition to lymphocytes and macrophages. Preliminary reports have appeared of tuberculin-like delayed hypersensitivity skin reactions following intradermal injection of *M. pneumoniae* antigens in patients [28]. More data are needed before this observation can be evaluated.

The role of cell–mediated immunity is of concern because animal data suggest that this response is more closely related to resistance to challenge than is serum antibody (Section V, D). Mediation of this effect could involve multiple pathways. A limited number of circulating thymus–derived (T) lymphocytes could be the repository of immunologic memory for prior *M. pneumoniae* infections. Such cells, on stimulation, could serve a "helper" function in the bone marrow–derived (B) lymphocyte response, could augment macrophage function through production of lymphokines, or could have direct cytotoxic effects on infected respiratory epithelial cells.

C. Protective Immunity and Reinfection

From the foregoing section, it is apparent that the nature of human immune responses that mediate protection against subsequent *M. pneumoniae* infections is unknown. Prior experience with the organism is reflected by serum antibodies, particularly of the IgG class, by secretory IgA from the respiratory mucosa, and by whether circulating leukocytes can or cannot be stimulated. It is known that reinfections can occur in the presence of serum antibodies, as evidenced by significant increases in titer upon exposure [29]. Under these circumstances, clinical disease is usually reduced or absent; however, second episodes of acute pneumonia have now been documented after an interim of 4 yr or more [30].

IV. Studies in Volunteers

A great deal of insight concerning *M. pneumoniae* disease in man has been derived from studies in volunteers. Early studies using sputa from natural cases as inocula established: (a) the communicable nature of the disease; (b) that the agent was nonbacterial; and (c) the relationship of cold agglutinins and *M. pneumoniae* antibodies (immunofluorescence) to the disease [11,31]. In later experiments it was found that the expression of the disease was inversely proportional to serum antibody status [32]. After *M. pneumoniae* was successfully grown in artificial media, Koch's postulates were fulfilled when the disease was produced in men inoculated with this material and the mycoplasma was again isolated in the laboratory [33]. Recently, volunteers were used to establish the presence of *M. pneumoniae*-specific 11S–IgA in secretions from the respiratory tract and to correlate this antibody with resistance to challenge [24].

Several candidate vaccines have been evaluated using volunteers [34].
Some killed–vaccine preparations have been deficient in antigenicity, or have
failed to confer adequate protective immunity [35]; others appear more promising [36]. The use of live attenuated vaccines in the respiratory tract may be
more successful, based on the rationale that local immune responses are of
primary importance in resisting reinfection. As with other live vaccines, problems may arise in finding organisms infectious for man, that are sufficiently
attenuated and stable in their properties.

Since natural *M. pneumoniae* disease is rarely fatal, and there are obvious
limitations to studies that can be done in volunteers, much work on disease
mechanisms has been conducted in experimental models. Information obtained
from these studies is summarized below.

V. Experimental Models of *M. pneumoniae* Disease

A number of experimental model systems have been used to gain insight about
the pathogenesis of *M. pneumoniae* disease [37]. Early in the search for the
agent of primary atypical pneumonia (PAP), Eaton and his colleagues [38] employed cotton rats and Syrian hamsters to show that pneumonic lesions were
regularly produced by intranasal inoculations of infected sputum. Histologically,
these lesions consisted of peribronchial and perivascular lymphoid infiltrates.
Attempts to pass the infection to mice, rabbits, and guinea pigs were unsuccessful. Later, Marmion and Goodburn [39] used the hamster model to study the
effect of gold salts on the PAP agent and suggested that it was a mycoplasma.

The hamster model was more fully studied by Dajani et al. [40] who described the course of the infection in the upper and lower respiratory tract.
Organisms were located by indirect fluorescence on the bronchial mucosal epithelium, and the peribronchial mononuclear cell infiltrate was shown to evolve
between days 7 and 24.

Although guinea pigs were long thought to be resistant on the basis of
Eaton's original studies, it has recently been shown that this animal can be infected intranasally with *M. pneumoniae* [41]. The course of infection and the
appearance of peribronchial infiltrates and intrabronchial exudates closely resemble the disease in the hamster. This animal model is particularly suited for
the study of delayed hypersensitivity in vivo and in vitro.

In addition to animal models, tracheal organ culture has proved to be particularly suited for studies of the effect of *M. pneumoniae* on ciliated epithelium.
Both hamster and fetal human tracheal rings have been used to show mode of
attachment, pathophysiologic effects, and ultrastructure of *M. pneumoniae*
organisms interacting with the respiratory epithelium in vitro.

A. Nature of Organism–Host Cell Relationship

Studies with isolated tracheal rings have shown that *M. pneumoniae* is unique among human oral mycoplasms in that it regularly produces ciliary inactivation and eventually destroys tracheal mucosal cells [42]. Fluorescent antibody and electron microscopic studies show that the organism attaches itself to the mucosal surface, but it does not invade intracellularly [43]. Human fetal tracheal organ cultures infected with *M. pneumoniae* revealed cytopathologic changes similar to those observed in hamster organ cultures [44].

Ultrastructural studies of *M. pneumoniae* in tracheal organ cultures show that the organism attaches itself to the epithelial cell by its specialized tip (Fig. 2). In selected sections, a microtubular structure projecting from the tip into the cytoplasm of the host cell can be seen. Studies are presently in progress to assay changes in the metabolism of host cells, which may be affected by this intimate parasitic association.

Further evidence that the pathogenicity of *M. pneumoniae* for tracheal epithelium relates to its close association with the mucosal cell is provided by experiments comparing a virulent strain with its avirulent, noncytadsorbing mutant obtained by multiple passage in broth cultures [45]. The parent strain was ciliotoxic, whereas the noncytadsorbing mutant had no effect on cilial function [42]. Since both virulent and avirulent strains produced H_2O_2, the inability to attach to the epithelium, rather than lack of this toxic factor, characterized the defective strain. Indeed, the intimate association of the tip with the host cell may allow H_2O_2 or other toxins the direct access necessary to produce cell damage.

The relevance of these in vitro studies with tracheal organ cultures was confirmed by experiments demonstrating a similar mode of attachment in vivo [46]. Exploiting this model should provide more information on the host-parasite interaction at the cellular level.

B. Experimental *M. pneumoniae* Disease in the Hamster

When inoculated intranasally with a broth culture of *M. pneumoniae,* the Syrian hamster develops a panrespiratory infection and bronchopneumonia. Figure 3 illustrates the course of the disease together with complement-fixation (CF) and growth-inhibition (GI) antibody responses. The infection reaches full expression between 7 and 14 days, with the pneumonic lesions following closely. Unlike Eaton's animals, which were infected with sputa or cotton–rat lung homogenates, hamsters infected with artificially cultivated *M. pneumoniae* show no gross lung lesions [39,40]. This discrepancy remains unexplained; preservation or enhancement of virulence by the inoculum of human sputum may have occurred, although the possibility of adventitious agents cannot be ruled out [38].

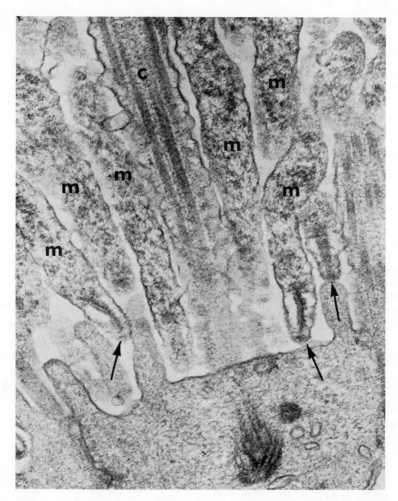

FIGURE 2 Mode of attachment of *M. pneumoniae* to hamster tracheal epithelium. Electron photomicrograph (70,000X) shows six filamentous organisms
(m) surrounding a cilium (c), and attached to the cell membrane by specialized
organelles (arrows). Section cut from tracheal ring in organ culture 72 hr after
inoculation. Produced through the courtesy of Dr. A. M. Collier.

The course of disease in the hamster model is similar to that of the typical
human case of *M. pneumoniae* pneumonia. The incubation period is shorter
than under natural conditions [10], but it is the same as seen in human volunteers [11]. Another similarity between human and animal disease is the persistance of colonization in the lower respiratory tract (Fig. 3) for up to 12 wk and
probably longer in the upper airways [40].

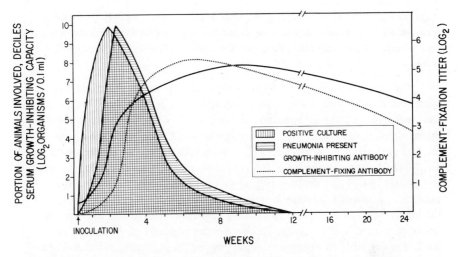

FIGURE 3 Experimental *Mycoplasma pneumoniae* infection of the Syrian hamster. Reprinted by permission from *Yale J. Biol. Med.,* **40**:436–443 (1968).

The appearance of CF and GI antibodies, commensurate with the onset and resolution of the pneumonia, is also similar to the pattern of the serum antibody response in man. However, the hamster has not been shown to form cold-hemagglutinating antibodies, nor is there any evidence of systemic illness in infected animals; this suggests that the absence of tissue-reactive antibodies may be one reason for the benign nature of *M. pneumoniae* disease in hamsters. A further characteristic of the hamster is the complete absence of bronchial lymphoid tissue [47] (See Chapter 2). We have never seen bronchial lymphoid-cell accumulations in normal animals, although occasional IgA-containing plasma cells can be found in the lamina propria [48]. Normal hamster lungs are bacteriologically sterile and remain free of mycoplasmas and viruses if the animals are appropriately housed. This apparently germ-free state of the hamster lung provides an unequivocally negative control for histologic studies, a situation unique among laboratory rodents [47].

To analyze the disease produced by *M. pneumoniae* in the hamster, the several components of this model will be discussed separately. These include the local tissue reaction in terms of pneumonic infiltrate and bronchial exudate, the humoral immune response—both local and systemic—and cellular immunity.

Immunopathologic Response

The peribronchial round-cell infiltrate, which is the microscopic hallmark of *M. pneumoniae* disease, consists of dense collections of plasmacytes, lympho-

cytes, and mononuclear cells (Fig. 4). The adjacent blood vessels are often surrounded by round cells. Upon close examination, the cellular infiltrate often is
seen to disrupt the muscularis mucosae and rarely extends into the epithelial
layer.

Indirect fluorescent staining of sections of lung for specific hamster immunoglobulins showed that most of the lymphoid cells, comprising the peribronchial infiltrates, contained immunoglobulin (Fig. 5 [48]). IgM predominated
during the first week and persisted throughout the 21-day period of observation,
but IgG accounted for nearly half of the immunoglobulin–positive plasmacytes
at 14 and 21 days. Surprisingly, IgA cells increased only minimally as compared
to IgM and IgG. These findings suggest that local antibody production is a
prominent feature of the immune response to *M. pneumoniae,* although not
predominantly IgA as expected according to present concepts of the "secretory
antibody system" [49]. Similar localized collections of IgM-producing cells
have been described in experimental pyelonephritis, suggesting such localized
immunologic activity may be not uncommon [50].

The role of immunoglobulin–negative lymphocytes in the peribronchial
infiltrate was not delineated, since no specific markers are available to differentiate hamster bone marrow–derived (B) and thymus–dependent (T) cells. However, the immunoglobulin–negativity of perivascular lymphocytes suggested that
they were a significant and discrete population of T cells [48]. Further evidence
of involvement of nonantibody producing lymphocytes was found when immune
animals were subjected to a challenge infection. As shown in Table 1, by the
third day an accelerated cellular response was seen in which perivascular small
lymphocytes predominated. This accelerated cellular response did not progress,
in contrast to the nonimmune animals undergoing infection for the first time.
After 10 days, the controls showed typical IgM and IgG plasmacytic infiltrates,
whereas cellular reactions in the challenge group were resolving. In contrast,
parenterally immunized animals failed to show the accelerated perivascular response, suggesting that prior localization of the antigen within the lung was
essential to the evolution of this response. This point may be significant in the
development of vaccines.

A regular feature of experimental as well as of natural *M. pneumoniae* disease are the polymorphonuclear and mononuclear phagocytes found within infected bronchi (Figs. 1 and 4). Ultrastructural localization of *M. pneumoniae*
has shown that these areas of tissue and bronchial cellular proliferation are contiguous to the most heavily parasitized epithelial cells (A. M. Collier, personal
communication). Figure 6 illustrates the sequence of cytologic changes within
the tracheobronchial tree during the course of experimental infection [51]. The
most obvious event is the appearance of polymorphonuclear leukocytes, which
are most numerous on day 15 at the peak of pneumonia. Since these cells are

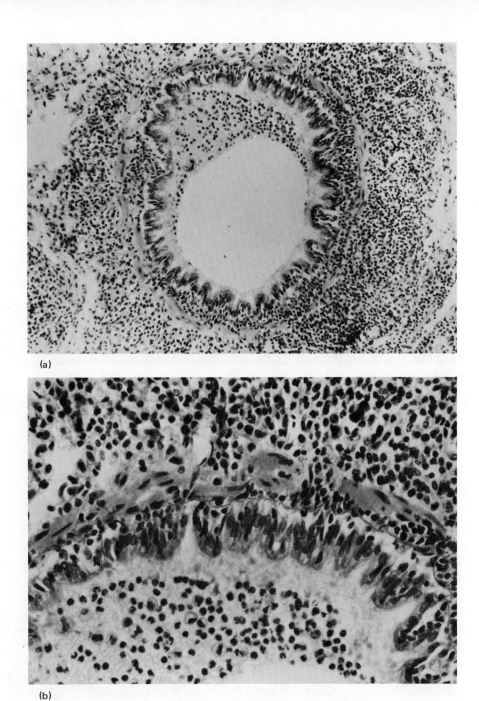

(a)

(b)

FIGURE 4 Histopathology of *M. pneumoniae* disease in the hamster. (a) Hematoxylin–eosin stained section showing peribronchial round–cell infiltrate and endobronchial exudate (40X). (b) Close–up showing lymphoid cells in lamina propria and polymorphonuclear and mononuclear phagocytes in lumen (100X).

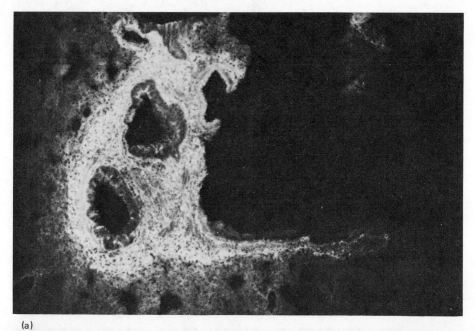

(a)

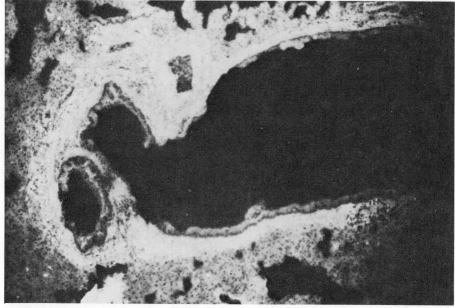

(b)

FIGURE 5 Frozen sections cut sequentially from *M. pneumoniae* infected hamster lung and stained by indirect fluorescence technique for immunoglobulin. (a) Anti–IgM; (b) Anti–IgG. (See reference [48]).

TABLE 1 Immunohistology of Lung Lesions in Immune Hamsters Following a Challenge Infection with *M. pneumoniae*

Immunization procedure	Lung cultures		Histopathology		Immunofluorescence	
	Pos./No.	Colony forming units/g	Pos./No.	Cell type[a]	Bronchial	Vascular
Three days after challenge[b]						
M-129-B7 i.n.[c]	5/6	$10^{3.3}$	5/6	SL		
				IgM	+	++
				IgG		+
PI 104166 i.p.[d]	5/5	$10^{5.6}$	4/5	IgM	+	+
Unimmunized controls	6/6	$10^{6.0}$	1/4	IgM	+	+
Ten days after challenge						
M-129-B7 i.n.	3/6	$10^{1.7}$	4/5	SL		
				IgM	+	+
PI 104166 i.p.	6/6	$10^{5.0}$	6/6	IgM		
				IgG	++	+
				IgA		
Unimmunized controls	5/6	$10^{5.2}$	5/6	IgM		
				IgG	++	+
				IgA		

[a]SL = immunoglobulin negative small lymphocytes; IgM, IgG, IgA designates cells with specific fluorescence for immunoglobulin class. Listed in order of prevalence in lesions.

[b]0.2 ml culture intranasally (i.n.) of *M. pneumoniae* strain M129-B7, in PPLO broth with fetal calf serum one month after immunization.

[c]Culture, 0.2 ml, in PPLO broth supplemented with horse serum.

[d]Five 0.2 ml intraperitoneal injections of concentrated, washed organisms grown in PPLO broth with human serum.

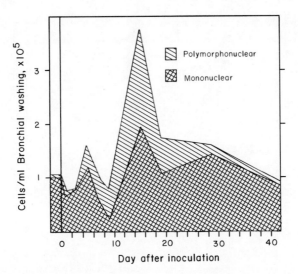

FIGURE 6 Endobronchial cytology during *M. pneumoniae* infection in hamsters. Saline lavage, 2 ml, was performed on six hamsters before and at each interval following intranasal infection. Animals developed pneumonic lesions as shown in Figure 3.

not ordinarily thought to divide after they leave the bone marrow, they must reach the bronchial lumen through the pulmonary vasculature, although they are rarely seen traversing from vessel to bronchus in fixed sections of tissue.

In addition to polymorphonuclear leukocytes, mononuclear cells contribute significantly to the exudate throughout the course of infection, peaking on day 15 but returning to normal by the sixth week. Plasma cells are not prominent within the exudate. Since immunofluorescent studies revealed no immunoglobulin-containing cells within the bronchial lumen, it would appear that antibody-producing cells are not part of the intraluminal reaction to *M. pneumoniae* [48].

Humoral Immune Response

The strict localization of *M. pneumoniae* to the respiratory epithelial surface and the obvious contiguous cellular activity described above strongly imply that much of the histopathology observed is an expression of the local immunologic reaction to the parasite. Products of this reactivity may be the source of antibodies in bronchial secretions and in serum. However, immunochemical analysis of bronchial washings has revealed only IgG and trace amounts of IgA [52]. When care was taken to preserve the biologic integrity of the mucosal epithelium to exclude serum antibody, the antibody in bronchial washings reacted in the GI assay but not in the CF test, suggesting it was probably IgA [53]. More direct evidence of antibody activity in infected bronchi was seen in the form of rosettes of epithelial cells surrounded by polymorphonuclear leukocytes [51]. This phenomenon was shown to require specific antibody and complement for in vitro reproduction. Rosettes reached maximum expression on day 14 in animals undergoing a primary infection, but appeared on day 3 in challenged immune hamsters. Thus, although direct evidence of a secretory antibody response in the hamster is lacking, these data strongly support the presence of *M. pneumoniae* antibody in secretions of infected animals.

As depicted in Figure 3, the serum antibody response in *M. pneumoniae* infected hamsters is similar to that seen in man. The immunoglobulin composition of these antibodies, in the experimental animal, differs in terms of the relative contributions of the three major classes of immunoglobulins [52]. While IgM is an early and significant part of the antibody response in man, in the hamster IgM antibody reactivity is generally undetectable—the measurable humoral response being comprised of IgG. Since only a small component of IgA-containing cells is demonstrable in the lamina propria of the lung, the absence of IgA antibody in the circulation is not surprising. On the other hand, the preponderance of IgM-containing plasmacytes in pulmonary infiltrates seems at odds with the absence of systemic IgM antibody. Slow or absent release from cells, failure of the IgM macromolecule to diffuse into the circulation, or inadequate detection methods are possible explanations.

Cellular Immunity

Systemic expressions of cellular immunity have been difficult to assay in the hamster. Although in vitro lymphocyte cultures have been successfully employed to detect reactivity to mitogens, to tumor viruses, and to several microbial antigens [54,55], experiments with *M. pneumoniae* antigens have been unsuccessful. The lack of an optimal culture system for nonhuman lymphocytes may contribute to our inability to demonstrate *M. pneumoniae*-sensitized cells by this method.

The only in vitro parameter of delayed hypersensitivity demonstrated in hamsters is migration-inhibition of macrophages [56,57]. Using cells from peritoneal exudate, Biberfeld [57] found that migration inhibitory factor (MIF) activity appears during the first week after infection and persists through the sixth week, thus paralleling the course of the pneumonia.

Hamsters, like mice, are difficult animals in which to demonstrate delayed skin-test reactions to antigens, including *M. pneumoniae*. Consequently, guinea

pigs were employed in an effort to study delayed hypersensitivity in vivo [58].
In parenterally immunized guinea pigs, skin-test reactions seem to correlate with
the appearance of sensitized lymphocytes, followed by serum antibody (Table 2).
Although there is little doubt that these data correlate with cell–mediated immunity to *M. pneumoniae,* they do not explain the role of delayed hypersensitivity within the infected lung.

While assay of MIF, or other lymphokines produced by tracheobronchial
cells, is feasible [59], a more direct approach is to study interactions between
alveolar macrophages and *M. pneumoniae* organisms. Preliminary work in this
area indicates that macrophages from normal guinea pigs require specific antibody to phagocytize *M. pneumoniae* in vitro [60]. Whether macrophages are
similarly influenced by mycoplasma immune lymphocytes or their soluble
products requires investigation. This area of research on parasite–host cell interactions would seem to be most promising in elucidating the nature of cell–
mediated immunity within the lung.

C. Effect of Immunosuppression on *M. pneumoniae* Disease in Hamsters

The experiments discussed in the foregoing sections raised questions as to the
role of T and B lymphocyte-mediated immunity in *M. pneumoniae* disease. The
work of Denny et al. [61] on *M. pulmonis* infection in thymectomized, irradiated, and antilymphocyte serum–treated mice suggested that thymus–dependent
immunity was important in limiting the infection to the lung, the spread of
mycoplasmas to other organs being directly proportional to the degree of immunosuppression. Accordingly, a similar approach was taken to study the role
of T cells in *M. pneumoniae*-infected hamsters [62].

Antithymocyte serum (ATS) was chosen as the simplest approach to
ablation of thymic–dependent immunity and the tratment deemed least likely
to alter other host defenses. Daily injections of ATS were shown to block peribronchial–perivascular infiltration, as shown in Table 3. The numbers of *M.
pneumoniae* organisms recovered from the lungs of immunosuppressed hamsters
were equal to or greater than those in untreated animals, depending upon
whether tracheobronchial lavage or ground lung was cultured [62]. In none of
these experiments was systemic invasion of *M. pneumoniae* detected, nor was
there microscopic evidence of epithelial-cell damage, suggesting that pathogenicity of the organisms was not being potentiated by immunosuppression.
There were relatively fewer intrabronchial polymorphonuclear leukocytes in
immunosuppressed animals, suggesting that these cells were somehow also subject to the influence of the local immune reaction to the mycoplasma.

TABLE 2 In vivo and in vitro Responses of Guinea Pigs to Immunization with *M. pneumoniae*, Key-hole Limpet Hemocyanin (KLH) and Tuberculin[a]

Response	Day tested (No. animals)			
	0 (6)	7 (2)	14 (2)	28 (2)
Intradermal reaction, 48 hr (mm)				
PPD, 0.005 mg	0	6	9	13
KLH, 0.2 mg	0	11	20	25
M. pneumoniae[b]	1–2	11	8	9
In vitro lymphocyte stimulation ratio[c]				
PHA	25.0	23.5	21.5	23.1
PPD	1.0	1.5	4.5	37.7
KLH	1.0	—	29.0	52.6
M. pneumoniae	1.0	16.7	12.0	20.5
M. pneumoniae serology[d]				
Complement-fixation	1:2	1:2	1:32	1:128
Growth-inhibition	0	1	2	4

[a]Footpad injection of 0.4 ml containing concentrated washed PI 104166 strain grown in human serum and KLH 1 mg/ml emulsified 1:1 in complete adjuvant H37Ra.
[b]Concentrated, 0.1 ml, washed Mac strain grown in horse serum medium.
[c][3H] thymidine uptake, antigen stimulated counts per minute per cell control counts [55].
[d]See reference 52.

TABLE 3 Effect of Antithymocyte Serum on Histology of *M. pneumoniae* Disease in Hamsters

| Treatment | No. animals | Colony forming U/g lung | Pulmonary histology[b] | |
			Intrabronchial exudate	Peribronchial infiltrate
ATS (rabbit)	4	$10^{6.9}$	1.8	0.4
ATS (rabbit)	6	$10^{6.5}$	1.5	0.2
ATS (pig)	5	$10^{6.8}$	0.7	0.5
Rabbit serum	6	$10^{6.3}$	2.5	2.3
None	6	$10^{6.2}$	2.2	2.2

[a]Serum, 0.1 ml, (intraperitoneal) daily from 2 days before infection until termination of experiment on day 14: see reference [62] for antithymocyte serum (ATS) preparation.
[b]Mean score of lesions: 1 to 3+.

To monitor more precisely the affects of ATS upon immune reactions in the hamster, intraperitoneal injections of sheep erythrocytes (SRBC) and whole *Brucella* organisms were included as examples of thymus–dependent (SRBC) and –independent (*Brucella*) antigens [63,64]. The SRBC antibody response was markedly limited by ATS, whereas *Brucella* agglutinin titers were reduced only slightly by this method of immunosuppression. These data, when compared with the effect of ATS on the localized response to *M. pneumoniae*, suggested that suppression of the B cell–derived plasmacyte infiltrate was due indirectly to blocking of a T–lymphocyte helper function rather than to direct suppression of B cells (Table 4).

Interpretation of these experiments is difficult because of limited information about various immunologic parameters in mycoplasma diseases. Further experiments employing selective immunosuppression and reconstitution are necessary to clarify the role of thymus– and bursal–equivalent regulation in immunity to *M. pneumoniae*. The increased virulence of *M. pulmonis* infections seen in immunosuppressed mice [61,65] and the effects of ATS in the hamster experiments cited above suggest the essential factor in resistance to mycoplasma infection is antibody produced cooperatively by B and T cells. A recent report that ablation of the bursa in chicks heightens susceptibility to *Mycoplasma synoviae* [66] further supports the contention that antibody is important in limiting infections by this class of microorganisms. In contrast, antibody appears to be less important in resistance to certain viruses and other intracellular parasites [67].

TABLE 4 Suppressive Effects of ATS on *M. pneumoniae* Pneumonia and Antibody Response to Parenteral Antigens

ATS treatment[a]	No. animals	Peribronchial infiltrate	Response to control antigens, $-\log_2$[b]		
			SRBC		*Brucella* agglutinins
			Hemagglutinins	Hemolysins	
Daily	10	0.3	0.5	2.4	4.9
None	12	2.3	4.2	6.5	5.5

[a]As in Table 3.
[b]Mean serum dilution end points on day 14 stimulated by intraperitoneal injections of sheep erythrocytes (SRBC) and *Brucella* organisms (Ring Test antigen, USDA) on days 0 and 10.

D. Protective Immunity and Reinfection

As mentioned in prior sections, reinfection of previously infected, but not parenterally immunized, hamsters results in an accelerated local cellular response. The significance of this localized immune reaction is suggested by studies in which resistance to challenge infection was greater in experimentally infected animals [52,53]. Evidence has been presented that local cellular activity resulting in both antibody production and an activated T-cell population occurs during reinfection of previously infected animals. Conversely, there was evidence of pulmonary sensitization following parenteral exposure to *M. pneumoniae* antigens (Table 1). Thus, whatever the mechanism of resistance to reinfection, all evidence indicates that prior antigenic stimulation of local respiratory immune tissues is the critical factor.

VI. Pathogenesis of *M. pneumoniae* Disease

In consideration of the foregoing discussion it is apparent that there are many gaps in our knowledge of the pathogenesis of *M. pneumoniae* disease as it occurs naturally or as it is reproduced experimentally. However, a coherent theory of the disease process can be developed, given the license to amalgamate available data, in the context of current concepts of immunology and immunopathology. The following discussion is an attempt to synthesize a unifying hypothesis, using material derived from these sources. Features of this hypothesis are depicted relative to disease stage in Figure 7.

At the time of initial exposure to *M. pneumoniae,* the normal lung is protected by several mechanisms. These include the structural integrity of the mucosal epithelium, its inherant ciliary activity, the presence of a mucus blanket

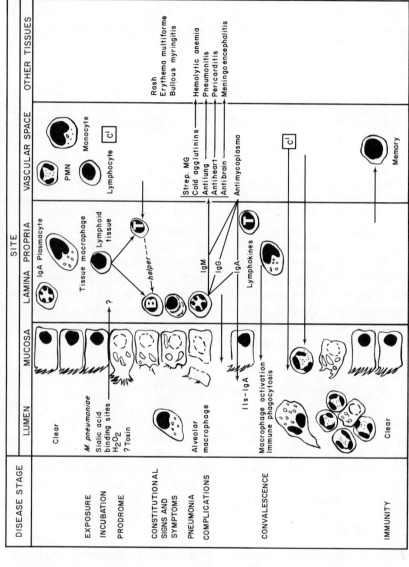

FIGURE 7 An hypothetical concept of the immunopathogenesis of *M. pneumoniae* disease. See text for discussion.

containing inhibitory substances, and the availability of alveolar macrophages. In the lamina propria are tissue macrophages and lymphoid cells, including a predominance of IgA-containing plasmacytes generated by previous antigenic stimuli. Lymphocytes responsive to new stimuli may be present within this population but many can be recruited from the vascular compartment, along with phagocytic cells and complement.

The organism has certain properties which allow it to overcome natural defense mechanisms protecting the tracheobronchial tree. Included are the minute size of the parasite, its inherent "waltzing" motility [3], and its possession of sialic acid binding sites enabling attachment to cell membranes by a differentiated organelle. The antigenic similarity between host and parasite (Section III, B, 2) probably delays recognition of the organisms as foreign. Intimately bound to host-cell membranes and situated amongst the cilia, the organism is then in a favorable environment to replicate. It is not clear how the organisms penetrate the mucus blanket and evade phagocytosis in order to reach their target cells. These are fruitful areas for investigation relevant to prevention of infection.

As shown by studies using tracheal organ cultures, the organisms replicate over the luminal surface of epithelial cells, which apparently supply the nutritional needs of the parasite. Host-cell injury is reflected by interference with cilial motion and cytopathologic changes within the cells. This may be mediated by the release of peroxide in close proximity to the cell membranes, nutritional deprivation of the cell, or elaboration of other toxic products by the organism. In organ cultures, there is a limited regenerative ability and an inability to mount inflammatory, or immune, or both responses. In the intact host, mucosal injury is probably more subtle, yet sufficient to allow penetration of organism products.

Absorbed toxic products may be responsible for early systemic manifestations of clinical disease, including headache, malaise, and fever. These products may also serve as the initial stimuli which set specific immune mechanisms in motion. The morphologic expression of this stimulation is mobilization and proliferation of lymphoid cells in the submucosa, representing division of antigen-responsive cells locally so that additional cells are recruited through the bloodstream. In accordance with current immunologic concepts, those small lymphocytes, which are thymus-derived, respond to stimuli generated by the infection; lymphokines are produced which would augment recruitment of additional cells and modify activity of macrophages and leukocytes in the area. Evidence is provided through immunosuppression experiments in *M. pneumoniae*-infected hamsters that T cells are also essential to initiate the B-cell response. Proliferation of the population of B cells is followed by maturation into plasmacytes, which sequentially synthesize antimycoplasma immunoglobulins of the major classes. The accumulation of lymphocytes and plasmacytes within the lamina propria constitutes the peribronchial infiltration characteristic of natural *M. pneumoniae* disease. Support for this concept is provided by observations of patients lacking a normal B–cell population and in whom there was severe illness without radiographic evidence of pneumonia [68].

The earliest immunoglobulin response, as detected in hyman serum or plasmacytes of infected hamster lungs, is IgM. Initially these antibodies must have relatively broad specificity, directed not only against mycoplasma antigens but against similar antigens found in host tissues and elsewhere in nature [69]. This explains the appearance, in some patients, of agglutinins for streptococcus-strain MG and the erythrocyte I antigen. IgM antibodies detected in complement–fixation procedures are probably directed at lipid or glycolipid constituents of normal tissues which resemble the lipid hapten of the mycoplasma [20]. These antibodies against heart, lung, and brain may mediate the autoimmune phenomena occasionally seen in severely ill patients. Since the antibodies occur frequently, but nonpulmonary complications are unusual, other factors—as yet undefined—must be operative in these instances.

Initial antimycoplasma antibodies are also of the IgM class and are detectable by agglutination and complement–fixation methods. As the immune response evolves, a greater part of serologic activity is comprised of IgG. While the plasmacytic peribronchial infiltrate may be the source of these antibodies initially, it is likely that regional lymph nodes also become involved in the generation of serum antibodies.

IgG, IgM, and IgA antibodies have been found in sputum from patients with *M. pneumoniae* disease. Since only 11 S IgA is a normal constituent of secretions from the respiratory tract, the data imply that other immunoglobulins are present as a result of transudation through the damaged mucosa. The possible role of these globulins in the bronchial lumen at the site of infection has been suggested earlier (Section II, C, 3). These immunoglobulins may serve to supplement the limited activity of secretory IgA by providing the mechanism for opsonization and lysis of organisms using complement [8,70].

Evidence from experimental disease, supported by limited observations in man (Fig. 1), indicates that large numbers of phagocytic cells occur in the endobronchial exudates coincident with the peak of the disease process. Presumably the interaction of mycoplasmas, antibodies, and complement provides a chemotactic stimulus for recruitment of polymorphonuclear leukocytes from the vascular space. Subsequently these phagocytes attack the opsonized microorganisms by surrounding infected epithelial cells. From in vitro models, evidence has also been provided that antibody augments phagocytosis by macrophages [60]. This could be due to an antitoxic effect on the organism, opsonization, or arming of the macrophage with antibody. Lymphokines from T cells in the submucosal area would also be expected to influence macrophage activity. Removal of mycoplasmas from epithelial cells and the elimination of cell debris seem to be accomplished by a combination of immune phagocytosis and mucociliary clearance.

During convalescence, exudates gradually diminish and disappearance of the peribronchial infiltrates is reflected by resolution within 1 to 2 wk of pneumonia seen by x-ray. Several more weeks may be required to terminate carriage of the organism, and for recovery from all clinical aspects of illness.

Convalescence is followed by a variable degree of immunity, as shown by challenge experiments in animals or volunteers, and evidence of anamnestic responses in partially immune individuals exposed during *M. pneumoniae* epidemics. This immunity is associated with the presence of *M. pneumoniae*-specific secretory IgA, a variety of serum antibodies principally of the IgG class, and circulating lymphocytes specifically responsive to the organisms. The function of each of these three components in mediating protective immunity is unknown. Presumably the IgA would constitute a first-line defense, since it would be available at the mucosal surface when re-exposure occurs. The duration of this response is unknown, but it is apparently short-lived since reinfection of individuals having only serum antibody (and presumably stimulable lymphocytes) does occur. Serum antibody perhaps aids in limiting the infection, since it is available at the mucosal surface after sufficient injury has occurred to allow transudation. In the experimental animal, this requires about 3 days after inoculation and is accompanied by the reappearance of submucosal cellular infiltrate; it is not known if this type of response occurs in man. Serum antibodies may persist for at least several years, finally becoming undetectable if reinfection has not intervened. Lymphocyte stimulability can be demonstrated up to 10 yr after *M. pneumoniae* disease [71], and may be present in antibody-negative subjects. This pool of circulating memory cells may have a role in resistance to challenge, by providing primed immunocytes for regeneration of the B-cell response and for macrophage activation. A variable degree of clinical illness may occur when a partially immune individual is challenged, depending directly upon the time since he was last infected and the level and quality of his persisting immunity.

VII. Conclusion

Mycoplasma pneumoniae, being a noninvasive respiratory mucosal parasite, offers a useful model for the study of host defense mechanisms in the lung. Progress in understanding this common infection of man can be expected as further understanding of immune processes—especially those acting on mucous surfaces—evolves. It is likely that there are common denominators concerning host–parasite relationships on other body surfaces, including the intestinal and genitourinary tracts. Definition of the basic mechanisms involved will provide a rational basis for intervention on behalf of the host.

References

1. R. M. Chanock, Mycoplasma infections of man, *N. Engl. J. Med.*, **273**: 1199–1206 (1965).
2. A. M. Collier and W. A. Clyde, Relationships between *Mycoplasma pneumoniae* and human respiratory epithelium, *Infect, Immun.*, **3**:694–701 (1971).
3. W. Bredt, Motility and multiplication of *Mycoplasma pneumoniae*, A phase contrast study, *Pathol. Microbiol.*, **32**:321–326 (1968).
4. O. Sobeslavsky, B. Prescott, and R. M. Chanock, Adsorption of *Mycoplasma pneumoniae* to neuraminic acid receptors of various cells and possible role in virulence, *J. Bacteriol.*, **96**:695–705 (1968).
5. O. Sobeslavsky, B. Prescott, W. D. James, and R. M. Chanock, Isolation and characterization of fractions of *Mycoplasma pneumoniae*, *J. Bacteriol.*, **91**:2126–2138 (1966).
6. B. L. Beckman and G. E. Kenny, Immunochemical analysis of serologically active lipids of *Mycoplasma pneumoniae*, *J. Bacteriol.*, **96**:1171–1180 (1968).
7. P. Plackett, Immunochemical analysis of *Mycoplasma pneumoniae:* Separation and chemical identification of serologically active lipids, *Aust. J. Exp. Biol. Med. Sci.*, **47**:171–195 (1969).
8. J. L. Gale and G. E. Kenny, Complement dependent killing of *Mycoplasma pneumoniae* by antibody: Kinetics of the reaction, *J. Immunol.*, **104**: 1175–1183 (1970).
9. N. Costea, V. J. Yakulis, and P. Heller, Inhibition of cold agglutinins (Anti-I) by *M. pneumoniae* antigens, *Proc. Soc. Exp. Biol. Med.*, **139**: 476–479 (1972).
10. H. M. Foy, J. T. Grayston, G. E. Kenny, E. R. Alexander, and R. McMahan, Epidemiology of *Mycoplasma pneumoniae* infection in families, *J.A.M.A.*, **197**:859–866 (1966).
11. Commission on Acute Respiratory Diseases. The transmission of primary atypical pneumonia to human volunteers. III. Clinical features, *Bull. Johns Hopkins Hosp.*, **79**:125–152 (1946).
12. J. F. Ph Hers, Fluorescent antibody technique in respiratory viral diseases, *Am. Rev. Respir. Dis.*, **88**:316–338 (1963).
13. A. M. Collier, Personal communication, (1973).
14. R. B. Couch, *M. Pneumoniae*. In *Viral and Mycoplasmal Infections of the Respiratory Tract*. Edited by V. Knight. Philadelphia, Lea and Febiger, 1973, pp. 217–235

15. W. S. Jordan and J. H. Dingle, *Mycoplasma pneumoniae* infections. In *Bacterial and Mycotic Infections of Man.* Edited by R. J. Dubos and J. G. Hirsch. Philadelphia, J. B. Lippincott, 1965, pp. 810–824.
16. J. C. Maisel, L. H. Babbitt, and T. J. John, Fatal *Mycoplasma pneumoniae* infection with isolation of organisms from lung, *J.A.M.A.,* **202**:287–290 (1967).
17. G. W. Fernald, W. A. Clyde, and F. W. Denny, Nature of the immune response to *Mycoplasma pneumoniae, J. Immunol.,* **98**:1028–1038 (1967).
18. C. Liu, Studies on primary atypical pneumonia, *J. Exp. Med.,* **106**:455–466 (1957).
19. J. V. Dacie. *The Haemolytic Anemias. Part 2. The Auto-Immune Haemolytic Anemias.* Second edition, New York, Grune and Stratton, 1962, pp. 493–499.
20. G. Biberfeld, Antibodies to brain and other tissues in cases of *Mycoplasma pneumoniae* infection, *Clin. Exp. Immunol.,* **8**:319–333 (1971).
21. G. Biberfeld, Distribution of antibodies within 19 s and 7 s immunoglobulins following infection with *Mycoplasma pneumoniae, J. Immunol.,* **100**:338–347 (1968).
22. G. Biberfeld, Antibody responses in *Mycoplasma pneumoniae* infection in relation to serum immunoglobulins, especially IgM, *Acta Pathol. Microbiol. Scand.,* **79**:620–634 (1971).
23. G. Biberfeld and G. Sterner, Antibodies in bronchial secretions following natural infection with *Mycoplasma pneumoniae, Acta Pathol. Microbiol. Scand.,* **79**:599–605 (1971).
24. H. Brunner, H. B. Greenberg, W. D. James, R. L. Horswood, R. B. Couch, and R. M. Chanock, Antibody to *Mycoplasma pneumoniae* in nasal secretions and sputa of experimentally infected human volunteers, *Infect. Immun.,* **8**:612–620 (1973).
25. B. G. Levinthal, C. B. Smith, P. P. Carbone, and E. M. Hersh, Lymphocyte transformation in response to *M. pneumoniae.* In *Proceedings of the Third Annual Leukocyte Culture Conference.* Edited by W. O. Rieke. New York, Appleton–Century–Crofts, 1969, pp. 519–529.
26. G. W. Fernald, In Vitro response of human lymphocytes to *Mycoplasma pneumoniae, Infect. Immun.,* **5**:552–558 (1972).
27. G. Biberfeld, Cell mediated immune response following *Mycoplasma pneumoniae* infection in man. II. Leukocyte migration inhibition, *Clin. Exp. Immunol.,* **17**:43–49 (1974).
28. H. Mizutani, H. Mizutani, T. Kitayama, A. Hayakawa, E. Nagayama, J. Kato, K. Nakamura, E. Tamura, and T. Isuchi, Delayed hypersensitivity in *Mycoplasma pneumoniae* infections, *Lancet,* **1**:186–187 (1971).
29. P. Steinberg, R. J. White, S. L. Fuld, R. R. Gutekunst, R. M. Chanock, and L. B. Senterfit, Ecology of *Mycoplasma pneumoniae* infections in marine recruits at Parris Island, S. C., *Am. J. Epidemiol.,* **89**:62–73 (1969).
30. H. M. Foy, C. G. Nugent, G. E. Kenny, R. McMahan, and J. T. Grayston, Repeated *Mycoplasma pneumoniae* pneumonia after 4½ years, *J.A.M.A.,* **216**:671–672 (1971).

31. W. A. Clyde, Jr., F. W. Denny, and J. H. Dingle, Fluorescent–stainable antibodies to the Eaton agent in human primary atypical pneumonia transmission studies, *J. Clin. Invest.,* **40**:1638–1647 (1961).

32. R. M. Chanock, D. Rifkind, A. M. Kravetz, V. Knight, and K. Johnson, Respiratory disease in volunteers infected with Eaton agent; A preliminary report, *Proc. Natl. Acad. Sci., USA,* **47**:887–890 (1961).

33. R. B. Couch, T. R. Cate, and R. M. Chanock, Infection with artificially propagated Eaton agent *(Mycoplasma pneumoniae), J.A.M.A.,* **187**:442–447 (1964).

34. R. M Chanock, Control of acute mycoplasmal and viral respiratory tract disease, *Science,* **169**:248–256 (1970).

35. C. B. Smith, W. T. Friedewald, and R. M. Chanock, Inactivated *Mycoplasma pneumoniae* vaccine, *J.A.M.A.,* **199**:353–358 (1967).

36. W. J. Mogabgab, Protective efficacy of killed *Mycoplasma pneumoniae* vaccine measured in large–scale studies in a military population, *Am. Rev. Respir. Dis.,* **108**:899–908 (1973).

37. W. A. Clyde, Jr., Models of *Mycoplasma pneumoniae* infection, *J. Infect. Dis.,* **127**:S69–S72 (1973).

38. M. D. Eaton, G. Meiklejohn, and W. van Herick, Studies on the Etiology of primary atypical pneumonia, *J. Exp. Med.,* **79**:649–668 (1944).

39. G. M. Goodburn and B. P. Marmion, A study of the properties of Eaton's primary atypical pneumonia organism, *J. Gen. Microbiol.,* **29**:271–290 (1962).

40. A. S. Dajani, W. A. Clyde, Jr., and F. W. Denny, Experimental infection with *Mycoplasma pneumoniae* (Eaton's agent), *J. Exp. Med.,* **121**:1071–1084 (1965).

41. H. Brunner, W. D. James, R. L. Horswood, and R. M. Chanock, Experimental *Mycoplasma pneumoniae* infection of young guinea pigs, *J. Infect. Dis.,* **127**:315–318 (1973).

42. A. M. Collier, W. A. Clyde, Jr., and F. W. Denny, Biologic effects of *Mycoplasma pneumoniae* and other mycoplasmas from man on hamster tracheal organ culture, *Proc. Soc. Exp. Biol. Med.,* **132**:1153:1158 (1969).

43. A. M. Collier, W. A. Clyde, Jr., and F. W. Denny, *Mycoplasma pneumoniae* in hamster tracheal organ culture: Immunofluorescent and electron microscopic studies, *Proc. Soc. Exp. Biol. Med.,* **136**:569–573 (1971).

44. A. M. Collier and W. A. Clyde, Jr., Relationships between *Mycoplasma pneumoniae* and human respiratory epithelium, *Infect. Immun.,* **3**:694–701 (1971).

45. R. P. Lipman and W. A. Clyde, Jr., The interrelationship of virulence cytadsorption, and peroxide formation in *Mycoplasma pneumoniae, Proc. Soc. Exp. Biol. Med.,* **131**:1163–1167 (1969).

46. A. M. Collier, Pathogenesis of *Mycoplasma pneumoniae* infection as studied in the foetal trachea organ culture. In *Pathogenic Mycoplasmas.* A CIBA Foundation Symposium, London. Amsterdam, Associated Scientific Publishers, 1972, p. 321.

47.   J. Bienenstock, N. Johnston, and D. Y. E. Perey, Bronchial lymphoid tissue. I. Morphologic characteristics, *Lab. Invest.*, **28**:686–692 (1973).
48.   G. W. Fernald, W. A. Clyde, Jr., and J. Bienenstock, Immunoglobulin-containing cells in lungs of hamsters infected with *Mycoplasma pneumoniae, J. Immunol.*, **108**:1400–1408 (1972).
49.   T. B. Tomasi, Jr., The concept of local immunity and the secretory system. In *The Secretory Immunologic System.* Edited by D. H. Dayton, Jr., P. A. Small, Jr., R. M. Chanock, H. E. Kaufman, and T. B. Tomasi. U.S. Government Printing Office, 1969, pp. 3–10.
50.   T. Miller and D. North, Studies of the local immune response to pyelonephritis in the rabbit, *J. Infect. Dis.*, **128**:195–201 (1973).
51.   W. A. Clyde, Jr., Immunopathology of experimental *Mycoplasma pneumoniae* disease, *Infect. Immun.*, **4**:757–763 (1971).
52.   G. W. Fernald, Immunologic aspects of experimental *Mycoplasma pneumoniae* infection, *J. Infect. Dis.*, **119**:255–266 (1969).
53.   G. W. Fernald and W. A. Clyde, Jr., Protective effect of vaccines in experimental *Mycoplasma pneumoniae* disease, *Infect. Immun.*, **1**:559–565 (1970).
54.   S. B. Singh and S. S. Tevethia, In vitro stimulation of hamster lymphocytes with concanavalin A., *Infect. Immun.*, **5**:339–345 (1972).
55.   G. W. Fernald and R. S. Metzgar, In Vitro studies of the response of hamster lymphocytes to phytohemagglutinin and antigenic stimulation, *J. Immunol.*, **107**:456–463 (1971).
56.   S. Arai, Y. Hinuma, K. Matsumoto, and T. Nakamura, Delayed hypersensitivity in hamsters infected with *Mycoplasma pneumoniae* as revealed by macrophage migration inhibition test, *Jpn. J. Microbiol.*, **15**:509–514 (1971).
57.   G. Biberfeld, Macrophage migration inhibition in response to experimental *Mycoplasma pneumoniae* infection in the hamster, *J. Immunol.*, **110**: 1146–1150 (1973).
58.   G. W. Fernald, *Mycoplasma pneumoniae* delayed hypersensitivity skin tests in guinea pigs, *Bacteriol. Proc.*, (1971), p. 103.
59.   R. H. Waldman and C. S. Henney, Cell–mediated immunity and antibody response in the respiratory tract after local and systemic immunization, *J. Exp. Med.*, **134**:482–494 (1971).
60.   D. A. Powell, W. A. Clyde, Jr., and G. W. Fernald, Interactions between alveolar macrophages and *Mycoplasma pneumoniae, J. Reticuloendothel. Soc.*, **15**:36a (1974).
61.   F. W. Denny, D. Taylor–Robinson, and A. C. Allison, The role of thymus-dependent immunity in *Mycoplasma pulmonis* infection of mice, *J. Med. Microbiol.*, **5**:327–336 (1972).
62.   G. Taylor, D. Taylor–Robinson, and G. W. Fernald, Reduction in the severity of *Mycoplasma pneumoniae* induced pneumonia in hamsters by immunosuppressive treatment with antithymocyte sers, *J. Med. Microbiol.*, 7:343–348 (1974).

63.   R. S. Kerbel and D. Eidinger, Variable effects of antilymphocyte serum on humoral antibody formation: Role of thymus dependency of antigen, *J. Immunol.*, **106**:917–926 (1971).

64.   B. T. Rouse and N. L. Warner, Depression of humoral antibody formation in the chicken by thymectomy and antilymphocyte serum, *Nature, New Biol.*, **236**:79–80 (1972).

65.   S. H. Singer, M. Ford, and R. L. Kirschstein, Respiratory diseases in cyclophosphamide treated mice, *Infect. Immun.*, **5**:953–956 (1972).

66.   T. H. Vardaman, K. Landreth, S. Whatley, L. J. Dreesen, and B. Glick, Resistance to mycoplasma synoviae is bursal dependent, *Infect. Immun.*, **8**:674–676 (1973).

67.   A. C. Allison, Immunity and immunopathology in virus infections, *Ann. Inst. Pasteur, Paris*, **123**:585–608 (1972).

68.   H. M. Foy, H. Ochs, S. D. Davis, G. E. Kenny, and R. R. Luce, *Mycoplasma pneumoniae* infections in patients with immunodeficiency syndromes: Report of four cases, *J. Infect. Dis.*, **127**:388–393 (1973).

69.   K. Lind, Production of cold agglutinins in rabbits induced by *Mycoplasma pneumoniae, Listeria monocytogenes,* or *Streptococcus* Mg, *Acta Pathol. Microbiol. Scand.*, **81**:487–496 (1973).

70.   H. Brunner, S. Razin, A. R. Kalica, and R. M. Chanock, Lysis and death of *Mycoplasma pneumoniae* by antibody and complement, *J. Immunol.*, **106**: 907–916 (1971).

71.   G. Biberfeld, P. Biberfeld, and G. Sterner, Cell–mediated immune response following *Mycoplasma pneumoniae* infection in man. I. Lymphocyte stimulation, *Clin. Exp. Immunol.*, **17**:29–41 (1974).

6

Respiratory Syncytial Virus

ROBERT H. PARROTT

George Washington University School
  of Health Sciences
Washington, D.C.

I. Introduction

The importance of respiratory syncytial (RS) virus as the major respiratory
disease pathogen of infancy and early childhood has been established beyond
question during the years since it was first recognized [1-3]. Some of the
findings from our studies emphasize the etiologic association and illness relationships; patterns of occurrence by time, sex, race and age; and factors influencing
pathogenesis and resistance to infection.

For purposes of this report, we will summarize our major findings and
those of others regarding RS viral disease and will state major unsolved questions.

A. Natural History

An epidemic of RS virus occurred in the Washington, D.C. area during each of
the 16 respiratory disease seasons between October 1957 and early 1970. There
were alternating short (7- to 12-month) and long (13- to 16-month) intervals
between peaks of successive epidemics (Fig. 1). Each RS viral epidemic lasted
approximately 5 months and its peak was closely associated in time with a

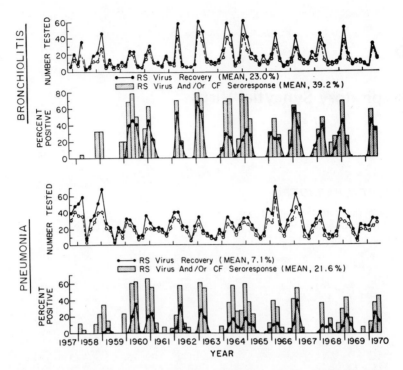

FIGURE 1 Respiratory syncytial (RS) virus infection in patients with bronchiolitis or pneumonia by 2-month intervals from October 1957–June 1970. ●——● Tested for RS virus; ○- - -○ tested by CF and for virus. Reprinted by permission from *Am. J. Epid.,* **98**:216–225 (1973).

dramatic increase in the number of infants and young children hospitalized with lower respiratory tract disease, especially bronchiolitis and pneumonia. Respiratory syncytial viral epidemics occurred primarily in the late fall, winter, or spring (Fig. 2). Overall, February and March were the peak months for RS viral disease.

B. Epidemiology

One of the most remarkable features of the epidemiology of RS viral disease in Washington, D.C. has been the consistent pattern of infection and disease. Other respiratory viruses have caused epidemics at irregular intervals, or have been endemic or have exhibited a mixed endemic–epidemic pattern, but RS virus is the only respiratory viral pathogen which has produced a sizable epidemic every year. Large annual variations in the impact of RS viral disease on the pediatric population served by Children's Hospital of Washington, D.C. were not observed.

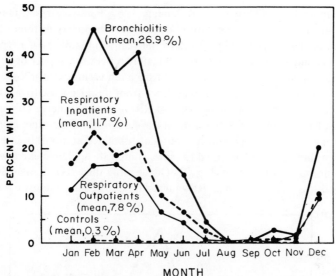

FIGURE 2 Frequency of respiratory syncytial (RS) virus recovery by month: Composite of observations from January 1960–June 1970. Reprinted by permission from *Am. J. Epidemiol,* **98**:216–225 (1973).

The number and proportion of infants and children admitted to the hospital for RS virus lower respiratory tract disease did not vary more than 2.7-fold. Also remarkable was the consistency with which RS virus produced the same clinical pattern of respiratory tract disease, especially bronchiolitis and pneumonia, year after year. These illnesses were barometers of RS viral infection in the community and when RS virus was at its epidemic peak, hospitalization for bronchiolitis and pneumonia soared.

C. Composite Outbreak

During the 1960–1970 period, yearly peaks of RS viral disease (the month when the highest percentage of pediatric respiratory disease patients yielded RS viral isolates) occurred in June 1960, January 1961, April 1962, February 1963, May

1964, December 1964, February 1966, January 1967, February 1968, February 1969, and April 1970. Since the outbreak peaks occurred in six different calendar months, data accumulated by month of the year would not show a typical RS virus epidemic wave, and could not adequately reflect the impact of RS virus on pediatric patients at monthly intervals during a representative outbreak. We were interested in accumulating the experience from the 11 consecutive outbreaks, since some aspects of the behavior of RS virus might emerge only after analysis of a large number of patients or, at least, a larger number than could be studied during one or two epidemics. Thus, data obtained at monthly intervals during the outbreaks were combined to plot a composite epidemic curve which showed a "normal" distribution (Fig. 3). Of the more than 1000 patients with respiratory disease who yielded an RS viral isolate during the composite outbreak,

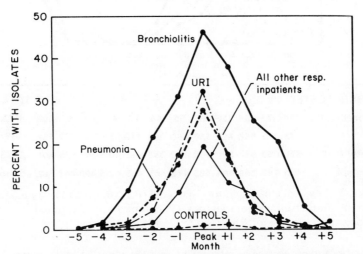

MONTHS IN RELATION TO MONTH WHEN RSV WAS MOST FREQUENTLY RECOVERED FROM ALL INPATIENTS AND OUTPATIENTS WITH RESPIRATORY TRACT DISEASE

NO. TESTED												TOTAL
Bronchiolitis	43	57	45	106	183	279	177	87	59	32	35	1103
Pneumonia	76	97	137	179	210	201	176	133	111	68	52	1440
Other in resp	181	160	233	200	190	165	142	124	124	104	87	1710
URI	479	478	582	652	781	660	622	586	560	319	276	5995
Control	340	367	473	413	564	500	527	462	459	360	352	4817

FIGURE 3 Frequency of recovery of respiratory syncytial (RS) virus from pediatric patients with respiratory disease and from controls, by month, during a composite of 11 consecutive epidemics (January 1960–June 1970). Reprinted by permission from *Am. J. Epidemiol.*, **98**:355–364 (1973).

40.1% shed virus during the peak epidemic month and 82.4% shed virus during the three midepidemic months. During the peak month of the composite epidemic, RS virus was recovered from 46.2% of all inpatients with bronchiolitis, from 33.6% of all inpatients with all forms of respiratory disease, and from 32.1% of all outpatients with respiratory disease. Control subjects free of respiratory disease rarely yielded RS virus. As indicated by the recovery of virus, or the development of serum complement fixation antibody, or both, 70.3% of patients with bronchiolitis and 56.4% of all inpatients with respiratory disease exhibited evidence of RS viral infection during the peak epidemic month. More than half of all hospitalized patients who yielded an RS virus isolate were less than 6 months of age. Among patients with bronchiolitis, about half of those with RS virus isolates were 3 months of age or younger.

D. Etiologic Association

Through the years, RS virus was recovered from 27% of 1179 inpatients with bronchiolitis and from 9% of 1547 patients with pneumonia, but only 0.3% of 5500 control subjects who were free of respiratory disease shed this virus. Based on virus recovery, or serum complement-fixation antibody response, or both, RS viral infection occurred in 43% of inpatients with bronchiolitis, 25% of inpatients with pneumonia, and 23% of all inpatients with acute respiratory tract disease.

These findings may represent an underestimation of the importance of RSV in infants, the individuals most often made seriously ill by the virus because the complement fixation and neutralization techniques do not efficiently detect infection in young infants.

E. Sex and Race

Clinical consequences of RS viral infection in infancy did not appear to be influenced by race. The same proportion of males and females with respiratory tract disease yielded RS virus; however, significantly more boys were admitted to the hospital for RS viral pneumonia, bronchiolitis, croup, and pharyngitis-bronchitis.

F. Risk

The behavior of RS virus in the pediatric population of Washington, D.C. has been discerned primarily through patterns of serious respiratory tract disease produced by this virus through a 15½-yr period. Although surveillance of seriously ill infants and children can serve as a barometer of the virus in the community, this type of study cannot, in itself, yield an estimate of the incidence of infection or risk of serious illness per infection. However, we found that approximately one-half of the infants tested during certain longitudinal viral studies were infected during their first RS viral epidemic, and almost all children were infected after living through two RS viral epidemics. These observations suggest that the risk of infection for previously uninfected infants and young children is extremely high. If one couples this information with the estimated size of the pediatric population served by Childrns's Hospital and the number of hospitalized patients with demonstrated RS viral infection, it is possible to derive a very crude estimate of the risk of serious RS virus bronchiolitis, i.e., severe enough to require admission to the hospital during primary infection. The crude estimate for the incidence of bronchiolitis requiring admission to the hospital per 1000 infants 0-12 months of age is 10 and for RS virus bronchiolitis the estimate is four. These data lead to a further estimate of one hospital admission for RS virus bronchiolitis per 100 primary RS viral infections during infancy. Of course, the toll of RS viral disease in infancy is considerably higher, since for every hospital admission for RS virus bronchiolitis there are many infants who develop respiratory disease almost as serious as that seen in the individuals admitted to the hospital.

II. Pathogenesis

A. Serum Antibody by Age

The occurrence of RS viral infection and disease during 11 consecutive yearly epidemics was examined with respect to patient-age and immunologic status. The peak incidence of RS virus bronchiolitis and pneumonia was observed at 2 months of age (Fig. 4). Thereafter, the incidence of these diseases decreased with increasing age, more rapidly for bronchiolitis than for pneumonia. Some years ago we observed that the level of serum neutralizing antibody by age during infancy resembled the age distribution of RSV bronchiolitis. This similarity prompted us to suggest that serum antibody might participate in an immunopathologic reaction in the lungs and that this reaction might contribute to the development and severity of bronchiolitis [4].

Recently, the level of neutralizing antibody by age in the sera of control infants and in the acute phase sera of infants with RS viral bronchiolitis or pneumonia was re-examined, using a larger collection of specimens than tested previously.

Each of the patients who had RS viral bronchiolitis or pneumonia during the first 3 months of life possessed neutralizing antibody in his serum during the acute phase of illness (Fig. 5). In most instances, the level of this antibody,

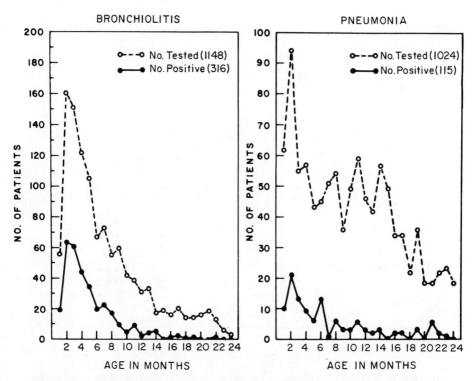

FIGURE 4 Occurence of respiratory syncytial (RS) virus bronchiolitis and pneumonia, by age, during the first 2 yr of life; infection detected by recovery of virus (January 1960–June 1970). Reprinted by permission from *Am. J. Epidemiol.*, **98**:289–300 (1973).

presumably of maternal origin, was moderately high. In contrast, 15 of 57 infants who developed RS viral bronchiolitis at 4 to 7 months of age lacked detectable antibody in their accute phase serum. The latter finding casts some doubt upon the essential role of serum antibody in RS viral bronchiolitis. Although the significance of serum antibody in the pathogenesis of disease may not be clear at this time, it is evident that relatively high levels of this type of antibody during the first 3 to 4 months of life do not protect the young infant from RS viral bronchiolitis or pneumonia. At this point, we are reluctant to dismiss completely the possibility that immunopathologic factors play an important role in RS viral bronchiolitis because of the strong suggestion, in the past, that an inactivated RS virus vaccine had potentiated the response of vaccinees to RS viral infection through an immunologic mechanism [5].

The serum complement–fixation antibody response to RS virus was impaired in infants 1 to 3 months of age. A delayed or decreased immunologic

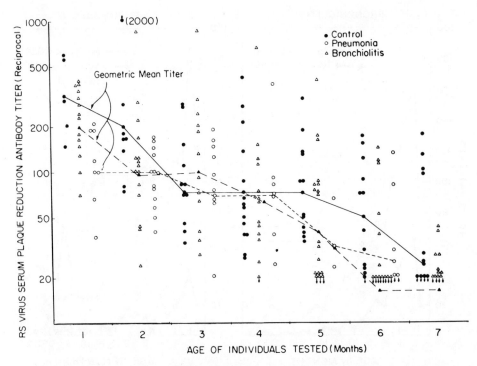

FIGURE 5 Titer of neutralizing antibody in serum of normal infants and in the acute-phase serum of infants with respiratory syncytial (RS) virus bronchiolitis or pneumonia, by age; neutralizing antibody determined by the plaque reduction technique. Reprinted by permission from the *Am. J. Epidemiol.*, **98**:289–300 (1973).

response or both could contribute to the increased severity of RS viral disease during early infancy. Recent studies of parainfluenza 1 (Sendai) virus in mice by Blandford and associates [6] have demonstrated an early immunologic response in the lungs several days before serum antibody was detected. If this type of early pulmonary immunologic response plays a role in the resolution of infection, which is likely, a delay, a decrease, or both, in response could lead to a more serious type of disease. One factor which might contribute to such an impaired response is immunologic suppression by maternally derived serum antibody. This type of immunologic suppression is known to affect the development of serum antibody, but it is not known whether local respitatory tract secretory antibody can be suppressed in a similar manner. The level of acute-phase serum neutralizing antibody was found to be inversely related to the height of the serum complement-fixing antibody response during convalescence, suggesting that maternally derived antibody may have suppressed the immunologic response of some infants.

B. Allergy

Gardner et al. postulated that the essential process in the pathogenesis of RS viral bronchiolitis is an allergic reaction which requires two infections with RS virus, whereas RS viral pneumonia does not require a sensitizing RS viral infection [7]. The question of one versus two infections in bronchiolitis is not merely of academic interest. Efforts to immunize infants with live attenuated RS virus have begun, and are being continued, with the expectation that protection rather than sensitization will result [8,9]. Several findings, particularly the constant age-distribution of patients with bronchiolitis throughout the RS viral epidemic, do not support the hypothesis that RSV bronchiolitis in infancy represents an "allergic" reaction to reinfection with the virus. In addition, levels of IgE in acute-phase sera of 160 infants with RSV bronchiolitis were not elevated when compared to age-matched controls.

C. Cell-mediated Immunity

In attempts to understand the apparent "sensitization" of individuals to RS virus after inactivated RS virus vaccine, we carried out in vitro lymphocyte transformation studies as a measure of cell-mediated immunity in infants who had received inactivated RSV vaccine and in a control group of infants. The findings strongly suggest that systemic RS virus-specific cell-mediated immunity developed after killed RS virus vaccine was administered and after natural RS viral infection. These findings suggest that cell-mediated immunity may be a factor in the altered response to natural infection, which occurred after inactivated RS virus vaccine was used. However, these findings also indicate that systemic cell-mediated immunity, along with serum antibody, is not sufficient to protect against RS virus infection.

D. Local Antibody

Stimulated by the observation that serum antibody was not protective in RS virus disease, evidence of a local immunologic response was sought. This effort was successful, and the development of neutralizing activity in nasal secretions was demonstrated in a significant proportion of infants and young children following natural or vaccine-induced infection with RS virus [10]. However, attempts to link local respiratory tract antibody with resistance and to define the level of local antibody which was protective have failed to date, because the nasal secretions of young infants contain a nonantibody inhibitor of RS virus. This inhibitor produces a low to moderate background of neutralizing activity in the secretions of infants which makes it difficult to identify young subjects who lack specific local respiratory tract antibody.

III.   Unresolved Questions

1. One of the major unresolved questions involves the *pathogenesis*
    of serious RS viral disease during early life and factors which
    favor life-threatening bronchiolitis in approximately 1 in 100
    infected infants. Are immunologic factors, such as poor anti-
    body response (local and systemic) or an Arthus–type reaction
    in the lung involving passively acquired serum antibody, impor-
    tant determinants of disease? One could also consider the pos-
    sibility that RS virus lymphocyte sensitization from the mother
    might be transferred to the infant before birth and might be
    involved in the pathogenesis of pulmonary disease. Recent
    evidence for the transfer of lymphocyte sensitization from
    mother to fetus has been presented [11,12].

2. What are the important determinants of *resistance* to RS viral
    infection and disease? Based on our observations, it is unlikely
    that serum neutralizing antibody plays an important role in
    protecting the host. By exclusion, it is likely that local respir-
    atory tract immunity is of prime importance. Although find-
    ings from studies in adult volunteers support this view, there
    are very few solid data concerning the function of local respir-
    atory tract RS virus antibody in infants and young children.
    The major barrier to better understanding in this area is the
    presence of a nonantibody inhibitor for RS virus in nasal secre-
    tions of infants and young children who appear to have escaped
    RS viral infection (as indicated by the absence of serum neu-
    tralizing antibody and by virtue of these individuals having
    been born after the last RS virus epidemic in the community).

References

1. H. W. Kim, J. O. Arrobio, C. D. Brandt, B. D. Jeffries, G. Pyles, J. L. Reid,
    R. M. Chanock, and R. H. Parrott, Epidemiology of respiratory syncytial
    virus infection in Washington, D.C. I. Importance of the virus in different
    respitatory tract disease syndromes and temporal distribution of infection,
    Am. J. Epidemiol., **98**:216–225 (1973).
2. R. H. Parrott, H. W. Kim, J. O. Arrobio, D. S. Hodes, B. R. Murphy, C. D.
    Brandt, E. Camargo, and R. M. Chanock, Epidemiology of respiratory
    syncytial virus infection in Washington, D.C. II. Infection and disease with
    respect to age, immunologic status, race, and sex, *Am. J. Epidemiol.,* **98**:
    289–300 (1973).

3. C. D. Brandt, H. W. Kim, J. O. Arrobio, B. C. Jeffries, S. C. Wood, R. M. Chanock, and R. H. Parrott, Epidemiology of respiratory syncytial virus infection in Washington, D.C. III. Composite analysis of eleven consecutive yearly epidemics, *Am. J. Epidemiol.,* **98**:355–364 (1973).

4. R. M. Chanock, Local antibody and resistance to acute viral respiratory tract disease. In *Proceedings Symposium on Secretory Immunologic System.* Washington, C.C., Government Printing Office, 1969, pp. 83–92.

5. H. W. Kim, J. G. Canchola, C. D. Brandt, G. Pyles, R. M. Chanock, K. E. Jensen, and R. H. Parrott, Respiratory syncytial virus disease in infants despite prior administration of antigenic inactivated vaccine, *Am. J. Epidemiol.,* **80**:422–434 (1969).

6. G. Blandford and R. B. Heath, Studies on the immune response and pathogenesis of Sendai virus infection of mice. I. The fate of viral antigens, *Immunology,* **22**:4 (1972).

7. P. S. Gardner, J. McQuillin, and S. D. M. Court, Speculation on pathogenesis in death from respiratory syncytial virus infection, *Br. Med. J.,* 327- 330 (1970).

8. H. W. Kim, J. O. Arrobio, G. Pyles, C. D. Brandt, E. Camargo, R. M. Chanock, and R. H. Parrott, Clinical and immunological response of infants and children to administration of low–temperature adapted respiratory syncytial virus, *Pediatrics,* **48**:745–755 (1971).

9. H. W. Kim, J. O. Arrobio, C. D. Brandt, P. Wright, D. Hodes, R. M. Chanock, and R. H. Parrott, Safety and antigenicity of temperature sensitive (TS) mutant respiratory syncytial virus (RSV) in infants and children, *Pediatrics,* **52**:56–63 (1973).

10. R. H. Parrott, H. W. Kim, J. A. Bellanti, J. O. Arrobio, J. Mills, C. D. Brandt, and R. M. Chanock, Development of nasal secretion neutralizing activity in infants and children following natural respiratory syncytial virus infection or administration of cold–adapted RS A2 virus. In *Proceedings Symposium on Secretory Immunologic System.* Washington, D.C., Government Printing Office, 1969, pp. 167–182.

11. S. Leikin, J. Whang–Peng, and J. J. Oppenheim, In vitro transformation of human cord blood lymphocytes by antigens. *Proceedings Fifth Leukocyte Culture Conference,* 1970, pp. 389–402.

12. E. J. Field and E. A. Caspary, Is maternal Lymphocyte sensitization passed to the child? *Lancet,* 337–341 (1971).

7

Interaction of *Pseudomonas* Bacteria with Antibodies and Cells in the Lung

HERBERT Y. REYNOLDS

National Institute of Allergy and Infectious Diseases
National Institutes of Health
Bethesda, Maryland

I. Introduction

Pseudomonas microorganisms are ubiquitous in the environment; yet they rarely cause illness in humans with competent immune defenses, even though bacteria may inhabit the gastrointestinal tract or colonize the skin. In contrast *Pseudomonas* infections, particularly of the respiratory tract, are frequent in people with chronic cardiopulmonary diseases [1,2] or in those receiving immunosuppressive therapy [3]. Such infections, in individuals with potentially impaired host defenses, do not always respond to optimal antibiotic treatment and often result in appreciable morbidity or death of the patient. Therefore, one might hope to find ways of improving host defenses in these susceptible people to enhance their resistance.

When bacteria, such as *Pseudomonas*, are inhaled or aerosolized into the respiratory tract, a significant portion of the inoculum is deposited in the

---

Portions of this manuscript were reprinted from the *Journal of Infectious Diseases,* November supplement 1974 by permission of the University of Chicago Press (Chicago).

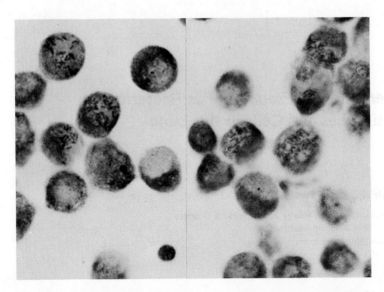

FIGURE 1 Wright–Giemsa stained rabbit alveolar macrophages attached to plastic dishes were photographed under oil emersion at 1100X. Some macrophages contain intracellular *Pseudomonas* opsonized with immune IgG antibody prepared from bronchial secretions.

terminal airway (alveolar spaces) where mucociliary removal and other means of mechanical clearance are not thought to be operative [4]. In the alveoli, clearance of particulate matter (size 0.5-3μm) and bacteriostasis is accomplished primarily by macrophages. As illustrated in Figure 1, if *Pseudomonas* organisms inoculated into the lower respiratory tract were completely ingested and contained within alveolar macrophages, intracellular killing would proceed and subsequent infection might be prevented. However, two intermediate events must occur: (a) efficient phagocytosis of the bacteria, which optimally requires opsonic antibody and (b) activation or stimulation of macrophages to kill intracellular bacteria. Potentially, both of these events can be manipulated in the host by altering his immune status either by active immunization with the microorganism or its products, or by previous infection with the agent.

Obviously, the interaction between bacteria and macrophages within the alveolar environment is complex, but in vitro methods do allow for individual assessment of several independent factors which together determine the rate and efficiency of macrophage phagocytosis. To dissect these further, we will discuss: (a) the kinds of antibodies produced in the lower respiratory tract and how the mode of active immunization can affect the class of immunoglobulin with antibody activity; (b) the relative opsonic efficiency of the resultant antibodies, particularly those obtained following intranasal immunization; and (c) the response of respiratory macrophages to effector substances (migration-inhibition factor) released by immune respiratory lymphocytes. The intention will be to evaluate the effect of each factor on promoting phagocytosis and killing of *Pseudomonas* by alveolar macrophages.

II. Materials and Methods

Details of the various methods can be found in three recent publications [5-7] but will be presented briefly here. New Zealand white rabbits (2-3 kg), culture-free of intranasal *Bordetella bronchiseptica* organisms, were immunized for intervals of 1 to 4 wk either intranasally or intramuscularly. The inoculum was either formalin-inactivated, whole-cell *Pseudomonas aeruginosa* vaccines or a lipopolysaccharide antigen, extracted with acid [8] from a strain of *Pseudomonas aeruginosa,* immunotype 2 [9] , which will be designated LPS-II. Following immunization, serum samples were obtained and intradermal skin testing done; when the animals were sacrificed, lungs and spleens were removed and skin was taken for histologic evaluation.

Intact lungs were lavaged with 150-ml of modified Hank's balanced salt solution (prepared without calcium and magnesium ions or phenol red). The respiratory cells were pelleted from the lavage fluid by centrifugation and after further washing were established in plastic dishes as cell cultures. McCoy's 5A media enriched with glutamine, 10% heat-inactivated fetal calf serum, and, in some instances, gentamicin sulfate ($5\mu g/ml$) was used. Cells were incubated in moist air and 5% CO_2 at $37^\circ C$.

The lavage fluid, after the respiratory cells were removed, was concentrated about 100-fold with positive pressure ultrafiltration, dialyzed against borate-saline buffer, adjusted to a final 1-ml volume, and designated concentrated bronchial secretions. These secretions were analyzed for a variety of components [5] , including hemagglutinative antibodies [10,11] , lipids, complement, immuno-globulins, and albumin. Bronchial secretions and serum were separated into size components in 10% to 40% linear sucrose density gradients by ultracentrifugation [5,12] . Various *Pseudomonas* antibodies were purified from bronchial secretions and serum by gel filtration, using the described procedures [5] .

To assess cellular immunity, the in vitro assay of inhibition of migration of alveolar macrophages from capillary tubes was used [7] . Immune lymphocytes were stimulated with LPS-II antigen to produce migration-inhibition factor

(MIF). For indirect MIF assays, non adherent lymphocytes (separated on wool-glass bead columns [13]) from the respiratory tract and spleen were stimulated in cell cultures.

For phagocytosis studies, IgA and IgG antibodies were used to opsonize viable [^{14}C] -labeled *Pseudomonas* organisms, which were then inoculated into macrophage cell monolayers. Total bacteria as ^{14}C counts in cell homogenates; viable bacteria as estimated by quantitative agar-pour plates; and phagocytic indexes, as calculated from Wright-Giemsa stained macrophage monolayers, were all measured. To evaluate the ability of lymphocyte-released MIF to activate immune alveolar macrophages, respiratory cells were obtained from rabbits intra-nasally immunized with LPS-II. A portion of the respiratory cell suspension was used in a direct MIF assay; the remaining cells were put into monolayer cultures. The design of the experiment was to stimulate half of the macrophage cell cultures with the LPS-II antigen; the other half served as nonstimulated controls. When there was discernible macrophage inhibition in the direct MIF assay, usually evident within 4 to 8 hr after stimulation, IgG opsonized viable [^{14}C] -labeled Type II *Pseudomonas* were added in a 10:1 ratio of bacteria per macrophages to the LPS-II stimulated and to the control macrophage monolayer cultures. There-after, phagocytic uptake of bacteria by the macrophages was measured as described above.

III. Results

A. Antibody Responses in Bronchial Secretions and Their Relationship to Route of Immunization

Immunization with whole-cell inactivated *Pseudomonas* vaccines [5] or with extracted lipopolysaccharide [7] will elicit specific antibody responses, which can be measured in serum and bronchial secretions by hemagglutination. Two groups of rabbits were immunized intranasally or intramuscularly with LPS-II for a 1- or 2-wk interval (three doese of antigen per week at the rate of 240μg/ dose intranasally and 20μg/kg intramuscularly); antibody titers in serum and bronchial secretions are given in Table 1. For serum specimens, total and 2-mercaptoethanol-resistant agglutinative titers are given to differentiate the proportions of macroglobulin (IgM) and IgG antibody present. Separation of IgM and IgG fractions in sera by gel filtration methods, previously used to identify agglutinative antibody activity in immune rabbit sera [5] , confirmed the reliability and specificity of these titers. For concentrated bronchial secre-tions, only total agglutinative titers were measured, because normal respiratory secretions lacked IgM immunoglobulin [5] . As shown in Table 1, serum anti-

TABLE 1 Antibody Response in Bronchial Secretions and Serum Following Intranasal or Intramuscular Immunization with LPS-II

	Nonimmunized controls	1 wk[a]	2 wk[b]	3 wk	4 wk
Intranasal					
Number rabbits	3	5	4	4	3
Bronchial secretions	<2[c] (0–2)	<2 (0–4)	2.8 (0–16)	8.0 (4–16)	12.7 (8–32)
Whole serum	2.5 (2–4)	111.4 (4–1024)	215.3 (64–1024)	1712.0 (1024–4096)	1290.2 (1024–2048)
Reduced serum[d]	<2 (0–2)	4.0 (2–8)	13.5 (4–256)	128.0 (32–256)	256.0 (128–512)
Intramuscular					
Number rabbits	3	3	5	5	3
Bronchial secretions	<2 (0–2)	<2 (0–2)	12.1 (4–32)	9.2 (4–32)	8.0 (4–16)
Whole serum	5.0 (4–8)	322.5 (256–572)	3104.2 (512–8192)	2048.0 (1024–4096)	645.1 (512–1024)
Reduced serum	<2 (0–2)	3.2 (2–4)	111.4 (16–512)	194.0 (64–512)	64.0 (32–128)

[a]After 3 doses LPS-II.
[b]After 6 doses LPS-II.
[c]Geometrical mean of hemagglutinative antibody titers for the group and titer range observed.
[d]Reduced with 2-mercaptoethanol.

body titers were detected at 1 wk, or after three doses of LPS–II, in both groups of immunized rabbits; but, antibody was principally confined to the IgM class. At 2 wk when the immunization course was completed, serum agglutinative titers in both IgM and IgG fractions were higher in rabbits immunized intramuscularly than in animals immunized intranasally. By the third week, serum titers were comparable in the two groups. Agglutination in bronchial secretions was not detected before 2 wk and generally was proportional to the serum IgG titer.

However, immunoglobulin classes in bronchial secretions with antibody activity for LPS–II were different, depending upon the route of immunization. Bronchial secretion specimens from rabbits, obtained 1 wk after intramuscular or intranasal immunization, were examined in sucrose density gradients. In Figure 2, a representative comparison of agglutinative activity and the quantitation of protein components in various gradient fractions are shown for bronchial secretions. The two gradients had comparable fraction numbers and the position of the 11 S and 7 S markers were identical. Agglutinative activity in bronchial secretions from an intranasally immunized rabbit was found in the IgA and IgG fractions, whereas in the bronchial specimen from the rabbit immunized intramuscularly agglutination was confined to the IgG fractions. Similar gradients showed agglutinative activity in serum specimens in both IgM and IgG fractions from rabbits immunized intramuscularly or intranasally.

Two points should be emphasized: (a) IgM antibody was not detected in the bronchial secretions separated as shown in Figure 2, because this immunoglobulin is not a constituent of normal bronchial secretions in rabbits [5] or humans [14,15], whereas an appreciable amount of serum agglutinative activity is found in the IgM fractions, and (b) complement activity is present in only small quantities in bronchial fluid and is thought to be a minor component in these secretions [5]. Therefore, it is apparent that the milieu of the normal respiratory tract is quite different from that of the intravascular space, and some of the options available for host–defense in the lungs are different.

The immune activity of these immunoglobulin fractions, as measured by agglutination, may be misleading. Agglutination is a secondary property of bacterial–antibody interaction, whereas antibodies in vivo probably have a primary action against bacteria either through fixation of complement to cause lysis or by functioning as an opsonin. Because complement components were present only in trace amounts in bronchial secretions, it was concluded that complement–mediated lysis is unlikely to be a principal mechanism for bacterial inactivation in the normal respiratory tract. Thus, the effectiveness of antibodies in bronchial secretions must be judged by opsonic activity. IgG and IgA immunoglobulins were isolated from immune bronchial secretions by gel–filtration chromatography before use in opsonic and phagocytosis studies.

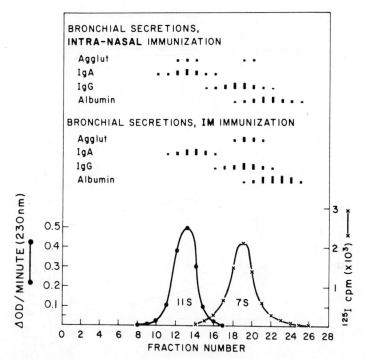

FIGURE 2   Bronchial secretions obtained from an intranasally and an intramuscularly (IM) immunized rabbit 1 wk after completed immunization with LPS–II were simultaneously spearated in sucrose density gradients by ultracentrifugation. Fractions from each gradient were comparable and the positions of the 11 S and 7 S markers were the same in each gradient. The position of the 11 S catalase marker (●) was determined enzymatically and is plotted as Δ OD/ min.; the radiodinated 7 S marker position (×) is shown as counts per minute (cpm). The relative concentrations of albumin, immunoglobulins, and hemagglutinative antibody activity in each gradient fraction are denoted by vertical bars. Reprinted by permission from *J. Clin. Invest.*, 53:1351–1358 (1974).

B.   Effectiveness of IgG and IgA Antibodies as Opsonins

An in vitro rabbit alveolar macrophage culture system, which has features borrowed from several systems previously described, was used to evaluate the effectiveness of opsonins in bronchial secretions in promoting phagocytosis and intracellular killing of *Pseudomonas* [6]. Figure 3 shows a comparison of the relative opsonic activity of IgG and IgA antibodies. IgG and IgA opsonins were separated chromatographically from pooled bronchial secretions obtained from rabbits immunized intranasally with killed whole–cell vaccine of *Pseudomonas aeruginosa.* The experiment was designed to challenge alveolar macrophage

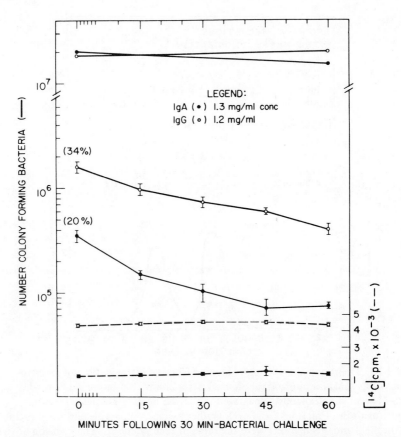

FIGURE 3 IgA and IgG opsonins, each with an agglutinative titer of 8 at the concentration used, were separated from pooled bronchial secretions obtained from rabbits immunized intranasally with *Pseudomonas*. Each dish contained 3×10^6 macrophages and was inoculated with 2×10^7 opsonized bacteria for a 30-min challenge period. Thereafter, cell homogenates were sampled for viable colony-forming bacteria (left ordinate) and for total [^{14}C] bacteria (right ordinate) during a 60-min period. Viability of the bacterial inocula mixed with the IgA and IgG opsonins is shown at the top of the figure. Reprinted by permission from *J. Immunol.*, **111**:369-380 (1973).

monolayers with viable opsonized [^{14}C]-labeled *Pseudomonas*. After a 30-min challenge period to allow phagocytosis, the excess bacteria were inactivated with gentamicin, $5\mu g/ml$, which was about twice the mean inhibitory concentration for the *Pseudomonas* strain; intracellular killing was measured during the next 60 min. Cell homogenates were sampled for viable colony-forming bacteria and for total [^{14}C]-labeled bacteria. The macrophage monolayers exposed to the IgG-opsonized bacteria had ^{14}C bacterial counts approximately threefold more than the TgA-challenged monolayers. This increased bacterial uptake was also reflected in the higher phagocytic index of the IgG-exposed group (34%). However, the contour of the killing curves, shown by the number of viable bacteria cultured from the monolayers, was essentially the same over the 60-min observation. The number of bacteria cultured from the IgA-challenged monolayers was consistently less at each time interval than that for the IgG-exposed monolayers because the macrophages ingested appreciably fewer bacteria.

Several conclusions can be drawn from these kinds of data. First, immune secretory IgA did not support phagocytosis to the same degree as did IgG and was judged to have less opsonic activity when compared at equal protein concentrations and comparable agglutinative activity. Second, once phagocytosis of the opsonized *Pseudomonas* occurred, intracellular killing of the organism proceeded at a rapid rate and apparently was not influenced by the immunoglobulin class of the opsonin. The primary function of the immune opsonin was to promote cellular phagocytosis, but after the bacteria had been internalized, the opsonin was no longer important. Third, the rate of intracellular killing of various gram-negative bacteria by macrophages is related to individual properties of the microorganism [16]. Different rates of intracellular killing for *Pseudomonas* species may be related to the organism's ability to secrete a mucoid slime layer or to other intrinsic properties of their cell walls.

C. Cellular Immunity in the Respiratory Tract

A variety of infectious agents [17-21], causing pulmonary infections in animal models, can produce cellular immunity or delayed hypersensitivity in the respiratory tract. Histologic studies of human lungs following fatal gram-negative bacterial pneumonia [1,22-24] have identified appreciable infiltrations of mononuclear cells. It has been suggested that the cellular response to these gram-negative infections might be an expression of delayed hypersensitivity. Recently, normal humans were shown to have delayed or tuberculin-like skin reactivity to a variety of bacterial endotoxins, which indicated that humans have preexisting or natural cellular immunity to these substances [25].

With this background, we anticipated that some evidence of cellular immunity should be detected in the rabbits, both systemically and in the respiratory tract, following immunization with LPS-II. If so, another variable in the *Pseudomonas*-opsonic antibody-alveolar macrophage interaction could be added. Intradermal skin testing with LPS-II antigen following immunization gave responses most compatible with an Arthus reaction due to the presence of circulating antibody to LPS-II. It was difficult to quantify a delayed "cellular"

component from the skin histology, even though minimal reactive doses of antigen were injected [25]. Therefore, an in vitro correlate of cellular immunity
[26], the release of MIF from antigen-stimulated immune lymphocytes, was
used.

As illustrated in Figure 4, the migration of macrophages lavaged from the
lungs of an intranasally immunized rabbit was inhibited when the immunizing
antigen, LPS-II, was added in nontoxic amounts to the respiratory cell mixture
(direct MIF assay). The respiratory cell suspensions usually contained about 7%
small lymphocytes [7]. Such inhibition was specific for respiratory cells recovered from intranasally immunized rabbits and was not found in control nonimmunized animals. Spleen-derived lymphocytes from intranasally immunized
rabbits, assayed with an indirect MIF assay, likewise had MIF reactivity. However, immunization by the intramuscular route was not effective in producing
respiratory-cell MIF activity but produced only spleen-associated activity [7].

The capacity of immune lymphocytes to produce MIF, obtained from
either the respiratory tract or spleen, disappeared within 2 to 3 wk after full
immunization had been achieved. Thus, the in vitro evidence of cellular immunity was transient following primary immunization with LPS-II. Booster

DIRECT MIF

Control   LPS (10 μg/ml)   LPS (25 μg/ml)

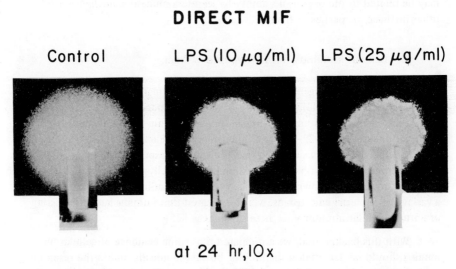

at 24 hr, 10x

FIGURE 4 Respiratory cells were lavaged from a rabbit 1 wk after completed
intranasal immunization with LPS-II. Macrophage migration from capillary
tubes in Sykes–Moore chambers was inhibited by two concentrations of LPS-II
added to the culture media for the direct MIF assay. At 24-hr, mean macrophage viability in each chamber was 83% ±0.6.

doses of antigen to restimulate MIF activity and to test the immunologic memory of lymphocytes for LPS-II were not done in these studies.

D. Interaction of Immune Lymphocytes, Alveolar Macrophages and Opsonized *Pseudomonas* Organisms

Although MIF, released from stimulated lymphocytes, would inhibit the mobility of respiratory macrophages, it was of interest to determine the total biologic effect on macrophages. To assess this, the following series of experiments was done. Rabbits, immunized intranasally for 2 wk with LPS-II, were sacrificed 1 wk later, when MIF activity in the respiratory cell-suspensions was anticipated to be maximal. A portion of the respiratory cell-suspension, obtained by bronchial lavage, was used in a direct MIF assay, as illustrated in Figure 4; the remaining cells were established in monolayer cultures. To half of the monolayers, LPS-II was added in a dose of $25\mu g/ml$ to the culture media and to the other half, the controls, a comparable volume of normal saline was added. LPS-II-stimulation of the monolayers continued until there was discernible inhibition of macrophage in the direct MIF assays. At this time, IgG opsonized [^{14}C]-labeled viable Type II *Pseudomonas* organisms were added to both groups of monolayers, and subsequent phagocytosis was evaluated during the succeeding 60-min interval.

In this series of experiments, cell monolayers were stimulated with LPS-II for intervals of 1 to 12 hr; however, macrophage inhibition by the direct MIF assay was usually evident in 4 to 8 hr. In Figure 5 a representative experiment is shown in which stimulation with LPS-II was continued for 6 hr. The phagocytic index at 30 min was slightly greater for LPS-stimulated monolayers than for the control, otherwise the two groups of monolayers reacted similarly to ^{14}C bacterial uptake and to viable bacteria cultured from the cell homogenatès. After the 15-min sampling, there was little increment in the number of viable bacteria cultured from the remaining cell monolayers, despite the continuous increase in the number of bacteria taken up by the cell layers, as illustrated by the ^{14}C counts. Once the immune opsonized-bacteria had been phagocytized, intracellular killing proceeded rapidly. The macrophage layers in both groups were able to attain an apparent equilibrium, which allowed intracellular killing to keep pace with further deposition and phagocytosis of bacteria from the liquid medium.

Under these experimental conditions, we have been unable to show that MIF stimulation is effective in significantly increasing *Pseudomonas* uptake or in accelerating intracellular killing by alveolar macrophages from immune rabbits. Our evidence of MIFs activity in the cellular interaction with macrophages is limited to inhibiting macrophage migration.

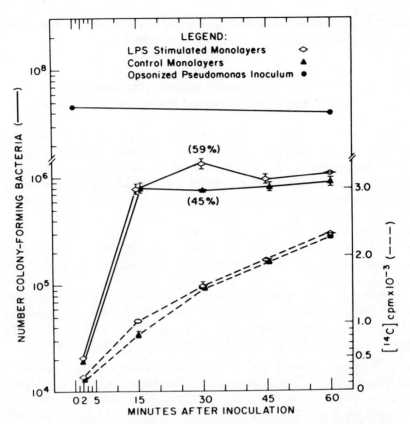

FIGURE 5 Respiratory cells were lavaged from the lungs of a rabbit 1 wk after immunization with LPS–II was completed. Culture dishes, which contained 2.8 × 10⁶ alveolar macrophages, were either stimulated with LPS–II at 25μg/ml in the supernatant (◊) or remained as nonstimulated controls (▲). After 6 hr incubation, by which time direct MIF assay with a portion of the original respiratory cell suspension was showing macrophage inhibition, an inoculum of IgG opsonized viable [¹⁴C] *Pseudomonas,* immunotype 2 was added to each culture dish at a 10:1 ratio of bacteria per cells. At intervals during the next 60–min, duplicate dishes from each group were measured for the number of colony-forming bacteria cultured from an 0.1–ml aliquot of the cell homogenates (left ordinate), and for total ¹⁴C bacteria in the remaining cell homogenates (right ordinate). The number of macrophages having phagocytized bacteria at 30 min is given in parentheses (phagocytic index). Viability of the bacterial inoculum (●) during the experiment is shown above the break in the log–scale for colony-forming bacteria.

IV. Discussion

Pseudomonads do not seem to be pathogenic or invasive for humans or animals with normal host immunity. Under usual circumstances, if *Pseudomonas* organisms are deposited in the alveolar spaces of the lung, pulmonary macrophages seem capable of containing the inoculum and averting infection. However, individuals with structural lung disease or with impaired function of the lymphoreticular system, due to specific disease involvement or immunosuppressive therapy, are particularly susceptible to *Pseudomonas* infections or to infections caused by other opportunistic microorganisms. In the susceptible individual, prior active immunization with *Pseudomonas* antigens may be desirable to induce additional humoral and cellular immunity, which could offer an advantage to the host in handling this infection.

Immunization can provide specific antibodies in the lower respiratory tract which coat or opsonize *Pseudomonas* and facilitate phagocytosis by alveolar macrophages. In this instance, however, the type of antibody elicited is important. IgG antibody, compared with secretory IgA antibody, at a comparable protein concentration, and agglutinating activity was better in supporting phagocytosis. Both parenteral and intranasal immunization successfully stimulated IgG antibody. This antibody may reach the respiratory secretions either by transudation from the intravascular space or by local synthesis in the submucosa of the respiratory tract [27].

Intranasal immunization, in contrast to the intramuscular route, provides several additional features which may be of advantage. First, secretory IgA (S-IgA) antibody is stimulated. The precise function of S-IgA in the lower lung has not been established. Its opsonic activity with this particular gram-negative bacterium was not as efficient as IgG; furthermore, bactericidal activity from S-IgA fixation of complement is an unsettled question [28-31] and may not be a lytic mechanism in normal lungs because of the small concentration of complement found in normal respiratory secretions [5,15]. However, S-IgA has been found to have viral neutralizing activity in secretions obtained from the upper respiratory tract [32] and from the intestine [33] and to neutralize cholera toxin [34]. It is likely that an important function of S-IgA is to prevent bacterial adherence to epithelial surfaces in the oropharynx [35] and thereby selectively regulate colonization of mucosal surfaces by microorganisms. Although the role of S-IgA antibody is still being defined, immunization regimens should include intranasal application of antigen in order to exploit the probability that S-IgA antibody protects against respiratory pathogens. Second, intranasal immunization will produce a population of immune lymphocytes capable of releasing an effector substance (MIF) upon appropriate antigenic challenge. At present, the origin of these sensitized lymphocytes is uncertain—whether they come from aggregates of bronchial-associated lymphoid tissue [36], from more distal portions of the airways [37], or are derived from circulating blood? Whole lung lavage unfortunately does not distinguish the level or depth in the respiratory tree from which the lymphocytes were recovered. Stimulated respiratory lymphocytes by direct MIF assay inhibited migration of rabbit alveolar macrophages, but they were capable of this function for only a brief interval of a few weeks after primary immunization. This phenomenon suggests that frequent contact with *Pseudomonas* antigens or antigen-persistence may be necessary to prolong the state of cellular hypersensitivity. If cellular hypersensitivity is a desirable host immune-defense, it is disappointing, with respect to the use of *Pseudomonas* vaccines in that frequent immunization or booster injections might be necessary. Finally, intranasal immunization potentially should enhance the bactericidal activity of immune alveolar macrophages, perhaps analogous to the accelerated killing of inhaled *Listeria monocytogenes* in the lungs of immunized mice [20]. In our in vitro studies, respiratory cells from intranasally immunized rabbits responded to stimulation with LPS-II by producing MIF, but this was not associated with a noticeable increase in phagocytosis or killing of IgG-opsonized viable *Pseudomonas* organisms. However, before the conclusion is reached that alveolar macrophages from immune animals have no enhanced responsiveness, in vitro conditions must be explored further to be certain they are optimal.

V. Summary

The development of humoral and cellular immunity in the lungs of rabbits was compared after intranasal and parenteral immunization with *Pseudomonas* antigens. The in vitro ability of respiratory antibodies and immune lymphocytes to increase the phagocytosis of *Pseudomonas* organisms by alveolar macrophages was studied to understand further the intricate interactions of bacteria, opsonins, and activated macrophages in the lower respiratory tract. Intranasal immunization induced both IgG and secretory IgA agglutinative antibodies in respiratory secretions; however, the opsonic activity of IgG seemed to be superior to that of IgA in promoting macrophage phagocytosis. Immune respiratory lymphocytes, recovered from intranasally immunized rabbits, inhibited the migration of alveolar macrophages when stimulated with the immunizing antigen in direct MIF assays. However, this capacity lasted only 2 to 3 wk and suggests that respiratory cellular immunity is transient after primary immunization and that frequent booster injections or persistent antigen contact may be necessary to maintain this cellular activity. In vitro activation of macrophages by immune lymphocytes did not increase macrophage phagocytosis of opsonized viable *Pseudomonas* or enhance bacterial killing compared with nonstimulated controls. Thus, immunization with *Pseudomonas* antigens, particularly by the intranasal route, produced specific respiratory antibodies and transient cellular or delayed hypersensitivity in the lungs. This offers the potential of improving alveolar macrophage function, which might augment natural host-defenses against *Pseudomonas* lung infections.

References

1. J. R. Tillotson and A. M. Lerner, Characteristics of nonbacteremic Pseudo-monas pneumonia, *Ann. Intern. Med.*, **68**:295–307 (1968).
2. H. D. Rose, M. G. Heckman, and J. D. Linger, *Pseudomonas aeruginosa* pneumonia in adults, *Am. Rev. Respir. Dis.*, **107**:416–422 (1973).
3. J. E. Pennington, H. Y. Reynolds, and P. P. Carbone, *Pseudomonas* pneu-monia, a retrospective study of 36 cases, *Am. J. Med.*, **55**:155–160 (1973).
4. G. M. Green, The J. Burns Amberson Lecture: In defense of the lung, *Am. Rev. Respir. Dis.*, **102**:691–703 (1970).
5. H. Y. Reynolds and R. E. Thompson, Pulmonary host defenses. I. Analysis of protein and lipids in bronchial secretions and antibody responses follow-ing vaccination with *Pseudomonas aeruginosa, J. Immunol.*, **111**:358–368 (1973).
6. H. Y. Reynolds and R. E. Thompson, Pulmonary host defenses. II. Inter-action of respiratory antibodies with *Pseudomonas aeruginose* and alveolar macrophages, *J. Immunol.*, **111**:369–380 (1973).
7. H. Y. Reynolds, R. E. Thompson, and H. B. Devlin, Development of cel-lullar and humoral immunity in the respiratory tract of rabbits to Pseudo-monas lipopolysaccharide, *J. Clin. Invest.*, **53**:1351–1358 (1974).
8. S. Hanessian, W. Regan, D. Watson, and T. H. Haskell, Isolation and char-acterization of antigenic components of a new heptavalent Pseudomonas vaccine, *Nature, New Biol.*, **229**:209–210 (1971).
9. M. W. Fisher, H. B. Devlin, and F. J. Gnabasik, New immunotype schema for *Pseudomonas aeruginosa* based on protective antigens, *J. Bacteriol.*, **98**:835–836 (1969).
10. J. G. Crowder, M. W. Fisher, and A. White, Type-specific immunity in pseudomonas disease, *J. Lab. Clin. Med.*, **79**:47–54 (1972).
11. K. F. Hubner and N. Gengozian, Depression of the primary immune response by dl–penicillamine, *Proc. Soc. Exp. Biol. Med.*, **118**:561–565 (1965).
12. H. Y. Reynolds and J. S. Johnson, Structural units of canine serum and secretory immunoglobulin A, *Biochemistry* **10**:2821–2827 (1971).
13. A. S. Rosenthal, J. M. Davie, D. L. Rosenstreich, and J. T. Blake, Depletion of antibody–forming cells and their precursors from complex cell popula-tions, *J. Immunol.*, **108**:279–281 (1972).
14. G. A. Falk, A. J. Okinaka, and G. W. Siskind, Immunoglobulins in the bronchial washings of patients with chronic obstructive pulmonary disease, *Am. Rev. Respir. Dis.*, **105**:14–21 (1972).

15. H. Y. Reynolds and H. H. Newball, Analysis of pretein components, lipids, and respiratory cells obtained from human lungs by bronchial lavage, *J. Lab. Clin. Med.,* **84**:559–573 (1974).

16. A. E. Jackson, P. M. Southern, A. K. Pierce, B. D. Fallis, and J. P. Sanford, Pulmonary clearance of gram–negative bacilli, *J. Lab. Clin. Med.,* **69**:833–841 (1967).

17. G. W. Fernald, W. A. Clyde, Jr., and J. Bienenstock, Immunoglobulin–containing cells in lungs of hamsters infected with Mycoplasma pneumoniae, *J. Immunol.,* **108**:1400–1408 (1972).

18. G. Biberfeld, Macrophage migration inhibition in response to experimental *Mycoplasma pheumoniae* infection in the hamsters, *J. Immunol.,* **110**: 1146–1150 (1973).

19. B. Galindo and Q. N. Myrvik, Migratory response of granulomatous alveolar cells from BCG–sensitized rabbits, *J. Immunol.,* **105**:227–237 (1970).

20. G. L. Truitt and G. B. Mackaness, Cell–mediated resistance to aerogenic infection of the lung, *Am. Rev. Respir. Dis.,* **104**:829–843 (1971).

21. E. Seravalli and A. Taranta, Release of macrophage migration inhibitory factor(s) from lymphocytes stimulated by streptococcal preparations, *Cell. Immunol.,* **8**:40–54 (1973).

22. P. F. Salmon, T. T. Tamlyn, and M. H. Grieco, *Escherichia coli* pneumonia. Case report, *Am. Rev. Respir. Dis.,* **102**:248–257 (1970).

23. J. R. Tillotson and A. M. Lerner, Characteristics of pneumonias caused by *Escherichia coli, N. Engl. J. Med.,* **277**:115–122 (1967).

24. S. Solomon, Primary Friedländer pneumonia: Report of 32 cases, *J.A.M.A.,* **108**:937–947 (1937).

25. S. E. Greisman and R. B. Hornick, Cellular inflammatory responses of man to bacterial endotoxin: A comparison with PPD and other bacterial antigens, *J. Immunol.,* **109**:1210–1222 (1972).

26. B. R. Bloom, In vitro approaches to the mechanism of cell–mediated immune reactions, *Adv. Immunol.,* **13**:101–208 (1971).

27. R. VanFurth and F. Aiuti, Immunoglobulin synthesis by tissues of the gastrointestinal and respiratory tracts. *Protides of Biological Fluids, Sixteenth Colloquim.* Edited by H. Peeters. London, Pergamon Press, 1969, pp. 479–484.

28. M. Adinolfi, A. A. Glynn, M. Lindsay, and C. M. Milne, Serological properties of IgA antibodies to *Escherichia coli* present in human colostrum, *Immunology,* **10**:517–526 (1966).

29. M. E. Kaplan, A. P. Dalmasso, and M. Woodson, Complement–dependent opsonization of incompatible erythrocytes by human secretory IgA, *J. Immunol.,* **108**:275–278 (1972).

30. D. S. Eddie, M. L. Schulkind, and J. B. Robbins, The isolation and biologic activities of purified secretory IgA and IgG anti-*Salmonella typhimurium* "O" antibodies from rabbit intestinal fluid and colostrum, *J. Immunol.,* **106**:181–190 (1971).

31. I. D. Wilson, Studies of the opsonic activity of human secretory IgA using an in vitro phagocytosis system, *J. Immunol.,* **108**:726–730 (1972).
32. J. A. Bellanti, M. S. Artenstein, and E. L. Buescher, Characterization of virus neutralizing antibodies in human serum and nasal secretions, *J. Immunol.,* **94**:344–351 (1965).
33. R. Keller and J. E. Dwyer, Neutralization of poliovirus by IgA coproantibodies, *J. Immunol.,* **101**:192–202 (1968).
34. N. F. Pierce and H. Y. Reynolds, Immunity of experimental cholera. II. Secretory and humoral antitoxin response to local and systemic toxoid administration, *J. Infect. Dis.,* **131**:383–389 (1975).
35. R. C. Williams and R. J. Gibbons, Inhibition of bacterial adherence by secretory immunoglobulin A: A mechanism of antigen disposal, *Science,* **177**:697–699 (1972).
36. J. Bienenstock, N. Johnston, and D. Y. E. Perey, Bronchial lymphoid tissue I. Morphologic characteristics, *Lab. Invest.,* **28**:686–692 (1973).
37. C. Nagaishi. In *Functional Anatomy and Histology of the Lung.* Baltimore, Md., University Park Press, 1971, p. 159.

8

The Role of Chemotaxis in the Inflammatory-immune Response of the Lung

JOHN I. GALLIN

National Institute of Allergy and Infectious Diseases
National Institutes of Health
Bethesda, Maryland

I. Introduction

Mobilization of leukocytes to the lung is central to normal pulmonary defenses against infections, tumors, or environmental factors, such as silica, coal, or asbestos. The pathologic manifestations of certain autoimmune, allergic and vasculitic disorders are also probably related in part to abnormal recruitment of leukocytes and release of their proteolytic enzymes. The process of directed leukocyte movement is known as chemotaxis, and agents which specifically attract leukocytes are chemotactic factors. The purpose of the present review is to define the known parameters of leukocyte chemotaxis and to describe how these parameters may interact to initiate and amplify the inflammatory-immune responses of the lung.

II. Methods

Although the ameboid movement of leukocytes has fascinated investigators for many years, it was not until 1962, when Boyden reported an in vitro technique for measuring chemotaxis by use of a micropore filter [1], that widespread studies of human leukotaxis were possible. A number of variations of the technique have evolved, but the principle remains unchanged. Leukocytes are placed in an upper compartment of a chamber, which is separated from a lower compartment by a micropore filter. A chemotactic stimulus is placed in the lower compartment and after incubation, the cells migrate through the filter towards the gradient of chemotactic factor. The number of cells reaching the bottom surface of the filter is used as a measure of chemotaxis. Using this chamber, it has been possible to evaluate the effects of numerous agents on leukocyte movement and the ability of different chemotactic factors to attract cells. Granulocyte, monocyte, lymphocyte, eosinophil, and pulmonary macrophage-migration have been studied with the technique. Despite the advantages, the classic Boyden method requires laborious filter-staining and microscopic counting (with observer subjectivity) and considerable variability. Recently, an improved radioassay of granulocyte chemotaxis employing chromium-51 labeled cells and a double micropore filter system has been developed [2,3]. Cells labeled with chromium-51 migrate through the upper and into the lower filter; chemotaxis is expressed as counts per minute (cpm) incorporated into the lower filter. This improved radioassay provides a rapid and objective assessment of chemotaxis.

An in vivo measure of leukocyte chemotaxis, using a Rebuck skin-window technique, is also available [4]. In this method, an abrasion is made in the skin, a glass slide is placed over the abrasion, and a qualitative measure of leukocytic infiltration is possible. In general there is good correlation between in vitro and in vivo techniques. The in vitro Boyden technique is more practical for rapid assessment of leukocyte function in large numbers of patients and for experiments designed to dissect the various components of the chemotactic response.

Using the above techniques, a number of patients have been described with disorders of chemotaxis [5-12], chemotactic factor generation [13-18], or containing serum inhibitors of chemotaxis [19-21]. Application of these methods to direct studies of pulmonary macrophages has been limited, largely because it is difficult to obtain adequate numbers of pulmonary cells from humans. However, as will be discussed, the clinical importance of chemotaxis to pulmonary defenses has been established through studies of patients with life-threatening pulmonary pathology and defective chemotaxis as their major host-defense defect.

III. Chemotactic Factors—Fluid Phase Components

Chemotactic factors have been isolated from plasma or serum through activation of fluid-phase components consisting of the complement [22-25], fibrinolytic [26], and kinin [27] generating systems as well as from leukocyte products

[28-34]. The following sections will review the mechanisms of formation of these chemotactic factors and their interrelationships in the inflammatory-immune response.

A. Complement Pathway

The complement system constitutes part of normal serum and is the best-studied of the chemotactic pathways contributing to the inflammatory response. The "classic" system consists of nine components or 11 proteins, which have been isolated, identified, and characterized functionally [24,35-37]. The nine components are designated C1, C2, C3, C4, C5, C6, C7, C8, and C9. C1, a macromolecular complex, consists of three serum proteins, C1q, C1r, and C1s, held together by calcium [37]. As shown in Figure 1, two major pathways of complement activation have been delineated. The classic pathway is activated by antigen-antibody complexes, which results in the conversion of C1 to activated $\overline{C1}$ [35]. Activated $\overline{C1}$ then catalytically assembles C3 convertase through its action of C4 and C2. The terminal complement components are then activated by C3 convertase. An "alternate" pathway can also be activated by antigen–antibody complexes or by endotoxin lipopolysaccharide [38-44]. In the alternate pathway, terminal complement components are activated by conversion of C3 proactivator to C3 activator, without a requirement for antibody or C1, C4, or C2 [38]. Recently, properdin [37], properdin convertase (the enzyme that activates properdin [45], a cleavage product of the thrid component of complement (C3b, [46]) and the enzyme that converts C3 proactivator to C3 activator (C3 proactivator convertase [47]) have been shown to be requirements for activation of the alternate complement pathway (Fig. 1), however, the precise mechanism of their interaction is not known. Products of C1 activation may also accelerate the alternate pathway and thereby further amplify the inflammatory response [48].

The major neutrophil chemotactic factor resulting from in vitro complement activation is a heat-stable small molecular weight (15,500) cleavage product of the fifth component of complement, designated C5a [49-51]. Small amounts of a cleavage product of the third component of complement (C3a), with a molecular weight of 6000, and a trimolecular complex of the fifth, sixth, and seventh compartments of complement ($\overline{C567}$) have also been reported [24,52]. The C3 fragment [53] and C5a [54] are also chemotactic for mononuclear cells. Chemotactic activity is more rapidly generated by the classic than by the alternate complement pathways in vitro, although there is no difference in the relative amount of activity resulting from activation of either pathway [3,55]. Moreover, either pathway appears to function independently, with quantitatively normal generation of chemotactic factors resulting despite complete absence or inhibition of the other complement pathway [3,55]. In addition to their chemotactic activity, C3a and

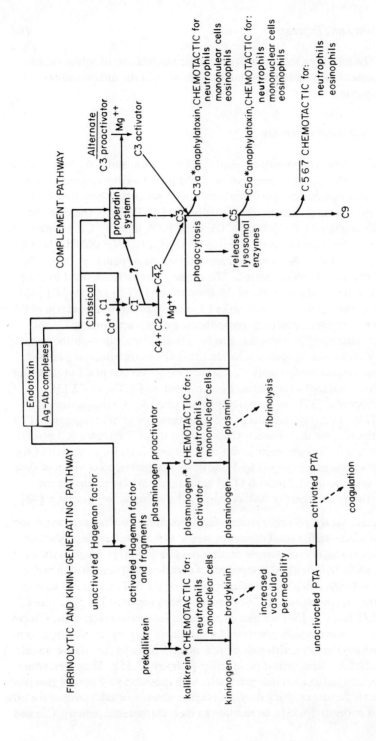

FIGURE 1 Schematic diagram of the generation of chemotactic factors by activation of fibrinolytic, kinin–generating, and complement pathways.

C5a have anaphylatoxic activity [46]; thus the biologic action of these molecules includes increased vascular permeability, which facilitates leukocyte emigration from the circulation.

An important regulatory mechanism of complement-associated chemotactic factor activity is through a C3a and C5a inactivator, which cleaves the C-terminal arginine from the C3a and C5a fragments [56]. Recently, Ward and Berenberg [21] demonstrated elevated levels of a chemotactic factor inactivator in Hodgkin's disease. It was postulated that the depressed delayed hypersensitivity associated with Hodgkin's disease was related, at least in part, to inadequate mobilization of leukocytes as a consequence of nonspecific inactivation of complement-derived, complement-independent, and lymphocyte-derived chemotactic factors by the excess chemotactic-factor inactivator [21]. The role of the chemotactic factor inactivator in pathologic states is currently under investigation in a number of laboratories.

B. Fibrinolytic and Kinin-generating Systems

In addition to complement activation, exposure of serum or plasma to endotoxins or contact with negatively charged surfaces, such as collagen, converts unactivated Hageman factor to activated Hageman factor and Hageman factor fragments. As shown in Figure 1, activated Hageman factor can initiate three different pathways: coagulation, fibrinolysis, and kinin-generation. The catalytic action of activated Hageman factor or Hageman factor fragments converts plasminogen proactivator to plasminogen activator, which then converts plasminogen to the fibrinolytic enzyme plasmin [57]. The active enzyme plasminogen-activator, is chemotactic for granulocytes [26], and we have recently found it to be chemotactic for mononuclear cells [58]. Activated Hageman factor, or Hageman factor fragments, also converts prekallikrein to kallikrein [59,60], the enzyme that digests kininogen to yield bradykinin (Fig. 1). The active enzyme kallikrein is also chemotactic for neutrophils [27] and for mononuclear cells [58]. Bradykinin increases vascular permeability and the increased vascular permeability caused by bradykinin may also localize these serum factors and leukocytes to sites of tissue injury.

In addition to the chemotactic activity of highly purified serum components of the fibrinolytic and kinin-generating systems, kaolin activation of serum yielded chemotactic activity, which could be distinguished from the complement-derived chemotactic factors [16]. Moreover, human plasma deficient in prekallikrein (Fletcher factor deficiency), which has a diminished rate of Hageman factor-activation and is incapable of generating kallikrein, possesses diminished chemotactic activity after kaolin activation, unless the absent substrate is added back to the plasma [16].

In vitro studies of the fibrinolytic enzyme, plasmin, have shown that it can activate the first component of complement [61] and cleave a chemotactic fragment off C3 [62]. This provides a tempting interrelation between the complement and fibrinolytic systems, however, the physiologic relevance of this to the in vivo situation has not been established.

IV. Cellular Derived Chemotactic Stimuli

In addition to fluid phase (plasma or serum)-derived chrmotactic factors, granulocytic and monocytic cellular products are apparently secreted as a result of exposure to chemotactic stimuli [63], phagocytosis [28,30,31,64], or antigen processing [33,34,54,65] to further amplify the inflammatory-immune response by either (a) being themselves chemotactic, (b) generating chemotactic activity from fluid-phase components, or (c) immobilizing leukocytes and preventing emigration away from inflammatory sites. The interrelating cell-derived factors amplifying inflammatory--immune responses are schematically summarized in Figure 2.

A. Granulocyte Products

Chemotactic Molecules

Granulocyte homogenates have been shown to contain a nondialyzable, heat-stable molecule chemotactic for granulocytes [29-31]. This cell-derived chemotactic factor may be released as a product of phagocytosis [29-31] and does not depend on serum factors for such release [31].

Exposure of leukocytes to endotoxin also results in the release of plasminogen activator [66]; however, the leukocyte-derived plasminogen activator has not yet been studied for chemotactic activity. In addition, a chemotactic factor specific for mononuclear cells has been isolated from rabbit neutrophils [32]. It has been proposed that this factor may account for monocyte infiltration of pneumonic inflammatory lesions following neutrophil invasion [32].

Other neutrophil products (proteases, or lysosomal enzymes, or both) are known to be released during phagocytosis [67,68]. One of these products is capable of directly cleaving C5 to C5a in vitro [69]. Ward and Zvaifler [64] recently showed that the enzyme responsible for this is also released from rabbit neutrophils following phagocytosis of rheumatoid factor. Dr Daniel Wright and I [70] have found that human neutrophils, phagocytizing latex particles, release a molecule capable of generating chemotactic activity from whole serum. On the

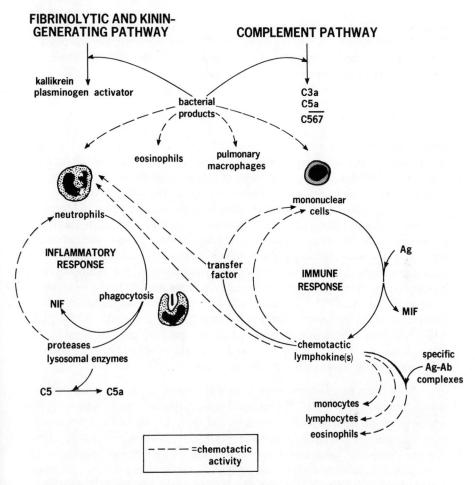

FIGURE 2 Schematic representation of the role of chemotaxis in the inter-relationships of inflammatory and immune responses.

basis of G–75 sephadex chromatography, at least part of the chemotactic activity generated in whole serum exposed to postphagocytic supernatants is the complement product C5a. Application of postphagocytic supernatants to human skin abrasions resulted in vivo acceleration of the inflammatory response (Wright and Gallin, unpublished observations).

In addition to releasing chemotactic factors or factors capable of activating other systems as a consequence of phagocytosis, granulocytes exposed to C5a release lysosomal enzymes [63,71] which may be important in the generation of chemotactic factors or may themselves be chemotactic. A neutrophil–immobilizing factor (NIF) has been isolated from neutrophils and mononuclear cells [72,73]. NIF inhibits chemotaxis and passive motility of neutrophils and eosinophils but not mononuclear cells [73]. It was postulated that NIF may be important in concentrating neutrophils at inflammatory sites [73].

B. Mononuclear Cell Products

Whereas the neutrophil is central to the inflammatory response, the mononuclear cell is central to the immune response. During antigen processing and the expression of cell-mediated immunity a number of immunologically specific and nonspecific processes occur that are analogous to events in the inflammatory response and serve to amplify the inflammatory-immune responses. As shown in Figure 2, exposure of human mononuclear cells (lymphocytes and monocytes) to specific antigen results in the release of chemotactic lymphokines. These lymphokines are nondialyzable (molecular weight about 40,000) heat-stable molecules chemotactic for mononuclear cells, neutrophils, and lymphocytes [65]. Treatment of lymphokines with antigen-specific immune complexes also yields an eosinophil chemotactic factor [74,75]. In addition, a distinct molecule, migration inhibitory factor (MIF), is released from lymphocytes on stimulation with antigen [72]. MIF inhibits the migration of pulmonary macrophages [76] and peripheral blood macrophages out of the capillary tubes and is thought to be important for localizing mononuclear cells at inflammatory-immune sites.

Stimulation of leukocytes with antigen also results in the release of antigen-specific transfer factor [77]. This material is dialyzable and can thereby be readily separated from larger contaminants and appears to be a critical mediator of antigen-specific delayed hypersensitivity [78]. It is receiving increasing attention as a therapeutic agent useful in reconstituting certain immune-deficiency states [79]. We recently showed that transfer factor contains a unique antigen-independent chemotactic factor with a molecular weight <5000 [34]. The chemotactic activity in transfer factor has potent in vivo and in vitro activity for granulocytes and somewhat less activity for mononuclear cells. This immunologically nonspecific biologic activity of transfer factor may play a critical role in the local cell recruitment necessary for adequately processing and amplifying the immunologically specific transfer-factor message [34] and, thereby, amplify subclinical inflammatory-immune responses. In this regard, the chemotactic activity in transfer factor could contribute to the phenomenon of "local" transfer of delayed allergy with transfer factor in patients with sarcoidosis [34].

Pulmonary macrophages are only weakly chemotactic [32], yet they respond to MIF [76]. Pulmonary macrophages are also capable of phagocytosis [80], although high oxygen tensions [80] are required for optimal phagocytosis. Studies of human pulmonary macrophages have been limited by difficulty in obtaining adequate numbers of cells.

V. Eosinophil Chemotaxis

The eosinophil is another chemotactically responsive leukocyte without major phagocytic or killing properties whose role in inflammation is not clear. However, a brief discussion is pertinent, since the eosinophil probably plays an important role in a number of parasitic and allergic inflammatory responses.

An eosinophil chemotactic-factor of anaphylaxis (ECF-A) has recently been recognized to exist preformed in human mast cells [81] and is released from human lung tissue sensitized with IgE antibody when challenged with antigen [82]. ECF-A has an estimated molecular weight of from 500 to 1000 and, although chemotactic for all leukocytes, preferentially attracts eosinophils from a mixed-leukocyte population [83]. C3a, C5a, and C$\overline{567}$ are also chemotactic for eosinophils [53,83]. Moreover, mixtures of C5a and ECF-A have been reported to synergistically increase the specificity of eosinophil chemoattraction [84]. A lymphokine has been demonstrated which, upon interaction with immune complexes, is preferentially chemotactic for eosinophils [75]. Recently, Clark, Gallin, and Kaplan have demonstrated that in low concentrations (10^{-6}-$10^{-8}\mu$), histamine *selectively* attracts eosinophils from mixed leukocyte populations (submitted for publication).

VI. Chemotactic Activity of
Products of Bacterial Growth
and Virus-Infected Tissues

The appearance of phagocytic and immunologically important leukocytes at the site of infectious lesions may be stimulated directly by products of bacterial growth, which are chemotactic for neutrophils [85-87], mononuclear cells [87], eosinophils [88], and alveolar macrophages [65]. They are relatively heat stable, have a molecular weight of less than 3600, and do not appear to be associated with structural components of the bacterial cell [87].

Not only are bacterial products chemotactic, but it has been postulated that leukotactic factors, elaborated as a result of virus infection of cells, may also play a protective role in vivo [89]. Infection of chick embryos with Newcastle disease virus or mumps virus and infection of monkey (BGM)-cell culture with mumps virus resulted in the elaboration of chemotactic activity for rabbit neutrophils and peripheral blood macrophages; no chemotactic activity was found in lysates of uninfected cells. Virus-infected cells also released material which was not itself chemotactic but could interact with human C3 or C5 to generate such activity [89]. In addition, leukocytes obtained from volunteers infected with *Mycoplasma pneumoniae* were shown to have acquired chemotactic activity to

mycoplasma [90]. Thus, direct products of bacterial, viral, or mycoplasma
infection can mobilize leukocytes to amplify the inflammatory–immune response.

VII. Mechanism of the Leukocyte Response to Chemotactic Factors

Although considerable knowledge has accumulated in recent years on the nature
of chemotactic factors, little is known about the mechanism by which leukocyte–
chemotactic factor interraction initiates the chemotactic process. It has been
demonstrated by Becker and Showell [91] that calcium and magnesium are required for optimal rabbit–neutrophil chemotaxis. Recently, we demonstrated
that optimal human neutrophil chemotaxis is also dependent on optimal calcium
and magnesium, with marked depression of chemotaxis resulting with excessive
or depressed divalent cation concentrations [92]. It has not yet been determined
if such ion dependency is clinically important in endocrine disorders of calcium
metabolism associated with increased infections, such as hypoparathyroidism
[93]. In addition to divalent cation requirements for optimal chemotaxis, an
association between calcium efflux and microtubule assembly on exposure of
neutrophils to chemotactic factors has recently been made [92,94]. Possibly
microtubule assembly results, at least in part, from lowered cytoplasm calcium
[94]. This microtubule assembly may be critical for imparting the net vector to
directed (chemotactic) motion [94]. Other factors, including cyclic AMP, ATP,
GTP, and cyclic GMP, which apparently influence both microtubule assembly
[95-97] and chemotaxis [98] are probably important. Furthermore, although
leukocyte chemotactic receptors have not yet been demonstrated, Becker and
Ward [99-101] have shown that membrane-associated serine esterases are essential for a normal chemotactic response. Moreover, neutrophils and mononuclear
cells apparently possess esterases with different chemical properties [32]. Ultimate illucidation of the biochemical–biophysical events associated with the
chemotactic process are necessary prior to a rational basis for therapeutic manipulation of leukocyte disorders.

VIII. Clinical Disorders of Chemotaxis and Their Association with Pulmonary Pathology

Patients with defects of either granulocyte [10] or mononuclear cell [102]
chemotaxis, or both [94], with recurrent pneumonia as a major clinical problem,
have been documented. Abnormal leukocyte locomotion has also been noted in
diabetes mellitus [5], Chediak-Higashi syndrome [6,103], rheumatoid arthritis
[7], agammaglobulinemia [8,94], the lazy leukocyte syndrome (abnormal

neutrophil spontaneous motility and neutrophil chemotaxis) [9], and in patients with pneumonia and recurrent *Trichophyton rubrum* infection [11]. Alcohol [104] and corticosteroid therapy [105], two agents associated with an increased incidence of pneumonia, also suppress in vivo leukocyte migration. Alveolar macrophage function has not yet been evaluated in the above clinical settings.

Inhibitors of the function of chemotactic factor have been described in cirrhosis [19], lupus erythematosus [16], and uremia [20]; it has not been determined if such inhibition reflects increased levels of normal inhibitors or the presence of circulating abnormal proteins. Diminished generation of chemotactic factors has been documented in deficiencies of the r fragment of the first [94], (C1r [106]) second [13,55], third [15], and fifth [24] components of compelment and in prekallikrein deficiency [17]. The relevance of these abnormalities to pulmonary pathophysiology has not yet been established.

IX. Conclusions and Speculations

Most studies of granulocyte chemotaxis have evolved since the advent of the in vitro Boyden chamber assay in 1962 [1]. Initial experiments characterizing the complement-related chemotactic factors suggested leukocyte chemotaxis was a phenomenon primarily related to the inflammatory response. However, the demonstration that products of the immune response, such as lymphokines and transfer factor, contain chemotactic factor activity provides evidence that the inflammatory response serves an important amplification role to the immune response [34].

With the demonstration of deposits of immune-complex and complement proteins in walls of blood vessels in experimental immunologic vasculitis [107] and the isolation, in peripheral tissues, of $\overline{C567}$ and C5a, after interaction of antigens, antibody, and complement [107], it is almost certain products of the complement system, reviewed in this chapter, are important in local inflammatory-immune processes in the lung. Although kallikrein- and plasminogen-activator are probably important amplifiers of local tissue inflammatory lesions, their precise role in pulmonary defenses has not been established. The pulmonary (alveolar) macrophage is actively phagocytic, has many immunologic properties similar to those of peripheral blood monocytes, but responds weakly to chemotactic stimuli [53]. Moreover, it is well-known that pulmonary inflammatory lesions are acutely invaded by neutrophils, followed later by mononuclear cells. Allergic reactions are characterized by eosinophil infiltration. Although chemotaxis is critical for such leukocyte mobilization, many questions remain unanswered. Does the phagocytizing pulmonary macrophage release chemotactic factors, neutrophil- or macrophage-immobilizing factors, or activate chemotactic-factor generating systems? Do pulmonary macrophages undergo chemotaxis under conditions of high oxygen-tension, as required for optimal pulmonary alveolar-macrophage phagocytosis? What role do bacteria or other noxious stimuli directly have in triggering the inflammatory-immune response in the lung? The fiberoptic bronchoscope and the availability of sophisticated chemotactic techniques should enable experiments designed to answer these questions of the mechanisms involved in the pulmonary inflammatory-immune response.

References

1. S. Boyden, The chemotactic effect of mixtures of antibody and antigen on polymorphonuclear leukocytes, *J. Exp. Med.,* **115**:463–466 (1962).
2. J. I. Gallin, R. A. Clark, and H. R. Kimball, Granulocyte chemotaxis: An improved in vitro assay employing ^{51}Cr-labeled granulocytes, *J. Immunol.,* **110**:233–240 (1973).
3. J. I. Gallin, Radioassay of granulocyte chemotaxis: Studies of human granulocytes and chemotactic factors. In *Chemotaxis, its Biology and Biochemistry.* Edited by E. Sorkin. Switzerland, Karger, Basel, 1974, pp. 146–160.
4. J. W. Rebuck and J. H. Crowley, A method for studying leukocyte functions in vivo, *Ann. N.Y. Adad. Sci.,* **59**:757–805 (1955).
5 A. J. Mowatt and J. Baum, Chemotaxis of polymorphonuclear leukocytes from patients with diabetes mellitus, *N. Engl. J. Med.,* **284**:621–627 (1971).
6. R. A. Clark and H. R. Kimball, Defective granulocyte chemotaxis in the Chediak–Higashi Syndrome, *J. Clin. Invest.,* **50**:2645–2652 (1971).
7. A. J. Mowatt and J. Baum, Chemotaxis of polymorphonuclear leukocytes from patients with rheumatoid arthritis, *J. Clin. Invest.,* **50**:2541–2549 (1971).
8. R. L. Steerman, R. Snyderman, S. L. Leikin, and H. R. Collen, Intrinsic defect of the polymorphonuclear leukocyte resulting in impaired chemotaxis and phagocytosis, *Clin. Exp. Immunol.,* **9**:839–852 (1971).
9. M. E. Miller, F. A. Oski, and H. B. Harris, Lazy leukocyte syndrome, *Lancet,* **1**:665–669 (1971).
10. R. A. Clark, R. K. Root, H. R. Kimball, and C. H. Kirkpatrick, Defective neutrophil chemotaxis and cellular immunity in a child with recurrent infections, *Ann. Intern. Med.,* **78**:515–519 (1973).
11. M. E. Miller, M. E. Norman, P. J. Koblenzer, and T. Schonauer, A new familial defect of neutrophil movement, *J. Lab. Clin. Med.,* **82**:1–8 (1973).
12. J. Baum, Chemotaxis in human disease. In *The Phagocytic Cell in Host Resistance.* New York, Raven Press, in press.
13. A. R. Page, H. Gewurz, R. J. Pickering, and R. A. Good, The role of complement in the acute inflammatory response, *Immunopathology,* **5**:221–228 (1967).

14. H. L. Keller and E. Sorkin, Chemotaxis of leukocytes, *Experientia,* 24: 641–652 (1968).

15. C. A. Alper, N. Abramson, R. B. Johnston, J. H. Jandl, and F. S. Rosen, Increased susceptibility to infection associated with abnormalities of complement mediated functions and of the thrid component of complement (C3), *N. Engl. J. Med.,* 282:349–358 (1970).

16. R. A. Clark, H. R. Kimball, and J. L. Decker, Neutrophil chemotaxis in systemic lupus erythematosis, *Ann. Rheum. Dis.,* 33:167–172 (1974).

17. A. P. Weiss, J. I. Gallin, and A. P. Kaplan, Fletcher factor deficiency: A diminished rate of Hageman factor activation caused by absence of prekallikrein with abnormalities of coagulation, fibrinolysis, chemotactic activity, and kinin generation, *J. Clin. Invest.,* 53:622–633 (1974).

18. M. E. Norman and M. E. Miller, Spontaneous chemotaxis in patients with glomerulonephritis and the nephrotic syndrome, *J. Pediatr.,* 83:390–398 (1973).

19. A. N. DeMeo and B. R. Andersen, Defective chemotaxis associated with a serum inhibitor in cirrhotic patients, *N. Engl. J. Med.,* 286:735–740 (1972).

20. G. Eknoyan, S. Hyde, C. Saenz, and R. Martin, Leukotaxis in renal failure: Demonstration of a dialyzable serum factor, *Am. Soc. Nephrol.,* 33 (abstr.).

21. P. A. Ward and J. A. Berenberg, Defective regulation of inflammatory mediators in Hodgkin's disease, *N. Engl. J. Med.,* 290:76–80 (1974).

22. R. Snyderman, H. Gewurz, and S. E. Mergenhagen, Interactions of the complement system with endotoxin lipopolysaccharide, *J. Exp. Med.,* 128: 259–275 (1968).

23. H. Gewurz, H. S. Shin, and S. E. Mergenhagen, Interactions of the complement system with endotoxin lipopolysaccharide: Consumption of each of the six terminal complement components, *J. Exp. Med.,* 128:1049–1057 (1968).

24. P. A. Ward, C. G. Cochrane, and H. J. Müller–Eberhard, The role of serum complement in chemotaxis of leukocytes in vitro, *J. Exp. Med.,* 122: 327–346 (1965).

25. V. J. Stecher and E. Sorkin, Studies on chemotaxis XII. Generation of chemotactic activity for polymorphonuclear leukocytes in sera with complement deficiencies, *Immunology,* 16:231–239 (1969).

26. A. P. Kaplan, E. J. Goetzl, and K. F. Austen, The fibrinolytic pathway of human plasma: II. The generation of chemotactic activity by activation of plasminogen proactivator, *J. Clin. Invest.,* 52:2591–2595 (1973).

27. A. P. Kaplan, A. B. Kay, and K. F. Austen, A prealbumin activator of prekallikrein. III. Appearance of chemotactic activity for human neutrophils by the conversion of human prekallikrein to kallikrein, *J. Exp. Med.,* 135: 81–97 (1972).

28. P. Phelps, Polymorphonuclear leukocyte motility in vitro. III. Possible release of a chemotactic substance after phagocytosis of urate crystals by polymorphonuclear leukocytes, *Arthritis Rheum.,* 12:197–204 (1969).

29.　J. F. Borel, H. U. Keller, and E. Sorkin, Studies on chemotaxis. XI. Effects on neutrophils of lysosomal and other subcellular fractions from leukocytes, *Int. Arch. Allergy Appl. Immunol.,* **35**:194–205 (1964).

30.　J. F. Borel, Studies on chemotaxis: Effect of subcellular leukocyte fractions on neutrophils and macrophages, *Int. Arch. Allergy Appl. Immunol.,* **39**:247–271 (1970).

31.　S. H. Zigmond and J. G. Hirsch, Leukocyte locomotion and chemotaxis: New methods for evaluation and demonstration of a cell–derived chemotactic factor, *J. Exp. Med.,* **137**:387–410 (1973).

32.　P. A. Ward, Chemotaxis of mononuclear cells, *J. Exp. Med.,* **128**:1201–1221 (1968).

33.　P. A. Ward, H. G. Remold, and J. R. David, The production by antigen-stimulated lymphocytes of a leukotactic factor distinct from migration inhibitory factor, *Cell. Immunol.,* **1**:162–174 (1970).

34.　J. I. Gallin and C. H. Kirkpatrick, Chemotactic activity in dialyzable transfer factor, *Proc. Natl. Acad. Sci. USA,* **71**:498–502 (1974).

35.　H. J. Müller–Eberhard, U. Hadding, and C. A. Calcott, Current problems in complement research, *Immunopathology,* **5**:179–188 (1967).

36.　J. F. Borel and E. Sorkin, Differences between plasma and serum mediated chemotaxis of leukocytes, *Experientia,* **25**:1333–1335 (1969).

37.　S. Ruddy, I. Gigli, and K. F. Austen, The complement system of man, *N. Engl. J. Med.,* **287**:489–495, 545–549, 592–596, 642–646 (1972).

38.　O. Götze and H. J. Müller–Eberhard, The C3–activator system: An alternate pathway of complement activation, *J. Exp. Med.,* **134**:90s–108s (1971).

39.　M. M. Phillips, R. Snyderman, and S. E. Mergenhagen, Activation of complement by endotoxin: A role for $\gamma 2$ globulins, C1, C4, and C2 in the consumption of terminal components by endotoxin–coated erythrocytes, *J. Immunol.,* **109**:334–341 (1972).

40.　J. J. Frank, J. May, T. Gaither, and L. Ellman, In vitro studies of complement function in sera of C4 deficient guinea pigs, *J. Exp. Med.,* **134**:176–189 (1971).

41.　J. E. May and M. M. Frank, Complement–mediated tissue damage: Contribution of the classical and alternate complement pathways in the Forssman reaction, *J. Immunol.,* **108**:1517–1525 (1972).

42.　A. L. Sandberg, R. Snyderman, M. M. Frank, and A. G. Osler, Production of chemotactic activity by guinea pig immunoglobulins following activation of the C3 complement shunt pathway, *J. Immunol.,* **108**:1227–1231 (1972).

43.　J. E. May, M. A. Kane, and M. M. Frank, Host defense against bacterial endotoxin-contribution of the early and late components of complement to detoxification, *J. Immunol.,* **109**:893–895 (1972).

44.　J. E. May, M. A. Kane, and M. M. Frank, Immune adherence by the alternate pathway, *Proc. Soc. Exp. Biol. Med.,* **141**:287–290 (1972).

45.　A. E. Stitzel and R. E. Spitzer, The utilization of properdin in the alternate pathway of complement activation: Isolation of properdin convertase, *J. Immunol.,* **112**:56–62 (1974).

46. C. G. Cochrane and H. J. Müller–Eberhard, The derivation of two distinct anaphylatoxin activities from the third and fifth components of human complement, *J. Exp. Med.*, **127**:371–386 (1968).

47. L. G. Humsicker, S. Ruddy, and K. F. Austen, Additional factors required for cobra venon induced activation of C3, *Fed. Proc.*, **31**:788 (1972) (abstr.).

48. J. E. May and M. M. Frank, A new complement–mediated cytolytic mechanism–the C1–bypass activation pathway, *Proc. Natl. Acad. Sci. USA*, **70**: 649–652 (1973).

49. R. Snyderman and S. E. Mergenhagen, Characterization of polymorphonuclear leukocyte chemotactic activity in serum activated by various inflammatory agents. In *Fifth International Symposium of the Canadian Society of Immunology.* Vol. 117. Edited by D. G. Ingramm. Karger, Basel, 1972.

50. R. Snyderman, H. S. Shin, J. K. Phillips, H. Gewurz, and S. E. Mergenhagen, A neutrophil chemotactic factor derived from C′5 upon interaction of guinea pig serum with endotoxin, *J. Immunol.*, **103**:413–422 (1969).

51. R. Snyderman, H. S. Shin, J. K. Phillips, H. Gewurz, and S. E. Mergenhagen, A polymorphonuclear leukocyte chemotactic activity in rabbit serum and guinea pig serum treated with immune complexes. Evidence for C5a as the major chemotactic factor, *Infect. Immun.*, **1**:521–525 (1969).

52. P. A. Ward, Chemotaxis of polymorphonuclear leukocytes, *Biochem. Pharmacol.*, **17**:99–105 (1968).

53. P. A. Ward, Chemotactic factors for neutrophils, eosinophils, mononuclear cells, and lymphocytes. In *Biochemistry of the Acute Allergic Reactions. Second International Symposium.* Edited by K. F. Austen and E. L. Becker. Oxford, 1971, pp. 229–242.

54. R. Snyderman, L. C. Altman, M. S. Hausman, and S. E. Mergenhagen, Human mononuclear leukocyte chemotaxis: A quantitative assay for humoral and cellular factors, *J. Immunol.*, **108**:887–860 (1973).

55. J. I. Gallin, R. A. Clark, and M. M. Frank, Human chemotactic factors generated by activation of the classical and alternate pathways, *Clin. Res.*, **21**:579 (1973) (abstr.).

56. V. A. Bokisch and H. J. Müller–Eberhard, Anaphylatoxin inactivator of human plasma: Its isolation and characterization as a carboxypeptidase, *J. Clin. Invest.*, **49**:2427–2436 (1970).

57. A. P. Kaplan and K. F. Austen, The fibrinolytic pathway of human plasma: Isolation and characterization of the plasminogen proactivator, *J. Exp. Med.*, **136**:1378–1393 (1972).

58. J. I. Gallin and A. P. Kaplan, Mononuclear cell chemotactic activity of kallikrein and plasminogen activator, *Fed. Proc.*, **33**:2383 (1974) (abstr.).

59. A. P. Kaplan and K. F. Austen, A prealbumin activator of prekallikrein, *J. Immunol.*, **105**:802–811 (1970).

60. A. P. Kaplan and K. F. Austen, A prealbumin activator of prekallikrein. II. Derivation of activators of prekallikrein from active Hageman factor by digestion with plasmin, *J. Exp. Med.*, **133**:696–712 (1970).

61. O. D. Ratnoff and G. B. Naff, The conversion of C'1s to C'1 esterase by plasmin and typsin, *J. Exp. Med.*, **125**:337–358 (1967).

62. P. A. Ward, A plasmin split product of C'3 as a new chemotactic factor, *J. Exp. Med.*, **126**:189–206 (1967).

63. I. M. Goldstein, M. Frai, A. G. Osler, and G. Weissman, Lysosomal enzyme release from human leukocytes: Mediation by the alternate pathway of complement activation, *J. Immunol.*, **111**:33–37 (1973).

64. P. A. Ward and N. J. Zvaifler, Quantitative phagocytosis by neutrophils. II. Release of the C5–cleaving enzyme and inhibition of phagocytosis by rheumatoid factor, *J. Immunol.*, **111**:1777–1782 (1973).

65. P. A. Ward, C. D. Offen, and J. R. Montgovery, Chemoattractants of leukocytes, with special reference to lymphocytes, *Fed. Proc.*, **30**:1721–1724 (1971).

66. I. M. Goldstein, B. Wünschmann, T. Astrap, and E. S. Henderson, Effects of bacterial endotoxin on the fibrinolytic activity of normal human leukocytes, *Blood*, **37**:447–453 (1971).

67. G. Weisman, R. B. Zurier, P. J. Spieler, and I. M. Goldstein, Mechanisms of lysosomal enzyme release from leukocytes exposed to immune complexes and other particles, *J. Exp. Med.*, **134**:149s–165s (1971).

68. D. G. Wright and S. E. Malawista, The mobilization and extracellular release of granular enzymes from human leukocytes during phagocytosis, *J. Cell. Biol.*, **53**:788–797 (1972).

69. P. A. Ward and J. H. Hill, C5 chemotactic fragments produced by an enzyme in lysosomal granules of neutrophils, *J. Immunol.*, **104**:535–543 (1970).

70. D. G. Wright and J. I. Gallin, Generation of chemotactic activity from human polymorphonuclear leukocytes during phagocytosis, *Fed. Proc.*, **33**:2382 (1974).

71. I. Goldstein, S. Hoffstein, J. Gallin, and G. Weissman, Mechanisms of lysosomal enzyme release from human leukocytes: Microtubule assembly and membrane fusion induced by a component of complement, *Proc. Natl. Acad. Sci. USA*, **70**:2916–2920 (1973).

72. E. J. Goetzl and K. F. Austen, A neutrophil–immobilizing factor derived from human leukocytes, Generation and partial characterization, *J. Exp. Med.*, **136**:1564–1580 (1972).

73. E. J. Goetzl, I. Gigli, S. Wasserman, and K. F. Austen, A neutrophil immobilizing factor derived from human leukocytes. II. Specificity of action on polymorphonuclear leukocyte mobility, *J. Immunol.*, **111**:938–945 (1973).

74. M. Torisu, T. Yoshida, P. A. Ward, and S. Cohen, Lymphocyte–derived eosinophil chemotactic factor. II. Studies on the mechanism of activation of the precursor substance by immune complexes, *J. Immunol.*, **111**:1450–1458 (1973).

75. J. R. David, Lymphocyte mediators and cellular hypersensitivity, *N. Engl. J. Med.*, **288**:143–149 (1973).

76. G. A. Warr and R. R. Martin, Response of human pulmonary macrophage to migration inhibition factor, *Am. Rev. Respir. Dis.*, **108**:371–373 (1973).

77. H. S. Lawrence and A. M. Pappenheimer, Transfer of delayed hypersensitivity to diphtheria toxin in man, *J. Exp. Med.*, **104**:321–335 (1956).

78. H. S. Lawrence, Transfer factor, *Adv. Immunol.*, **11**:195–266 (1969).

79. C. H. Kirkpatrick and J. I. Gallin, Treatment of infectious and neoplastic diseases with transfer factor, *Oncology*, **29**:46–73 (1974).

80. A. B. Cohen and M. J. Cline, The human alveolar macrophage: Isolation, cultivation in vitro, and studies of morphologic and functional characteristics, *J. Clin. Invest.*, **50**:1390–1398 (1971).

81. S. I. Wasserman, E. J. Goetzl, and K. F. Austen, Preformed eosinophil chemotactic factor of anaphylaxis, *J. Immunol.*, **112**:351–358 (1974).

82. A. B. Kay and K. F. Austen, The IgE midiated release of an eosinophil leukocyte chemotactic factor from human lung, *J. Immunol.*, **107**:899–902 (1971).

83. A. B. Kay, D. J. Stechschulte, and K. F. Austen, An eosinophil leukocyte chemotactic factor of anaphylaxis, *J. Exp. Med.*, **133**:602–619 (1971).

84. A. B. Kay, H. S. Shin, and K. F. Austen, Selective attraction of eosinophils and synergism between eosinophil chemotactic factor of anaphylaxis (ECF-A) and a fragment cleaved from the fifth component of complement (C5a), *Immunology*, **24**:969–976 (1973).

85. H. Harris, Mobilization of defensive cells in inflammatory tissue, *Bacteriol. Rev.*, **24**:3–15 (1960).

86. H. M. Keller and E. Sorkin, Studies on chemotaxis V. On the chemotactic effect of bacteria, *Int. Arch. Allergy*, **31**:505–517 (1967).

87. P. A. Ward, I. H. Lepow, and L. J. Newman, Bacterial factors chemotactic for polymorphonuclear leukocytes, *Am. J. Pathol.*, **52**:725–736 (1968).

88. P. A. Ward, Chemotaxis of human eosinophils, *Am. J. Pathol.*, **54**:121–128 (1969).

89. P. A. Ward, S. Cohen, and T. D. Flanagan, Leukotactic factors elaborated by virus-infected tissues, *J. Exp. Med.*, **135**:1095–1103 (1972).

90. R. Martin, W. Glenn, R. Couch, and V. Knight, Chemotaxis of human leukocytes: Responsiveness to mycoplasma pneumoniae, *J. Lab. Clin. Med.*, **81**:520–529 (1973).

91. E. L. Becker and H. J. Showell, The effect of Ca^{2+} and Mg^{2+} on the chemotactic responsiveness and spontaneous motility of rabbit polymorphonuclear leukocytes, *Z. Immun. Forsch.*, **143**:466–476 (1972).

92. J. I. Gallin and A. S. Rosenthal, The regulatory role of divalent cations in human granulocyte chemotaxis: Evidence for an association between calcium exchanges and microtubule assembly, *J. Cell. Biol.*, **62**:594–609 (1974).

93. R. M. Blizzard and J. H. Gibbs, Candidiasis: Studies pertaining to its association with endocrinopathies and pernicious anemia, *Pediatrics*, **42**:231–237 (1968).

94. J. I. Gallin, Abnormal chemotaxis: Cellular and humoral components.

In *The Phagocytic Cell in Host Resistance*. Edited by J. A. Bellanti and P. H. Dayton. New York, Raven Press, 1975, pp. 227–248.

95.   R. W. Berry and M. M. Shelanski, Interactions of tubulin with vinblastin and guanosine triphosphate, *J. Mol. Biol.*, 71:71–80 (1972).

96.   M. L. Shelanski, F. Gaskin, and C. R. Cantor, Assembly of microtubules in the absence of added nucleotide, *Proc. Natl. Acad. Sci. USA*, 70: 765–768 (1973).

97.   M. L. Shelanski, Chemistry of the filaments and tubules of brain, *J. Histochem. Cytochem.*, 21:529–539 (1973).

98.   R. D. Estensen, H. R. Hill, P. G. Quie, J. Hogan, and N. D. Goldberg, Cyclic GMP and cell movement, *Nature*, 245:458–460 (1973).

99.   P. A. Ward and E. L. Becker, Mechanisms of the inhibition of chemotaxis by phosphonate esters, *J. Exp. Med.*, 127:1001–1020 (1967).

100.   E. L. Becker and P. A. Ward, Partial biochemical characterization of the activated esterase required in the complement–dependent chemotaxis of rabbit polymorphonuclear leukocytes, *J. Exp. Med.*, 127:1021–1030 (1967).

101.   E. L. Becker and P. A. Ward, Esterases of the polymorphonuclear leukocyte capable of hydrolyzing acetyl DL–phenyl–alanine β–naphthyl ester, *J. Exp. Med.*, 129:569–584 (1969).

102.   R. Snyderman, L. C. Altman, A. Frankel, and M. Blaese, Defective mononuclear leukocyte chemotaxis: A previously unrecognized immune dysfunction, *Ann. Intern. Med.*, 78:509–513 (1973).

103.   J. I. Gallin, J. A. Klimerman, G. A. Padgett, and S. M. Wolff, Defective mononuclear cell chemotaxis in the Chediak Higashi Syndrome of humans, mink, and cattle, *Blood*, 45:863–870 (1975).

104.   R. G. Brayton, P. E. Stokes, M. S. Schwartz, and D. B. Louria, Effect of alcohol and various diseases on leukocyte mobilization, phagocytosis, and intracellular killing, *N. Engl. J. Med.*, 282:123–128 (1970).

105.   C. R. Bishop, J. W. Athens, D. R. Boggs, H. R. Warner, G. E. Cartwright, and M. M. Wintrobe, Leukokinetic studies. XIII. A nonsteady state kinetic evaluation of the mechanism of cortisone–induced granulocytosis, *J. Clin. Invest.*, 47:249–260 (1968).

106.   N. K. Day, H. Geiger, R. Stroud, M. de Bracco, B. Mencado, D. Windhorst, and R. A. Good, C1r deficiency: An inborn error associated with cutaneous and renal disease, *J. Clin. Invest.*, 51:1102–1108 (1972).

107.   P. A. Ward, Complement derived leukotactic factors in pathological fluids, *J. Exp. Med.*, 134:109s–113s (1971).

Part II

CONTRIBUTIONS OF IMMUNOLOGIC PROCESS
TO DEFENSE OF THE LUNG

9

Experimental Infections of the Lung

DAVID C. DALE

National Institute of Allergy and Infectious Diseases
National Institutes of Health
Bethesda, Maryland

I. Introduction

Experimental infections of the lower respiratory tract have been studied extensively in an attempt to understand the pathogenicity of microorganisms and the mechanisms of host-resistance to infections. This review will emphasize:

1. Methods for producing and studying experimental pulmonary infections;

2. Basic pathophysiologic concepts derived from studies of experimental pneumonia; and

3. Areas of current and proposed investigation.

A categoric review of the species specificities of individual pathogens or the spectrum of pneumonia in individual species has not been attempted; recent reviews of this information are available and are cited in the reference list [1-3].

II. Methods of Infection

Controlled inoculation of microorganisms into the pulmonary tract is possible by three basic approaches:

1. Organisms are inoculated by transtracheal injection or instilled through an endotracheal tube in an anaesthetized animal. The advantages of this route are that a specific quantity of organisms can be directly delivered to a specified level of the respiratory tract and that simultaneous with the inoculation, a bronchus can be plugged, [4], the vocal cords can be anesthetized, [5], or gelatin or mucus can be instilled [6] to enhance the pathogenicity of an organism of relatively low virulence. These mechanical modifications of the host are also the simplest methods for simulating some abnormalities which predispose humans to pulmonary infections. The chief disadvantages of direct tracheal or bronchial inoculation are (a) anesthesia is an unnatural situation for the acquisition of an infectious agent and (b) there is greater opportunity for animal to animal variation in the inoculation procedure than with intranasal or aerosol challenge.

2. Intranasal inoculation of viruses [7] and some bacteria [8] has been studied for many years. This method assumes that some of the inoculum will be aspirated or that the upper respiratory infection will spread to the trachea and lungs. In general, normal animals can not be easily infected with bacteria by this method except with virulent organisms.

3. Aerosolization of bacteria and viruses has been used widely, particularly for small animals [1,9]. This method is advantageous for uniform exposure of groups of animals and is applicable to a wide variety of viruses, bacteria, and fungi. The number of viable organisms delivered to target tissues is best assessed by quantitative cultures of the tissues after a specific time of exposure to the aerosol.

The probability that the inoculated organisms will cause an infection can be increased by a variety of preinoculation manipulations of the host. These include exposure to cold [10], noxious gases [11], cigarette smoke [1], ethanol [1], radiation [12], thymectomy [13], and various immunosuppressive [14] and anti-inflammatory drugs [15].

III. Basic Concepts from Experimental Studies

Experimental studies have been addressed to several kinds of questions:

1. Is an organism pathogenic or what is its relative pathogenicity compared to similar organisms?

2. What pathologic lesions does the organism cause?

3. What are the mechanisms of bacterial–viral synergism to cause more severe pulmonary disease in combined infections?

4. What are the critical factors of pulmonary–host resistance?

5. Which modes of therapy are most effective for experimental infections?

Methods most often applied to answer these questions are survival statistics, histologic examination of autopsy tissues, and cultures of target tissues for the inoculated organisms. Recently, investigators have sought to study the factors involved in host–resistance in a more dynamic fashion by serial electron micros-copy studies [16,17], bronchial lavage techniques [18,19], studies of turnover rates of radioisotope-tagged mononuclear cells [19], and bacterial clearance rates measured under various conditions, using radiolabeled microorganisms [1,20].

It is well known that within many bacterial species there are wide variations of pathogenicity for a given animal host. This conclusion is based in part on studies of experimental pneumonia. For instance, studies of pneumococcal pneu-monia in dogs helped to establish that organisms with thick capsules and of cer-tain serotypes are more virulent [21]. Similarly, studies in pigs support the ob-servation in man that encapsulated strains of *Hemophilus* are more virulent than nonencapsulated organisms [22]. Recently, the pathogenicity of different strains of *Pseudomonas aeruginosa,* for mice, was compared with respect to their in vitro production of elastase, hemolysin, lecithinase, and protease in an attempt to assess the virulence factors for this ubiquitous organism [9]. The mice were exposed to a standard aerosolized inoculum and rates at which the bacteria were cleared from the lungs were measured. Only the strains producing extracellular lecithinase increased in numbers in the mouse lung.

The pathogenicity of *Salmonella* and other intracellular organisms seems to correlate with the microbes' capacity to survive inside leukocytes after phago-cytosis. In experimental *Salmonella cholerasuis* pulmonary infection in pigs, studies by electron microscopy indicate that after several days of containment in neutrophils and pulmonary macrophages, intact organisms are released from the cells and the debris of the leukocytes and bacteria plus the surrounding tissue necrosis lead to microabscess formation [8,16].

Tubercule bacilli also remain intact for prolonged periods in pulmonary macrophages following experimental infections [23], and the typical pathologic lesions of caseous necrosis are related to the release of toxic materials from intracellular organisms.

For *Mycoplasma,* a host of viruses, and a variety of other organisms, animal inoculation studies have been used to study pathogenicity of organisms isolated from human infections in attempts to establish animal models of human disease. In general, experimental studies of organisms isolated from naturally acquired animal infections are more useful for experimental studies than are human pathogens. Mycoplasmal pneumonia can be induced in pigs [24], dogs [25], mice [26], calves [27], sheep [28], and hamsters [29]. Adenovirus infections have been recently studied in dogs [29,30], herpes–virus infections in calves [31], influenzal pneumonia in mice [32], and picornavirus infections in cats [33]. Considerable attention has also been addressed recently to studies of *Pneumocystis carinii* pneumonia [34] in rats.

Pathologic processes which follow pulmonary inoculation of many microbes closely mimic naturally acquired infections. The advantage of studying an experimental process pathologically is to study its time course. The pyogenic bacteria, for example *Diplococcus pneumoniae,* evoke an acute inflammatory response. This type of infection has provided an excellent opportunity to study the diapedesis of neutrophils across capillary walls [35]. The healing of infections, with abscess formation in which mononuclear cells and plasma cells accumulate, has also been recently studied. Because the accumulation of mononuclear cells and plasma cells correlates temporally with clearance of bacteria, it has been inferred that cellular immunity and, possibly, locally active humoral immunity, are key events for the recovery of the host. In contrast to this pathologic reaction, experimental mycoplasmal infections do not lead to accumulations of plasma cells but only to a peribronchial mononuclear inflammatory response [13]. Most experimental viral infections in animals, as in man, cause edema of the alveolar septae, peribronchiolar and perivascular accumulation of lymphocytes, and varying degrees of injury to the tracheobronchial epithelial cells [30].

Injury to the ciliary epithelium lining the lower respiratory tract, caused by virus infections, is a well–recognized predisposing factor to bacterial superinfection. Since the classic studies of Shope [37], repeated investigations have confirmed that viral respiratory–tract infections make animals far more susceptible to severe bacterial pneumonia [36,38]. After viral infections, bacteria are not cleared normally from the lower respiratory tract because the virus damages the mechanical clearing-action of respiratory-tract epithelium and consequent stasis allows for bacterial multiplication. Breaks in the mucosal surface may also allow submucosal penetration of bacteria [36].

Host-defense factors of the lung have been reviewed extensively in other chapters of this volume. In these chapters, emphasis has been given to cellular and humoral factors, which can be measured in normal pulmonary tissues. In most infections of the lung, however, phagocytic cells as well as opsonins, humoral mediators of inflammation, and other factors are recruited from the blood to compose the pulmonary inflammatory response. These are undoubtedly the limiting host-defense factors in many clinical and experimental infections.

Recent studies of experimental *Pseudomonas* pneumonia in leukopenic dogs illustrate how blood granulocytes can be the limiting factor for recovery from an experimental infection [12]. Dogs were given low-dose total body irradiation to make them gradually leukopenic. This radiation dose did not reduce the number of pulmonary macrophages or lymphocytes recoverable by bronchial lavage. It was observed that susceptibility to infection was inversely related to the blood granulocyte count. In addition, the experimentally infected dogs treated with gentamicin alone (1.7 mg/kg-8 hr) did not clear the inoculated *Pseudomonas* from the lung. In contrast, if the dogs were given blood granulocytes and the same dose of gentamicin they uniformly cleared the inoculated bacteria [12].

Another aspect of pulmonary host-defense analyzable in an experimental infection is the source and renewal rates of the pulmonary macrophage population. Labeling studies employing tritiated thymidine and marrow transplantation indicate that alveolar macrophages are derived from the bone marrow, traverse the blood as monocytes, and may undergo a limited number of mitoses before becoming typical pulmonary macrophages [19]. These cells can be exfoliated after ingestion of inoculated organisms and are recoverable by bronchial lavage.

In animals treated with adrenocorticosteroids, in vivo studies indicate that the efficacy of containment and killing of inoculated microorganisms by pulmonary macrophages is reduced [15,39]. Several studies suggest that the phagocytized bacteria or fungi are not killed but survive inside the phagocyte and in turn kill the phagocytic cell [15,40]. Thus, these experimental studies suggest that the critical factor in infections of animals receiving corticosteroids is the failure of macrophage bacteriocidal function.

The relative importance of a number of other host-defense factors has been evaluated in experimental pulmonary infections. Thymectomized mice are more susceptible to *Mycoplasma pulmonis* infection that are normal mice [13]. Histologically, they do not develop the normal mononuclear cellular response. It has been proposed that this is a model for pulmonary infection, with normal local

responses of granulocytes but defective cellular immunity. Similarly antilymphocyte globulin has been used to increase the susceptibility of guinea pigs to *Candida*
infections [41]. It has been reported that cyclophosphamide reduces lethality
for an experimental viral pneumonia, presumably by decreasing the inflammatory
response to the virus [42]. Whether this somewhat surprising result can be related
to the size of the inoculum or to the dose of cyclophosphamide is not clear from
the published report.

IV. Current and Proposed Research

Two main areas of research on experimental pulmonary infections are particularly
important to the practice of human medicine. First, further in vivo studies are
needed to better define the critical host–defense factors in various types of infections. For instance, can the susceptibility to certain kinds of pulmonary infections
in patients receiving corticosteroids and immunosuppressive drugs be related to
failure of containment and elimination of the microorganism because of a failure
of macrophage function? What are the quantitative aspects of local cellular immunity and to what degree are they altered by drugs and diseases affecting cellular
responses? Quantitative approaches must be applied to make experimental studies
more directly relevant to human disease.

Second, further research is needed on the treatment of experimental infections. For instance, studies are not in progress to compare various antibiotic
regimens in the treatment of *Pseudomonas* pneumonia in leukopenic dogs [43].
These studies should provide some guidelines for directing human research on
treating leukopenic patients with *Pseudomonas* infections. Studies of the treatment of many other experimental infections, particularly fungal and viral infections, could also be of great value. The study of treatment of animal diseases
should also include investigations of methods to reconstitute defective host–
defense mechanisms, to modify the inflammatory response, to reduce mortality
from an excessive host response, and to correlate tissue levels of antimicrobial
agents with blood levels to better guide chemotherapy of infections. Continued
study of experimental pulmonary infections should continue to provide valuable
insights for understanding pulmonary infections in man.

References

1. R. Rylander, Pulmonary defense mechanisms to airbourne bacteria, *Acta.
   Physiol. Scand., Suppl.,* **306**:9–89 (1968).
2. F. W. Denhy, W. A. Clyde, Jr., and W. P. Glexen, *Mycoplasma pneumoniae*
   disease: Clinical spectrum, pathophysiology, epidemiology, and control,
   J. Infect. Dis., **123**:74–92 (1971).

3. J. H. Darbyshire and D. H. Roberts, Some respiratory virus and mycoplasma infections of animals, *J. Clin. Pathol.*, **21**:Supp 2:61–87 (1968).
4. P. N. Coryllos and G. L. Birnbaum, Lobar pneumonia considered as pneumococcic lobar atelectasis of the lung: Bronchscopic investigation, *Arch. Surg.*, **18**:190–241 (1929).
5. E. E. Terrel, O. H. Robertson, and L. T. Coggeshall, Experimental *Pneumococcus* lobar pneumonia in the dog. I. Method of production and course of the disease, *J. Clin. Invest.*, **12**:393–432 (1933).
6. O. H. Robertson and J. P. Fox, The relationship of infecting dosage, leucocytic response, bacteremia, and extent of pulmonary involvement to the outcome of experimental lobar pneumonia in the dog, *J. Exp. Med.*, **69**: 229–246 (1939).
7. M. Degre and L. A. Glasgow, Synergistic effect in viral–bacterial infection. I. Combined infection of the respiratory tract in mice with parainfluenza virus and *Hemophilus influenza, J. Infect. Dis.*, **118**:449–462 (1968).
8. A. Baskerville, C. Dow, W. L. Curran, and J. Hanna, Ultrastructure of phagocytosis of *Salmonella cholera-suis* by pulmonary macrophages in vivo, *Br. J. Exp. Pathol.*, **53**:641–647 (1972).
9. P. M. Sourthern, B. B. Mays, A. K. Pierce, and J. P. Sanford, Pulmonary clearance of *Pseudomonas aeruginosa, J. Lab. Clin. Med.*, **76**:548–559 (1970).
10. W. D. Won and H. Ross, Relationship of low temperature to mouse resistance to infection with *Klebsiella* pneumonia, *Aerosp. Med.*, **42**:642–645 (1971).
11. G. A. Fairchild, J. Roan, and J. McCarroll, Atmosphere pollutants and the pathogenesis of viral respiratory infection: Sulfur dioxide and influenza infection in mice, *Arch. Environ. Health*, **25**:174–182 (1972).
12. D. C. Dale, H. Y. Reynolds, J. E. Pennington, T. W. Pitts, and R. G. Graw, Granulocyte transfusion therapy of experimental *Pseudomonas* pneumonia, *J. Clin. Invest.*, **54**:664–671 (1974).
13. F. W. Denny, D. Taylor–Robinson, and A. C. Allison, The role of thymus dependent immunity in *Mycoplasma pulmonis* infections of mice, *J. Med. Microbiol.*, **5**:327–336 (1972).
14. S. H. Singer, M. Ford, and R. L. Kirschstein, Respiratory disease in cyclophosphamide–treated mice with mycoplasmal infections, *Infect. Immunol.*, **5**:953–956 (1972).
15. L. I. Linaris and L. Friedman, Experimental paracoccidioidomycosis in mice, *Infect. Immunol.*, **5**:681–687 (1972).
16. A. Baskerville, C. Dow, W. L. Curran, and J. Hanna, Further studies on experimental bacterial pneumonia: Ultrastructural changes produced in the lungs by *Salmonella cholera-suis, Br. J. Exp. Pathol.*, **54**:90–98 (1973).
17. M. J. Finegold, Pneumonic plague in monkeys. An electron microscopic study, *Am. J. Pathol.*, **54**:167–185 (1969).
18. Q. N. Myrvik, E. S. Leake, and B. Fariss, Studies on pulmonary alveolar macrophages from the normal rabbit: A technique to procure them in a high state of purity, *J. Immunol.*, **86**:128–132 (1961).

19. G. P. Velo and W. G. Spector, The origin and turnover of alveolar macrophages in experimental pneumonia, *J. Pathol.,* **109**:7–19 (1973).

20. G. M. Green and W. H. Kass, The role of the alveolar macrophage in the clearance of bacteria from the lung, *J. Exp. Med.,* **119**:164–175 (1964).

21. J. F. Gaskell, Pathology of the lung, *Lancet,* **2**:951–957 (1927).

22. T. W. A. Little and J. D. J. Harding, The comparative pathogenicity of two porcine *Haemophilus* species, *Vet. Rec.,* **88**:540–545 (1971).

23. J. J. Merckx, A. L. Brown, and A. G. Karlson, An electron–microscope study of experimental infections with acid–fast bacilli, *Am. Rev. Respir. Dis.,* **89**:485–496 (1964).

24. W. P. Switzer, Response of swine to *Mycoplasma hyopneumoniae* infection, *J. Infect. Dis.,* **127**:Suppl.:559–560 (1973).

25. D. Armstrong, V. Morton, M. H. Friedman, L. Steger, and J. G. Tully, Canine pneumonia associated with *Mycoplasma* infection, *Am. J. Vet. Res.,* **33**:1471–1478 (1972).

26. J. R. Lindsey and H. Cassell, Experimental *Mycoplasma pulmonis* infection in pathogen–free mice. Models for study mycoplasmosis of the respiratory tract, *Am. J. Pathol.,* **72**:63–84 (1973).

27. S. L. Furlong and G. S. Cotton, Identity of mycoplasmas from sheep pneumonia in Queensland and Victoria, *Aust. Vet. J.,* **49**:215–216 (1973).

28. A. S. Dajani, W. A. Clyde, Jr., and F. W. Denny, Experimental infection with *Mycoplasma pneumoniae* (Eaton's Agent), *J. Exp. Med.,* **121**:1071–1084 (1965).

29. N. G. Wright, H. Thompson, and H. J. Cornwall, Canine adenovirus pneumonia, *Res. Vet. Sci.,* **12**:162–167 (1971).

30. A. M. Cole, Experimental adenovirus pneumonia in calves, *Vet. J.,* **47**:306–311 (1971).

31. S. A. Monhanty, M. G. Lillie, A. L. Ingling, and R. C. Hammond, Effects of an experimentally induced herpesvirus infection in calves, *J. Am. Vet. Med. Assoc.,* **161**:1008–1011 (1972).

32. L. N. Ayer, D. F. Tierney, and D. Imagawa, Shortened survival of mice with influenza when given oxygen at one atmosphere, *Am. Rev. Respir.,* **107**:955 (1973).

33. E. A. Holzinger and D. E. Kahn, Pathological features of picornavirus infections in cats, *Am. J. Vet. Res.,* **31**:1623–1630 (1970).

34. J. K. Frenkel, J. T. Good, and J. A. Shultz, Latent pneumocystis infection of rats, relapses and chemotherapy, *Lab. Invest.,* **15**:1559–1577 (1966).

35. C. G. Loosli and R. F. Baker, Acute experimental pneumococcal (Type 1) pneumonia in the mouse. The migration of leukocytes from the pulmonary capillaries into the alveolar spaces as revealed by the electron microscope, *Trans. Am. Clin. Climatol. Assoc.,* **74**:15–28 (1962).

36. M. Degre and L. A. Solberg, Synergistic effect in viral–bacterial infection. 3. Histopathological changes in the trachea of mice following viral and bacterial infection, *Acta. Pathol. Microbiol. Scand., Sect. B,* **79**:129–136 (1971).

37. R. E. Shope, Swice influenza. III. Filtration experiments and etiology, *J. Exp. Med.,* **54**:373–385 (1931).

38. P. B. Spradbrow and A. M. Cole, The production of calf pneumonia with *Escherichia coli* and a bovine picornavirus, *J. Comp. Pathol.,* **81**:551–555 (1971).

39. D. K. Sandhu, R. S. Sandhy, V. N. Damodaran, and H. S. Randhawa, Effect of cortisone on bronchopulmonary aspergillosis in mice exposed to spores of various aspergillus species, *Sabouraudia,* **8**:32–38 (1970).

40. H. S. Hsu, Cellular basis of cortisone–induced host susceptibility to tuberculosis, *Am. Rev. Respir. Dis.,* **100**:677–684 (1969).

41. H. Grubek, D. Szymanska, E. Trenkner, D. Weyman–Rzucidlo, and M. Okon, Effect of anti–lymphocytic serum on experimental infection with Candida albicans in guinea pigs, *Acta Microbiol. Pol., Ser. A,* 221–30 (1970).

42. S. H. Singer, P. Noguchi, and R. L. Kirschstein, Respiratory diseases in cyclophosphamide–treated mice. II. Decreased virulence of PR8 influenza virus, *Infect. Immunol.,* **5**:957–960 (1972).

43. D. C. Dale, H. Y. Reynolds, J. E. Pennington, R. Elin, and R. G. Graw, (1974). Unpublished data.

10

Immunodeficiency and Pulmonary Disease

STEPHEN H. POLMAR

Case Western Reserve School of Medicine
Cleveland, Ohio

I. Introduction

The immune system, in its broadest sense, consists of a series of inter-relating specific and nonspecific host-defense mechanisms. The absence or dysfunction of any one or more of these mechanisms usually results in an increased susceptibility to infection, primarily of the skin, and of the gastrointestinal and respiratory tracts. In the past, the term *immunodeficiency disease* has been used to denote defects related to the function of the lymphoid system, i.e., antibody deficiency and delayed hypersensitivity defects. However, recent observations of increased susceptibility to respiratory-tract infections in patients with leukocyte dysfunction syndromes and complement deficiencies emphasizes the need to include these disorders in any consideration of the immunologic bases of respiratory-tract infection. Therefore, for purposes of this discussion, the term immunodeficiency will refer to abnormal function of leukocytes and the complement system as well as to defects in antibody synthesis and cell-mediated (delayed hypersensitivity) immunity.

Supported in part by grants from The National Institute of Arthritis and Metabolic Diseases (AM 08305-11) and the Cleveland Chapter of the National Cystic Fibrosis Research Foundation (United Torch of Cleveland).

Acute, recurrent, and chronic respiratory tract infection is a significant cause of morbidity and mortality in most patients with immunodeficiency disorders. The classic forms of immunodeficiency disease (X-linked agammaglobulinemia [Bruton], DiGeorge syndrome, severe combined immunodeficiency syndrome [Swiss type]) have been extensively discussed in the medical literature and present little difficulty in diagnosis [1,2]. Although these entities will be used as prototypes, emphasis will be placed upon related disorders the diagnoses of which are more difficult and are often missed, especially if immune function is evaluated only superficially. Where possible, immunopathogenetic mechanisms will be stressed, since it is only by understanding the mechanism of disease that intelligent approaches to therapy can be undertaken.

Good [3] has called the immunodeficiency diseases *experiments of nature.* Indeed, clinical observations and laboratory studies of patients with these disorders have stimulated thought and guided research leading to much of our current knowledge of the ontogeny of immunologic competence and the function of host-defense mechanisms in general. In many respects, the less severe and more limited forms of immunodeficiency associated with specific target organs and restricted spectra of infection may be more informative than the generalized defects seen in many of the classic immunodeficiency states. In these disorders, cause and effect relationships may be discerned more readily. In this regard, it is hoped that insights gained from the study of pulmonary disorders associated with immunodeficiency will stimulate the development of our understanding of respiratory tract immunity.

II. Antibody Deficiency Syndromes

Antibodies represent a major bulwark of the body's defense against encapsulated, high-grade pathogens, such as pneumococci, *Hemophilus influenzae,* streptococci, and meningococci and play an important role in the prevention of viral infection. IgG antibodies provide most of the antibacterial, antiviral, and antitoxin properties of serum and interstitial fluids; they are potent opsonins, and facilitate polymorphonuclear leukocyte chemotaxis and phagocytosis through activation of the complement system. IgM antibodies are potent bacterial agglutinins, facilitating clearance of intravascular bacteria by the reticuloendothelial system, and are also efficient activators of the complement system. IgA is the major antibacterial and antiviral antibody of the mucous membranes. The protective roles of IgD and IgE are not as yet well-established.

To evaluate antibody-mediated immunity immunoglobulin levels in serum (and sometimes secretions) must be measured and the antibody response to specific antigens assessed. Immunoelectrophoresis and radial diffusion are generally available for quantitating serum immunoglobulins. Antibodies produced by prior immunization or infection may be assessed by the Schick test, and antibody titers to polio, diphtheria, rubella, rubeola, ASO, and other antigens can be determined. The patient's response to new immunization may be studied by immunization with a killed bacterial vaccine, such as typhoid vaccine. If abnormalities are found, lymph node architecture should be evaluated for germinal center formation and plasma cells.

A. Antibody Deficiency with Immunoglobulin Deficiency

X-linked agammaglobulinemia (X-LA) is the most extreme form of antibody deficiency syndrome. Patients lack the ability to produce all immunoglobulin classes as well as antibodies. Lymph nodes lack germinal centers and plasma cells but retain their paracortical thymus-dependent lymphocyte (T cell) mantle. Their peripheral blood lacks lymphocytes bearing surface immunoglobulins (B cells) [4,5]. The onset of clinical disease is usually between 6 and 12 months of life, shortly after the disappearance of maternal IgG. As one would expect, these patients are extremely susceptible to recurrent infection with encapsulated bacterial pathogens, but infection with most gram-negative bacteria, viruses, and fungi are rare. Recurrent pneumonias and bronchitis occur early in life, often progressing to bronchiectasis. Chronic sinusitis occurs somewhat later in childhood, further complicating pulmonary management. *Pneumocystis carinii* pneumonitis has also been reported in these patients [6-9]. Meningitis, sepsis, otitis, septic arthritis, and cellulitis are also common problems.

Most patients with X-linked agammaglobulinemia are treated with intramuscular injections of pooled alcohol-precipitated gamma globulins, yet in spite of apparently adequate immunoglobulin replacement, many patients develop progressive sinopulmonary disease. Buckley [10] has treated X-LA patients with plasma transfusions which she felt controlled infection better than did intramuscular injections of gamma globulin. This improvement was thought to be due to the higher immunoglobulin and antibody levels achieved with plasma therapy. However, failure of immunoglobulin replacement alone to arrest progressive pulmonary disease in some patients may be related to other serum protein deficiencies. Kohler and Müller-Eberhard [11] and Gewurz *et al.* [12] have reported C1q deficiencies among X-LA patients as well as in some other immunodeficiency states. It is possible that part of the improvement in clinical status, with plasma therapy, may be the result of replacing deficient complement components.

There are other forms of agammaglobulinemia that resemble the X-linked form both in immunologic deficits and clinical manifestations. Congenital agammaglobulinemia may occur sporadically or may be familial but not sex-linked. In some patients agammaglobulinemia or severe hypogammaglobulinemia develops later in childhood or in adult life. Upper and lower respiratory tract infections are a prominent and constant part of the clinical picture in these disorders. Chronic bronchitis, sinusitis, and otitis as well as recurrent pneumonias occur in most patients. In the adult acquired form of agammaglobulinemia, malabsorption, intestinal giardiasis, and autoimmune disorders are observed frequently [13].

Immunodeficiency with hyper-IgM (dysgammaglobulinemia Type IV) has many features in common with the congenital agammaglobulinemias [14,15]. Recurrent bacterial infections, including bronchitis, pneumonia, bronchiectasis, sinusitis, and otitis are common. *Pneumocystis carinii* pneumonitis also occurs in these patients [9]. Fungal and unusual viral infections are rare. Hepatospleno-megaly, hemolytic anemia, thrombocytopenia, neutropenia, and pancytopenia occur with some regularity. Normal or elevated levels of IgM are present in serum, but IgG and IgA are absent. This dysgammaglobulinemia illustrates the useless-ness of serum protein electrophoresis in the diagnosis of immunoglobulin defi-ciencies since, in this entity, serum electrophoresis is often normal, whereas the IgA and IgG deficiency is readily detected by immunoelectrophoresis and radial diffusion quantitation. Response to immunization is variable, patients produce antibody to some antigens but not to others. Immunologic memory is impaired and booster responses are not observed, but cell-mediated immunity is intact. Lymph nodes and tonsils are generally enlarged, but few lymphoid follicles are seen, germinal centers are absent, and plasma cells are decreased in number or absent [14,15]. Immunodeficiency with hyper-IgM is often inherited as an X-linked recessive trait, but may occur sporadically as well. This immunode-ficiency has also been reported in association with intrauterine viral infections, such as rubella [16,17]. Patients show a good response to immunoglobulin replacement therapy.

Increased susceptibility to bacterial infections is generally not attributed to hypogammaglobulinemia unless the serum IgG level is less than 200 mg/100 ml. The selective IgG subclass deficiencies are an important exception to this general rule [18,19]. The IgG class of immunoglobulins is made up of four subclasses IgG1, IgG2, IgG3, and IgG4, which comprise 65%, 23%, 8%, and 4% of the total IgG, respectively. Subclasses differ in antigenic composition, chemical structure, biologic properties, as well as antibody spectrum [20]. For example, IgG1, IgG2, and IgG4 have biologic half lives of 21 days, while IgG3 has a half life of only 8 days. IgG1 and IgG3 fix complement efficiently, IgG2 only slightly, and IgG4 not at all. Rh antibodies are usually of the IgG1 and IgG3 subclasses, but never of the IgG2 class, whereas antibodies to polysaccharide antigens are usually of the IgG2 class. Therefore, a deficiency of one or more of the IgG subclasses could result in significant antibody deficiency in the absence of markedly reduced total IgG levels.

Patients with IgG subclass deficiencies have normal or elevated levels of IgM and IgA, but IgG levels are below the lower limit of normal for age but usually above 200 mg/100 ml [18,19]. Lymph node architecture, germinal centers, and plasma cells are normal. The spectrum of infection in these patients is very similar to that of the X-linked agammaglobulinemics. Recurrent pyogenic infection with pneumococci, *Hemophilus influenzae,* streptococci, and staphylococci occur frequently, but fungal and unusual viral infections are not seen. Chronic bronchitis, recurrent pneumonia, bronchiectasis, sinusitis, and otitis are prominent features of the clinical picture. As one would expect, immunoglobulin replacement has been found effective in controlling infection in these patients [19].

The significance of IgA and IgE deficiency in the pathogenesis of respiratory tract disease has been an area of controversy during recent years. This topic is discussed in detail in Section II, C.

B. Antibody Deficiency Without Immunoglobulin Deficiency

Patients with antibody deficiency and normal immunoglobulin levels serve to emphasize the inadequacy of employing only immunoelectrophoresis, quantitative immunoglobulin determinations, or both, in screening for humoral immunodeficiency. Blecher *et al.* [21], Buckley *et al.* [22], and Davis [23] have described patients with normal or elevated immunoglobulin levels who did not produce antibodies to many antigens to which they were exposed either by immunization or infection. Complement levels and leukocyte function studies were normal in all patients, and cell-mediated immunity was normal in two patients [21,23] but defective in the two patients reported by Buckley [22]. Recurrent and persistent pneumonias, abscesses (including lung abscesses), bronchiectasis, otitis, and chronic dermatitis were salient clinical features in this immunodeficiency. Recognition of this entity is especially important, since patients respond well to immunoglobulin replacement therapy [23].

C. IgE Deficiency, IgA Deficiency and Pulmonary Disease

The question of the significance of IgA deficiency in the pathogenesis of pulmonary disease is intimately related to the question of the significance of IgE deficiency, especially since some immunodeficiencies in which sinopulmonary disease classically occurs, such as ataxia telangiectasia, manifest both IgA and IgE deficiencies [24]. Selective IgE deficiency will be discussed first, followed by a consideration of IgA deficiency with and without IgE deficiency.

Although the role of IgE in the mediation of immediate hypersensitivity reactions is well-established, the function of IgE in protective immunity is less well-defined. Initial suggestions for a protective role for IgE in respiratory tract immunity were based on observations of chronic sinopulmonary disease in two patients with apparent IgE deficiency [25]. IgE deficiency was diagnosed by lack of reaction in reverse cutaneous anaphylaxis tests with intradermal injections of anti-IgE. However Levy and Chen [26] described a healthy individual with isolated IgE deficiency and subsequently Gleich *et al.* [27] and Polmar *et al.* [28], using sensitive double antibody radioimmunoassay techniques, described an additional nine asymptomatic IgE-deficient individuals (IgE levels less than 15 ng/ml). On the basis of these data, one must conclude that IgE deficiency alone does not usually predispose individuals to respiratory infection [28,29]. It is debatable whether selective IgE deficiency should be considered an immunodeficiency disease or merely a variant of normal

Selective IgA deficiency is defined as a serum IgA level less than 5 mg/100 ml, with no other immunoglobulin deficiency, normal antibody production, and intact cell-mediated immunity [30]. Almost all such individuals lack detectable secretory and serum IgA. Selective IgA deficiency is the most frequently observed immunodeficiency and may occur sporadically, show an autosomal dominant or recessive inheritance pattern, or be found in association with intrauterine viral infection, such as the rubella syndrome [16,30]. Diseases most frequently associated with IgA deficiency include autoimmune disorders (rheumatoid arthritis, systemic lupus erythematosus, and thyroiditis), recurrent respiratory tract infections, and allergic disorders [30]. Respiratory problems common among IgA-deficient patients include frequent mild viral upper respiratory tract infections, recurrent otitis media, sinusitis, bronchitis, bronchospasm, and asthma associated with viral infections and recurrent pneumonia. Emphysema and bronchiectasis occur in more severely affected patients. In general the respiratory tract disease of IgA deficiency is milder than in most antibody deficiency syndromes, and obstruction is a prominent feature of virtually all types of upper and lower respiratory tract disease in these patients.

However, many IgA-deficient individuals are entirely healthy [31,32] and indeed IgA deficiency occurs in 1 out of 500 normal individuals [33]. Therefore, other factors must be operative, determining which IgA-deficient individuals will suffer recurrent respiratory infection and which will not. Ammann, Roth, and Hong's [34] report of a mentally retarded child with combined IgA and IgE deficiency and recurrent sinopulmonary infections suggested that the combination of IgA and IgE deficiency might result in greater susceptibility to respiratory tract infection than IgA deficiency alone. This concept gained support from studies on patients with ataxia telangiectasia by Ammann and his collaborators [24]. In this study IgE deficiency was diagnosed by the absence of a wheal and flare reaction to an intradermal injection of anti-IgE (reverse cutaneous anaphylaxis test). In the 16 patients with ataxia telangiectasia studied, there appeared to be a correlation between the combined deficiency of IgA and IgE and the presence of sinopulmonary disease. However, most of the patients with IgE-deficient ataxia telangiectasia were lymphopenic and had varying degrees of cell-mediated immunodeficiency as well.

However, Polmar and collaborators [28] studied serum IgE levels in 44 patients with ataxia telangiectasia and found no significant correlation between IgE deficiency or combined IgE-IgA deficiency and sinopulmonary disease. Depression of delayed hypersensitivity appeared to be the single factor most closely correlated with predisposition to respiratory tract disease, but even this correlation was not statistically significant.

Schwartz and Buckley [35] and Polmar *et al.* [28] provided additional evidence against the association of combined IgA and IgE deficiency and increased susceptibility to respiratory infection. Schwartz and Buckley did not observe IgE deficiency among IgA-deficient patients with recurrent infection. Polmar and collaborators found that 70% of IgA-deficient patients who were not IgE deficient had recurrent respiratory infection, whereas all those with combined IgA and IgE deficiency were asymptomatic.

The striking association between IgE and respiratory tract infection in IgA-deficient patients may explain the prominence of obstructive symptomatology observed in these patients. In the absence of secretory IgA antibodies, synthesis of IgE may be excessively stimulated by bacterial or viral antigens. In the presence of such IgE antibodies relatively minor bacterial or viral infections might trigger immediate hypersensitivity reactions, resulting in local conditions (e.g., transudation of fluid, mucosal congestion, and bronchospasm) conducive to the growth of pathogenic microorganisms as well as for the destruction of respiratory tract tissues.

Autoimmune diseases are prominent among IgA-deficient patients [30]. In this disease group, idiopathic pulmonary hemosiderosis has been reported in four patients with selective IgA deficiency [30,36,37]. However, Matsaniotis *et al.* [38] found elevated serum IgA levels in 11 patients with idiopathic pulmonary hemosiderosis; IgA deficiency was not observed. Primary pulmonary hemosiderosis with cow's milk sensitivity and multiple circulating precipitins to cow's milk proteins has been described by Heiner and Sears [39]. Precipitating antibodies to cow's milk proteins occurs in 50% of IgA-deficient patients. However, this form of pulmonary hemosiderosis is rare among IgA-deficient patients [30]. IgA deficiency was not observed in two patients with Heiner's syndrome studied by Huntley *et al.* [40] nor in six patients with this same disease in our laboratory [41].

III. Cell-mediated Immunodeficiency Syndromes

Lymphoid stem cells differentiating under the influence of the thymus acquire the capability to mediate cutaneous delayed hypersensitivity, graft rejection, and graft–vs–host reactions. The major effector cell is the small thymic-dependent lymphocyte (T cell). This cell is capable of killing other cells through the release of cytotoxins or may recruit and activate cells, such as macrophages, through the release of migration inhibition factor and other lymphokines. These cell-mediated immune mechanisms are the major bodily defense mechanisms against fungal as well as intracellular bacterial and viral infections.

Cell-mediated immunity is more difficult to evaluate than humoral immunity because cell-mediated immune reactions are difficult to quantitate. Partial cell-mediated immunodeficiencies are particularly difficult to evaluate, since the characteristics of T-lymphocyte subpopulations are still poorly defined. Clinically, cell-mediated immunity may be assessed by the absolute peripheral blood small lymphocyte count and cutaneous delayed hypersensitivity tests to ubiquitous antigens (e.g., Candida, trichophyton, PPD, streptokinase-streptodornase, histoplasmin). Sensitization and challenge with 2,4-dinitro-1-chlorobenzene (DNCB) can be used, if other skin tests are negative. T lymphocytes form a dense cellular mantle under germinal centers of lymph nodes, and the absence or diminution of this cell population is associated with cell-mediated immunodeficiency. Proliferative responses of peripheral blood lymphocytes to nonspecific mitogens, such as phytohemagglutinin and conconavalin A, and to allogeneic cells, correlated with cell-mediated immunity, as does the production of migration inhibition factor (MIF).

Salient clinical features of patients with cell-mediated immunodeficiency vary with the severity and completeness of their defect. For this discussion, these immunodeficiencies will be divided into two groups: (a) those manifesting virtually a complete absence of cell-mediated immune functions (Di George Syndrome and severe combined immunodeficiency syndromes) and (b) those manifesting restricted or partial cell-mediated immunodeficiency (ataxia telangiectasia, chronic mucocutaneous candidiasis, and other partial deficiency states).

A. Di George Syndrome and Severe Combine Immunodeficiency Syndromes

Lymphoid stem cells, destined to differentiate into immunologically competent T lymphocytes require the inductive influence of the thymus. Embryologic events interfering with the development of the third and fourth pharyngeal pouch anlage result in aplasia, hypoplasia, or other anomalies of structures that arise from these pharyngeal pouches (i.e., thymus, parathyroids, aortic arch, external ear, and nasomedial parts of the face). Di George syndrome, which results from just such an embryologic accident, is characterized by absence or hypoplasia of the thymus and parathyroids, with neonatal hypocalcemic tetany and marked cell-mediated immunodeficiency [42]. Abnormalities of the face, low-set ears, anomalies of the aortic arch, and tetrology of Fallot are part of the classic syndrome. Such patients lack a thymic shadow on x-ray studies, but do not manifest lymphopenia. They lack cutaneous delayed hypersensitivity reactions, cannot be sensitized to DNCB, and do not show blastogenic responses to T-cell mitogens. Immunoglobulin levels and antibody synthesis are usually normal. Such patients suffer recurrent candidal infections, recurrent pneumonias (including pneumocystis), chronic diarrhea, and fail to thrive. Thus, pulmonary infections are just part of a syndrome complex, and these patients usually come to medical attention because of neonatal hypocalcemia before recurrent infection becomes a problem. Fetal thymus transplantation has reconstituted cell-mediated immune functions in some of these children [43,44].

Severe combined immunodeficiency syndrome probably consists of a group of immunopathologic entities, all of which result from either the complete absence of or abnormalities in the development of the lymphoid stem cells. Autosomal recessive (Swiss-type agammaglobulinemia) and X-linked recessive (thymic alymphoplasia) forms exist. Patients lack thymus shadows, are lymphopenic, and are devoid of cell-mediated as well as humoral immune functions. Onset of disease is usually within the first few months of life (mean onset 2 to 3 months), and the infections seen are the result of cell-mediated immune deficiency. Although oral candidiasis, chronic dermatitis, chronic diarrhea, and sepsis occur in greater than 50% of such patients, 89% or more have pneumonias or other pneumopathies [45]. Hitzig [45] described a characteristic intractable pertussoid cough in these patients. Bronchopneumonia is a constant or repetitive event. Giant cells pneumonias due to measles, and overwhelming infections with viruses (cytomegalovirus, adenovirus) and fungi (candida, aspergillus) occur commonly. The most characteristic pneumopathy in severe combined immunodeficiency is *pneumocystis carinii* pneumonitis [46]. Pneumocystis infection is present at the time of death in most of these patients. Walzer and collaborators [9] found that 60% of patients under 1 yr of age, with *pneumocystis carinii*

pneumonitis, had severe combined immunodeficiency. Onset of pneumonitis
may be abrupt or relatively insidious. Patients are usually afebrile and physical
findings are slight, but cyanosis is frequently impressive and disproportionate to
the dearth of pulmonary physical findings. Arterial O_2 saturations may be extremely low, consistent with an "alveolar–capillary block" syndrome [7], chest
roentograms may show either a diffuse interstitial infiltrate radiating from the
hila, or a diffuse alveolar pattern with air bronchograms. There is relative
sparing of the lung periphery and bases, and hilar adenopathy is absent [7].
Definitive diagnosis is made by the identification of *pneumocystis carinii* cysts
in Giemsa or Methenamine silver–stained lung biopsies [7,47]. Cysts may
sometimes be identified in sputum, tracheal aspirates, and bronchial washings
or brushings.

While the Di George syndrome signals its presence early, with neonatal
hypocalcemia, facial, ear, and sometimes cardiac anomalies, severe combined
immunodeficiency syndromes may present some differential diagnostic problems.
Entities with prominent pulmonary or gastrointestinal involvement or both, such
as cystic fibrosis, coeliac disease, and intestinal lymphangiectasia, may be confused with severe combined immunodeficiency and vice versa. Persistent lymphopenia should suggest the diagnosis, which may then be confirmed by in vitro
lymphocyte studies. Absence of the thymic shadow on x–ray films in an ill
infant is not diagnostic, since the thymus rapidly shrinks under stress [46].

Early diagnosis of severe combined immunodeficiency is especially important, since many of these patients can be saved. Immunologic reconstitution
with histocompatible bone marrow cells is the treatment of choice [48]. In some
cases in which a histocompatible marrow donor was not available, transfer factor
and plasma therapy have been useful, with some successes reported [49].

B. Partial Cell–Mediated Immunodeficiencies

Implication of cell–mediated immunodeficiency in the pathogenesis of pulmonary
disease is frequently obscured by the association of humoral and cellular defects
in many patients with chronic pulmonary disease. Chronic sinopulmonary disease,
including bronchitis, recurrent pneumonias, bronchiectasis, and sinusitis, occur in
patients with cell–mediated immunodeficiency and acquired agammaglobulinemia
[13,50,51], IgA deficiency [52], and in patients with ataxia telangiectasia
[53,54].

There are, however, a number of lines of evidence suggesting that even partial cell–mediated immunodeficiency may be important in the pathogenesis of
chronic pulmonary disease. As mentioned earlier, many patients with ataxia
telangiectasia have IgA or IgE deficiency or both and varying degrees of cell-

mediated immunodeficiency [24,28]. There is a general correlation between the severity of sinopulmonary disease and the severity of both humoral and cellular immunodeficiency [54]. There is, however, no correlation between IgA and IgE deficiency and sinopulmonary disease, whereas there does appear to be some correlation between cell-mediated immunodeficiency and sinopulmonary disease in these patients [28].

Chronic bronchitis, recurrent pneumonias, and bronchiectasis are not infrequently observed among patients with chronic mucocutaneous candidiasis [55,56]. In this syndrome, *Candida albicans* infection is limited to the skin, nails, mucous membranes, and, occasionally, the oropharynx and esophagus. Candidal pulmonary disease or infection of other organs does not occur. Polymorphonuclear leukocyte function, immunoglobulin and anticandidal antibody synthesis, and complement levels are normal. Cell-mediated immunodeficiency is usually present but may vary in severity. Some patients show complete cutaneous anergy, unresponsiveness to DNCB sensitization, absence of lymphocyte proliferation with candida as well as nonspecific mitogens, and fail to produce MIF. However, in other patients only suboptimal proliferative responses or MIF production to candida antigen are observed, while all other parameters of cell-mediated immunity are normal [55]. One patient with candidiasis and chronic pulmonary disease showed absence of lymphocyte cytotoxin production and monocyte unresponsiveness to autologous and heterologous MIF [56]. The association of cell-mediated immunodeficiency with chronic pulmonary disease in these patients might be fortuitous. Alternatively, it may be an important clue, suggesting that cell-mediated immunodeficiency, even if only partial, may significantly compromise pulmonary immunologic defense mechanisms.

We have recently begun to study a group of patients with chronic sinopulmonary disease and partial cell-mediated immunodeficiency. These patients range in age from 10 to 22 yr, all have histories of chronic bronchitis, with onset during the first 3 yr of life, progressing to bronchiectasis. Chronic sinusitis was present after age 7, but acute pneumonias rarely occurred. All patients studied have normal serum immunoglobulin, antibody and complement (CH_{50}) levels, normal nitroblue tetrazolium reduction, and myeloperoxidase staining. All patients lacked delayed hypersensitivity to candida, trichophytin, streptokinase-streptodornase, PPD, and histoplasmin but reacted weakly to DNCB sensitization and challenge, although one patient required repeated sensitizations. Some of these patients have shown 10%-20% of the normal thymidine uptake after stimulation with Conconavalin A. More detailed studies of cell-mediated immune function are in progress.

There are a number of possible explanations for the apparent association of partial cell-mediated immunodeficiency and chronic lung disease. In such patients T lymphocytes may be unable to terminate chronic low-grade viral or intracellular bacterial infections resulting in slow but progressive destruction of lower respiratory tract tissues. However, the pulmonary alveolar macrophage appears to be the most important cell responsible for maintaining sterility in the lower respiratory tract [57] and it would seem most likely that in such patients function of this cell must be compromised. Sensitized lymphocytes are capable of activating pulmonary alveolar macrophages, probably through the secretion of lymphokines [57]. For example, macrophages activated by BCG–sensitized lymphocytes efficiently kill intracellular bacterial parasites such as *Listeria monocytogenes* [57]. In the absence of functional T–cells, the function of pulmonary alveolar macrophages may be significantly compromised, resulting in chronic lower respiratory tract infection.

IV. Phagocyte Dysfunction Syndromes

Phagocytosis and intracellular killing of bacteria and other pathogens is an important line of primary defense against infection as well as the ultimate means to dispose of most pathogens. While phagocytosis is the most primitive defense mechanism, the more "sophisticated" immune mechanisms, antibody, complement, and cell–mediated immunity, act primarily to enhance the efficiency of phagocytic cells. Phagocyte function consists of four basic processes: chemotaxis, opsonization, ingestion, and intracellular killing. Defects in any one of these processes results in increased susceptibility to infection and, frequently, respiratory tract infection as well. Serum proteins, such as complement components, play an important role in enhancing chemotaxis and opsonization. The deficiency of these proteins results in phagocyte dysfunction and susceptibility to infection. Similarly, serum factors may inhibit chemotaxis, opsonization, and intracellular killing of bacteria, resulting in an increased frequency of infection. Intrinsic defects in the phagocyte itself also results in increased susceptibility to infection. Examples of these types of phagocyte dysfunctions are described in the following sections.

A. Defective Intracellular Killing (Chronic Granulomatous Disease)

Chronic granulomatous disease (CGD) is characterized by recurrent and chronic suppurative granulomatous infections caused by low–grade pathogens. Patients are uniquely susceptible to infection by catalase–producing bacteria (*Staphylococci, E. coli, Aerobacter, Klebsiella*) but not susceptible to catalase–negative bacteria (streptococci, diplococci). Onset of disease occurs in infancy, with chronic eczema, skin abcesses, adenitis, liver abcesses, and osteomyelitis.

Recurrent and chronic pulmonary infection is a prominent feature of this disease. Extensive parenchymal infiltration with hilar adenopathy, as well as broncho-pneumonias, lobar pneumonias, pleural effusion, empyema, pulmonary abcesses, and right middle lobe atelectasis occur. Infections respond extremely slowly to appropriate antibiotics. "Encapsulated pneumonias," round homogenous parenchymal densities, are characteristically observed in CGD [58].

Intracellular killing of bacteria by iodination requires H_2O_2, myeloperoxidase and iodide. CGD leukocytes are defective in activation of the hexose monophosphate shunt following phagocytosis, such that H_2O_2 is not produced and intracellular bacterial killing is impaired. CGD cells cannot reduce nitroblue tetrazolium and this finding serves as a simple screening test for this entity [59]. Complement levels and cell-mediated immunity are normal and immunoglobulin levels are elevated. At the present time there is no definitive treatment for this disease.

B. Complement Deficiencies and Phagocyte Dysfunction

Complement components play important roles in host defense, both through the mediation of inflammatory reactions as well as the enhancement of phagocyte related functions, chemotaxis and opsonization. When IgG or IgM antibody to a bacterial pathogen is present and antibody-antigen complexes form, the complement system is activated starting with C1. C1 sequentially interacts with C4, C2, C3, C5, C6, C7, C8, and C9 (classic pathway). Activation of C3 results in cleavage of this molecule into two active fragments, C3a and C3b. C3a promotes polymorphonuclear leukocyte chemotaxis, while C3b adheres to bacterial cell walls forming a specific site for attachment to phagocyte cell membranes, thus significantly enhancing phagocytosis. Cleavage of C5 also produces chemotactic and opsonic fragments. In the absence of specific antibody, the complement system cannot be activated in the classic manner described above. Activation of an alternate pathway (the properdin system) may be initiated by lipopolysaccharides (endotoxin) in the absence of specific antibody. The alternate pathway joins the complement cascade at the C3 level and thus retains much of the biologic activity of the complement system, even though C1, C4, and C2 are bypassed.

Patients with C3 and C5 deficiencies have been described [60,61]. Alper and coworkers [60] described a patient with Kleinfelter's syndrome, a deficiency of C3, and a history of recurrent pneumonias, streptococcal and meningococcal sepsis, acute and chronic otitis, sinusitis, and mastoiditis. The patient's serum did not enhance phagocytosis of antibody-sensitized pneumococci and did not induce chemotaxis when incubated with antibody–antigen complexes. The total hemolytic complement level (CH_{50}) was also markedly depressed, 15 U/ml. The C3 deficiency in this patient was due to hypercatabolism of this complement component. C3 deficiency has been reported in a 15–yr–old girl with a similar spectrum of infection, but in her case the deficiency was due to a lack of synthesis rather than to hypercatabolism [62]. Patients with C5 dysfunction have been reported [61]. The clinical picture in these patients is dominated by chronic seborrheic dermatitis, diarrhea, and wasting (Leiner's syndrome). Although respiratory infections do occur, they are a relatively minor part of this syndrome.

Patients with sickle–cell anemia show an increased susceptibility to pneumococcal meningitis, septicemia, and pneumonia. Functional asplenia may, in part, explain the propensity for pneumococcal bacteremia observed in these patients. In addition, Winkelstein and Drachman [63] observed that the serum of patients with sickle–cell anemia were deficient in pneumococcal opsonins. In normal individuals and in patients with sickle–cell anemia antipneumococcal antibody titers are low, thus limiting opsonization through the classical pathway. While serum of normal individuals is capable of opsonizing pneumococci by activation of the alternate pathway, Johnston and coworkers [64] have shown that the serum of patients with sickle–cell disease is deficient in one of the components of the alternate pathway and is incapable of opsonizing pneumococci. The degree to which this impairment in phagocytosis contributes to recurrent pneumococcal infection, as well as the exact nature of the alternate pathway defect, remains to be elucidated.

C.   Inhibitors of Phagocyte Function

Increased susceptibility to infection may result from the presence of a humoral inhibitor of phagocyte function. Two patients with a serum inhibitor of neutrophil chemotaxis have been described [65,66]. Both patients had recurrent skin infection, purulent rhinitis, otitis media, recurrent pneumonia, and bronchitis. One patient also had disseminated cytomegalovirus infection [66]. Antibody and cell–mediated immunity, intracellular bacterial killing, and NBT tests were normal, but the Rebuck skin window showed absence of a polymorphonuclear leukocyte response. Serum from these patients was found to inhibit chemotaxis of their own as well as normal polymorphonuclear leukocytes. Normal plasma was found to contain an antagonist. Plasma transfusion corrected the defect in the Rebuck skin window response and resulted in a marked decrease in the susceptibility of these patients to infection.

Serum inhibitors of phagocyte function may effect cells other than poly-morphonuclear leukocytes. Boxerbaum and coworkers [67] described an inhibitor of pulmonary alveolar macrophage function in the serum of patients with cystic fibrosis. This factor inhibits both the phagocytosis and intracellular killing of *Pseudomonas* by rabbit pulmonary alveolar macrophages. This inhibitor is specific for *Pseudomonas* and does not inhibit the function of polymorphonuclear leukocytes. The inhibitor is extremely labile and is, as yet, poorly characterized. The relative importance of this factor in the pathogenesis of lung disease in cystic fibrosis has not as yet been determined.

V. Concluding Remarks

Clearly, a wide variety of defects in host–defense mechanisms result in increased susceptibility to respiratory tract infections and recurrent or chronic pulmonary disease. The spectrum of pulmonary manifestations of these immunodeficiency disorders is rather limited, and one frequently finds great difficulty in correlating a specific clinical picture to a specific immune defect in most cases. However, accurate diagnosis and an understanding of the pathogenesis of disease is essential before rational therapy can be instituted.

The diseases described in the preceding sections should serve to emphasize the need for establishing symbiotic relationships between pulmonary disease specialists and immunologists. Adequate assessment of immunologic competence must become an integral part of the evaluation of patients with recurrent or chronic pulmonary infections. When immunologic defects are identified, replacement or reconstitutive therapy may be life saving. However, when irreversible pulmonary damage has occurred, immunologic therapy may have a rather limited beneficial effect on the overall clinical course of patients. Thus, major emphasis must be placed upon early diagnosis, both by pulmonary specialist and immunologist, followed by immunologic therapy and preventive pulmonary care.

References

1. R. A. Gatti and R. A. Good, The immunological deficiency diseases, *Med. Clin. North Am.,* **54**:281–307 (1970).
2. E. R. Stiehm and V. A. Fulginiti. *Immunologic Disorders in Infants and Children.* Philadelphia, W. A. Saunders, 1973, pp. 145–330.
3. R. A. Good, W. D. Biggar, and B. H. Park, Immunodeficiency diseases of man. In *Progress in Immunology.* Edited by B. Amos. New York, Academic Press, 1972, pp. 699–722.

4. H. M. Grey, E. Rabellino, and B. Pirofsky, Immunoglobulins on the surface of lymphocytes. IV. Distribution in hypogammaglobulinemia, cellular immune deficiency, and chronic lymphatic leukemia, *J. Clin. Invest.*, **50**: 2368–2375 (1971).

5. M. D. Cooper, A. R. Lawton, and D. E. Bockman, Agammaglobulinaemia with B lymphocytes. Specific defect of plasma–cell differentiation, *Lancet*, 2:791–794 (1971).

6. B. A. Burke, L. J. Krovetz, and R. A. Good, Occurrence of Pneumocystitis carinii pneumonia in children with agammaglobulinemia, *Pediatrics*, **28**: 196–205 (1961).

7. J. B. Robbins, Pneumocystitis carinii pneumonitis. A review, *Pediatr. Res.*, 1:131–158 (1967).

8. D. G. Jose, R. A. Gatti, and R. A. Good, Eosinophilia with pneumocystis carinii pneumonia and immune deficiency syndromes, *J. Pediatr.*, **79**: 748–754 (1971).

9. P. D. Walzer, M. G. Schultz, K. A. Western, and J. B. Robbins, Pneumocystis carinii pneumonia and primary immune deficiency diseases of infancy and childhood, *J. Pediatr.*, **82**:416–422 (1973).

10. R. H. Buckley, Plasma therapy in immunodeficiency diseases, *Am J. Dis. Child.*, **124**:376–381 (1972).

11. P. F. Kohler and H. J. Müller–Eberhard, Complement–immunoglobulin relation: Deficiency of C′-1q associated with impaired immunoglobulin G synthesis, *Science*, **163**:474–475 (1968).

12. H. Gewurz, R. J. Pickering, C. L. Christian, R. Snyderman, S. E. Mergenhagen, and R. A. Good, Decreased C′-1q protein concentration and agglutinating activity in agammaglobulinaemia syndromes: An inborn error reflected in the complement system, *Clin. Ex. Immunol.*, **3**:437–445 (1968).

13. S. D. Douglas, L. S. Goldberg, and H. H. Fudenberg, Clinical serologic and leukocyte function studies on patients with idiopathic "acquired" agammaglobulinemia and their families, *Am. J. Med.*, **48**:48–53 (1970).

14. F. S. Rosen, S. V. Kevy, E. Merler, C. A. Janeway, and D. Gitlin, Recurrent bacterial infections and dysgamma–globulinemia: Deficiency of 7 S gamma–globulins in the presence of elevated 19 S gamma globulin. Report of two cases, *Pediatrics*, **28**:182–195 (1961).

15. E. R. Stiehm and H. H. Fudenberg, Clinical and immunologic features of dysgammaglobulinemia type I. Report of a case diagnosed in the first year of life, *Am. J. Med.*, **40**:805–815 (1966).

16. J. F. Soothill, K. Hayes, and J. A. Dudgeon, The immunoglobulins in congenital rubella, *Lancet*, 1:1385–1388 (1966).

17. R. N. Schimke, C. Bolano, and C. H. Kirkpatrick, Immunologic deficiency in the congenital rubella syndrome, *Am. J. Dis. Child.*, **118**:626–633 (1969).

18. W. D. Terry, Variations in the subclasses of IgG. In *Immunologic Deficiency Diseases in Man*. Birth Defects Orig. Art. Ser. Vol. 4. No. 1. Edited by D. Bergsma. New York, The National Foundation, 1968, pp. 357–363.

19. P. H. Schur, H. Borel, E. W. Gelfand, C. A. Alper, and F. S. Rosen, Selective gamma G globulin deficiencies in patients with recurrent pyogenic infections, *N. Engl. J. Med.,* **283**:631–634 (1970).

20. W. J. Yount, M. M. Dorner, H. G. Kunkel, and E. A. Kabat, Studies on human antibodies. VI. Selective variations in subgroup composition and genetic markers, *J. Exp. Med.,* **127**:633–646 (1968).

21. T. E. Blecher, J. F. Soothill, M. A. Voyce, and W. H. C. Walker, Antibody deficiency syndrome: A case with normal immunoglobulin levels, *Clin. Exp. Immunol.,* **3**:47–56 (1968).

22. R. H. Buckley, B. B. Wray, and E. Z. Belmaker, Extreme hyperimmunoglobulinemia E and undue susceptibility to infection, *Pediatrics,* **48**: 59–70 (1972).

23. S. D. Davis, Antibody deficiency diseases. In *Immunologic Disorders of Infants and Children.* Edited by E. R. Stiehm and V. A. Fulginiti. Philadelphia, W. B. Saunders, 1973, pp. 193–194.

24. A. J. Ammann, W. A. Cain, K. Ishizaka, R. Hong, and R. A. Good, Immunoglobulin E deficiency in ataxia–telangiectasia, *N. Engl. J. Med.,* **281**:469–472 (1969).

25. W. A. Cain, A. J. Ammann, R. Hong, K. Ishizaka, and R. A. Good, IgE deficiency associated with chronic sinopulmonary infection, *J. Clin. Invest.,* **48**:12A–13A (1969).

26. D. A. Levy and J. Chen, Healthy IgE–deficient person, *N. Engl. J. Med.,* **283**:541–542 (1970).

27. G. J. Gleich, A. K. Averbeck, and H. A. Swedlund, Measurement of IgE in normal and allergic serum by radioimmunoassay, *J. Lab. Clin Med.,* **77**: 690–698 (1971).

28. S. H. Polmar, T. A. Waldmann, S. T. Balestra, M. C. Jost, and W. D. Terry, Immunoglobulin E in immunologic deficiency diseases. I. Relation of IgE and IgA to respiratory tract disease in isolated IgE deficiency, IgA deficiency, and ataxia telangiectasia, *J. Clin. Invest.,* **51**:326–330 (1972).

29. S. H. Polmar, T. A. Waldmann, and W. D. Terry, IgE in immunodeficiency, *Am. J. Pathol.,* **69**:499–512 (1972).

30. A. J. Ammann and R. Hong, Selective IgA deficiency: Presentation of 30 cases and a review of the literature, *Medicine,* **50**:223–236 (1971).

31. J. H. Rockey, L. A. Hansen, J. F. Heremans, and H. G. Kunkel, Beta–2A aglobulinemia in two healthy men, *J. Lab. Clin. Med.,* **63**:205–212 (1964).

32. L. S. Goldberg, E. V. Barnett, and H. H. Fudenberg, Selective absence of IgA: A family study, *J. Lab. Clin. Med.,* **72**:204–212 (1968).

33. R. Bachmann, Studies on the serum gamma–A–globulin level. 3. The frequency of A–gamma–A–globulinemia, *Scand. J. Clin. Lab. Invest.,* **17**: 316–320 (1965).

34. A. J. Ammann, J. Roth, and R. Hong, Recurrent sinopulmonary infections, mental retardation, and combined IgA and IgE deficiency, *J. Pediatr.,* **77**: 802–804 (1970).

35. D. P. Schwartz and R. H. Buckley, Serum IgE concentrations and skin reactivity to anti–IgE antibody in IgA–deficient patients, *N. Engl. J. Med.,* **284**:513–517 (1971).

36. W. C. Levin, S. E. Ritzman, M. E. Haggard, R. G. Gregory, and J. A. Reinarz, Selective A–Beta–2–A–Globulinemia, *Clin. Res.,* **11**:694 (1963).
37. I. Krieger and J. A. Brough, Gamma–A deficiency and hypochronic anemia due to defective iron mobilization, *N. Engl. J. Med.,* **276**:886–894 (1967).
38. N. Matsaniotis, A. Constantopoulous, and J. Karpouzas, Immunoglobulin levels in idiopathic pulmonary hemosiderosis, *Lancet,* **2**:1078 (1969).
39. D. C. Heiner and J. W. Sears, Chronic respiratory disease associated with multiple circulating precipitins to cow's milk, *Am. J. Dis. Child.,* **100**:500–502 (1960).
40. C. C. Huntley, J. B. Robbins, A. D. Lyerly, and R. H. Buckley, Characterization of precipitating antibodies to ruminant serum and milk proteins in humans with selective IgA deficiency, *N. Engl., J. Med.,* **284**:7–10 (1971).
41. T. F. Boat, V. Whitman, S. H. Polmar, C. F. Doershuk, R. C. Stern, and L. W. Matthews, Upper airway obstruction and heart failure in patients with Heiner's Syndrome, *Pediatr. Res.,* **8**:465 (1974).
42. A. M. Di George, Congenital absence of the thymus and its immunologic consequences: Concurrence with congenital hypoparathyroidism. In *Immunologic Deficiency Diseases in Man.* Edited by D. Bergsma and R. A. Good. National Foundation Birth Defects Orig. Art. Ser. Vol. 4, No. 1. Baltimore, Williams and Wilkins Company, 1968, pp. 116–121.
43. W. W. Cleveland, B. J. Fogel, W. T. Brown, and H. E. M. Kay, Foetal thymic transplant in a case of Di George's syndrome, *Lancet,* **2**:1211–1214 (1968).
44. C. S. August, F. S. Rosen, R. M. Filler, C. A. Janeway, B. Markowski, and H. E. M. Kay, Implantation of a foetal thymus, restoring immunological competence in a patient with thymic aplasia (Di George's syndrome), *Lancet,* **2**:1210–1211 (1968).
45. W. H. Hitzig, Congenital thymic and lymphocytic deficiency syndromes. In *Immunologic Disorders in Infants and Children.* Edited by E. R. Stiehm and V. A. Fulginiti. Philadelphia, W. B. Saunders Company, 1973, pp. 218–228.
46. J. A. Kirkpatrick, M. A. Capitano, and R. M. Pereira, Immunologic abnormalities: Roentgen observations, *Radiol. Clin. North Am.,* **10**:245–259 (1972).
47. S. Stone, Interstitial plasma cell pneumonia (pneumocystis carinii pneumonia). In *Disorders of the Respiratory Tract in Children.* Vol. I. Edited by E. Kendig. Philadelphia, W. A. Saunders, 1972, pp. 254–258.
48. R. A. Gatti, H. J. Meuwissen, H. D. Allen, R. Hong, and R. A. Good, Immunological reconstitution of sex–linked lymphopenic immunological deficiency, *Lancet,* **2**:1366–1369 (1968).
49. A. S. Levin, L. E. Spitler, and H. H. Fudenberg, Transfer factor therapy in immune deficiency states, *Annu. Rev. Med.,* **24**:175–208 (1973).
50. C. H. Kirkpatrick and W. E. Ruth, Chronic pulmonary disease and immunologic deficiency, *Am. J. Med.,* **41**:427–439 (1966).
51. W. L. Koop, J. S. Trier, E. R. Stiehm, and P. Foroozan, "Acquired" agammaglobulinemia with defective delayed hypersensitivity, *Ann. Intern. Med.,* **69**:309–317 (1968).

52. J. I. Tennenbaum, R. L. St. Pierre, and G. J. Cerilli, Chronic pulmonary disease associated with an unusual dysgammaglobulinaemia, *Clin. Exp. Immunol.*, 3:983–988 (1968).

53. G. Karpati, A. H. Eisen, F. Andermann, H. L. Bacal, and P. Robb, Ataxia-telangiectasia: Further observations and report of eight cases, *Am. J. Dis. Child.*, 110:51–63 (1965).

54. D. E. McFarlin, W. Strober, and T. A. Waldmann, Ataxia–telangiectasia, *Medicine*, 51:281–314 (1972).

55. C. H. Kirkpatrick, R. R. Rich, and J. E. Bennett, Chronic mucocutaneous candidiasis: Model building in cellular immunity, *Ann. Intern. Med.*, 74:955–978 (1971).

56. J. S. Louie and L. S. Goldberg, Lymphocyte–monocyte defect associated with anergy and recurrent infections, *Clin. Exp. Immunol.*, 11:469–474 (1972).

57. Q. N. Myrvik, Function of the alveolar macrophage in immunity, *J. Reticuloendothiel. Soc.*, 11:459–468 (1972).

58. J. J. Wolfson, P. G. Quie, S. D. Laxdal, and R. A. Good, Roentgenologic manifestations in children with a genetic defect of polymorphonuclear leukocyte function. Chronic granulomatous disease of childhood, *Radiology*, 91:37–48 (1968).

59. D. G. Nathan, R. L. Baehner, and D. K. Weaver, Failure of nitro blue tetrazolium reduction in the phagocytic vacuoles of leukocytes in chronic granulomatous disease, *J. Clin. Invest.*, 48:1895–1904 (1969).

60. C. A. Alper, N. Abramson, R. B. Johnston, Jr., J. H. Jandl, and F. S. Rosen, Increased susceptibility to infection associated with abnormalities of complement–mediated functions and of the third component of complement (C3). *N. Engl. J. Med.*, 282:350–354 (1970).

61. J. C. Jacobs and M. E. Miller, Fatal familial Leiner's disease: A deficiency of the opsonic activity of serum complement, *Pediatrics*, 49:225–232 (1972).

62. C. A. Alper, H. R. Colten, F. S. Rosen, A. R. Rabson, G. M. MacNab, and J. S. S. Gear, Homozygous deficiency of C3 in a patient with repeated infections, *Lancet*, 2:1179–1181 (1972).

63. J. A. Winkelstein and R. H. Drachman, Deficiency of pneumococcal serum opsonizing activity in sickle–cell disease, *N. Engl. J. Med.*, 279:459–466 (1968).

64. R. B. Johnston, S. L. Newman, and A. G. Struth, An abnormality of the alternate pathway of complement activation in sickle–cell disease, *N. Engl. J. Med.*, 288:803–808 (1973).

65. C. W. Smith, J. C. Hollers, E. Dupree, A. S. Goldman, and R. A. Lord, A serum inhibitor of leukotaxis in a child with recurrent infections, *J. Lab. Clin. Med.*, 79:878–885 (1972).

66. R. B. Soriano, M. A. South, A. S. Goldman, and C. W. Smith, Defect of neutrophil mobility in a child with recurrent bacterial infections and disseminated cytomegalovirus infection, *J. Pediatr.*, 83:951–958 (1973).

67. B. Boxerbaum, M. Kagumba, and L. W. Matthews, Selective inhibition of phagocytic activity of rabbit alveolar macrophages by cystic fibrosis serum, *Am. Rev. Respir. Dis.*, 108:777–783 (1973).

11

Asthma and Atopic Hypersensitivity

CHARLES H. KIRKPATRICK

National Institute of Allergy and Infectious Diseases
National Institutes of Health
Bethesda, Maryland

I. Introduction

Asthma, a common form of intermittent airways obstruction, has been defined by the American Thoracic Society as a disease characterized by increased responsiveness of the trachea and bronchi to various stimuli and manifested by a widespread narrowing of the airways that changes in severity either spontaneously or as a result of therapy [1]. By avoiding mention of specific etiologic agents or provocative events, this definition illustrates that the physiologic abnormalities in subjects with asthma are rather constant and that a common denominator in these patients is exaggerated responses of the airways to a variety of factors, such as inhaled pollen granules; dusts, danders, and noxious chemicals; ingested drugs and foodstuffs; psychologic disturbances; exertion; environmental and climatic changes; and infections.

In many patients acute episodes are precipitated by exposure to antigens, and recent research has defined many of the relationships between immunologic reactions and the release of mediators directly responsible for the functional abnormalities. In other patients, especially those in whom acute asthma is precipitated by infections or drugs, such as aspirin, the mechanisms of airways obstruction are poorly understood.

In spite of the heterogeneity of factors that provoke episodes of asthma, several lines of evidence suggest that there may be a common pathway that leads to the physiologic abnormalities, and that this pathway may be activated or triggered by a variety of stimuli. For instance, physiologic studies during acute asthma have demonstrated qualitatively similar abnormalities, including diffuse obstruction, especially in the small airways [2-5], nonuniform ventilation [6], and regional changes in ventilation–perfusion ratios [7]. In severe attacks there may be hypoxia and cyanosis. It is noteworthy that the pattern of physiologic changes during acute episodes is apparently unrelated to the etiology of the attack.

The pathologic changes in the lungs of patients with asthma are also remarkably similar from patient to patient. The reversible episodes of airways obstruction have at least three components: (a) widespread spasm of bronchial smooth muscle, (b) edema of bronchial mucosa, and (c) occlusion of airways by mucus [8]. Histologically, there may be hypertrophy of bronchial smooth muscle, hyperplasia of mucous glands, thickening of bronchial basement membranes, and infiltration of peribronchial tissues and intraluminal debris with eosinophils [9].

A third characteristic suggestive of a common pathway in the pathogenesis of asthma is the extraordinary sensitivity of patients with asthma to the bronchoconstrictive effects of inhaled histamine and methacholine (mecholyl, acetyl-β-methyl choline) [10-12]. In fact, this response is so typical that Spector and Farr [13] stated that a positive mecholyl response in an asymptomatic patient is highly suggestive that he has reversible obstructive airways disease; a negative test should suggest other diagnoses.

This chapter will review selected immunologic and pharmacologic aspects of asthma. Since most cases of asthma occur in allergic or atopic persons, emphasis will be placed on the immunologic characteristics of the atopic state. Because of its possible contribution to the hypothetical "common pathway" in asthma, the hypothesis that atopic patients have an imbalance of partial blockade of responses of the autonomic nervous system will be considered. The mechanisms of immunologic release of pharmacologic mediators in asthma (and probably other allergic diseases) and their control at the cellular level are reviewed in Chapter 21.

II. The Atopic Patient

The term "atopy" was introduced by Coca and Cooke [14] to designate a population of patients in which disorders, such as allergic rhinitis, asthma, and atopic dermatitis, were common. Genetic studies of allergic diseases and reaginic (IgE) antibody synthesis are reviewed in detail in Chapter 20 and will be mentioned only briefly here. It is well known that allergic disorders cluster in families, but the mode of genetic transmission is unclear.´ Interpretation of family studies is complicated by the fact that members of the same pedigree often show considerable variability in both the clinical expression and severity of allergic diseases [15]. However, a genetic predisposition to allergy is supported by several studies, including the survey by Schwartz [16] of the incidence of allergic diseases and other illnesses in families of patients with asthma, which showed that allergic rhinitis, vasomotor rhinitis, and eczema (in females) occurred with significantly increased frequencies. There were no statistically significant associations between asthma and migraine, gastrointestinal allergy, epilepsy, or a number of skin diseases. Other family studies have examined the incidence of allergy among identical and fraternal twins. In general, the prevalence of allergic disorders among dizygotic twins was the same as that among ordinary siblings, whereas concordance for allergic diseases among monozygotic twins was more common. The literature review reported by Schade [17] showed that 59% of monozygotic twins, but only 12% of dizygotic twins, were concordant for atopy. Recently, Edfors-Lubs [18] reported a study of 7000 twin-pairs in which somewhat lower concordance numbers (number of concordant pairs per number of pairs in which the disease occurred in one or both members) were found. The values for monozygotic and dizygotic twin-pairs for asthma was 19 and 4.8, respectively; for allergic rhinitis, 21.4 and 13.7; and for eczema, 15.5 and 4.0. Thus, although genetic factors contribute to the predisposition for the development of allergic diseases, they apparently do not dictate which disorder will be expressed by the patient.

A second characteristic of atopic patients is a unique antibody response to inhaled antigens, a phenomenon that has been studied in depth by Salvaggio and coworkers [19-22]. Atopic patients responded to intranasal immunizations with protein (ribonuclease, tetanus toxoid, or hemocyanin) and carbohydrate (dextran) antigens by producing high titers of skin-sensitizing antibodies [19-22]. In contrast, immediate-type responses to skin tests were rarely observed in normal subjects immunized by the same schedule. When the same antigens were given parenterally, both atopics and controls had similar antibody responses, an observation that argued against the possibilities that control subjects were constitutionally unresponsive to the antigens or „processed" the antigens along nonimmunologic pathways [23,24]. Subsequent experiments showed that differences between the two groups were not due to differences in the permeability of mucous membranes to antigens [25].

Recently, it has been reported that atopic subjects responded to intranasal immunizations with tetanus toxoid with lower IgA, but higher IgE antibodies than controls [26]. Moreover, Taylor and coworkers [27] reported that children with IgA deficiency frequently develop infantile eczema, and Buckley and Dees [28] noted an increased frequency of milk antibodies in patients with IgA deficiency. These observations are compatible with Salvaggio's suggestion that an important component of the pathogenesis of certain atopic bypersensitivities may be the inability of atopic subjects to synthesize adequate amounts of secretory IgA antibodies to protect mucous membranes from inhaled antigens.

Presumably, the same phenomenon applies to ingested antigens. Indeed, studies of the fate of inhaled pollen granules have shown that essentially all of the granules were deposited on the oropharyngeal mucosa and then swallowed. Only soluble pollen extract and perhaps fragments of pollen granules actually entered the airways [29,30].

A. Biologic Aspects of IgE

The critical role of IgE antibodies in the pathogenesis of many allergic diseases has been established by a variety of observations. Surveys of allergic patients have shown that serum [31-39] and respiratory secretions [39-41] from most patients with allergic asthma or atopic dermatitis contain significantly elevated concentrations of IgE whereas serum IgE is often normal in patients with rhinitis without asthma or atopic dermatitis and in patients with intrinsic or infectious asthma. Curiously, serum from patients with urticaria may contain low concentrations of IgE [32]. Seasonal exposures of atopic patients to environmental antigens induce synthesis of IgE antibodies [37,39], and the same antigens that provoke symptoms cause immediate-type wheal and flare responses when injected into the skin of allergic subjects. Finally, IgE antibodies passively sensitize leukocytes and lung fragments for antigen-dependent release of histamine and slow-reacting substance of anaphylaxis.

A prognostic relationship of IgE-mediated skin reactions to the subsequent development of clinical allergy has been suggested by the observations of Hagy and Settipane [42]. When college students were scratch-tested as freshman and reinterviewed as seniors, 4.7% had developed new symptomatic allergies. The most common disorder was seasonal hayfever and the occurrence of this disorder was significantly more frequent in subjects who were scratch-test positive when tested as asymptomatic freshmen. Hayfever developed in 18 of 108 (16.7%) skin-test positive students, but in only 9 of 506 (1.8%) skin-test negative subjects. There were no relationships between skin-test responses and the subsequent development of nonseasonal rhinitis or asthma, although the numbers of new cases of these disorders were small. These observations illustrate the association between reaginic antibody responses and clinical disorders and that synthesis of reaginic antibodies may precede the onset of symptomatic allergy.

Finally, recent studies indicated that the capacity of patients with ragweed pollenosis to develop reaginic antibodies is influenced by genetic factors and may be linked to genetic determinants for histocompatibility (HL-A) antigens [43-45]. Levine *et al.* [43] found that IgE antibody production to ragweed antigen E, by members of successive generations, was associated with certain haplotypes, although not necessarily with the same HL-A antigens. Marsh and coworkers [44] reported a strong correlation between HL-A7 and reaginic antibody responses to the ragweed antigen RA 5.

Sullivan *et al.* [46] demonstrated IgE molecules on the membranes of blood basophils by electron microscopy, and Ishizaka and coworkers [47] reported that the numbers of IgE molecules on basophils from normal donors was significantly less than the number on basophils from atopic subjects (17,857 ±2719 vs. 25,700 ±3266 molecules per cell, $P = <0.05$). The mean number of IgE molecules bound per cell was not a function of the serum IgE concentration, and after the cell receptors were saturated by incubating the cells with an IgE myeloma protein, there was no significant difference between the mean number of molecules bound by cells from normal and atopic subjects. Thus, in the "resting state," cells from atopic patients have a greater number of basophilic receptor sites occupied by IgE. The potential biologic significance of this finding is illustrated by the fact that there is a rough inverse relationship between the mean number of IgE molecules on cells and the concentration of anti-IgE required for maximal histamine release [47], suggesting that cells from atopic subjects may be partially "primed" for histamine release by the increased numbers of IgE molecules on cell membranes.

While little is known about the regulation of IgE antibody synthesis in man, it has been the subject of intense study in rodents. As with other antibody classes, optimal synthesis of IgE antibodies depends on the dose and schedule of immunization of antigen and on critical interactions between thymus-derived T cells and bone marrow-derived B cells [48-50]. Tada and coworkers [51-53] reported that the synthesis of IgE-like homocytotropic antibodies in rats is prolonged and enhanced if the animals are irradiated, splenectomized, thymectomized, or treated with one of several immunosuppressive drugs shortly before immunization. The enhancing effect of thymectomy was noted only with animals operated on as young adults; neonatally thymectomized rats were poor antibody producers. Synthesis of IgE antibodies could be terminated by administering 7 S γG serum from intact rats immunized with the same antigen [54], or by infusing thymocytes or spleen cells from donors immunized with the homologous hapten-carrier combination or the homologous carrier alone [55]. Cells from animals immunized with the homologous hapten on a different carrier were not effective. Thus, the thymus appears to be essential for maturation of this immune response in early life and for regulating homocytotropic antibody synthesis in mature animals.

In subsequent experiments Tada *et al.* [56,57] found that IgE production could be terminated by administering a soluble extract of thymus cells from immune animals. The composition of the active material is unknown, but the activity was sensitive to digestion with trypsin and pronase but resistant to deoxyribonuclease and ribonuclease. The activity of the extract was removed by absorption with hapten–carrier or carrier alone, but not by antisera to rat immunoglobulins. The mechanism of the suppressive effect is also unclear, but from measurements of the rate of decay of serum antibody titers Tada *et al.* [57] suggested that the extract affects antibody-secreting cells rather than undifferentiated precursor cells.

Conceivably, these observations on the modulating effects on IgE synthesis of cells, cell extracts, or specific antisera, may have application in treating certain allergic diseases. For example, specific immunotherapy may stimulate production of IgG antibodies that, in turn, could suppress IgE synthesis (Chapter 22).

B. Non–IgE Reaginic Antibodies

Many rodents have two classes of homocytotropic antibodies: one analogous to IgE and the second residing in a subclass of IgG. The IgG antibodies are relatively resistant to denaturation by heat and will interact with antigens to cause anaphylaxis soon after passive administration to nonallergic animals These properties are in contrast to IgE antibodies, which are heat-labile and have a latent period before they passively sensitize normal animals [58].

Although the reaginic activity in most allergic patients is IgE antibody, there is also evidence implicating non–IgE antibodies. For example, not all allergic patients have elevated levels of serum IgE. Specific IgE antibodies connot be identified in the sera of some patients with asthma who have positive responses to inhaled antigens and in some in whom attacks cannot be prevented by disodium cromoglycate (DSCG), a drug that effectively inhibits IgE–mediated histamine release.

In 1966 Reid *et al.* [59] reported skin-fixing antibody activity in the IgG fraction of several atopic sera. This report preceded the discovery of IgE, and it is unclear if their preparations also contained IgE. Subsequently, Parish [60] described an IgG–like skin sensitizing antibody in the serum of some allergic patients. This antibody sensitized monkey skin for cutaneous anaphylaxis at 2 and 4 hr, but not 24 hours after intradermal injection. The activity remained in sera after heating at 56°C for 2 hr, and active fractions from DEAE chromatographically-fractionated sera contained IgG but no detectable IgE. Recently, Bryant *et al.* [61] confirmed these observations in a group of skin-test positive patients with asthma who were not protected from antigenic challenges by DSCG. By passive cutaneous anaphylaxis, it was shown that the reaginic activity in the serum of eight of the patients was heat-stable and had a short latent period. This activity, too, was in the IgG-containing fractions from chromatographic columns.

These observations suggest that some allergic patients possess a non-IgE antibody that may react with antigen to cause release of histamine. Parish [60] suggested that antibodies of this type may contribute to tissue changes in chronic allergic reactions, such as hypersensitivity pneumonitis or vasculitis. It is uncertain whether they are directly related to acute allergic reactions, such as asthma or allergic rhinitis, but it is conceivable that this immune response may characterize a subpopulation of patients with a unique pathogenesis and in whom different therapeutic schedules may be required.

C. Cell-mediated Immunity

There is no direct evidence that cell-mediated immunity is involved in the pathogenesis of asthma or most other acute allergic diseases. Indeed, they are considered prototypes of the Type 1 allergic responses mediated by reaginic antibodies. However, in some cases of asthma and hypersensitivity pneumonitis, sensitizing exposures have elicited both humoral and cell-mediated immune responses. Brostoff and Roitt [62] reported that delayed cutaneous responses to grass extracts could be demonstrated in pollen-sensitive patients if the antigen and an antihistamine were injected together. This phenomenon was not found in a recent study of patients with ragweed pollenosis [63]. However, several laboratories have shown that blood lymphocytes from patients with pollenosis or hypersensitivity pneumonitis will respond to antigens in vitro with enhanced DNA synthesis and lymphokine production [63-70], even when the patients did not show delayed cutaneous reactions to the same antigens [63,69,70]. In some cases treatment with specific immunotherapy was accompanied by reduced antigen-induced blastogenic responses [66-69].

The clinical significance of these observations is unclear. Experiments described in Chapters 3, 4, and 7 show that immunization of animals via the respiratory tract may be followed by both humoral and cellular immune responses in the lung, but only feeble systemic immune responses. Allergic humans apparently have a more complex immune response to inhaled environmental antigens. In addition to the humoral (predominantly IgE) responses discussed earlier, they apparently develop some components of cell-mediated immunity. Future experiments should determine whether these responses involve T or B lymphocytes or both and should identify the role of these responses in the pathogenesis of or resistance to immunologic lung diseases.

III. Immunopathology of Asthmatic Lungs

In addition to the previously described bronchial edema, hyperplasia of mucous glands and tissue eosinophilia [8,9], it has been shown that immunoglobulins may be deposited in the lungs of asthmatic patients. In their report, McCarter and Vasquez [71] noted that 50% of tissues from nonasthmatic controls also had similar deposits and they concluded that deposition of gamma globulins was nonspecific. Callerame et al. [72,73] studied the classes of immunoglobulins in basement membranes and infiltrating cells in mainstem bronchi of 18 asthmatics. IgM was identified in the basement membranes of 11; IgG and IgA were each present in seven specimens; C3 and fibrinogen were rarely found; and IgE was never detected in the basement membrane. Control tissues from uninflamed areas did not contain immunoglobulins.

Mononuclear cells containing immunoglobulins occurred in clusters among the submucous glands and just below the basement membranes. Cells staining for each of the immunoglobulin classes were identified, although IgE cells were least frequent. However, immunoglobulin-containing cells were also common in tissues from subjects who were not asthmatic and the frequency of these cells was directly related to the intensity of the inflammatory response in the tissues.

A similar study of autopsy specimens from patients with asthma gave different results [74]; IgE was detected in the epithelium and basement membranes of small bronchi and bronchioles and in intraluminal mucus; deposits containing IgE were observed more frequently than other immunoglobulins.

The importance of immunoglobulins in these tissues is currently unclear. Presumably IgE antibodies in the epithelium could interact with inhaled antigens, although, as discussed above, only small amounts of inhaled particulate antigens reach the lower airways [29,30]. A more complex model of allergic inflammation, based on experiments in rabbits, has been proposed by Cochrane [75]. According to this model, antigenic stimulation results in the production of both circulating antigen-antibody complexes and IgE-like homocytotropic antibodies. The interaction of an antigen with antibody-coated basophils leads to the release of a platelet aggregating factor. The platelets, in turn, release a vasoactive substance that allows circulating immune complexes to deposit in tissues, with the subsequent production of local inflammatory responses. A similar sequence in the lungs of patients with asthma could account for the variety of immunoglobulins observed in pulmonary tissues.

A. Autonomic Mechanisms in Asthma

The airways of many animals are controlled by the autonomic nervous system. In general, cholinergic stimulation causes bronchoconstriction, whereas adrenergic stimulation causes bronchodilation. In fact, cholinergic fibers in the vagus mediate the bronchoconstrictive effects of many stimuli. Inhaled histamine has a direct effect on smooth muscle, but in dogs much of the bronchoconstrictive activity of histamine is indirect and transmitted by the vagus [76]. In laboratory animals and some patients with asthma the severity of bronchoconstriction following antigen–induced histamine release is markedly reduced by cholinergic blockade or by vagotomy [77-80]. Even in normal subjects stimulation of sensory receptors in the larynx or airways, by nonantigenic irritating particles or chemicals, may cause coughing and bronchoconstriction, and this response can be prevented by vagotomy or atropine [81-84]. In patients with asthma the threshold at which these bronchoconstrictive responses are elicited are far lower than in normal subjects, and these responses, too, are susceptible to cholinergic blockade [85].

Direct sympathetic innervation of the airways is limited and apparently directed at inhibiting cholinergic stimuli [86]. The main source of adrenergic activity on the airways is the circulating catecholamines, which interact with β-adrenergic receptors to produce bronchodilation.

Szentivanyi [87] has suggested that a common denominator, leading to bronchoconstriction in asthma, could be decreased responsiveness to β-adrenergic stimuli. This hypothesis derived from experiments in mice that had been rendered exquisitely sensitive to the lethal effects of histamine and serotonin by pretreatment with *Bordetella pertussis* vaccine. Subsequent experiments showed that a similar state of histamine hypersensitivity could be produced by treating the mice with β-adrenergic blocking drugs. As a corollary to this hypothesis, Szentivanyi also postulated that the β-adrenergic receptor was the enzyme adenyl cyclase.

The potential relationship of this hypothesis to human asthma prompted a number of investigations of autonomic responses in subjects with asthma. Cookson and Reed [88] reported that asthmatics responded to β-agonists with less hyperglycemia and less peripheral vasodilatation than do controls. In other studies subjects with asthma responded to stimulation with β-agonists with subnormal increments of blood glucose [89-91], lactate [91], free fatty acids [92, 93], decreased eosinopenia [94], or bradycardia [92,95], although these findings have not always been confirmed [96]. Moreover, McNeill [97] reported that the β-adrenergic blocker, propranolol, caused acute bronchoconstriction in patients with asthma. Each of these observations is compatible with the notion that subjects with asthma have an imbalance in adrenergic responses, most likely in the form of partial blockade of the β-adrenergic receptors. With respect to the initial model in the pertussis vaccine-treated mice, Sen and coworkers [98] recently reported that normal children had increased cutaneous responses to histamine and decreased vasopressor and hyperglycemic responses to epinephrine shortly after they received routine immunizations with diphtheria–pertussis–tetanus (DPT) vaccine. Similar effects were not seen in children immunized with diphtheria–tetanus (DT) vaccine.

Some of the physiologic changes in asthmatics may be related to chronic therapy with sympathomimetic drugs [91]. Nelson and associates [99,100] reported similar abnormalities in normal volunteers after the administration of ephedrine or epinephrine, and these effects persisted for many hours after treatment with the drugs ceased.

Studies with blood leukocytes from patients with asthma have provided additional support for autonomic imbalance. Stimulation of these cells with β-agonists in vitro has produced increments of cellular cyclic adenosine monophosphate (CAMP) that are significantly less than those observed with cells from normal subjects [101,102]. CAMP is the product of activity of the enzyme adenyl cyclase and these observations are also compatible with Szentivanyi's β-adrenergic blockade theory. In general, the impaired responses were most striking in patients with active, severe asthma, but minimal or absent in patients with asthma of recent onset or asthma that was inactive. In fact, studies with identical twins showed that impaired β-adrenergic responses were present only in the symptomatic sibling [103]. These clinical observations, together with Szentivanyi's mouse data suggest that impaired autonomic responses in patients with asthma are acquired rather than congenital. It is also of interest that the abnormality in CAMP synthesis is less marked in patients with asthma who are receiving steroid therapy [101,102] and that a similar defect in leukocyte CAMP synthesis could not be produced in normal subjects by administering ephedrine for 2 wk [102].

B. Asthma and Respiratory Infections

It is well-known that acute episodes of asthma may be provoked by respiratory infections. Although the sputum often appears purulent, cultures usually yield normal respiratory flora rather than a recognized pathogen. This has prompted the suggestion that patients with asthma may be "allergic" to bacterial products, either from the normal flora or from foreign organisms that were not detected. Direct evidence for bacterial allergy in these patients is essentially nil and attempts to treat patients by desensitization with bacterial vaccines have had questionable benefits.

One mechanism through which microorganisms may predispose asthma to an acute episode has been described by Reed and associates [11,104]. Significant increases in the bronchoconstrictive responses to methacholine aerosols were noted both during acute respiratory infections and following immunization with killed influenze vaccine. These observations assume special significance in view of recent evidence that many asthma-provoking infections are due to viruses. In one report 58 of 139 episodes of wheezing were associated with identifiable viruses; respiratory syncytial and parainfluenzae, Type II viruses, were most frequently isolated [105]. In a prospective study of somewhat older children, 42 of 61 episodes of asthma were coincident with a symptomatic respiratory infection [106]. Rhinoviruses were the most commonly identified agent.

The mechanism of exacerbation of asthma during acute respiratory infections is unclear. Recent studies [107,108] have shown that even mild upper respiratory infections may cause obstruction of small airways, which persists long after the causative episode has resolved. Thus, it seems probable that acute episodes of asthma during infection may be precipitated through several mechanisms. Acute infections may increase the production of mucus, which partially occludes the airways. The threshold for bronchoconstrictive stimuli may be decreased through some activity in microbial material, and, finally, even mild upper respiratory tract infections may be accompanied by the obstruction of small airways.

IV. Concluding Comments

A goal of this chapter has been to review some of the immunologic and physiologic components of atopic hypersensitivities. Atopic patients differ from normal subjects in that they respond to environmental antigens, especially those encountered on mucous membranes, by producing reaginic antibodies. In most cases these antibodies are IgE immunoglobulins, but in some patients IgG reagins may be important. A consequence of this antibody synthesis is sensitization of mast cells for antigen-induced release of mediators, which, in turn, elicit physiologic components of the diseases. The possibility that atopic patients may also be deficient in production of secretory IgA antibodies, which would "protect" against transmembrane sensitization, is currently uncertain.

In addition to the immunologic component, many patients with asthma are unusually sensitive to the bronchoconstrictive activities of histamine and cholinergic agonists, and some evidence indicates that excessive cholinergic activity may render mast cells more susceptible to antigen-mediated mediator release.

Finally, some patients with asthma apparently have a partial blockade of β-adrenergic responses, a phenomenon which could compound the effects of excessive cholinergic activity. The evidence for β-blockade is most pronounced during acute asthmatic episodes and in the most severely ill patients, but it is unclear whether the phenomenon is a consequence of the event that provoked the acute asthmatic episode or is itself a pre-existing or inciting factor.

References

1. American Thoracic Society. Chronic bronchitis, asthma, and pulmonary emphysema: A statement by the Committee on Diagnostic Standards for nontuberculous respiratory diseases, *Am. Rev. Respir. Dis.,* **85**:762–768 (1962).

2. G. Levine, E. Housley, P. MacLeod, and P. T. Macklem, Gas exchange abnormalities in mild bronchitis and asymptomatic asthma, *N. Engl. J. Med.,* **282**:1277–1282 (1970).

3. D. J. Hill, L. I. Landau, and P. D. Phelan, Small airway disease in asymptomatic asthmatic adolescents, *Am. Rev. Respir. Dis.,* **106**:873–880 (1972).

4. E. R. McFadden, R. Kiser, and W. J. DeGroot, Acute bronchial asthma. Relations between clinical and physiologic manifestations, *N. Engl. J. Med.,* **288**:221–225 (1973).

5. K. N. V. Palmer and G. R. Kelman, A comparison of pulmonary function in extrinsic and intrinsic bronchial asthma, *Am. Rev. Respir. Dis.,* **107**:940–945 (1973).

6. E. R. McFadden and H. A. Lyons, Airway resistance and uneven ventilation in bronchial asthma, *J. Appl. Physiol.,* **25**:365–370 (1968).

7. J. L. Ohman, W. Schmidt-Nowara, M. Lawrence, H. Kazemi, and F. C. Lowell, The diffusing capacity in asthma. Effect of airflow obstruction, *Am. Rev. Respir. Dis.,* **107**:932–939 (1973).

8. B. Rose and M. Rademaker, The pathogenesis of bronchial asthma. In *Immunological Diseases.* Edited by M. Samter. Boston, Little, Brown and Co., 1971, pp. 859–877.

9. B. S. Cardell and R. S. B. Pearson, Death in asthmatics, *Thorax,* **14**:341–352 (1959).

10. J. J. Curry, Comparative action of acetyl beta-methyl choline and histamine on the respiratory tract in normals, patients with hay fever, and subjects with bronchial asthma, *J. Clin. Invest.,* **26**:430–438 (1947).

11. C. D. Parker, R. E. Bilbo, and C. E. Reed, Methacholine aerosol as test for bronchial asthma, *Arch. Intern. Med.,* **115**:452–458 (1965).

12. J. F. Cade and M. C. F. Pain, Role of bronchial reactivity in aetiology of asthma, *Lancet,* **2**:186–188 (1971).

13. S. L. Spector and R. S. Farr, Bronchial inhalation procedures in asthmatics, *Med. Clin. North Am.,* **58**:71–84 (1974).

14. A. F. Coca and R. A. Cooke, On the classification of the phenomena of hypersensitiveness, *J. Immunol.,* 8:163–182 (1923).
15. W. B. Sherman, The atopic diseases—introduction. In *Immunologic Diseases.* Edited by M. Samter. Boston, Little, Brown and Company, 1971, pp. 767–774.
16. M. Schwartz, Heredity in Bronchial Asthma, *Acta Allergol., Supp.* 2:1–288 (1952).
17. H. Schade, Allergische Krankeiten. In *Humangenetik, Ein Kurzes Handbuch. Bank III/1.* Edited by P. E. Becker. Stuttgart, Georg Thieme Verlag, 1964, pp. 551–606.
18. M. L. Edfors–Lubs, Allergy in 7,000 twin pairs, *Acta Allergol.,* 26:249–285 (1971).
19. J. E. Salvaggio, J. J. A. Cavanaugh, F. C. Lowell, and S. Leskowitz, A comparison of the immunologic responses of normal and atopic individuals to intranasally administered antigen, *J. Allergy,* 35:62–69 (1964).
20. J. Salvaggio, R. Waldman, M. H. Fruchtman, F. M. Wigley, and J. E. Johnson, Systemic and secretory antibody response of atopic and non-atopic individuals to intranasally administered tetanus toxoid, *Clin. Allergy,* 3:43–49 (1973).
21. J. Salvaggio, E. Castro–Murillo, and V. Kundur, Immunologic response of atopic and normal individuals to Keyhole limpet hemocyanin, *J. Allergy,* 44:344–354 (1969).
22. J. Salvaggio, E. H. Kayman, and S. Leskowtiz, Immunologic responses of atopic and normal individuals to aerosolized dextran, *J. Allergy,* 38:31–40 (1966).
23. S. Leskowitz and F. C. Lowell, A comparison of the immunologic responses of normal and allergic individuals, *J. Allergy,* 32:152–161 (1961).
24. J. Salvaggio and S. Leskowitz, A comparison of the immunologic responses of normal and atopic individuals to parenterally injected alum–precipitated protein antigen, *Int. Arch. Allergy,* 26:264–279 (1965).
25. K. Karakitas, J. Salvaggio, and K. P. Mathews, Comparative nasal absorption of allergens in atopic and nonatopic subjects, *J. Allergy Clin. Immunol.,* 53:93 (1974) (abstr.).
26. B. Butcher, G. Leslie, and J. Salvaggio, Secretory immunologic response of atopic and nonatopic individuals to topically applied antigen, *J. Allergy and Clin. Immunol.,* 53:115 (1974) (abstr.).
27. B. Taylor, A. P. Norman, H. A. Orgel, C. R. Stokes, M. W. Turner, and J. F. Soothill, Transient IgA deficiency and pathogenesis of infantile atopy, *Lancet,* 2:111–113 (1973).
28. R. H. Buckley and S. C. Dees, Correlation of milk precipitins with IgA deficiency, *N. Engl. J. Med.,* 281:465–469 (1969).
29. A. F. Wilson, H. S. Novey, R. A. Berke, and E. L. Surprenant, Deposition of inhaled pollen, pollen extract in human airways, *N. Engl. J. Med.,* 288:1056–1058 (1973).
30. W. W. Busse, C. E. Reed, and J. H. Hoehne, Where is the allergic reaction in ragweed asthma? II. Demonstration of ragweed antigen in airborn

particles smaller than pollen, *J. Allergy Clin. Immunol.*, **59**:289–293 (1972).

31. S. G. O. Johansson, Raised levels of a new immunoglobulin class (IgND) in asthma, *Lancet*, **2**:951–953 (1967).

32. S. G. O. Johansson, H. H. Bennich, and T. Berg, The clinical significance of IgE, *Prog. Clin. Immunol.*, **1**:157–181 (1972).

33. L. L. Henderson, H. H. Swedlund, R. G. Van Dellen, J. P. Marcoux, H. M. Carryer, G. A. Peters, and G. J. Gleich, Evaluation of IgE tests in an allergy practice, *J. Allergy Clin. Immunol.*, **48**:361–365 (1971).

34. T. Foucard, T. Berg, S. G. O. Johansson, and B. Wahren, Virus serology and serum IgE levels in children with asthmatoid bronchitis, *Acta Paediatr. Scand.*, **60**:621–629 (1970).

35. C. B. S. Wood and J. Oliver, Serum IgE in asthmatic children. Relationship to age, sex, eczema, and skin sensitivity tests, *Arch. Dis. Child.*, **47**: 890–896 (1972).

36. E. Spitz, E. W. Gelfand, A. L. Sheffer, and K. F. Austen, Serum IgE in clinical immunology and allergy, *J. Allergy Clin. Immunol.*, **49**:337–347 (1972).

37. L. M. Lichtenstein, K. Ishizaka, P. S. Norman, A. B. Sobotka, and B. M. Hill, IgE antibody measurements in ragweed hay fever. Relationship to clinical severity and the results of immunotherapy, *J. Clin. Invest.*, **52**: 472–482 (1973).

38. S. P. Stone, S. A. Muller, and G. J. Gleich, IgE levels in atopic dermatitis, *Arch. Derm.*, **108**:806–811 (1973).

39. J. W. Yunginger and G. J. Gleich, Seasonal changes in serum and nasal IgE concentrations, *J. Allergy and Clin. Immunol.*, **51**:174–186 (1973).

40. K. Ishizaka and R. W. Newcomb, Presence of γE in nasal washings and sputum from asthmatic patients, *J. Allergy*, **49**:197–204 (1970).

41. R. H. Waldman, C. Virchow, and D. S. Rowe, IgE levels in external secretions, *Int. Arch. Allergy*, **44**:242–248 (1973).

42. G. W. Hagy and G. A. Settipane, Prognosis of positive allergy skin tests in an asymptomatic population. A three year follow up of college students, *J. Allergy*, **48**:200–211 (1971).

43. B. B. Levine, R. H. Stember, and M. Fotino, Ragweed hay fever: Genetic control and linkage to HL–A haplotypes, *Science*, **178**:1201–1203 (1972).

44. D. G. Marsh, W. B. Bias, S. H. Hsu, and L. Goodfriend, Association of the HL–A7 cross–reacting group with a specific reaginic antibody response in allergic man, *Science*, **179**:691–693 (1973).

45. M. N. Blumenthal, D. B. Amos, H. Noreen, N. R. Mendell, and E. J. Yunis, Genetic mapping of the Ir locus in man: Linkage to second locus of HL–A, *Science*, **184**:1301–1303 (1974).

46. A. L. Sullivan, P. M. Grimley, and H. Metzger, Electron microscopic localization of immunoglobulin E on the surface membrane of human basophils, *J. Exp. Med.*, **134**:1403–1416 (1971).

47. T. Ishizaka, C. S. Soto, and K. Ishizaka, Mechanisms of passive sensitization. III. Number of IgE molecules and their receptor sites on human basophil granulocytes, *J. Immunol.*, **111**:500–511 (1973).

48.   D. Katz and B. Benacerraf, The regulatory influence of activated T cells on B cell responses to antigen, *Adv. Immunol.*, **15**:1–94 (1972).

49.   H. Okudaira and K. Ishizaka, Reaginic antibody formation in the mouse. III. Collaboration between hapten–specific memory cells and carrier–specific helper cells for secondary antihapten antibody formation, *J. Immunol.*, **111**:1420–1428 (1973).

50.   T. Kishimoto and K. Ishizaka, Regulation of antibody response *in vitro*. V. Effect of carrier–specific helper cells on generation of hapten–specific memory cells of different immunoglobulin classes, *J. Immunol.*, **111**:1–9 (1973).

51.   T. Tada, M. Taniguchi, and K. Okumura, Regulation of homocytotropic antibody formation in the rat. II. Effect of X–irradiation, *J. Immunol.*, **106**:1012–1018 (1971).

52.   K. Okumura and T. Tada, Regulation of homocytotropic antibody formation in the rat. III. Effect of thymectomy and splenectomy, *J. Immunol.*, **106**:1019–1025 (1971).

53.   M. Taniguchi and T. Tada, Regulation of homocytotropic antibody formation in the rat. IV. Effects of various immunosuppressive drugs, *J. Immunol.*, **107**:579–585 (1971).

54.   T. Tada and K. Okumura, Regulation of homocytotropic antibody formation in the rat. I. Feedback regulation by passively administered antibody, *J. Immunol.*, **106**:1002–1011 (1971).

55.   K. Okumura and T. Tada, Regulation of homocytotropic antibody formation in the rat. VI. Inhibitory effect of thymocytes on the homocytotropic antibody response, *J. Immunol.*, **107**:1682–1689 (1971).

56.   T. Tada, K. Okumura, and M. Taniguchi, Regulation of homocytotropic antibody formation in the rat. VIII. An antigen–specific T cell factor that regulates anti–hapten homocytotropic antibody response, *J. Immunol.*, **111**:952–961 (1973).

57.   K. Okumura and T. Tada, Regulation of homocytotropic antibody formation in the rat. IX. Further characterization of the antigen–specific inhibitory T cell factor in hapten–specific homocytotropic antibody response, *J. Immunol.*, **112**:783–791 (1974).

58.   K. J. Bloch and J. L. Ohman, The stable homocytotropic antibodies of guinea pig, mouse, and rat; and some indirect evidence for the *in vivo* interaction of homocytotropic antibodies of two different rat immunoglobulin classes at a common receptor on target cells. In *Biochemistry of the Acute Allergic Reactions.* Edited by K. F. Austen and E. L. Becker. Philadelphia, F. A. Davis Co., 1971, pp. 45–61.

59.   R. T. Reid, P. Minden, and R. S. Farr, Reaginic activity associated with IgG immunoglobulin, *J. Exp. Med.*, **123**:845–858 (1966).

60.   W. E. Parish, Short–term anaphylactic IgG antibodies in human sera, *Lancet,* **2**:591–592 (1970).

61.   D. H. Bryant, M. W. Burns, and L. Lazarus, New type of allergic asthma due to IgG "reaginic" antibody, *Br. Med. J.*, **4**:589–592 (1973).

62.   J. Brostoff and I. Roitt, Cell–mediated (delayed) hypersensitivity in patients with summer hay fever, *Lancet,* **2**:1269–1272 (1969).

63. R. E. Rocklin, H. Pence, H. Kaplan, and R. Evans, Cell–mediated immune response of ragweed–sensitive patients to ragweed antigen E, *J. Clin. Invest.*, **53**:735–744 (1974).

64. S. H. Young, J. Zimmerman, and E. Smithwick, The in vitro response of human lymphocytes challenged by ragweed antigen, *Pediatrics*, **42**:976–979 (1968).

65. R. N. Maini, D. C. Dumonde, J. A. Faux, F. E. Hargreave, and J. Pepys, The production of lymphocyte mitogenic factor and migration–inhibition factor by antigen–stimulated lymphocytes of subjects with grass pollen allergy, *Clin. Exp. Immunol.*, **9**:449–465 (1971).

66. M. N. Blumental, J. Hallgren, and E. Yunis, In vitro functions of lymphocytes in human atopy, *J. Allergy*, **47**:107 (1971) (abstr.).

67. A. Malley, M. S. Wilson, M. Barnett, and F. Perlman, Site of action of antigen D immunotherapy in grass–sensitive patients, *J. Allergy*, **47**:111 (abstr.).

68. S. Romagnani, G. Biliotti, A. Passalera, and M. Ricci, In vitro lymphocyte response to pollen extract constituents in grass pollen–sensitive individuals, *Int. Arch. Allergy*, **44**:40–50 (1973).

69. J. A. Anderson, S. R. Lane, W. A. Howard, S. Leiken, and J. J. Oppenheim, The effect of hyposensitization on alternaria–induced lymphocyte blastogenesis, *Cell. Immunol.*, **10**:442–449 (1974).

70. V. L. Moore, J. N. Fink, J. J. Barboriak, L. L. Ruff, and D. P. Schlueter, Immunologic events in pigeon breeders' disease, *J. Allergy Clin. Immunol.*, **53**:319–328 (1974).

71. J. H. McCarter and J. J. Vasquez, The bronchial basement membrane in asthma: Immunohistochemical and ultrastructural observations, *Arch. Pathol.*, **82**:328–335 (1966).

72. M. L. Callerame, J. J. Condemi, M. G. Bohrud, and J. H. Vaughn, Immunologic reactions of bronchial tissues in asthma, *N. Engl. J. Med.*, **284**:459–464 (1971).

73. M. L. Callerame, J. J. Condemi, K. Ishizaka, S. G. O. Johansson, and J. H. Vaughn, Immunoglobulins in bronchial tissues from patients with asthma, with special reference to IgE, *J. Allergy*, **47**:187–197 (1971).

74. M. A. Gerber, F. Paronetto, and S. Kochwa, Immunohistochemical localization of IgE in asthmatic lungs, *Am. J. Pathol.*, **62**:339–352 (1971).

75. C. G. Cochrane, Mechanisms involved in the deposition of immune complexes in tissues, *J. Exp. Med.*, **134**:75s–89s (1971).

76. M. A. DeKock, J. A. Nadel, S. Zwi, H. J. H. Colebatch, and C. R. Olsen, New method for perfusing bronchial arteries: Histamine bronchoconstriction and apnea, *J. Appl. Physiol.*, **21**:185–194 (1966).

77. I. H. Itkin and S. C. Anand, The role of atropine as a mediator blocker of induced bronchial obstruction, *J. Allergy*, **45**:178–186 (1970).

78. D. Y. C. Yu., S. P. Galant, and W. M. Gold, Inhibition of antigen–induced bronchoconstriction by atropine in asthmatic patients, *J. Appl. Physiol.*, **32**:823–000 (1972).

79. J. E. Mills, H. Sellick, and J. G. Widdicombe, Vagal deflation reflexes mediated by lung irritant receptors. In *Breathing. Hering-Breuer Centenary Symposium.* Edited by R. Porter. London, J. and A. Churchill, Ltd., 1970, pp. 77–92.

80. W. M. Gold, G. F. Kessler, and D. Y. C. Yu, Role of vagus nerves in experimental asthma in allergic dogs, *J. Appl. Physiol.*, 33:719–725 (1972).

81. J. A. Nadel and J. G. Widdicombe, Reflex effects of upper airway irritation on total lung resistance and blood pressure, *J. Appl. Physiol.*, 17:861–865 (1962).

82. H. Sellick and J. G. Widdicombe, Stimulation of lung irritant receptors by cigarette smoke, carbon dust, and histamine aerosol, *J. Appl. Physiol.*, 31: 15–19 (1971).

83. J. G. Widdicombe, D. C. Kent, and J. A. Nadel, Mechanism of bronchoconstriction during inhalation of dust, *J. Appl. Physiol.*, 17:613–616 (1962).

84. J. A. Nadel, H. Salem, B. Tamplin, and Y. Tokiwa, Mechanism of bronchoconstriction during inhalation of sulfur dioxide, *J. Appl. Physiol.*, 20:164–167 (1965).

85. B. G. Simonsson, F. M. Jacobs, and J. A. Nadel, Mechanism of changes in airway size during inhalation of various substances in asthmatics: Role of the autonomic nervous system, *Am. Rev. Respir. Dis.*, 95:873–874 (1967).

86. G. A. Cabezas, P. D. Graf, and J. A. Nadel, Sympathetic versus parasympathetic nervous regulation of airways of dogs, *J. Appl. Physiol.*, 31: 651–655 (1971).

87. A. Szentivanyi, The beta–adrenergic theory of the atopic abnormality in bronchial asthma, *J. Allergy*, 42:203–232 (1968).

88. D. V. Cookson and C. E. Reed, A comparison of the effects of isoproterenol in the normal and asthmatic subject, *Am. Rev. Respir. Dis.*, 88: 636–643 (1963).

89. S. D. Lockey, J. A. Glennon, and C. E. Reed, Comparison of some metabolic responses in normal and asthmatic subjects to epinephrine and glucagon, *J. Allergy*, 40:349–354 (1967).

90. S. Inoue, Effects of epinephrine on asthmatic children, *J. Allergy*, 40: 337–348 (1967).

91. E. Middleton and S. R. Finke, Metabolic response to epinephrine in asthma, *J. Allergy*, 42:288–299 (1968).

92. C. H. Kirkpatrick and C. Keller, Impaired responsiveness to epinephrine in asthma, *Am. Rev. Respir. Dis.*, 96:692–699 (1967).

93. A. A. Mathé and P. H. Knapp, Decreased plasma free fatty acids and urinary epinephrine in bronchial asthma, *N. Engl. J. Med.*, 281:234–238 (1969).

94. C. E. Reed, M. Cohen, and T. Enta, Reduced effect of epinephrine on circulating eosinophils in asthma and after beta–adrenergic blockade or *Bordetella pertussis* vaccine, *J. Allergy*, 46:90–102 (1970).

95. E. P. Cohen, T. L. Petty, A. Szentivanyi, and R. E. Priest, Clinical and pathological observations in fatal bronchial asthma, *Ann. Intern. Med.*, 62: 103–109 (1965).

96. M. H. Grieco, R. N. Pierson, and F. X. Pi–Sunyer, Comparison of the circulatory and metabolic effects of isoproterenol epinephrine and meth-oxamine in normal and asthmatic subjects, *Am. J. Med.*, **44**:863–872 (1968).
97. R. S. McNiell, Effect of a beta–adrenergic blocking agent, propanolol, on asthmatics, *Lancet*, **2**:1101–1102 (1964).
98. D. K. Sen, S. Arora, S. Gupta, and R. K. Sanyal, Studies of adrenergic mechanisms in relation to histamine sensitivity in children immunized with *Bordetella pertussis* vaccine, *J. Allergy Clin. Immunol.*, **54**:25–31 (1974).
99. H. S. Nelson, The effect of ephedrine on the response to epinephrine in normal men, *J. Allergy Clin. Immunol.*, **51**:191–198 (1973).
100. H. S. Nelson, J. W. Black, L. B. Branch, B. Pfuetze, H. Spaulding, R. Summers, and D. Wood, Subsensitivity to epinephrine following the administration of epinephrine and ephedrine to normal individuals, *J. Allergy Clin. Immunol.*, **55**:299–309 (1975).
101. P. J. Logsdon, E. Middleton, and R. G. Coffey, Stimulation of leukocyte adenyl cyclase by hydrocortisone and isoproterenol in asthmatic and non-asthmatic subjects, *J. Allergy Clin. Immunol.*, **50**:45–56 (1972).
102. C. W. Parker and J. W. Smith, Alterations in cyclic adenosine monophos-phate metabolism in human bronchial asthma. I. Leukocyte responsive-ness to B–adrenergic agents, *J. Clin. Invest.*, **52**:48–59 (1973).
103. C. J. Falliers, R. R. de A. Cardoso, H. N. Bane, R. Coffey, and E. Middleton, Discordant allergic manifestations in monozygotic twins: Genetic identity versus clinical, physiologic, and biochemical differences, *J. Allergy*, **47**:207–219 (1971).
104. J. J. Ouellette and C. E. Reed, Increased response of asthmatic subjects to metacholine after influenza vaccine, *J. Allergy*, **36**:558–563 (1965).
105. K. McIntosh, E. F. Ellis, L. S. Hoffman, T. G. Lybass, J. J. Eller, and V. A. Fulginiti, The association of viral and bacterial respiratory infec-tions with exacerbations of wheezing in young asthmatic children, *J. Pediatrics*, **82**:578–590 (1973).
106. T. E. Minor, E. C. Dick, A. N. DeMeo, J. J. Ouellette, M. Cohen, and C. E. Reed, Viruses as precipitants of asthmatic attacks in children, *J.A.M.A.*, **227**:292–298 (1974).
107. J. J. Picken, D. E. Niewoehner, and E. H. Chester, Prolonged effects of viral infections of the upper respiratory tract upon small airways, *Am. J. Med.*, **52**:738–746 (1972).
108. W. W. Fridy, R. H. Ingram, J. C. Hierholzer, and M. T. Coleman, Airways function during mild viral respiratory illnesses, *Ann. Intern. Med.*, **80**:150–155 (1974).

12

Hypersensitivity Pneumonitis

JORDAN N. FINK

The Medical College of Wisconsin
Milwaukee, Wisconsin

I. Introduction

Probably the most common hypersensitivity lung disease occurring in man is asthma, usually caused by sensitivity to antigens indigenous to the patient's environment. In patients with asthma, an alteration in their autonomic nervous system can often be demonstrated by insufflation with certain pharmacologic mediators. The insufflation of histamine or acetylcholine into the airways of such individuals will usually result in measurable bronchospasm, which is readily reversible. Furthermore, insufflation challenge, using an aerosol of the specific antigen, will usually reproduce the patient's symptoms within several minutes. Those asthmatics sensitive to environmental antigens may also demonstrate elevated levels of the skin-sensitizing antibody, immunoglobulin E. This antibody can be demonstrated by an immediate wheal and flare reaction when the appropriate antigen is applied to scarified skin.

Recent evidence has indicated that other immunologic processes, involving certain antigens that combine with antibodies of the IgG class, which, unlike

Supported by Specialized Center of Research (SCOR) Grant HL 15389 from the National Heart and Lung Institute.

IgE, precipitate with the specific antigen or fix complement, may play a role in the genesis of other hypersensitivity respiratory diseases. When the antigens inhaled are part of certain biologic dusts, the respiratory disorders induced are termed "hypersensitivity pneumonitis" or "extrinsic allergic alveolitis." These diseases differ from asthma in that they involve the alveolar and interstitial tissues as well as the middle and terminal airways.

Hypersensitivity pneumonitis is the result of immunologic reactions to a variety of inhaled organic dusts. The disease may present in a number of clinical forms, depending on such factors as the immunologic response of the patient, the duration and amount of exposure to the inhaled dust, and the nature of that dust [1-16].

II. Etiology of Hypersensitivity Pneumonitis

The inhalation of any of a number of inhaled organic dusts has been associated with sensitization and the subsequent development of a hypersensitivity pneumonitis (Table 1). The dusts may be derived from animal proteins, as in bird handlers' disease where the inhaled proteins are dried avian (pigeon, parakeet, budgerigar) materials [1-5], or in pituitary snuff takers' disease when pituitary powder containing bovine or porcine serum proteins are inhaled [6]. Other common sources of dusts, which may act as antigens and hypersensitivity pneumonitis, include vegetable materials contaminated with a variety of saprophytic fungi. Such reactions are seen in the diseases farmer's lung [7,8], mushroom handlers' lung [9], or bagassosis [10]. In these disorders, the inhaled dusts are usually contaminated with one of the thermophilic actinomycetes identified as *Micropolyspora faeni, Thermoactinomyces vulgaris* or *T. sacharii* [7-11]. These ubiquitous organisms thrive best at 45° to 60°C, the temperatures usually reached during the decomposition process of vegetation. Thermophilic organisms are, in fact, most likely responsible for the actual process of decay of the vegetable material. This is probably accomplished by the release, from the organisms, of a variety of proteolytic enzymes as well as other substances that allow decomposition by other saprophytic organisms. Recently, thermophilic actinomycetes have been found unassociated with a specific occupation, such as farming, but residing in air-conditioning or forced-air heating systems of commercial or residential buildings [12,13]. About 15% of the individuals exposed to those contaminated environments develop symptoms of hypersensitivity pneumonitis similar to farmer's lung or bagassosis [12].

Other inhaled fungal materials may also cause a hypersensitivity pneumonitis. Woodworkers inhaling large amounts of wood dust contaminated with a saprophytic fungi, such as *Alternaria* species [14], or inhaling redwood dust

TABLE 1 Etiologic Agents in Hypersensitivity Pneumonitis

Disease	Exposure	Antigen
Farmer's lung	Moldy vegetable compost	*Micropolyspora faeni*
Mushroom worker's lung		*Thermoactinomyces vulgaris*
Bagassosis		*Thermoactinomyces saccharii*
Humidifier or air-conditioner lung	Contaminated forced air system	
Maple bark stripper's lung	Moldy bark	*Cryptostroma corticale*
Malt worker's lung	Moldy malt	*Aspergillus clavatus*
Sequoiosis	Moldy redwood dust	*Aureobasidium pulliulans*
Paprika splitter's lung	Paprika dust	*Mucor stolonifer*
Wheat weevil disease	Wheat flour weevils	*Sitophilus granarius*
Cheese worker's lung	Cheese mold	*Penicillium caseii*
Suberosis	Moldy cork	*Penicillium sp.*
Bird breeder's lung	Pigeons, parakeets, budgerigars etc.	Avian proteins
Pituitary snuff lung	Porcine, bovine pituitary	Porcine, bovine proteins

containing *Graphium sp* [15], workers removing the bark from maple logs and exposed to the spores of *Cryptostroma corticale* [16], individuals working in cheese-producing factories in which spores of *Penicillium caseii* may be inhaled [1], or brewers working in malt factories where spores of *Aspergillus clavatus* may contaminate the environment, also may become sensitized and develop a similar illness [1]. It is likely that, as exposure to newly recognized antigens increases, the number of inhaled organic dusts recognized as capable of sensitizing individuals will grow.

III. Clinical Features

The clinical features of these disorders probably depend on the antigenicity of the organic dust, the immunologic responses of the patient to the inhaled dust, and the intensity and frequency of the patient's exposure to that dust. Features of the ensuing clinical illness are usually similar, regardless of the type or nature of the inhaled offending dust. Thus, hypersensitivity pneumonitis should be considered a respiratory disease syndrome with a broad spectrum of clinical features rather than as separate specific illnesses.

A. The Acute Form

The most easily distinguished and probably most common form of hypersensitivity pneumonitis results from intermittent exposure to one of the antigenic organic dusts. The patient becomes sensitized to the dust, after a variable period of exposure, by inhalation at work or home. Respiratory and systemic symptoms of dyspnea, cough, fever, chills, malaise, and myalgia occur explosively about 4 to 6 hr after the dust is inhaled [1-16]. Although the symptoms may persist for up to 12 hr, the patient recovers spontaneously from each acute attack. Each time the patient exposes himself to the dust, the acute episode recurs. The extent and degree of the attack seem to depend on the amount of exposure and the sensitivity of the patient to the specific antigenic dust. Frequent or severe attacks are also associated with a variable degree of anorexia and chronic weight loss. Symptoms often suggest an acute viral illness, such as influenza, and many patients have received appropriate therapy for recurrent respiratory infections rather than for their allergic lung disease.

Physical examination of the patient during the acute episode reveals an acutely ill, toxic-appearing, dyspneic patient [1-16]. Prominent are bibasilar end-inspiratory moist rales that appear early and persist throughout the attack. The findings disappear within 12 to 18 hr after the attack begins, and the patient remains asymptomatic between attacks as long as he avoids exposure. A leukocytosis up to 25,000 white blood cells, with a marked shift to the left, may be seen during the acute episode. Eosinophilia is variable and may be as high as 10%. These laboratory abnormalities also usually return to normal after the acute episode subsides. Elevated levels of all of the immunoglobulins are often seen in the serum of sensitive patients, but IgE levels are within normal limits, unless the patients have typical allergic rhinitis or asthma in addition to hypersensitivity pneumonitis [17].

Changes in pulmonary function that occur after exposure may be of several types. The response that seems to be the most common occurs at the 4- to 6-hr period and appears to involve peripheral airways. There is a decrease in forced vital capacity and one-second forced expiratory volume, with little change in the ratio of the two values or in expiratory flow rates. These demonstrable changes reach a peak at about 6 hr and function returns to normal as other clinical features improve. Other detectible abnormalities include a decrease in gas transfer capacity reflecting disturbances in ventilation–perfusion relationships, and a decrease in compliance, indicating an increase in lung stiffness [1,7,18].

The other type of response observed occurs as a two-stage reaction [1,18]. There is an immediate asthmatic type reaction, as demonstrated by a decrease in forced vital capacity, forced expiratory flow volume, as well as expiratory flow rates. Such patients may have dyspnea, with slight wheezing, reflecting involvement of the lower airways. This immediate type of response is then followed by the late 4- to 6-hr reaction [1]. Chest x-ray examinations may be within normal limits, as between attacks, or may demonstrate peripheral bibasilar infiltrations, with occasional nodular lesions suggestive of interstitial or alveolar involvement [1,3]. Both pulmonary function and chest x-ray abnormalities return to normal when exposure is avoided, providing irreversible tissue damage has not occurred as a result of repeated insults to the pulmonary parenchyma. Corticosteroids may be necessary and effective as adjunct therapy to reverse clinical abnormalities.

B. Chronic Form

In some cases of hypersensitivity pneumonitis, irreversible pulmonary damage may occur. Fibrosis with irreversible pulmonary insufficiency may be seen in some patients inhaling dusts from parakeets, budgerigars (lovebirds), or in long-standing cases of farmer's lung [1-18]. These patients may develop restrictive ventilatory impairment, marked diffusion defects, and "stiff" lungs that do not respond either to prolonged avoidance or corticosteroid therapy. Granulomas form among interstitial fibrosis. Alveolar wall thickening due to the infiltration of lymphocytes, plasma cells, and some eosinophils, has also been demonstrated in biopsies from some of these patients [1,4].

In some patients with the chronic form of pigeon breeders' disease, farmer's lung, or bagassosis, pulmonary function tests have shown elevation of residual volumes, diminished flow rates, and loss of pulmonary elasticity, abnormalities suggestive of emphysema [7,10,18]. Examination of lung biopsies from these cases has revealed obstructive bronchiolitis with the destruction of alveolar air sacs [4,7,10]. These severely ill patients do not respond to therapy with bronchodilators, corticosteroids, or even prolonged avoidance of exposure and, as a result of the disease, have a permanent respiratory impairment [1,7,18].

IV. Laboratory Findings

A. Roentgenographic Features

The most consistent pattern observed on chest x-ray films of patients with hypersensitivity pneumonitis has been a combination of fine, sharp nodulations, reticulation or honeycombing throughout the pulmonary fields, and coarsening of bronchovascular markings [1-16]. These roentgenographic features are consistent with an interstitial process (Fig. 1). During acute attacks, soft, patchy, ill-defined parenchymal densities with a tendency to coalesce may be seen in the lung fields. In the chronic phase of the disease, the appearance of a fibrotic pulmonary process, with diffuse interstitial involvement, may be seen. Unfortunately, there are no specific chest roentgenographic features that enable the physician to distinguish one type of hypersensitivity pneumonitis from another, or from the large number of pulmonary diseases that present with interstitial or alveolar involvement. Thus, a knowledge of the history and other clinical features are important in evaluating the chest x-ray of a patient suspected of having hypersensitivity pneumonitis.

B. Pathologic Features

The demonstrable histologic features of the lung that occur in hypersensitivity pneumonitis depend on the stage of the disease at the time the lung biopsy is obtained [1,4,8,10]. Early in mushroom picker's lung, farmer's lung, or other lung disease due to vegetable dust inhalation, lymphocytes can be seen to infiltrate the alveolar walls, and the alveolar spaces may contain plasma cells and engorged alveolar macrophages. Histiocytes that contain foamy cytoplasm may be demonstrated in clusters surrounded by large numbers of lymphocytes and their presence may be unique for this group of diseases [4]. In pigeon breeders' disease, due to the inhalation of serum proteins, the foam cells are more prominent and may occupy an interstitial as well as an intra-alveolar position. In

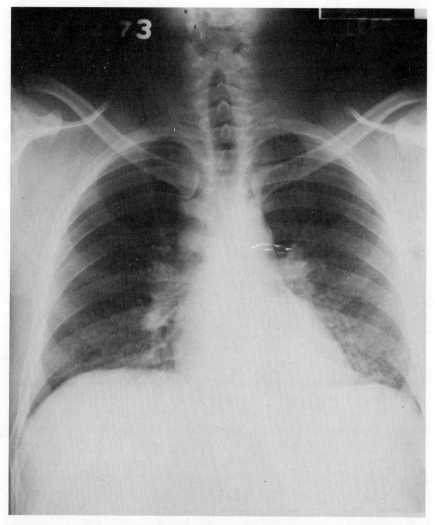

FIGURE 1 Chest x-ray of patient with recurrent acute attacks of pigeon breeders' disease demonstrating interstitial nodular infiltrations.

these hypersensitivity lung diseases some sarcoid-like granulomata that show foci of central necrosis may be found within lymphoid infiltrates. Scattered Langhans-type giant cells are present in varying numbers [1,4] (Fig. 2).

In the more severe or chronic cases, fibrotic areas may be seen in alveolar interstitial position and may be associated with destruction of lung parenchyma [1,4,7]. There may be interspersed lymphocytes and plasma cells, but these

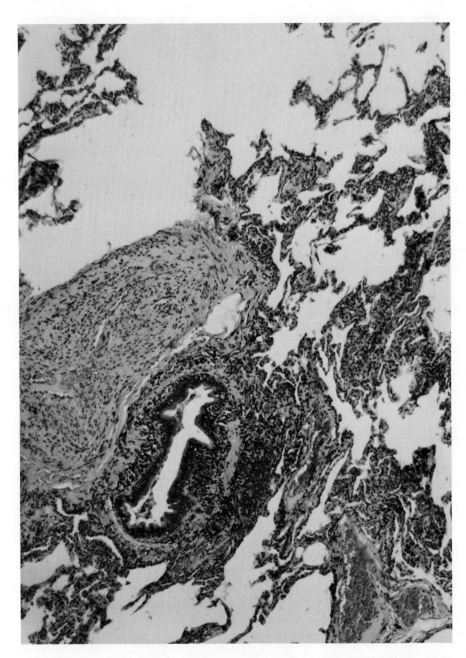

FIGURE 2 Lung biopsy of patient with hypersensitivity pneumonitis due to inhalation of thermophilic actinomycetes demonstrating interstitial and peri-bronchial lymphocytic infiltrations and early giant cell formations.

cells are less prominent than in the acute form of hypersensitivity pneumonitis. The collagen-thickened walls of the bronchioles may be generally infiltrated by lymphocytes, and their lumens may be obstructed by granulation tissue [4]. These features may suggest severe interstitial fibrosis or obliterative bronchiolitis. Honeycombing or cystic changes may be associated with dense fibrosis, and there may be features of centrilobular emphysema [1,4,7].

C. Immunologic Features

The characteristic immunologic feature of hypersensitivity pneumonitis is the occurrence of precipitins against the specific offending antigen [1-16]. Serum antibodies may be demonstrated by gel-diffusion techniques (Fig. 3). Precipitins can be demonstrated in the serum of most sick patients, but up to 50% of asymptomatic individuals exposed to the same organic dusts also have demonstrable precipitating antibodies in their sera [1,5]. Thus, precipitating antibody to a given antigen in a patient's serum must be considered in light of the clinical

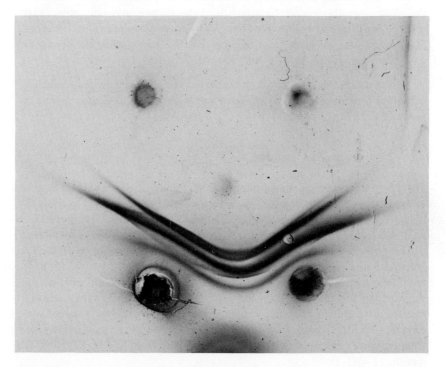

FIGURE 3 Immunodiffusion studies of sera from patients with pigeon breeders' disease (lower wells) and nonexposed individuals (upper wells) against pigeon serum (center well).

features of that patient's illness as well as the nature of his environmental exposure.

More recently, several groups of investigators have demonstrated cell-mediated immunity to organic dust antigens in patients with hypersensitivity pneumonitis [19,20]. Whether this type of hypersensitivity is important in the pathogenesis of these diseases remains to be elucidated. In pigeon breeders' disease, where inhaled serum proteins can be implicated in the etiology, skin tests with the serum may be of value. An immediate wheal and flare (Type I) reaction may be demonstrated by the intradermal injection of dilute protein [1,2]. This reaction is followed by a late (4-6 hr, Type III) skin reaction resembling the Arthus phenomenon. The late reaction begins with erythema and edema and may progress to central necrosis, but it usually subsides within 24 hr. Examination of biopsies of such skin reactions have demonstrated mild polymorphonuclear and plasma-cell infiltration of the area surrounding the vessels—lesions consistent with an Arthus–type reaction [1]. This reaction may also occur in the patient's lung, following the inhalation of antigen, but there is as yet no clear evidence implicating precipitating antibodies in the genesis of these diseases. Precipitating antibodies, so characteristic of this disease, may only reflect exposure to the antigen and immunization by inhalation. Recent evidence suggests, in fact, that such antibodies may be protective and may prevent the disease in well, but immunologically reactive, individuals [20].

No reliable reagents are yet available for skin testing individuals inhaling nonserum protein organic dust antigens, and other means of diagnosis must be used.

D. Experimental Features

The recent use of animal models has provided methods whereby the pathogenesis of hypersensitivity pneumonitis can be studied. Richerson [21] selectively immunized guinea pigs and rabbits, which induce Type III humoral or Type IV cell-mediated hypersensitivity to soluble protein antigens. Challenge of pulmonary tissue of sensitized animals has induced different lesions, depending on the immune response of the animals. In those animals selectively sensitized for humoral responses, challenge was followed by a hemorrhagic alveolitis and capillaritis, suggestive of the Arthus phenomenon. On the other hand, in animals selectively sensitized for cellular responses, challenge was followed by interstitial infiltrative disease, with little intraalveolar reaction. These latter lesions more closely resembled the lesions described in patients with biopsy–proven hypersensitivity pneumonitis [1,4,7].

Our group has used the monkey to evaluate the role of Type III humoral and Type IV cellular hypersensitivity in the pathogenesis of these diseases [22].

Monkeys passively sensitized with monkey serum, containing high titers of precipitating antibodies, to pigeon serum proteins were subsequently challenged by insufflation with pigeon serum. Within 6 hr the animals developed respiratory distress and fever. Examination of the lungs revealed hemorrhagic alveolitis. Immunofluorescent studies demonstrated the presence of antigen, immunoglobulin, and complement—all indicative of an immune complex, Type III, inflammatory process, but unlike human lesions.

Similar respiratory symptoms could be reproduced 6 hr after monkeys passively sensitized with large numbers of cells obtained from pigeon serum sensitized monkeys were challenged. Examination of these monkey lungs revealed, as in Richerson's experiments, interstitial involvement with round cells—lesions suggestive of the human disease. In these monkey lungs, no immunoglobulin or complement components could be detected by immunofluorescence.

These experimental findings suggest that cell-mediated rather than humoral-mediated mechanisms may be more important in the genesis of hypersensitivity pneumonitis. The experimental studies in animals, however, are acute experiments, and chronic exposure studies will be necessary to further clarify the problem. It may indeed be that the reaction is a mixed one, with several immunologic mechanisms being involved.

V. Diagnosis

The diagnosis of hypersensitivity pneumonitis may be made by an appropriate and detailed environmental history, specific laboratory and serologic studies, and a trial of avoidance and re-exposure to the environment containing the suspected organic dust. Because the chronic or more insidious form of the disease may be difficult to diagnose, lung biopsy may be necessary in some patients.

On occasion, the diagnosis may be confirmed by cautiously exposing the patient to the suspected antigen or environment and observing the clinical response. This procedure should be carried out during an asymptomatic period. The patient may enter the suspected environment (barn, coop, or other area) and then brought to the hospital where he is observed for the next 8 hr for characteristic signs or symptoms. Corticosteroids may be necessary therapy if an acute attack ensues.

A search for environmental antigens, which may possibly be inhaled by the patient, may also be necessary. Various dusts or liquids (humidifier, furnace) in the patient's home or working area should be cultured in various microbiologic media conducive to the growth of a variety of mesophilic or thermophilic organisms. Extracts of the dusts, as well as extracts of cultured organisms obtained from collected dusts, should be prepared for gel diffusion studies in searching for possible antigens.

VI. Therapy

Avoiding the offending antigen is the most important measure in the tratment of hypersensitivity pneumonitis. Therefore, the offending antigen or environment must be identified. The use of masks or filters capable of removing dusts, appropriate ventilation of working areas, a change in residential forced-air systems, or even changing occupations may be necessary therapeutic measures.

Drug therapy is indicated in these disorders when the offending antigen cannot be avoided. Antihistamines or bronchodilators usually have no effect on the acute symptoms, and the response to cromolyn sodium is variable. The response to corticosteroids, however, is often dramatic. These drugs may also be used to abort acute attacks, but they should not replace avoidance as therapy.

The ultimate prognosis depends on the degree to which the disease can be reversed once avoidance, drug therapy, or both has been instituted. If pulmonary fibrosis has not been too severe, clinical abnormalities are most likely reversible. With irreversible lung damage, however, the necessary therapy may be that associated with treatment of patients with progressive pulmonary insufficiency. Thus, most important in the treatment of hypersensitivity pneumonitis, are early detection of clinical illness, identification of the offending antigen in the environment, and avoidance of that antigen.

References

1. J. Pepys, Hypersensitivity disease of the lungs due to fungi and other organic dusts. In *Monographs in Allergy, No. 4.* Basel, Switzerland, S. Karger, 1969.
2. J. N. Fink, A. J. Sosman, J. J. Barboriak, D. P. Schleuter, and R. A. Holmes, Pigeon breeders' disease—A clinical study of a hypersensitivity pneumonitis, *Ann. Intern. Med.,* **68**:1205–1219 (1968).
3. J. D. Unger, J. N. Fink, and G. Unger, Pigeon breeders' disease—Roentgenograph lung findings in a hypersensitivity pneumonitis, *Radiology,* **90**: 683–687 (1968).
4. G. T. Hensley, J. C. Garancis, G. D. Cherayil, and J. N. Fink, Lung biopsies of pigeon breeders' disease, *Arch. Pathol.,* **87**:572–579 (1969).
5. J. J. Barboriak, A. J. Sosman, and C. E. Reed, Serologic studies in pigeon breeders' disease, *J. Lab. Clin. Med.,* **65**:600–604 (1965).
6. J. Pepys, P. A. Jenkins, P. J. Lachmann, and W. E. Mahon, An iatrogenic

auto–antibody: Immunological responses to pituitary snuff in patients with diabetes insipidus, *Clin. Exp. Immunol.,* **1**:377–389 (1966).

7. H. A. Dickie and J. Rankin, Farmer's lung: An acute granulomatous interstitial pneumonitis occurring in agricultural workers, *J.A.M.A.,* **167**:1069–1076 (1958).

8. D. A. Emanuel, F. J. Wenzel, C. I. Bowerman, and B. R. Lawton, Farmer's lung. Clinical pathologic and immunologic study of twenty–four patients, *Am. J. Med.,* **37**:392–401 (1964).

9. L. S. Bringhurst, R. N. Byrne, and J. Gershon–Cohen, Respiratory disease of mushroom workers, *J.A.M.A.,* **171**:15–18 (1959).

10. H. A. Buechner, A. L. Prevatt, J. Thompson, and O. Butz, Bagassosis–A review with further historical data, studies of pulmonary function, and results of adrenal steroid therapy, *Am. J. Med.,* **25**:234–247 (1958).

11. T. Cross, A. M. Maciver, and J. Cacey, The thermophilic actinomycetes in moldy hay, *J. Gen. Microbiol.,* **50**:351–359 (1968).

12. J. N. Fink, E. F. Banaszak, W. H. Thiede, and J. J. Barboriak, Interstitial pneumonitis due to hypersensitivity to an organism contaminating a heating system, *Ann. Intern. Med.,* **74**:80–83 (1971).

13. E. F. Banaszak, W. H. Thiede, and J. N. Fink, Hypersensitivity pneumonitis due to contamination of an air–conditioner, *N. Eng. J. Med.,* **283**: 271–276 (1970).

14. D. P. Schlueter, J. N. Fink, and G. T. Hensley, Wood pulp workers' disease: A hypersensitivity pneumonitis caused by *Alternaria, Ann. Intern. Med.,* **77**:907–914 (1972).

15. H. I. Cohen, T. C. Merigan, J. C. Kosek, and F. Eldridge, A granulomatous pneumonitis associated with redwood sawdust inhalation, *Am. J. Med.,* **43**:785–794 (1967).

16. D. A. Emanuel, F. J. Wenzel, and B. R. Lawton, Pneumonitis due to *Cryptostroma corticale* (maple bark disease), *N. Engl. J. Med.,* **274**:1413–1418 (1966).

17. R. Patterson, J. N. Fink, J. J. Pruzansky, C. Reed, M. Roberts, R. Slavin, and C. R. Zeiss, Serum immunoglobulin levels in pulmonary allergic aspergillosis and certain other lung diseases, with special reference to immunoglobulin E, *Am. J. Med.,* **54**:16–22 (1973).

18. D. P. Schlueter, J. N. Fink, and A. J. Sosman, Pulmonary functions in pigeon breeders' disease, *Ann. Intern. Med.,* **70**:457–470 (1969).

19. J. R. Caldwell, D. E. Pierce, C. Spencer, R. Leder, and R. H. Waldman, Immunologic mechanisms in hypersensitivity pneumonitis, *J. Allergy Clin. Immunol.,* **52**:225–230 (1973).

20. V. L. Moore, J. N. Fink, J. J. Barboriak, L. C. Ruff, and D. P. Schlueter, Immunologic events in pigeon breeders' disease, *J. Allergy Clin. Immunol.,* **53**:319–328 (1974).

21. H. B. Richerson, F. H. Cheng, and S. C. Bauserman, Acute experimental hypersensitivity pneumonitis in rabbits, *Respir. Dis.,* **104**:568–575 (1971).

22. G. T. Hensley, J. N. Fink, and J. J. Barboriak, Hypersensitivity pneumonitis in the monkey, *Arch. Pathol.,* **97**:33–38 (1974).

13

Pulmonary Vasculitis

ANTHONY S. FAUCI

National Institute of Allergy and Infectious Diseases
National Institutes of Health
Bethesda, Maryland

I. Introduction

Vasculitis is a clinicopathologic phenomenon characterized by inflammation of
blood vessels, most often small arterioles, venules, and capillaries [1]. The inflammation consists of infiltration in and around the vascular endothelium and
wall by granulocytes or mononuclear cells, or both. These cells may then release
substances that damage the vessels. The process may smoulder and remain low
grade, or it may progress to acute fibrinoid necrosis of the involved vessels. A
wide variety of diseases can have vasculitis as a part of their clinical picture.
Most of these disorders have a common feature—they are known or suspected of
having an hypersensitivity or allergic component.

Pulmonary vasculitis can be a part of systemic or disseminated vasculitis,
or it can be the principal feature of certain diseases. In the present chapter, the
pathophysiologic mechanisms, clinical features, associated diseases, and treatment of pulmonary vasculitis will be discussed.

II. Mechanisms of Pulmonary Vasculitis

The pathophysiologic mechanisms of vasculitis in general and, particularly, pulmonary vasculitis can best be described in the context of the four types of allergic reactions classified by Coombs and Gell [2]. The Type III (immune-complex) reaction is the prototypic allergic reaction associated with vascular damage, although other types, particularly Type II (direct cytotoxic) and Type IV (delayed or cell-mediated hypersensitivity) reactions have also been implicated. In addition, many experimental and clinical disorders manifest significant overlap in two or more of these types of allergic reactions [2]. Although Type I reactions (IgE dependent, immediate hypersensitivity) result in the release of vasoactive materials, true vasculitis usually is not a feature of these reactions.

Cochrane and Dixon [3] outlined the pathophysiologic events associated with antigen–antibody complex–induced vascular damage, particularly in the animal serum sickness model. In brief, circulating soluble immune complexes larger than 19 S, formed in antigen excess, are trapped passively by capillary basement membranes or arterial internal elastic laminae, and complement is activated. Increased vascular permeability caused by the release of vasoactive amines from clumped platelets appears to be important in the localization of complexes in vessels. Various components of complement are chemotactic for polymorphonuclear leukocytes [4], causing them to infiltrate the site of the involved vessel. In addition, activated complement components may be involved in the release of lysosomal enzymes from the polymorphonuclear leukocytes [5], causing damage to both the wall of the vessel and the surrounding parenchyma.

Vasculitis can also be an important component of Type IV (cell-mediated hypersensitivity) reactions. The mechanism of vessel-wall damage in this type of reaction has been reviewed by Waksman [6]. Antigens react with sensitized lymphocytes, which then release macrophage inhibitory factor (MIF), causing an accumulation of monocytes that evolve into macrophages. These macrophages release lysosomal hydrolases, which damage vessel walls and the surrounding parenchyma. The progression from accumulation of mononuclear cells, through infiltration by macrophages and epithelioid cells, and the formation of a typical granulomatous inflammatory response has been well-described [7].

The enormous and complex pulmonary vascular network, the heavy concentration of vasoactive cells, as well as the unique relationship that exists in the respiratory tract between man's external and internal environment, establish the lung as an organ of prime importance in hypersensitivity disease in general, and vasculitis in particular [8]. Immune complexes or sensitized lymphocytes can arrive at the pulmonary vascular network through the circulation, while sensitizing antigens can reach the respiratory tract from the environment. These mechanisms of pulmonary vasculitis are outlined in Figures 1 and 2.

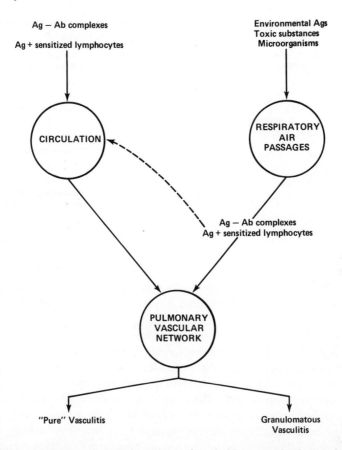

FIGURE 1 Diagrammatic representation of probable events in the mechanism of pulmonary vasculitis. Circulating antigen–antibody complexes (Ag–Ab) or antigen plus sensitized lymphocytes reach the pulmonary vasculature through the circulation. In addition, antigens can gain access through respiratory passages and form complexes or react with sensitized lymphocytes. These then can reach the pulmonary vessels directly or perhaps recirculate and deposit through the circulation. Pure vasculitis or granulomatous reaction in association with vasculitis can then occur.

III. Diseases with Pulmonary Vasculitis

A. Those Associated with Disseminated Vasculitis

Virtually any disease characterized by disseminated vasculitis can potentially have pulmonary vasculitis as either a predominant or minor feature. In most cases, actual vasculitis in the lung was not documented and it was difficult to

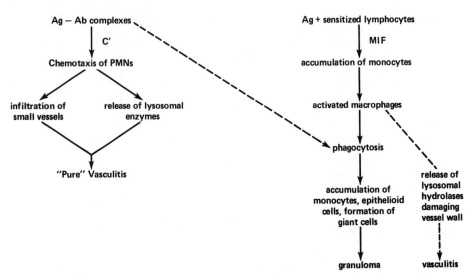

FIGURE 2 Illustration of possible mechanisms in the production of vasculitis, with or without granuloma formation. See text for description of events.

obtain tissue. However, it is reasonable to assume, in cases of disseminated vasculitis in which vascular inflammation and damage is documented in easily accessible tissues, such as skin, that associated pulmonary infiltrates also are caused by vasculitis. Such an association has been confirmed in some cases of serum sickness in humans [9]. The concept of antigen combining with antibody to form circulating immune complexes (Type III allergic reaction), or of antigen reacting with sensitized lymphocytes (Type IV reaction) is hypothetical, for in many disorders the offending antigen has not been identified. However, there are well-studied cases in which immune complexes and complement have been identified in the vascular lesions in several diseases. This subject has recently been reviewed by McCombs [8]. Although immune-complex deposition has not been extensively studied in the lungs in human diseases, it is highly likely, in diseases with disseminated vasculitis, that widespread deposition of immune complexes occurs to a greater or lesser degree in all small vessels, including pulmonary vessels.

Table 1 lists several diseases in which pulmonary vasculitis is seen as part of a broader, disseminated vasculitic process. This is in contrast to other diseases, which will subsequently be discussed, in which the pulmonary vasculitis is a principal feature of the disease, often in association with granulomata.

Immune complex deposition has been convincingly demonstrated in rheumatoid arthritis [10], systemic lupus erythematosus [11], and serum sickness [12]. Similar findings have also been reported in periarteritis nodosa [13].

TABLE 1   Diseases in Which Pulmonary Vasculitis is Associated with Disseminated Vasculitis

Serum sickness

Drug–induced hypersensitivity states

Systemic lupus erythematosus and other collagen vascular diseases

Vasculitic stage of rheumatoid arthritis

Vasculitis associated with tumors, especially lymphoproliferative diseases

Potentially, any disorder in which disseminated vasculitis occurs

Over the years, much confusion has arisen regarding the classification of periarteritis nodosa. Rose and Spencer [14] attempted to divide this disorder into two main categories, with and without lung involvement. "Classic" periarteritis nodosa is characterized by necrotizing nodular lesions in large muscular arterioles, near their bifurcations. The pulmonary circulation and spleen are usually spared. Periarteritis nodosa with lung involvement differs from this group in that a respiratory illness initiates and frequently dominates the disease. There is blood and tissue eosinophilia and granulomatous arteritis in several organs. Asthma is not usually found in these patients. It is different from Loeffler's pneumonia, which characteristically does not have angiitis [15] and also differs from allergic granulomatosis, which will be discussed below. It is generally accepted that periarteritis nodosa is an expression of a hypersensitivity state. The etiologic agent or agents involved are unknown.

Small vessel vasculitis accompanying a serum sickness–like syndrome is seen with a variety of drug hypersensitivity states, including reactions to sulfonamide, penicillin, busulfan and several others [8,16]. Of particular note is a lupus–like syndrome that can be associated with prolonged administration of hydralazine [17], as well as procainamide [18]. Drug hypersensitivity vasculitis has been referred to as *microscopic periarteritis nodosa* because of the predominant involvement of small vessels [19]. However, this entity is probably distinct from true periarteritis nodosa [15] and should be considered a related but separate entity.

Systemic vasculitis accompanying lymphoproliferative disorders is well known [16], although the antigens involved are not clearly defined.

B. Pulmonary Granulomatous Vasculitis

Of particular interest in the study of pulmonary vasculitis are those disorders in which granuloma formation consistently accompanies the vascular inflammation. In these disorders the lung is the principal and often the only organ system

TABLE 2   Diseases in Which Pulmonary Granulomatous Vasculitis is the Principal Feature of the Disorder

Wegener's granulomatosis
Periarteritis nodosa with lung involvement[a]
Allergic granulomatosis
Lymphomatoid granulomatosis

[a]See Rose and Spencer [14].

extensively involved. Table 2 lists those disorders in which pulmonary vasculitis together with granuloma formation are the predominant features of the disease. The etiologies of these disorders are obscure. However, it appears that Type IV (cell-mediated) allergic reactions play a predominate role in pathogenesis. Despite the prevalence of granuloma formation, which is one of the hallmarks of Type IV reactions, Type III (immune complex) reactions may also play an important role in such diseases as Wegener's granulomatosis, which will be discussed below. In addition, under appropriate conditions immune complexes themselves, acting as foreign bodies, may give rise to granulomatous reactions [20].

Wegener's granulomatosis is a disorder characterized by a clinicopathologic triad of (a) necrotizing, granulomatous, small vessel vasculitis involving the upper and lower respiratory tracts, (b) focal glomerulitis which may progress to fulminant glomerulonephritis, and (c) disseminated vasculitis to a greater or lesser degree [21,22]. A limited form of this disease, sparing the kidneys, has been described [23]. Although still an uncommon disease, it is probably not nearly as rare as was formerly thought when cases were unrecognized or confused with other disorders. Wegener's granulomatosis is a distinct clinical entity, and the diagnostic, clinical, and pathologic features of this disease have recently been reviewed [24]. The pathogenesis of this disease remains unclear. It has been suggested for some time that it is caused either by sensitization to the microbial flora of the upper respiratory tract with subsequent crossreaction with respiratory tract tissue, or by an "autoimmune" reaction to respiratory tract tissues which have been altered by endogenous microbial flora, exogenous drugs, irritating chemicals, or environmental factors [24,25]. The histopathologic lesions in both the upper and lower respiratory tracts are characterized by necrotizing granulomatous inflammation and vasculitis, suggesting predominantly a Type IV (cell-mediated) allergic reaction. However, Type III immune complex deposition has been demonstrated in some of the glomerular lesions of Wegener's granulomatosis both by immunofluorescent techniques [24] and by electron microscopy [26]. The precise relationship between these two types of reactions in Wegener's granulomatosis remains unclear at present, but it is safe to say that the disease has at least some features of both types of reactions.

The subjective and objective clinical patterns of the pulmonary granulomatous vasculitis of Wegener's granulomatosis have been extensively studied in a series of patients followed at the National Institute of Allergy and Infectious Diseases [24]. Of the 18 patients studied, all had pulmonary disease. Ten patients had tissue diagnoses of their pulmonary lesions. Of these 10 patients, 7 had necrotizing granulomata with vasculitis and 3 had necrotizing granulomata without demonstrable vasculitis on the specimens examined. Figures 3, 4, and 5 show the typical histopathologic pictures of lung biopsies in Wegener's granulomatosis. Surprisingly, the pulmonary lesions were frequently asymptomatic, especially early in the course of the disease. However, cough, hemoptysis, vague chest discomfort, and pleuritic pain were commonly seen. Less frequently, severe pulmonary symptoms and impaired pulmonary function were noted. Secondary infection of pulmonary lesions in Wegener's granulomatosis as well as in other necrotizing vasculitides is rare [27]. The radiologic manifestations of pulmonary granulomatous vasculitis are numerous and diversified [24]. Solitary or multiple nodular densities, either poorly defined or sharply circumscribed, are seen most often. They vary in size from 1 cm to more than 9 cm, may be unilateral, but more commonly involve both lungs. Cavitation is quite common. Focal areas of atelectasis adjacent to infiltrates are uncommon, as are pleural effusions. Mediastinal lymph node enlargement is rare, and calcium deposition is not seen. Figure 6 shows a typical chest roentgenogram of a patient with Wegener's granulomatosis. Of particular interest is the fact that these infiltrates, although often progressive, may be fleeting and transient, appearing and disappearing in different lung fields even before appropriate therapy was instituted.

Churg and Strauss [28], and some years later Churg [29], described an uncommon granulomatous inflammation and vascular necrosis involving primarily the lungs, heart, skin, and nervous system. They called the disorder *allergic granulomatosis*. Unlike Wegener's granulomatosis, it is found predominantly in patients with an allergic background and characteristically, high levels of blood eosinophilia are found. It is distinct from Loeffler's pneumonia in which vasculitis is not characteristic [15]. It differs also from periarteritis nodosa with lung involvement. Allergic granulomatosis is seen in patients with asthma [28,29], whereas asthma is uncommon in periarteritis nodosa [14].

Recently, an entity termed *lymphomatoid granulomatosis* has been reported by Liebow and his colleagues [30]. They described 40 patients with a proliferative lymphoreticular disease associated with a necrotizing granulomatous vasculitis involving predominantly the lungs. The lymphoreticular process usually spares the lymph nodes, spleen, and bone marrow. However, 13% of their patients progressed to a disseminated atypical lymphoma. The question remains whether this entity is a secondary hypersensitivity reaction to the presence of a primary lymphoma, which is kept in check by the allergic reaction, or

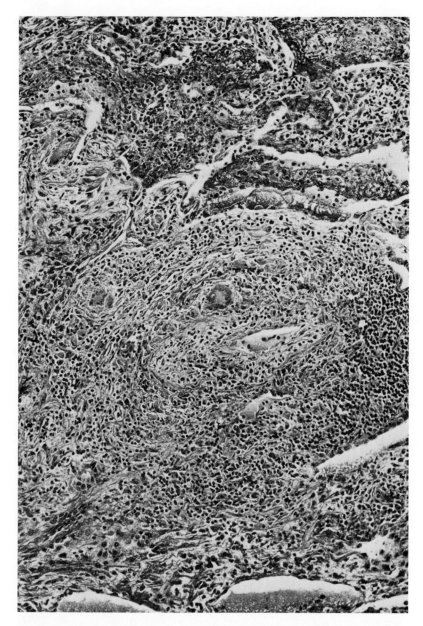

FIGURE 3 Photomicrograph of a lung biopsy in a 36–yr–old–man with Wegener's granulomatosis. Typical granulomatous inflammation with multi-nucleated giant cells are seen. Hematoxylin and eosin stain. Original magnification 95X.

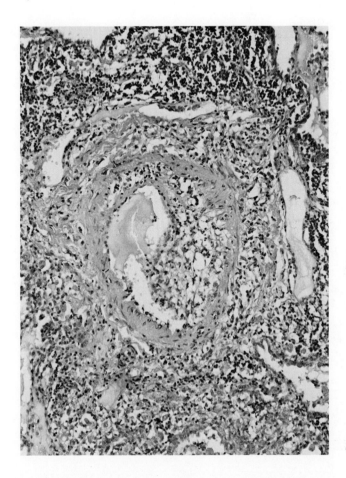

FIGURE 4 Photomicrograph of a lung biopsy in a 41–yr–old–man with Wegener's granulomatosis. Vasculitis of an arteriole with dense perivascular infiltration by mononuclear cells together with subintimal and vessel wall involvement are seen. Hematoxylin and eosin stain. Original magnification 140X.

whether the necrotizing granulomatous vasculitis with lymphoreticular proliferation is a response to an unidentified antigen, and the process subsequently progresses to a lymphoma. Clarification awaits further long–term study of this disorder.

Rarely, vasculitis is seen in the granulomata of sarcoidosis [31,32] and in the infectious granulomata of tuberculosis [33].

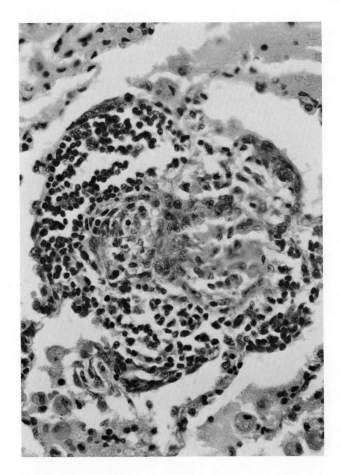

FIGURE 5 Photomicrograph of a lung biopsy of a 36–yr–old man with
Wegener's granulomatosis (same patient as in Fig. 3). Vasculitis involving
alveolar capillary is seen. Hematoxylin and eosin stain. Original magnification 350X.

IV. Treatment

A. Corticosteroids

The mainstay of treatment for pulmonary vasculitis is the same as that for systemic vasculitis, namely corticosteroids [16]. However, responses vary depending on the underlying disease process with which the pulmonary vasculitis is
associated, i.e., lupus erythematosus, periarteritis nodosa, and others.

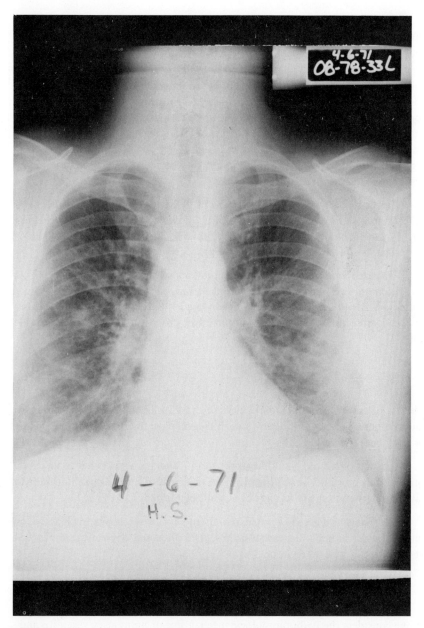

FIGURE 6 Chest roentgenogram of 34–yr–old man with Wegener's granulomatosis. Diffuse and nodular infiltration is seen. Lung biopsy showed granulomatous vasculitis.

In drug hypersensitivity vasculitis, recognition and discontinuation of the offending agent may be sufficient in itself to cause remission of disease. However, in these instances, a relatively brief course of corticosteroid therapy frequently hastens recovery [16]. The situation is somewhat unusual with rheumatoid arthritis. Diffuse vasculitis sometimes accompanies rheumatoid arthritis [34]. Although corticosteroids are a highly effective mode of therapy in refractory rheumatoid arthritis, they have been implicated as a precipitating or aggravating factor in the vasculitis of this disease [35]. In such a situation, each case must be carefully and individually considered to try to determine whether the arteritis is related to corticosteroid therapy or whether it is part of the natural acceleration of the disease itself.

In the case of vasculitis associated with lymphoproliferative disorders and other tumors, corticosteroid is also the drug of choice [16]. Appropriate therapy directed at the tumor itself, when feasible, is, of course, necessary to remove the probable source of the hypersensitivity reaction.

The pulmonary vasculitis and granulomata of allergic granulomatosis respond quite favorably to corticosteroid therapy [16,29]. In contrast, although temporary improvement of pulmonary disease is sometimes noted with the use of corticosteroids in Wegener's granulomatosis, progression of disease is the rule [36,37].

B. Cytotoxic Agents

The use of cytotoxic agents, particularly cyclophosphamide, has been shown to induce dramatic long-term remissions in Wegener's granulomatosis, even in cases of advanced disease [24,38].

In lymphomatoid granulomatosis, steroid therapy is reported to increase survival, but mortality is still high [32]. The effect of other agents in this possibly heterogeneous entity has not been well established.

Mechanisms whereby corticosteroids and cytotoxic agents, such as cyclophosphamide, suppress the vasculitic processes discussed above are complex and, at present, not well understood.

C. Mechanisms of Therapeutic Effects

If one considers the pathophysiologic mechanisms of pulmonary vasculitis and granuloma formation, as outlined in Figures 1 and 2, areas where corticosteroids or cytotoxic agents, or both potentially exert their therapeutic effects can be appreciated. The immediate effects of corticosteroids on the disease process are probably due, at least in part, to interference with the migration of granulocytes and monocytes into and around the inflammatory site, which, in this case, is a small blood vessel. In experimental situations, corticosteroids have been shown to impede the migration of granulocytes and monocytes into inflammatory sites [39], to interfere with granulocyte chemotaxis [40] and phagocytosis by macrophages [41], and to block the ability of macrophages from responding to MIF produced by immune lymphocytes [42]. In addition, in human studies, a single dose of 400 mg of hydrocortisone caused a transient lymphocytopenia and monocytopenia, probably as a result of a redistribution of cells between body compartments [43]. All of these mechanisms have the immediate effect of preventing offending cells from entering the site of immunologic involvement, where they can amplify the inflammatory response.

Corticosteroids have been shown to stabilize lysosomal membranes [44]. This property of these agents can impair the release of lysosomal enzymes from granulocytes and activated macrophages. These enzymes, as mentioned above, are damaging to the vascular endothelium and vessel wall. Corticosteroid administration also results in decreased production and increased catabolism of immunoglobulins [45] and complement [46], two of the main factors in the pathogenesis of immune complex vasculitis. Whether or not this is of clinical significance is uncertain at present. In addition, corticosteroids added to in vitro cultures of lymphocytes interfere with mitogen–induced blastogenesis [47,48]. The in vivo significance of this demonstration has not been well worked out, but this ability of corticosteroids to interfere with lymphocyte proliferation has obvious potential clinical import in lymphocyte-mediated disease.

The effects of cytotoxic agents, such as cyclophosphamide or azathioprine, are less immediate than those of corticosteroids and are more involved with suppression of the production or proliferation of offending cells [49] than with migration and circulation of these cells.

Cyclophosphamide, as an example of a cytotoxic immunosuppressive agent, has come to be an effective therapeutic agent in the treatment of certain hypersensitivity diseases [50]. Some of the most dramatic results from this agent are seen with its use in Wegener's granulomatosis [24,38]. Careful study [51,52] of various parameters of immune responsiveness has demonstrated that with doses of cyclophosphamide inducing and maintaining disease remission in Wegener's granulomatosis, the following occurs: (a) absolute lymphocytopenia and monocytopenia, (b) a proportionally greater decrease in circulating bursa-equivalent (B) lymphocytes than thymus–derived (T) lymphocytes, (c) intact mitogen–induced in vitro lymphocyte blastogenic responses, (d) decreased in vitro lymphocyte blastogenic responses to certain common antigens (streptokinase-streptodornase and tetanus toxoid), with established cutaneous delayed hypersensitivity remaining intact, (e) suppression of primary induction of delayed hypersensitivity and antibody response to a new foreign antigen (Keyhole limpet hemocyanin), and (f) decrease of elevated serum immunoglobulin levels to normal.

The exact relationship of this type of immune suppression to the ability of this agent to induce disease remission is still speculative. It may be the suppression of only one paricular factor that is specific for the disease process, or more likely, it may be a combination of several. Intensive ongoing investigation with this and other hypersensitivity diseases in several centers will hopefully elucidate this perplexing problem.

V. Summary

Pulmonary vasculitis can be a manifestation of several different disorders. The common feature is an infiltration of small vessels of the pulmonary vascular network by granulocytes, or monocytes, or both, with subsequent damage to the vessel endothelium and wall by enzymes released from the cells. Granulomata may or may not be a part of the process. Although several disorders can have pulmonary vasculitis, the clinicopathologic feature, which is probably common to all, is a hypersensitivity reaction, either a Type III or a Type IV reaction, or a combination of the two. The antigens responsible for the hypersensitivity reaction have not yet been identified in most of these disorders.

Corticosteroid therapy is effective in many instances, but this is quite variable depending on the primary disease process. Cyclophosphamide and other cytotoxic agents have proven highly effective in some disorders with pulmonary vasculitis, particularly Wegener's granulomatosis.

References

1. R. P. McCombs, J. F. Patterson, and H. E. McMahan, Syndromes associated with "allergic" vasculitis, *N. Engl. J. Med.,* **255**:251–261 (1956).
2. R. R. A. Coombs and P. G. H. Gell, The classification of allergic reactions underlying disease. In *Clinical Aspects of Immunology.* Chapter 13. Edited by P. G. H. Gell and R. R. A. Coombs. Philadelphia, F. A. Davis Co., 1968, pp. 317–337.
3. C. G. Cochrane and F. J. Dixon, Cell and tissue damage through antigen–antibody complexes. In *Textbook of Immunopathology.* Vol I. Edited by P. A. Miescher and H. J. Müller–Eberhard. New York, Grune and Stratton, 1968, pp. 94–110.
4. P. A. Ward, C. G. Cochrane, and H. J. Müller–Eberhard, The role of serum

complement in chemotaxis of leukocytes in vitro, *J. Exp. Med.,* **122**:327–346 (1965).

5. G. Weissman and P. Dukor, The role of lysosomes in immune responses, *Adv. Immunol.,* **12**:283–331 (1970).

6. B. H. Waksman, Delayed (cellular) hypersensitivity. In *Immunological Diseases.* Chapter 13. Vol. 1. Edited by M. Samter. Boston, Little, Brown and Co., 1971, pp. 220–252.

7. W. G. Spector and G. B. Ryan, The mononuclear phagocyte in inflammation. In *Mononuclear Phagocytes.* Chapter 13. Edited by R. Van Furth. Philadelphia, F. A. Davis Co., 1970, pp. 219–232.

8. R. P. McCombs, Diseases due to immunologic reactions in the lung, *N. Engl. J. Med.,* **286**:1186–1194 (1972).

9. E. Clark and B. I. Kaplan, Endocardial, arterial, and other mesenchymal alterations associated with serum disease in man, *Arch. Pathol.,* **24**:458–475 (1937).

10. H. G. Kunkel, H. J. Müller–Eberhard, H. H. Fudenberg, and T. B. Tomasi, Gamma globulin complexes in rheumatoid arthritis and certain other conditions, *J. Clin. Invest.,* **40**:117–129 (1961).

11. D. Koffler, P. H. Shur, and H. G. Kunkel, Immunological studies concerning the nephritis of systemic lupus erythematosus, *J. Exp. Med.,* **126**: 607–624 (1967).

12. F. J. Dixon, J. D. Feldman, and J. J. Vazquez, Experimental glomerulonephritis. The pathogenesis of a laboratory model resembling the spectrum of human glomerulonephritis, *J. Exp. Med.,* **113**:899–920 (1961).

13. F. Paronetto and L. Strauss, Immunocytochemical observations in periarteritis nodosa, *Ann. Intern. Med.,* **56**:289–296 (1962).

14. G. A. Rose and H. Spencer, Polyarteritis nodosa, *Q. J. Med.,* **26**:43–81 (1957).

15. D. Alarcon–Segovia and A. L. Brown, Classification and etiologic aspects of necrotizing angiitides: An analytic approach to a confused subject with a critical review of the evidence for hypersensitivity in polyarteritis nodosa, *Mayo Clin. Proc.,* **39**:205–222 (1964).

16. R. P. McCombs, Systemic "allergic" vasculitis, *J.A.M.A.,* **194**:1059–1064 (1965).

17. D. Alarcon–Segovia, K. G. Wakim, J. W. Worthington, and L. E. Ward, Clinical and experimental studies on the hydralazine syndrome and its relationship to systemic lupus erythematosus, *Medicine,* **46**:1–33 (1967).

18. J. M. Kaplan, H. L. Wochtel, S. E. Czarnecki, and J. J. Sampson, Lupus–like illness precipitated by procainamide hydrochloride, *J.A.M.A.,* **192**: 444–447 (1965).

19. P. M. Zeek, Periarteritis nodosa and other forms of necrotizing angiitis, *N. Engl. J. Med.,* **248**:764–772 (1953).

20. F. J. Dixon, J. J. Vazquez, W. O. Weigle, and C. G. Cochrane, Pathogenesis of serum sickness, *Arch. Pathol.,* **65**:18–28 (1958).

21. G. C. Godman and J. Churg, Wegener's granulomatosis: Pathology and review of the literature, *Arch. Pathol.,* **58**:533–553 (1954).

22.   J. Fahey, E. Leonard, J. Churg, and G. Godman, Wegener's granulomatosis, *Am. J. Med.*, **17**:168–179 (1954).

23.   C. B. Carrington and A. A. Liebow, Limited forms of angiitis and granulomatosis of Wegener's type, *Am. J. Med.*, **41**:497–527 (1966).

24.   A. S. Fauci and S. M. Wolff, Wegener's granulomatosis: Studies in eighteen patients and a review of the literature, *Medicine*, **52**:535–561 (1973).

25.   I. M. Blatt, H. S. Seltzer, P. Rubin, A. C. Furstenberg, J. H. Maxwell, and W. J. Schull, Fatal granulomatosis of the respiratory tract (lethal midline granuloma–Wegener's granulomatosis), *A.M.A. Arch. Otolaryngol.*, **70**: 707–757 (1959).

26.   R. G. Horn, A. S. Fauci, A. S. Rosenthal, and S. M. Wolff, Renal biopsy pathology in Wegener's granulomatosis, *Am. J. Pathol.*, **74**:423–433 (1974).

27.   D. C. Levin, Pulmonary abnormalities in the necrotizing vasculitides and their rapid response to steroids, *Radiology*, **97**:521–526 (1970).

28.   J. Churg and L. Strauss, Allergic granulomatosis, allergic angiitis, and periarteritis nodosa, *Am. J. Pathol.*, **27**:277–301 (1951).

29.   J. Churg, Allergic granulomatosis and granulomatous–vascular syndromes, *Ann. Allergy*, **21**:619–628 (1963).

30.   A. A. Liebow, C. R. B. Carrington, and P. J. Friedman, Lymphomatoid granulomatosis, *Human Pathol.*, **3**:457–558 (1972).

31.   E. Bottcher, Disseminated sarcoidosis with a marked granulomatous arteritis, *Arch. Pathol.*, **68**:419–423 (1959).

32.   A. A. Liebow, Pulmonary angiitis and granulomatosis, *Am. Rev. Respir. Dis.*, **108**:1–18 (1973).

33.   M. G. Bohrod, Periarteritis nodosa–like lesions in tuberculous meningitis, *N. Y. State J. Med.*, **48**:275–276 (1948).

34.   F. R. Schmid, Arteritis in rheumatoid arthritis, *Am. J. Med.*, **30**:56–83 (1961).

35.   J. W. Kemper, A. H. Baggenstoss, and C. H. Slocumb, The relationship between therapy with cortisone to the incidence of vascular lesions in rheumatoid arthritis, *Ann. Intern. Med.*, **46**:831–851 (1957).

36.   D. Hollander and R. T. Manning, The use of alkylating agents in the treatment of Wegener's granulomatosis, *Ann. Intern. Med.*, **67**:393–398 (1967).

37.   H. L. Israel and A. S. Patchefsky, Wegener's granulomatosis of lung: Diagnosis and treatment, *Ann. Intern. Med.*, **74**:881–891 (1971).

38.   S. N. Novack and C. M. Pearson, Cyclophosphamide therapy in Wegener's granulomatosis, *N. Engl. J. Med.*, **284**:938–942 (1971).

39.   D. R. Boggs, J. W. Athens, G. E. Cartwright, and M. M. Wintrobe, The effect of adrenal glucocorticosteroids upon the cellular composition of inflammatory exudates, *Am. J. Pathol.*, **44**:763–773 (1964).

40.   P. A. Ward, The chemosuppression of chemotaxis, *J. Exp. Med.*, **124**: 209–226 (1964).

41.   E. Wiener, Y. Marmary, and Z. Curelaru, The in vitro effect of hydrocortisone on the uptake and intracellular digestion of particulate matter by macrophages in culture, *Lab. Invest.*, **26**:220–226 (1972).

42. J. E. Balow and A. S. Rosenthal, Glucocorticoid suppression of macrophage migration inhibitory factor, *J. Exp. Med.,* **137**:1031–1041 (1973).

43. A. S. Fauci and D. C. Dale, The effect of in vivo hydrocortisone on subpopulations of human lymphocytes, *J. Clin. Invest.,* **53**:240–246 (1974).

44. G. Weissman. In *Lysosomes in Biology and Pathology.* Vol. 1. Edited by J. T. Dingle and H. B. Fell. Amsterdam and London, North Holland Publishing Co., 1969, p. 276.

45. W. T. Butler and R. D. Rossen, Effects of corticosteroids in man. I. Decreased serum IgG concentration caused by 3 or 5 days of high doses of methylprednisolone, *J. Clin. Invest.,* **52**:2629–2640 (1973).

46. J. P. Atkinson and M. M. Frank, Effect of cortisone therapy on serum complement components, *J. Immunol.,* **111**:1061–1066 (1973).

47. P. C. Nowell, Inhibition of human leukocyte mitosis by prednisolone in vitro, *Cancer Res.,* **21**:1518–1521 (1961).

48. D. H. Heilman, M. R. Gambrill, and J. P. Leichner, The effect of hydrocortisone on the incorporation of tritiated thymidine by human blood lymphocytes cultured with phytohemagglutinin and pokeweed mitogen, *Clin. Exp. Immunol.,* **15**:203–212 (1973).

49. A. E. Gabrielsen and R. A. Good, Chemical suppression of adaptive immunity, *Adv. Immunol.,* **6**:91–228 (1967).

50. A. D. Steinberg, P. H. Plotz, S. M. Wolff, V. G. Wong, S. G. Agus, and J. L. Decker, Cytotoxic drugs in treatment of nonmalignant diseases, *Ann. Intern. Med.,* **76**:619–642 (1972).

51. A. S. Fauci, S. M. Wolff, and J. S. Johnson, Effect of cyclophosphamide on the immune response in Wegener's granulomatosis, *N. Engl. J. Med.,* **285**:1493–1496 (1971).

52. A. S. Fauci, D. C. Dale, and S. M. Wolff, Cyclophosphamide and lymphocyte subpopulations in Wegener's granulomatosis, *Arthritis Rheum.,* **17**:355–362 (1974).

14

Drug-induced Hypersensitivity Disease of the Lung

EDWARD C. ROSENOW III

Mayo Medical School
Rochester, New York

I. Introduction

A. *Primum Non Nocere* (above all, do no harm)

Drug-induced disease is the most common single iatrogenic illness and is a problem that is increasing because we are living in a drug-taking society. An adverse drug reaction may be defined as any unintended or undesired consequence of drug therapy. Such reactions account for 2% to 5% of all hospital admissions; 15% to 30% of all hospitalized patients have drug reactions [1,2]. This chapter reviews the mechanisms of drug reactions, their possible relationship to the induction of pulmonary disease with emphasis on the immune reaction, and specific drug-induced pulmonary reactions that conceivably could be based on hypersensitivity. The lung is infrequently recognized as the target of a drug reaction; only recently has the importance of this problem been emphasized [3–7]. Much more is known about cutaneous, blood, liver, and renal diseases induced by drugs [8–11].

Approximately 25% of all drug-induced diseases are thought to be on an "allergic" or hypersensitivity basis and this probably is a reasonably accurate percentage for drug-induced pulmonary disease. Therefore, all drug reactions should not be lumped under the term *allergic reaction* (until recently, this term was used to imply almost any type of adverse drug reaction). Brown's classification of adverse drug reactions in 1955 is still valid [12]. In this chapter, hypersensitivity to drugs is synonymous with drug allergy—it requires the established or assumed presence of antibodies or sensitized lymphocytes.

II. Types of Adverse Reactions

A. Reactions That Occur in Any Person

1. *Overdosage.* The reaction to the drug is directly related to absolute overdosage, according to previously determined pharmacologic criteria. The reaction also can result from accumulation of the drug due to organ failure that prevents metabolism or excretion of the drug at normal rates (indirect overdosage).

2. *Side-effects.* These are undesirable but unavoidable pharmacologic actions of the drug (for example, sedative effect of antihistaminic drugs).

3. *Secondary effects.* These are indirect but not inevitable consequences of the primary action of the drug (for example, immune suppression by corticosteroids given for anti-inflammatory purposes).

4. *Drug interaction.* One or more drugs may inhibit, alter, enhance, or otherwise affect the biotransformation of another drug.

B. Reactions That Occur in Susceptible Persons (Genetically Predetermined?)

1. *Intolerance.* This untoward effect represents a qualitatively normal but quantitatively increased pharmacologic effect of the drug (for example, digitalis toxicity on "usual" therapeutic dose).

2. *Idiosyncrasy.* The adverse reaction is qualitatively abnormal and does not correspond to the usual pharmacologic actions of the drug; some of these reactions are definitely genetically predetermined (for example, hemolytic anemia in patients with glucose-6-phosphate dehydrogenase [G-6-PD] deficiency).

3. *Allergy or hypersensitivity.* An immune response in the patient leads to the formation of specific antibodies or sensitized lymphocytes. However, the demonstration of these antibodies or lymphocytes is not conclusive evidence that an allergic reaction has taken place.

The intolerant, idiosyncratic, and allergic reactions to drugs are, for the most part, unpredictable, at least with our current state of knowledge about drug reactions. Currently, it is not possible clinically to subclassify drug reactions into one of these groups. There are a number of problems related to the diagnosis of drug-induced allergic disease, the main one being the lack of suitable in vivo and, particularly, in vitro methods of detecting and confirming the reaction, which basically requires the detection of antibodies or sensitized lymphocytes to the antigenic determinant of the drug. The ideal would be to have in vitro screening methods for detecting the susceptible person *before* the drug is given and the reaction occurs.

III. Diagnosis of Allergic Drug Reactions

A. Methods Used

There are in vivo and in vitro methods available to evaluate some allergic drug reactions after they occur (see below), but these are almost never helpful in allergic drug-induced pulmonary reactions. Many drug reactions are not recognized because they are mild and transient or because the new symptoms are attributed to the disease for which the drug is being given. Also, the interval between the administration of the drug and the onset of clinical symptoms or findings may be so long that neither the patient nor the physician recognizes the correlation. To complicate the situation further, more often than not the patient is taking more than one drug that might be capable of inducing a drug reaction. Unfortunately, only a minority of drug reactions are reported in any detail, which limits the collection of data that might increase our knowledge about this problem. To add to the difficulties, there appears to be no suitable animal model for studying the idiosyncratic, intolerant, or allergic drug reaction—the experimental inbred animals used in sensitivity studies usually produce a predictable result because of genetic homogeneity, which is not the case in man.

A hypersensitivity or allergic reaction is a reaction between an antigen and its specific antibody or sensitized lymphocytes; not all such reactions are clinically significant, nor does the presence of these antibodies or lymphocytes imply that a reaction must occur. However, the definitive diagnosis rests on the demonstration of these antibodies or lymphocytes. Currently, this is not possible or practical in most drug allergy conditions, with the exception of penicillin allergy, which only rarely causes pulmonary disease (a Type I reaction of anaphylaxis with edema and bronchospasm). The diagnosis of drug allergy must then be inferred or assumed on the basis of the following [2,9].

1. *Observed reactions do not resemble known pharmacologic effects of the drug.* What determines the end-organ of a drug reaction or why one drug is a "neurotoxin" and another a "hemotoxin" or "hepatotoxin" is not known. The "shock organ" may be an innocent bystander in drug antigen–antibody reactions. On the other hand, if the antigenic determinants conjugate to noncirculating components of tissue, the tissue may become part of the antigen. It is assumed that the observed reaction and manifestations are due to the release of substances, such as kinins, SRS-A, histamine, serotonin, cytotoxins, and other polypeptides, from the antigen–antibody reaction or disruption of sensitized lymphocytes. In the lung it would appear that different substances are released in different situations, depending on the drug and on the patient. These substances can (a) alter vascular permeability to cause pulmonary edema and pleural effusion; (b) cause bronchospasm; (c) produce hypersecretion of mucus; (d) induce cellular infiltration (eosinophils, lymphocytes, and so forth); (e) cause granuloma formation; or (f) possibly, cause nearneoplastic changes in the Type II alveolar cell, as seen with busulfan of cyclophosphamide. Clinical and morphologic responses to antigen–antibody reactions, toxic reactions, and idiosyncrasies may be identical. The only way to separate them is to demonstrate antibodies or sensitized lymphocytes.

2. *There is a latent period.* This usually is 7 to 10 days but may be as short as hours or as long as weeks after therapy begins. The fact that significant nonanaphylactic reactions can begin within hours after the first dose of a drug may be due to a crossreaction from previously administered drugs, with similar antigenic determinants producing subclinical sensitization.

3. *Once a reaction has occurred, it generally recurs after the same or a closely related drug is readministered, often in minute doses.*

4. *Reactions may occur only in a minority of persons receiving the drug.* This may be genetically predetermined. As will be discussed below, the biologic degradation of the drug may

form a metabolite that, when combined with a macromolecule, forms a hapten–protein conjugate and becomes an antigen. It is the biologic degradation or transformation that may be genetically predetermined, and in a small proportion of the population a particular metabolite is formed that becomes a potential antigen. If the hypersensitivity drug reaction occurred in every patient who took the drug, the drug would not be tolerable for clinical use. Atopic persons are not necessarily more prone to drug reactions, with the possible exception of Type I reactions, and even this is uncertain. However, some persons react maximally to minimal stimulation and vice versa; the former may be the case with atopic persons.

5. *Pathologic changes are rarely characteristic.* The lung reacts to a multitude of injurious agents in a limited manner, and these are nonspecific, with one exception—the bizarre appearance of the Type II alveolar cell that occurs in response to busulfan or cyclophosphamide (this has not been proved to be a hypersensitivity type of reaction).

B. Classification and Mechanisms

A classification of hypersensitivity drug reactions is the same for any immune reaction. (See Preface in Gell and Coombs [11] for classification of immune reactions.) However, not enough is known about most drug reactions to permit categorization of each one into a specific immune mechanism. This is particularly true of drug-induced pulmonary hypersensitivity disease. A few hypersensitivity drug reactions can be subclassified into various types. Penicillin can almost be called the *universal antigen* because it can cause all four types of immune response, truly a diverse antigen. Other examples are as follows.

Type 1. Anaphylactic. Sera, antitoxins, hormones, penicillin, procainamide, and many other substances can cause this reaction.

Type 2. Cytotoxic. The reaction produces agglutination and, in the presence of complement, lysis of the target cell, which usually is an erythrocyte, leukocyte, or platelet; quinidine is a common example of drugs that produce this type.

Type 3. Arthus phenomenon. This occurs with low molecular-weight drugs, such as penicillin, sulfa, and *p*-aminosalicylic acid (PAS), as well as with heterologous sera.

Type 4. Delayed hypersensitivity. Contact dermatitis from topically applied penicillin is an example of this reaction (there is some question as to whether this is a true example of a Type IV reaction) [13].

Drugs fall into the category of simple chemicals—that is, organic compounds with a molecular weight less than 1000. For a simple chemical to become an antigen and induce the host to synthesize specific antibodies or sensitize lymphocytes (an immune response), presumably it must first bind irreversibly to tissue macromolecules through covalent bonding [2,9,14,15]. These macromolecules are usually proteins. This then is a hapten-protein conjugate that contains the antigenic determinant. Only a few drugs, such as insulin, other organ extracts, and foreign antisera, are complete antigens in the sense that they are capable of inducing sensitization without bonding to another protein [16]; these are high molecular-weight proteins of animal source. The resultant immunologic response is primarily directed against the simple chemical group that serves as the antigenic determinant, although some reactivity may be directed against the protein carrier. How or why the antigenic determinant stimulates the formation of antibody or sensitizes lymphocytes is not well known but is under intensive study [17,18].

The ability of an antigen of any kind to stimulate an immune response, in general, depends on several features [16]. First, it must be foreign to the host, or at least recognized as foreign. Second, it should have a molecular weight of more than 6000 or be able to bind irreversibly with a macromolecule. There is a general correlation between molecular weight and immunogenicity. Low molecular-weight polypeptides (<6000) are considerably less immunogenic than are larger polypeptides but occasionally can produce antibody if given repeatedly and, especially, if administered in complete adjuvant [16]. The ability to cross-react with previously or subsequently administered drugs is important in that many drugs are given for only short periods that are not long enough to stimulate an immune response. If the immune response had been initiated, but not completed previously, by a drug with an antigenic determinant, the subsequent administration of that drug or one with a similar antigenic determinant may bring about the immune response. Finally, it must be certain that impurities or additives with the drug preparation, such as polylysine, dextran, or other macromolecular substances, are not stimulating an allergic reaction or simulating one by nonallergic stimulation of the release of histamine, kinins, and so forth.

The antigenic determinants of allergenic drugs other than penicillin have not yet been identified; until this is done, the proper haptenic reagents needed for meaningful studies on the immunologic mechanisms of individual drugs cannot be prepared. One of the main reasons it is difficult to identify antigenic determinants may be that the drug does not form the antigenic determinant of the protein conjugate in most cases but rather a metabolite or degradation product of the drug does. Most drugs do not appear to be capable of irreversible covalent bonding with a protein. Metabolites or degradation products are more reactive and capable of binding firmly to tissue or serum proteins to form a complete antigen. Use of the unaltered drug for testing to detect sensitivity would not be expected to show an immunologic response resulting from a drug metabolite. More work like that of Eisner and Shahidi [19] in detecting an antibody to a metabolite must be done to remove the problem of clinical detection of drug allergy from the realm of suspicion to that of positive identification.

C. Diagnosis of Drug Allergy

History

Currently, this is the most common and, unfortunately, usually the only method of implicating a hypersensitivity reaction as the cause of the patient's problem. However, the suspicion that a drug reaction may be occurring arises only if the clinician considers the possibility. It cannot be overemphasized that a detailed drug history must be taken. It is not enough to ask only what the patient was taking at the time of the reaction; one must inquire specifically about drugs that could account for the clinical picture. This has been a particular problem with the nitrofurantoins in our experience; the patient may be taking this drug so matter-of-factly for mild chronic urinary tract symptoms that he or she no longer thinks of it as a drug.

It is just as important to find out about drugs used in the past, including the history of previous drug reactions; there may be no apparent relationship between previous use of drugs or drug reactions and the current problem, but as more is learned about drug reactions of all kinds, the possibility of crossreactions may become more evident. Furthermore, in regard to the possibility of allergic drug reactions, the history of associated symptoms, such as fever or rash, and the temporal relationship to the ingestion or administration of the drug may lend additional support to the possibility of a hypersensitivity reaction.

In Vivo Testing

Miniature tissue lesions can be produced by the injection of a specific antigen into the skin. The most common of these tests are the scratch or prick test, the intracutaneous test, and the patch test; the last is used mainly in contact allergy. The scratch and intracutaneous tests primarily detect an antibody belonging to the IgE class. These tests are rarely helpful in diagnosing most drug allergies, except to penicillin, and are almost never helpful in drug-induced pulmonary hypersensitivity reactions. When the exact antigenic determinant (metabolic or degradation product) is unknown, appropriate antigen for testing cannot be prepared.

The most definitive method of confirming a suspected drug as the cause of the patient's symptoms is the rechallenge or provocative test. In rare situations— for example, because the drug is needed as a therapeutic agent and there is no noncrossreacting acceptable substitute—it is essential to determine whether a patient is reactive to a drug. Otherwise, this procedure is unwarranted and dangerous; if it needs to be done, it should be done under strictest precautions.

In Vitro Testing

Detecting hypersensitivity drug reactions through in vitro tests avoids the dangers of in vivo challenges, but many such tests are difficult to perform and may not correlate with the clinical situation. In vitro detection of drug-induced antibodies can be divided into three categories: (a) physicochemical, (b) serologic, and (c) in vitro live-cell tests [20]. Only brief mention of the various types of tests available will be given here. None of these has come into widespread clinical use because of technical problems, lack of appropriate antigen, and, most often, the poor results that have been obtained for what was thought to be an allergic reaction. The level of circulating antibody in serum may be too low to cause a detectable serologic reaction; on the other hand, to demonstrate an antibody against a drug does not necessarily confirm a hypersensitivity drug reaction. Another problem with antibody detection is the interval between the last dose of the drug and the test. Very little is known about this relationship. It will vary, of course, with different types of drugs and there probably is considerable individual variation.

The most popular and most successful of the in vitro tests has been the serologic tests; these include agglutination, complement-fixation reactions, and immunofluorescence. As with other in vivo and in vitro methods, none of these has been of value in drug-induced pulmonary hypersensitivity reactions. There has been little or no evaluation of IgE or serum complement in drug-induced pulmonary disease.

Detection of live-cell changes in vitro include the basophil degranulation test, histamine release test, and lymphocyte transformation test (LTT). The LTT and the detection of migration inhibitory factor (MIF) may have real potential, but results have varied [20-24].

D. Drugs Possibly Associated With Pulmonary Hypersensitivity Reactions

Table 1 lists the drugs that I think *may* cause a pulmonary hypersensitivity reaction. As of this time, no antibody or sensitized lymphocyte against any of these drugs or their metabolites has been demonstrated, with the exception of antibodies against leukocytes after a blood transfusion and against pituitary snuff. It is only by inference that I can prepare such a table. I cannot even use the process of elimination, because there is no information available regarding a possible genetic variant that would explain an idiosyncratic or intolerant response mimicking an allergic reaction. Even the assay of serum or tissue concentration of a drug would be helpful in detecting an overdose from improper metabolism or excretion of the suspected drug, but this is almost never available, particularly in reports of adverse drug reactions in pulmonary disease. This could be the situation in busulfan, cyclophosphamide, bleomycin, methotrexate, or chronic nitrofurantoin reactions.

Some pulmonary drug reactions are occasionally accompanied by eosinophilia, which frequently is noted in allergic reactions. These include reactions to nitrofurantoin (acute type of reaction), methotrexate, pituitary snuff, and the drugs associated with the pulmonary infiltration-eosinophilia (PIE) syndrome. Bronchospasm is another reaction that has been associated with hypersensitivity states, but it can occur in the absence of demonstrable allergic manifestations. The drugs associated with the induction of bronchospasm are nitrofurantoin (acute reaction), pituitary snuff, aspirin, propranolol, and drugs associated with the PIE syndrome. Of course, many anaphylactic reactions include bronchospasm. Finally, drugs that induce systemic lupus erythematosus probably do so on a hypersensitivity basis.

Nitrofurantoin

This probably is the most commonly reported drug known to produce pulmonary disease. There appears to be two modes of reaction—acute and chronic [25-36]. The mechanisms probably are different because the two types of reaction are totally dissimilar. If it is assumed that the reactions are on an immune basis, it is possible that the acute and chronic are two different types of immune reactions, such as Type II or III for the acute form and Type IV for the chronic. This is purely speculation. It is interesting to postulate, however, that the difference between the two reactions is an individual variation, possibly on a genetic basis.

TABLE 1   **Drugs Known to Produce Pulmonary Disease**

Antibiotics	Neuroactive and Vasoactive Agents
Nitrofurantoin[a]	Methysergide[a]
Sulfonamides[a]	Diphenylhydantoin
Penicillin[a]	Hexamethonium,[a] mecamylamine,
Neomycin	pentolinium
Streptomycin	Propranolol
Kanamycin	
Gentamicin	Inhalants
Polymyxin B	Oxygen
Colistin	Mineral oil
	Isoproterenol
Chemotherapeutic Agents	Cromolyn sodium
Busulfan, cyclophosphamide[a]	Acetylcysteine
Methotrexate[a]	Polymyxin B
Bleomycin[a]	
Procarbazine[a]	Intravenous
Melphalan[a]	Blood[a]
	Lymphangiograms
Analgesics (including illicit drugs)	Particulate matter
Heroin[a]	
Methadone[a]	Miscellaneous
Propoxyphene[a]	Drugs that induce systemic lupus
Hashish	erythematosus[a]
Marihuana	Hydrochlorothiazide[a]
Aspirin	Chlordiazapoxide[a]
Indomethacin	Anticoagulants
	Vitamin D, calcium, inorganic
Endocrine Agents	phosphate
Corticosteroids	
Oral contraceptives	
Pituitary snuff[a]	

[a]Possibly through a hypersensitivity mechanism

The acute type of nitrofurantoin reaction is characterized by the onset of fever, chills, dyspnea, and cough 3 to 10 days after the course of therapy is initiated, but onset may be within a few hours. (The fact that the reaction can begin within a few hours after the first dose argues against an allergic reaction; when this has occurred, it is possible that this drug had been taken by the patient in the past or that this was a crossreaction.) The pulmonary response appears to be pulmonary edema, although this has not been proved; there has not been a report of biopsy in the acute type of reaction nor has there been a report of a death. Moist rales are heard. The chest roentgenogram usually shows a pattern consistent with noncardiac pulmonary edema, but the changes may be minimal, particularly in comparison to the presence of widespread rales.

Remission usually occurs within 24 to 48 hr after the drug intake is discontinued. The onset and remission appear to be too rapid for the response to be an acute interstitial pneumonitis, and pulmonary edema is favored. Also, the finding of pleural effusion tends to support the theory that this is a form of pulmonary edema, probably on the basis of increased permeability of the alveolar capillary basement membrane. Eosinophilia can occur, as can bronchospasm or anaphylactic reaction. It is not uncommon for the patient to present with a history of several episodes of the acute reaction before the diagnosis is made, the nitrofurantoin being inadvertently discontinued during each illness. However, it also is characteristic for the latent interval to decrease with each episode.

The symptoms and the findings of fever, eosinophilia, rapid onset, typical latent period, and positive response to a small rechallenge dose favor the theory that the acute nitrofurantoin pulmonary reaction is a hypersensitivity drug reaction. There has been one report [21] or an in vitro test being used in a case of nitrofurantoin drug reaction.

Illustrative Case 1

> A 51-yr-old woman had had "four pneumonias" in a 6-month period, with fever, cough, and dyspnea each time. In each episode the chest roentgenogram was similar to that in Figure 1, with bilateral infiltrates at the bases. With each hospitalization, her regular medications, including nitrofurantoin which has been started 1 wk prior to her first episode, were discontinued. Within a short time after admission, her symptoms were relieved and the chest roentgenogram cleared. She resumed taking her regular medication shortly after each dismissal. It was not until her fourth "pneumonia" that the correlation between the nitrofurantoin therapy and the onset of illness was recognized. There was an eosinophilia (8%) at her last admission. Results of pulmonary function studies at the time of her last admission and 6 wk later during a follow-up visit are shown in Table 2.

The pulmonary function data in Case 1 show a combination of restrictive and obstructive lung disease; the obstructive element is not always present and has been given little recognition in the cases reported, but it does occur.

The chronically induced phase has none of the secondary features of the acute phase—no pleural effusion, fever, eosinophilia, or bronchospasm [33-36]. The cough and dyspnea begin insidiously 6 months to a number of years after the patient starts taking nitrofurantoin on a more or less regular basis. The roentgenographic pattern is that of an interstitial pneumonitis and fibrosis (Fig. 2).

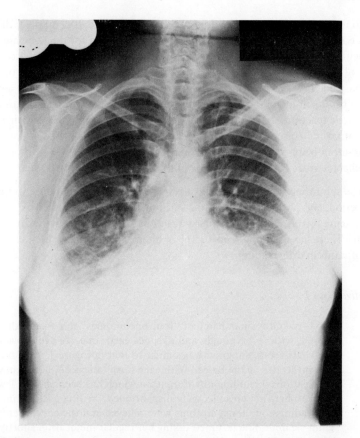

FIGURE 1   Acute nitrofurantoin pneumonitis, showing bilateral basilar infiltrates and probable bilateral pleural effusions. Appearance returned to normal within 1 wk after discontinuing nitrofurantoin therapy.

TABLE 2   Pulmonary Function Studies in 51-Yr-Old Woman With Acute Nitrofurantoin Pneumonitis

Variable	Normal	On admission	At 6-wk follow-up
Vital capacity (liters)	2.4	1.8	2.7
Total capacity (liters)	4.1	2.6	3.6
Maximal breathing capacity (liters/min)	67	77	104
Maximal mid-expiratory flow (liter/s)	>1.5	0.8	2.8
D_{CO} (SS) (ml/min-mm Hg)	12	6	12

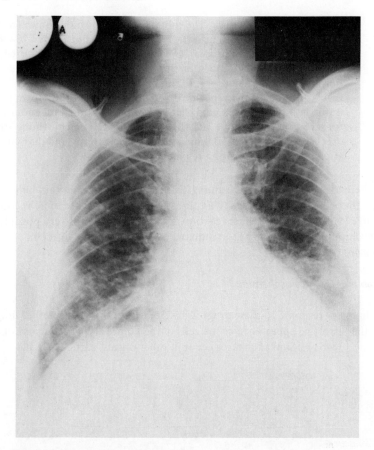

FIGURE 2 Chronic nitrofurantoin pneumonitis. There is a diffuse interstitial process bilaterally that cleared completely 3 months after discontinuation of the nitrofurantoin regimen and start of corticosteroid therapy.

Velcro-type rales may be heard on auscultation, particularly at the bases. Clubbing has not been reported. Histologically, the changes are the same as those seen in classic interstitial pneumonitis and fibrosis (CIPF), which has been reported [37] to have some immunologic features.

Illustrative Case 2

A 65-yr-old man had had cough and dyspnea for 1 yr. There was no history of fever, chills, night sweats, or nitrofurantoin therapy. There were no other medical problems. Velcro-type rales were evident on auscultation of the lungs. The thoracic roentgenogram showed a diffuse interstitial process (Fig. 2). Pulmonary function studies revealed a moderate restrictive process. An open lung biopsy was reported as showing "marked chronic interstitial pneumonitis with interstitial fibrosis" (Fig. 3), a nonspecific finding. Shortly after this, the patient was questioned specifically about taking "a little brown pill" (nitrofurantoin), and he said that he had been taking it on and off for several years without knowing the name of the medication. An excellent response was obtained with steroid therapy and discontinuation of the nitrofurantoin regimen.

There are no characteristic features of the chronic nitrofurantoin lung reaction that point to a hypersensitivity disease; however, because there is good supportive evidence that the acute reaction is an allergic one, it is very possible that the chronic reaction also has an immune basis, albeit with a different mechanism.

Busulfan and Cyclophosphamide

The pulmonary response to these drugs is different from that to any other drugs in that the histologic appearance of the cells in the lung is atypical and almost neoplastic [38–51]. Similar changes occur in other organs, particularly the

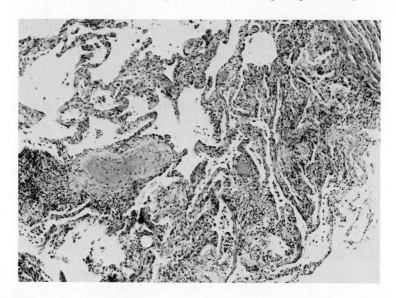

FIGURE 3 Chronic nitrofurantoin pneumonitis and fibrosis, showing significant cellular infiltration of interstitium. There was little fibrotic reaction in this case. (Hematoxylin and eosin; 70X.)

genitourinary system. There are at least two known cases of carcinoma of the lung in patients receiving these drugs (along with typical histologic changes of these drugs) [3,43]. Clinically, the patient has subacute onset of cough, dyspnea, and fever beginning, on the average, 3 to 4 yr after he starts to take the drug for a hematologic disorder. The initial impression is that the patient has leukemic infiltration of the lungs or an opportunistic infection. Scattered rales may be heard. The chest roentgenogram (Fig. 4) shows a combined acinar and interstitial pattern. A pleural effusion has been reported in some cases. Laboratory data are of little value; pulmonary function studies show a restrictive pattern.

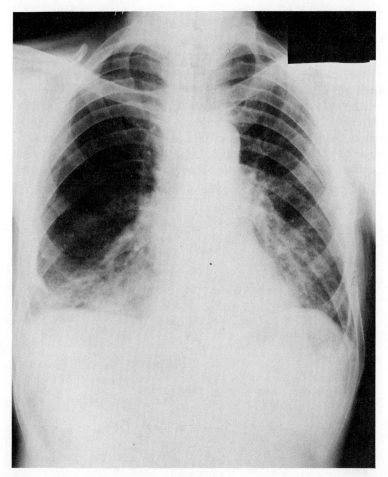

FIGURE 4 Busulfan lung, showing a diffuse intraalveolar and interstitial process in both lungs, particularly at the base but also evident in left upper lobe. It is not uncommon for this process to occur somewhat asymmetrically, at least in the early stages.

Illustrative Case 3

This 71-yr-old man was referred to our clinic with a diagnosis of chronic myelogenous leukemia made 3 yr ago at another institution. He had been started on busulfan therapy and eventually received a total of 1200 mg. Six months prior to this admission, cough and dyspnea developed; more recently, he had daily fevers (up to 39.4°C). The thoracic roentgenogram on admission is shown in Figure 4. His course was rapid deterioration during 1 wk. Only at autopsy was the correct diagnosis of busulfan lung made. Histologically, the Type II alveolar cell takes on a bizarre appearance; the bronchial epithelial cell also shows similar but less abnormal changes, and a fibrotic reaction takes place (Fig. 5).

With the help of the clinical history, our cytologists have been able to diagnose busulfan or cyclophosphamide lung on several occasions from sputum or bronchial washings because of the characteristic appearance of the Type II alveolar cell. There is no way, at this time, of knowing whether or not this is a hypersensitivity reaction. There are limited ways in which the lung can react in response to a hypersensitivity reaction, and in no other known hypersensitivity reaction involving the lungs do these bizarre atypical cells appear. For this reason,

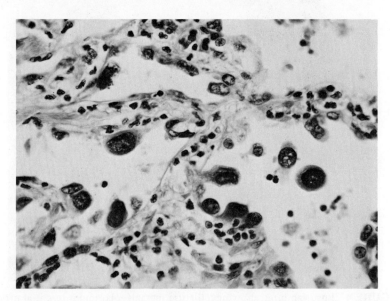

FIGURE 5 Busulfan lung, showing marked atypia of the Type II pneumocytes as well as significant changes in epithelial cells. (Hematoxylin and eosin; 400X.)

it is possible that the busulfan lung is not a hypersensitivity reaction. However, the regular occurrence of fever does suggest an allergic mechanism. Corticosteroids are frequently of little or no benefit, and the patient dies even though the drug has been discontinued. There is one case report [52] of a pulmonary reaction to melphalan, with histologic changes similar to those with busulfan.

Methotrexate

In the lungs of patients receiving methotrexate for acute lymphatic leukemia or psoriasis, changes occur 10 days to 6 months after therapy has been initiated; there is acute onset of fever, cough, and dyspnea [53-58]. There have been only a few reports of the histologic findings because most signs and symptoms reverse when the drug is discontinued and steroid therapy is started. Histologic features vary from "granulomatous reaction" to "changes similar to the busulfan lung, without the bizarre, atypical cells." Most authors, for various reasons, think that methotrexate lung is a hypersensitivity reaction, possibly because it responds rapidly to steroids. However, it is interesting that the onset occurs within several days after methotrexate therapy is started in some patients and months afterward in others, apparently related to the amount of drug taken per week. Again, as with other drugs discussed here, this reaction does not occur in every patient who takes the drug, including those who have been taking it for years. There have been no reported in vitro studies with this drug. Cirrhosis and low-grade hepatitis are other complications of methotrexate therapy [57].

Methysergide

This drug produces a "fibrotic" reaction in the lungs, pleura, heart, and retroperitoneal space in a small percentage of patients who take it for vascular headaches [59-63]. The apparent pulmonary fibrosis is usually at least partially reversible after the drug intake is discontinued, an unusual occurrence for fibrotic reactions in the lung. The onset of dyspnea is insidious; there may be no cough and rales or friction rub usually are not heard. The chest roentgenogram (Fig. 6) reveals a ground-glass appearance over the lower half of the lung fields, most likely due to pleural thickening. Pleural effusion can occur, but in my experience with three patients, pleural changes have been limited to a fibrotic reaction. There are no other manifestations of an allergic reaction, such as fever, eosinophilia, or rash.

Drug-Induced Systemic Lupus Erythematosus (SLE)

This is an important aspect of drug-induced pulmonary hypersensitivity disease because the more that is learned about the mechanism of this disease the better

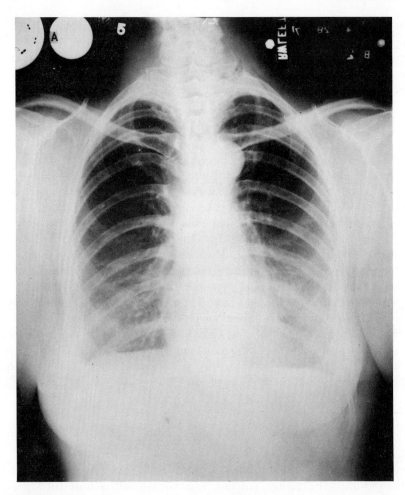

FIGURE 6 Methysergide lung. Ground–glass appearance is typical of pleural thickening seen in this drug–induced pulmonary disease. There also is evidence of pleural effusion. In this patient, there was no free fluid seen on decubitus films. There also may be an interstitial fibrotic process but it is less pronounced than the pleural fibrosis.

other aspects of drug-induced disease [64-69] will be understood. One theory is that these drugs only unmask a propensity to SLE that was already there. On this basis, it is possible that drug reactions of any kind occur only in certain persons predisposed to them. The reaction is primarily dose-related; it does not occur as early as within a few days or weeks after the drug is started. Therefore, it is of utmost importance to identify such persons and *prevent* drug reactions.

TABLE 3   Drugs That Induce Systemic Lupus Erythematosus

Procainamide	Aminosalicylic acid
Hydralazine	Griseofulvin
Isoniazid	Phenylbutazone
Diphenylhydantoin	Methylthiouracil
Mephenytoin	Propylthiouracil
Trimethadione	Reserpine
Primidone	Methyldopa
Ethosuximide	Oral contraceptives
Penicillin	Digitalis
Sulfonamides	Gold
Tetracycline	Thiazides
Streptomycin	Guanoxan
Isoquinazepon	Practolol
Penicillamine	

Table 3 lists most of the drugs that have been reported to produce the SLE syndrome.

Drug-induced SLE is different from that which usually occurs spontaneously in that there is less renal and cutaneous and more pleuropulmonary reaction in drug-induced SLE [69]. Also, the disease usually, but not always, remits after the drug is discontinued. A change in serum complement is not involved, but antibodies to denatured DNA, nucleohistone, and erythrocyte membranes are demonstrable. It may be that these drugs combine with nuclear macromolecules or other potential autoantigens to render them more immunogenic.

The thoracic roentgenogram and pleuropulmonary histologic changes in drug-induced SLE are nonspecific and not diagnostic; they are similar to those seen in spontaneously occurring SLE.

Illustrative Case 4

A 48-yr-old man had been taking procainamide (1.0 g per day) and an indeterminate amount of hydralazine (Apresoline) for 6 months for arrhythmia and hypertension. On admission he reported having had nonanginal chest pains, cough, dyspnea, orthopnea, fever, and arthralgias for 6 wk. The LE clot test was positive; assay for antinuclear antibody (ANA) was negative. Laboratory data were: hemoglobin, 10.5 g/100 ml; creatinine, 1.0 mg/ 100 ml; and sedimentation

rate, 110 mm in 1 hr (Westergren). Urinalysis revealed grade 2
proteinuria (0.5 g/24 hr) and an occasional cast. The chest roentgenogram (Fig. 7) showed pleural and pericardial effusion, a diffuse infiltration at the bases, and "atelectasizing pneumonitis."
The drugs were discontinued, and corticosteroid therapy produced
marked improvement. The corticosteroid regimen was discontinued after 6 months, with no recurrence of symptoms; the chest
roentgenogram was negative.

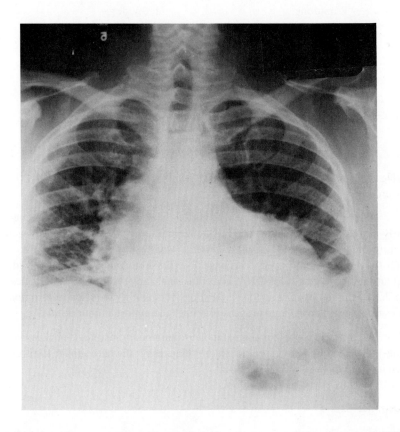

FIGURE 7 Procainamide–induced SLE, showing many of the changes of SLE,
both spontaneous and drug–induced. Cardiomegaly is due to large pericardial
effusion. Pleural effusion is present as well. The lung parenchyma demonstrates
an interstitial pneumonitis plus areas of atelectasizing pneumonitis. Roentgenographic appearance returned to normal within 3 months of discontinuation of
procainamide therapy and start of corticosteroid regimen.

Heroin, Methadone, and Propoxyphene

Pulmonary edema produced by the oral or intravenous administration of these drugs may be solely on the basis of depression of the respiratory center, with hypoxia, as postulated by some; however, pulmonary edema does not accompany all situations of acute respiratory center depression and hypoxia, a good example being barbiturate intoxication [70-77]. There must be some other unexplained mechanism, possibly a hypersensitivity reaction. There have been no reports that pulmonary edema recurred in survivors of the first episode when they returned to the habit, but such recurrence would be expected on the premise that, once the person is sensitized, administration of a small amount of the drug should precipitate a reaction. However, in this situation more than in any other so far mentioned, contaminants may play a significant role in whatever causes the pulmonary edema.

Leukoagglutinins

Noncardiac normovolemic pulmonary edema can be associated with whole-blood transfusion [78-80]. Antibodies to leukocytes have been demonstrated, and it is postulated that these produce a hypersensitivity pneumonitis. An abrupt onset (within minutes of starting the transfusion) of chills, fever, tachycardia, dyspnea, and cough is usual. The infiltration seen on the thoracic roentgenogram clears within 48 to 96 hr. The clinical course and roentgenologic findings are similar to those in the acute nitrofurantoin reaction. The donors in most cases are multiparous females.

Other Drugs

A number of drugs have been associated with the induction of bronchospasm; however, in none of these cases has there been a definite association with an allergic reaction. The bronchospasm related to aerosolized isoproterenol, cromolyn sodium, polymyxin B, and other drugs probably is brought on by a direct irritative effect or, as in the case of isoproterenol, by a metabolite that is a weak antagonist of β-adrenergic receptors. The increased airway resistance associated with propranolol apparently is mediated by the autonomic nervous system. The bronchoconstriction related to acetylsalicylic acid was thought for years to be on an immune basis, but now there is evidence that its effects may be mediated by direct stimulation of humoral receptors [81-83]. Inhalation of pituitary snuff can produce either bronchospasm or an extrinsic allergic alveolitis, with demonstrable antibodies in the serum against the extract [84-86].

Three cases of acute pulmonary reaction after the ingestion of hydrochlorothiazide have been reported [87,88]. A similar reaction after an overdose
(intravenously) of chlordiazepoxide (Librium) also has been noted [89]. Recently, several reports have implicated procarbazine in a hypersensitivity pulmonary reaction [90-92]; the symptoms began acutely or subacutely and were
similar to those of nitrofurantoin pulmonary reaction. Bleomycin produces a
severe, frequently fatal, pulmonary pneumonitis-fibrosis in a small percentage
of the patients who take this drug [93-95]. It has always been thought that the
pulmonary side-effects of bleomycin were due to toxic effects rather than to a
hypersensitivity reaction and that, if the doses were kept to less than 300 to 400
mg, the chances for pulmonary complications would be minimized. There are
no secondary effects, such as eosinophilia or fever; the changes can be reproduced in dogs [96]. Sulfonamides and other drugs have been known to be
related to the induction of a vasculitis as well as the pulmonary infiltration-
eosinophilia syndrome [97-99]; this has been thought to be on an allergic basis,
but there is little evidence in the form of demonstrated antibodies or sensitized
lymphocytes against these drugs.

References

1. K. L. Melmon, Preventable drug reactions: Causes and cures, *N. Engl. J. Med.,* **284**:1361-1368 (1971).
2. R. D. DeSwarte, Drug allergy. In *Allergic Diseases: Diagnosis and Manage-ment.* Edited by R. Patterson. Philadelphia, J. B. Lippincott Co., 1972, pp. 393-494.
3. E. C. Rosenow, III, The spectrum of drug–induced pulmonary disease, *Ann. Intern. Med.,* **77**:977-991 (1972).
4. P. D. B. Davies, Drug–induced lung disease, *Br. J. Dis. Chest,* **63**:57-70 (1969).
5. M. E. Whitcomb, Drug–induced lung disease, *Chest,* **63**:418-422 (1973).
6. A. Brettner, E. R. Heitzman, and W. G. Woodin, Pulmonary complications of drug therapy, *Radiology,* **96**:31-38 (1970).
7. G. Ansell, Radiological manifestations of drug–induced disease, *Clin. Radiol.,* **20**:133-148 (1969).
8. M. Samter and C. W. Parker. *Hypersensitivity to Drugs.* Vol. 1. New York, Pergamon Press, 1972.
9. A. L. De Weck, Drug reactions. In *Immunological Diseases.* Vol. 1. Second edition. Edited by M. Samter. Boston, Little, Brown, and Com-pany, 1971, pp. 415-440.
10. L. H. Criep. *Clinical Immunology and Allergy.* Second edition. New York, Grune & Stratton, 1969, pp. 148-176; 179-187.
11. J. F. Ackroyd and A. J. Rook, Allergic drug reactions. In *Clinical Aspects of Immunology.* Second edition. Edited by P. G. H. Gell and R. R. A. Coombs. Philadelphia, F. A. Davis Company, 1968, pp. 693-755.

12. E. A. Brown, Problems of drug allergy, *J.A.M.A.,* **157**:814–819 (1955).

13. H. F. Dvorak and M. C. Mihm, Jr., Basophilic leukocytes in allergic contact dermatitis, *J. Exp. Med.,* **135**:235–254 (1972).

14. H. Remmer and R. Schüppel, The formation of antigenic determinants. In *Hypersensitivity to Drugs.* Vol. 1. Edited by M. Samter and C. W. Parker. New York, Pergamon Press, 1972, pp. 67–89.

15. M. Samter, Hypersensitivity to drugs: Definition and scope. In *Hypersensitivity to Drugs.* Vol. 1. Edited by M. Samter and C. W. Parker. New York, Pergamon Press, 1972, pp. 3–9.

16. R. Hoigné, Therapeutic agents that are complete antigens. In *Hypersensitivity to Drugs.* Vol. 1. Edited by M. Samter and C. W. Parker. New York, Pergamon Press, 1972, pp. 23–65.

17. B. B. Levine, Immunochemical mechanisms of drug allergy, *Annu. Rev. Med.,* **17**:23–38 (1966).

18. N. R. Shulman, Immunologic reactions to drugs (editorial), *N. Engl. J. Med.,* **287**:408–409 (1972).

19. E. V. Eisner and N. T. Shahidi, Immune thrombocytopenia due to a drug metabolite, *N. Engl. J. Med.,* **287**:376–381 (1972).

20. B. N. Halpern, Antibodies produced by drugs and methods for their detection. In *Hypersensitivity to Drugs.* Vol. 1. Edited by M. Samter and C. W. Parker. New York, Pergamon Press, 1972, pp. 113–147.

21. R. E. Rocklin and J. R. David, Detection *in vitro* of cellular hypersensitivity to drugs, *J. Allergy Clin. Immunol.,* **48**:276–282 (1971).

22. B. Halpern, N. T. Ky, and N. Amache, Diagnosis of drug allergy *in vitro* with the lymphocyte transformation test, *J. Allergy Clin. Immunol.,* **40**: 168–181 (1967).

23. T. Han, P. L. Chawla, and J. E. Sokal, Sulfapyridine–induced serum-sickness–like syndrome associated with plasmacytosis, lymphocytosis, and multiclonal gamma–globulinopathy, *N. Engl. J. Med.,* **280**:547–548 (1969).

24. I. Sarkany, Clinical and laboratory aspects of drug allergy, *Proc. R. Soc. Med.,* **61**:891–894 (1968).

25. E. J. Hailey, H. W. Glascock, Jr., and W. F. Hewitt, Pleuropneumonic reactions to nitrofurantoin, *N. Engl. J. Med.,* **281**:1087–1090 (1969).

26. H. L. Israel and P. Diamond, Recurrent pulmonary infiltration and pleural effusion due to nitrofurantoin sensitivity, *N. Engl. J. Med.,* **266**:1024–1026 (1962).

27. D. C. F. Muir and J. A. Stanton, Allergic pulmonary infiltration due to nitrofurantoin, *Br. Med. J.,* **1**:1072 (1963).

28. M. J. Murray and R. Kronenberg, Pulmonary reactions simulating cardiac pulmonary edema caused by nitrofurantoin, *N. Engl. J. Med.,* **273**:1185–1187 (1965).

29. W. G. Strauss and L. M. Griffin, Nitrofurantoin pneumonia, *J.A.M.A.,* **199**: 765–766 (1967).

30. C. J. DeMasi, Allergic pulmonary infiltrates probably due to nitrofurantoin, *Arch. Intern. Med.,* **120**:631–634 (1967).

31. T. M. Nicklaus and A. B. Snyder, Nitrofurantoin pulmonary reaction: A
     unique syndrome, *Arch. Intern. Med.,* **121**:151–155 (1968).
32. M. A. Glueck and M. L. Janower, Nitrofurantoin lung disease: Clues to
     pathogenesis, *Am. J. Roentgenol. Radium Ther. Nucl. Med.,* **107**:818–
     822 (1969).
33. E. C. Rosenow, III, R. A. DeRemee, and D. E. Dines, Chronic nitrofuran-
     toin pulmonary reaction, *N. Engl. J. Med.,* **279**:1258–1262 (1968).
34. R. B. David, H. A. Andersen, and G. B. Stickler, Nitrofurantoin sensitivity:
     Report of a child with chronic inflammatory lung disease, *Am. J. Dis.
     Child.,* **116**:418–421 (1968).
35. K. S. Israel, R. E. Brashear, H. M. Sharma, et al., Pulmonary fibrosis and
     nitrofurantoin, *Am. Rev. Respir. Dis.,* **108**:353–356 (1973).
36. I. Ruikka, T. Vaissalo, and H. Saarimaa, Progressive pulmonary fibrosis
     during nitrofurantoin therapy, *Scand. J. Respir. Dis.,* **52**:162–166 (1971).
37. R. A. DeRemee, E. G. Harrison, Jr., and H. A. Andersen, The concept of
     classic interstitial pneumonitis–fibrosis (CIP–F) as a clinicopathologic
     syndrome, *Chest,* **61**:213–220 (1972).
38. H. Oliner, R. Schwartz, F. Rubio, Jr., et al., Interstitial pulmonary fibrosis
     following busulfan therapy, *Am. J. Med.,* **31**:134–139 (1961).
39. B. E. Heard and R. A. Cooke, Busulfan lung, *Thorax,* **23**:187–193 (1968).
40. W. A. Littler, J. M. Kay, P. S. Hasleton, et al., Busulphan lung, *Thorax,*
     24:639–655 (1969).
41. E. Leake and W. G. Smith, Diffuse interstitial pulmonary fibrosis after
     busulphan therapy, *Lancet,* **2**:432–434 (1963).
42. R. V. Smalley and R. L. Wall, Two cases of busulfan toxicity, *Ann. Intern.
     Med.,* **64**:154–164 (1966).
43. K.-W. Min and F. Györkey, Interstitial pulmonary fibrosis, atypical epi-
     thelial changes, and bronchiolar cell carcinoma following busulfan therapy,
     Cancer, **22**:1027–1032 (1968).
44. W. A. Burns, W. McFarland, and M. J. Matthews, Busulfan–induced pul-
     monary disease: Report of a case and review of the literature, *Am. Rev.
     Respir. Dis.,* **101**:408–413 (1970).
45. R. H. Kirschner and J. R. Esterly, Pulmonary lesions associated with
     busulfan therapy of chronic myelogenous leukemia, *Cancer,* **27**:1074–
     1080 (1971).
46. Case Records of the Massachusetts General Hospital, (Case 40–1971), *N.
     Engl. J. Med.,* **285**:847–855 (1971).
47. I. G. Koss, M. R. Melamed, and K. Mayer, The effect of busulfan on
     human epithelia, *Am. J. Clin. Pathol.,* **44**:385–397 (1965).
48. W. A. Littler and C. Ogilvie, Lung function in patients receiving busulfan,
     Br. Med. J., **4**:530–532 (1970).
49. H. J. Woodliff and L. R. Finlay-Jones, Busulfan lung, *Med. J. Aust.,* **2**:
     719–722 (1972).
50. A. E. Rodin, M. E. Haggard, and L. B. Travis, Lung changes and chemo-
     therapeutic agents in childhood: Report of a case associated with cyclo-
     phosphamide therapy, *Am. J. Dis. Child.,* **120**:337–340 (1970).

51.   A. A. Topilow, S. P. Rothenberg, and T. S. Cottrell, Interstitial pneumonia after prolonged treatment with cyclophosphamide, *Am. Rev. Respir. Dis.,* **108**:114–117 (1973).

52.   B. W. Codling and T. M. H. Chakera, Pulmonary fibrosis following therapy with melphalan for multiple myeloma, *J. Clin. Pathol.,* **25**:668–673 (1972).

53.   A. M. Clarysse, W. J. Cathey, G. E. Cartwright, et al., Pulmonary disease complicating intermittent therapy with methotrexate, *J.A.M.A.,* **209**: 1861–1864 (1969).

54.   I. R. Schwartz and M. K. Kajani, Methotrexate therapy and pulmonary disease, *J.A.M.A.,* **210**:1924 (1969).

55.   Acute Leukemia Group B, Acute lymphocytic leukemia in children: Maintenance therapy with methotrexate administered intermittently, *J.A.M.A.,* **207**:923–928 (1969).

56.   G. C. Goldman and S. L. Moschella, Severe pneumonitis occurring during methotrexate therapy: Report of two cases, *Arch. Dermatol.,* **103**:194–197 (1971).

57.   D. J. Filip, G. L. Logue, T. S. Harle, et al., Pulmonary and hepatic complications of methotrexate therapy of psoriasis, *J.A.M.A.,* **216**:881–882 (1971).

58.   M. E. Whitcomb, M. I. Schwarz, and D. C. Tormey, Methotrexate pneumonitis: Case report and review of the literature, *Thorax,* **27**:636–639 (1972).

59.   J. R. Graham, H. I. Suby, P. R. LeCompte, et al., Fibrotic disorders associated with methysergide therapy for headache, *N. Engl. J. Med.,* **274**: 359–368 (1966).

60.   J. R. Graham, Cardiac and pulmonary fibrosis during methysergide therapy for headache, *Am. J. Med. Sci.,* **254**:1–12 (1967).

61.   R. P. Bays, Pleuropulmonary fibrosis following therapy with methysergide maleate: Two case reports, *J. L. State Med. Soc.,* **120**:426–427 (1968).

62.   W. Hindle, E. Posner, M. T. Sweetnam, et al., Pleural effusion and fibrosis during treatment with methysergide, *Br. Med. J.,* **1**:605–606 (1970).

63.   A. Kok-Jensen and O. Lindeneg, Pleurisy and fibrosis of the pleura during methysergide treatment of hemicrania, *Scand. J. Respir. Dis.,* **51**:218–222 (1970).

64.   D. Alarcón-Segovia, K. G. Wakim, J. W. Worthington, et al., Clinical and experimental studies on the hydralazine syndrome and its relationship to systemic lupus erythematosus, *Medicine* (Baltimore), **46**:1–33 (1967).

65.   D. Alarcón-Segovia and D. G. Alarcón, Pleuro–pulmonary manifestations of systemic lupus erythematosus, *Dis. Chest,* **39**:7–17 (1961).

66.   W. St. C. Symmers, So–called 'collagen diseases' as a manifestation of sensitivity to drugs. In *Drug-Induced Diseases.* Edited by L. Meyler and H. M. Peck. Springfield, Illinois, Charles C. Thomas, 1962, pp. 123–136.

67.   S. L. Lee, I. Rivero, and M. Siegel, Activation of systemic lupus erythematosus by drugs, *Arch. Intern. Med.,* **117**620–626 (1966).

68.   R. B. Byrd and B. Schanzer, Pulmonary sequelae in procaine amide induced lupus-like syndrome, *Dis. Chest,* **55**:170–172 (1969).

69.   S. E. Blomgren, J. J. Condemi, and J. H. Vaughan, Procainamide–induced lupus erythematosus: Clinical and laboratory observations, *Am. J. Med.,* 52:338–348 (1972).

70.   D. B. Louria, T. Hensle, and J. Rose, The major medical complications of heroin addiction, *Ann. Intern. Med.,* 67:1–22 (1967).

71.   A. D. Steinberg and J. S. Karliner, The clinical spectrum of heroin pulmonary edema, *Arch. Intern. Med.,* 122:122–127 (1968).

72.   J. L. Duberstein and D. M. Kaufman, A clinical study of an epidemic of heroin intoxication and heroin–induced pulmonary edema, *Am. J. Med.,* 51:704–714 (1971).

73.   S. Katz, A. Aberman, U. I. Frand, et al., Heroin pulmonary edema: Evidence for increased pulmonary capillary permeability, *Am. Rev. Respir. Dis.,* 106:472–474 (1972).

74.   J. M. Kjeldgaard, G. W. Hahn, J. R. Heckenlively, et al., Methadone–induced pulmonary edema, *J.A.M.A.,* 218:882–883 (1971).

75.   A. L. Goldman and R. W. Enquist, Methadone pulmonary edema, *Chest,* 63:275–276 (1973).

76.   I. J. Bogartz and W. C. Miller, Pulmonary edema associated with propoxyphene intoxication, *J.A.M.A.,* 215:259–262 (1971).

77.   F. S. Tennant, Jr., Complications of propoxyphene abuse, *Arch. Intern. Med.,* 132:191–194 (1973).

78.   J. S. Thompson, C. D. Severson, M. J. Parmely, et al., Pulmonary "hypersensitivity" reactions induced by transfusion of non–HL–A leukoagglutinins, *N. Engl. J. Med.,* 284:1120–1125 (1971).

79.   H. N. Ward, Pulmonary infiltrates associated with leukoagglutinin transfusion reactions, *Ann. Intern. Med.,* 73:689–694 (1970).

80.   J. P. Byrne, Jr. and J. A. Dixon, Pulmonary edema following blood transfusion reaction, *Arch. Surg.,* 102:91–94 (1971).

81.   B. Giraldo, M. N. Blumenthal, and W. W. Spink, Aspirin intolerance and asthma: A clinical and immunological study, *Ann. Intern. Med.,* 71:479–496 (1969).

82.   M. Samter and R. F. Beers, Jr., Intolerance to aspirin: Clinical studies and consideration of its pathogenesis, *Ann. Intern. Med.,* 68:975–983 (1968).

83.   A. M. Yurchak, K. Wicher, and C. E. Arbesman, Immunologic studies on aspirin: Clinical studies with aspiryl–protein conjugates, *J. Allergy Clin. Immunol.,* 46:245–253 (1970).

84.   J. Pepys. *Hypersensitivity Diseases of the Lungs Due to Fungi and Organic Dusts.* Basel, S. Kerger AG, 1969, pp. 112–117.

85.   W. E. Mahon, D. J. Scott, G. Ansell, et al., Hypersensitivity to pituitary snuff with miliary shadowing in the lungs, *Thorax,* 22:13–20 (1967).

86.   L. O. Harper, R. G. Burrell, N. L. Lapp, et al., Allergic alveolitis due to pituitary snuff, *Ann. Intern. Med.,* 73:581–584 (1970).

87.   C. Beaudry and L. LaPlante, Severe allergic pneumonitis from hydrochlorothiazide, *Ann. Intern. Med.,* 78:251–253 (1973).

88. A. D. Steinberg, Pulmonary edema following ingestion of hydrochloro-thiazide, *J.A.M.A.*, **204**:825–827 (1968).
89. S. Richman and R. D. Harris, Acute pulmonary edema associated with librium abuse: A case report, *Radiology*, **103**:57–58 (1972).
90. S. E. Jones, M. Moore, N. Blank, et al., Hypersensitivity to procarbazine (Matulane) manifested by fever and pleuropulmonary reaction, *Cancer*, **29**:498–500 (1972).
91. J. J. Lokich and W. C. Moloney, Allergic reaction to procarbazine, *Clin. Pharmacol. Ther.*, **13**:573–574 (1972).
92. V. A. Dohner, H. P. Ward, and R. E. Standord, Alveolitis during procar-bazine, vincristine, and cyclophosphamide therapy, *Chest*, **62**:636–639 (1972).
93. R. A. Rudders and G. T. Hensley, Bleomycin pulmonary toxicity, *Chest*, **63**:626–628 (1973).
94. A. L. Horowitz, M. Friedman, J. Smith, et al., The pulmonary changes of bleomycin toxicity, *Radiology*, **106**:65–68 (1973).
95. F. Perez–Guerra, L. E. Harkleroad, R. E. Walsh, et al., Acute bleomycin lung, *Am. Rev. Respir. Dis.*, **106**:909–913 (1972).
96. R. W. Fleischman, J. R. Baker, G. R. Thompson, et al., Bleomycin–induced interstitial pneumonia in dogs, *Thorax*, **26**:675–682 (1971).
97. G. R. Jones and D. N. S. Malone, Sulphasalazine induced lung disease, *Thorax*, **27**:713–717 (1972).
98. D. S. Fiegenberg, H. Weiss, and H. Kirshman, Migratory pneumonia with eosinophilia: Associated with sulfonamide administration, *Arch. Intern. Med.*, **120**:85–89 (1967).
99. W. St. C. Symmers, The occurrence of angiitis and of other generalized diseases of connective tissues as a consequence of the administration of drugs, *Proc. R. Soc. Med.*, **55**:20–28 (1962).

15

Eosinophilia and the Lung

ERIC A. OTTESEN

National Institute of Allergy and Infectious Diseases
National Institutes of Health
Bethesda, Maryland

I. Introduction

Pulmonary eosinophilia is a generic term for an array of clinical and pathologic entities that have at least two features in common: (a) pulmonary infiltration and (b) an increased number of eosinophil leukocytes in the lung alone or in both the lung and peripheral blood. The presentations of these various states as well as the agents that cause them are numerous, diverse, and still only incompletely delineated despite the contributions of many observers who have offered both detailed case descriptions and thoughtful schematic frameworks for classifying these eosinophilic syndromes.

Concurrent with the accumulation of clinical information about these conditions, studies of the eosinophil leukocyte itself—its structure, function, kinetics, and mechanisms of response—have been pursued by individuals in many different laboratories. Recently, a number of new findings have provided further insights into the pathogenesis of these conditions. It is our purpose to review these new laboratory observations and to relate them to the various clinical syndromes that make up the pulmonary eosinophilia complex.

II. Clinical States

In 1952 Crofton and his colleagues [1] reviewed the subject of clinical pulmonary eosinophilia and offered a classification scheme that has been utilized
extensively since then [2–4]. They divided the complex into the following five
descriptive syndromes: (a) simple pulmonary eosinophilia (Loeffler's syndrome),
(b) prolonged pulmonary eosinophilia, (c) tropical eosinophilia, (d) pulmonar
eosinophilia with asthma, and (e) pulmonary eosinophilia associated with periarteritis nodosa. As even these authors emphasized, distinctions among these
groups of entities may be both arbitrary and sometimes vague. Still the scheme
has proven valuable in approaching this subject in the past, and its clinical and
pathologic features will be reviewed, at least briefly, here.

A. Simple Pulmonary Eosinophilia
   (The Loeffler Syndrome)

Simple pulmonary eosinophilia, as described originally by Loeffler [5], was
defined by Crofton *et al.* [1] as a condition of essentially asymptomatic or
minimally symptomatic individuals who demonstrated peripheral blood eosinophilia, transient migratory pulmonary infiltrates seen on chest radiographs, and
spontaneous resolution of these findings within 1 month. The radiographic "infiltrates," which may be unilateral or bilateral, have a patchy distribution but are
found predominantly at the pleural surfaces and most often in the upper lung
fields. It is generally agreed that the syndrome probably represents an allergic
response to a variety of causative agents [1,2,6].

Foremost among these agents are the tissue–invading parasitic helminths.
Both human and nonhuman parasites can produce this picture in man. Though
numerous instances of pulmonary infiltration and peripheral blood eosinophilia
have been ascribed to parasitic causes, among the human parasites only *Ascaris
lumbricoides* [7] and *Strongyloides stercoralis* [8] have been extensively documented as producing this syndrome. Among the nonhuman parasites, the dog
and cat ascarids, *Toxacara canis* and *T. cati,* may evoke simple pulmonary eosinophilia as part of the visceral larva migrans syndrome [9], and the dog hookworm
Ancylostoma braziliense may do so as a feature of cutaneous larva migrans [10].

Certain drugs, such as *p*–aminosalicylic acid [11], sulfonamides [12], and
chlorpropamide [13], along with chemicals, such as nickel carbonyl [14], have
also been implicated in producing Loeffler pneumonia. In some instances, however, these conditions may not satisfy the strict criteria of simple pulmonary
eosinophilia, as they are "self-limited" only after the offending agent has been
withdrawn and, in addition, may cause symptoms and pulmonary damage far
more severe than the designation *Loeffler syndrome* is meant to imply.

There are also idiopathic causes of this syndrome, with clinical features resembling those already described but for which etiologic associations are still unknown.

B. Prolonged Pulmonary Eosinophilia

Several features distinguish this group of diseases from that of simple pulmonary eosinophilia. First, the duration of illness is prolonged, generally greater than 1 month, and second, the clinical symptoms in these diseases are more severe than those of the Loeffler syndrome. Fever, night sweats, weight loss, cough, and even dyspnea often accompany the prolonged pulmonary eosinophilias.

A variety of diseases may express themselves with this general picture—for example, parasitic [15], fungal [16], or bacterial [17] infections; hypersensitivity pneumonitities [18]; and drug allergies [19]. In addition, Carrington *et. al.* [20] recently delineated a group of patients with chronic eosinophilic pneumonia who presented with histories of prolonged and severe symptoms that included fever, night sweats, weight loss, and dyspnea. Most had peripheral blood eosinophilia, and their pulmonary function tests showed evidence of restrictive lung disease. Roentgenographically there were characteristic dense and progressive infiltrates at the periphery of the lungs, without segmental or lobar distribution. These resolved rapidly with corticosteroid therapy but recurred in the same locations, if therapy was unsuccessful.

Though the pathologic findings in all types of pulmonary eosinophilia appear to be remarkably similar [2], studies of the prolonged pulmonary eosinophilias have provided the most thorough and detailed descriptions of this pulmonary pathology [2,20]. Characteristically, the alveoli are filled with a mixture of eosinophils, large and often vacuolated mononuclear cells, and occasionally multinucleate giant cells. The interstitium is generally edematous and infiltrated predominantly with eosinophils, but mononuclear and plasma cells may be found as well. Occasionally, in some of the distal air spaces there are masses of eosinophils, described by Liebow [2] as "eosinophilic abscesses." Necrosis may be evident in the centers of these masses, and sometimes a granulomatous response surrounds the eosinophils. Finally, there may even be minimal microangiitis in associated small blood vessels, but generally this is not a prominent feature of the prolonged eosinophilic pneumonias.

C. Tropical Eosinophilia

Though isolated cases of tropical eosinophilia have been observed since the turn of the century, the syndrome was first well-delineated by Frimodt-Möeller and

Barton [21] and later by Weingarten [22]. As defined by Donohugh [23], the
syndrome is characterized by the following: (a) pulmonary symptoms persistent
for weeks or months, progressing from simple cough to significant dyspnea, and
often accompanied by attacks of paroxysmal, nocturnal asthma; (b) the nonspecific systemic symptoms of malaise, fatigue, weight loss, and low-grade fever;
(c) a peripheral blood eosinophilia of 2000 eosinophils per cubic millimeter and
generally even greater than $4000/mm^3$; (d) high levels of antibody to filarial
antigen; and (e) clinical improvement after treatment with antifilarial chemotherapy. The chest x-ray film may show diffuse, bilateral, miliary mottling with
increased hilar markings, more prominent toward the bases, which may progress
to patchy areas of consolidation.

A history of recent residence in the tropics is characteristic, but for years
there was only circumstantial evidence to suggest filaria as the causative agent of
this syndrome. Then, in 1960 Webb *et al.* [24] and later Danaraj *et al.* [25]
presented detailed biopsy series that demonstrated microfilaria in the nodular
pulmonary lesions of these patients. When found within the nodules, the parasites were surrounded either by necrotic tissue or eosinophilic leukocytes. Granulomatous responses composed of epithelioid histiocytes, fibroblasts, multinucleate giant cells, and eosinophils were found both around microfilaria and in
areas in which no parasites could be demonstrated. These granulomas appeared
generally well within lung parenchyma and away from the bronchial tree. Interstitial infiltrates, too, were observed, and the cell types found included eosinophils, lymphocytes, macrophages, and plasma cells. A similar exudative response
also was seen in the surrounding alveolar spaces.

Classically, filarial infection with overt microfilaremia does not involve the
lung, and it is still unclear just which species of filaria actually produce this picture of tropical eosinophilia. The epidemiologic and pathologic data, taken
together, suggest that in the appropriate setting the human filarial parasites
Wuchereria bancrofti and *Brugia malayia* may be involved [26]; experimental
infection with nonhuman filarids will also produce the syndrome [27], but it is
unclear whether they are a significant cause of the naturally occurring disease.
The important point to be emphasized here, however, is that in tropical eosinophilia there is little or no microfilaremia; rather, it appears that the host has been
able to sequester and contain the larval worms in the pulmonary parenchyma.
By localizing this major defense mechanism in one tissue, the host is able to limit
the extent of infection but, at the same time, subjects himself directly to the
pulmonary damage and consequent symptoms that characterize this syndrome.

D. Pulmonary Eosinophilia With Asthma

Segregation of pulmonary eosinophilias on the basis of whether or not asthma—
the reversible, widespread narrowing of bronchial airways—is a feature of the

clinical presentation is perhaps the least defensible aspect of the classification by Crofton *et al.* [1]. In fact, in many of the conditions leading to pulmonary eosinophilia, clinical asthma is manifest at some point in time. Moreover, many of the mechanisms by which eosinophilia itself develops (discussed in Section IV below) are "allergic" or immunologic in nature, and it is just these types of reactions that are responsible for generating much of what is recognized as clinical asthma (see Chapter 11).

Clearly, however, asthma is more prominent with some forms of pulmonary eosinophilia than with others. Foremost among these conditions must be the syndrome of allergic bronchopulmonary aspergillosis, described first in 1925 [28] and regarded by Pepys and Simon [29] as both the most common complication of long-standing asthma in Great Britain and as a frequent cause of pulmonary eosinophilia with asthma in other areas as well. Manifestations of the disease derive from a local, primarily noninvasive colonization of segments of the bronchial airways with species of *Aspergillus*. Growing in the tough sputum plugs characteristic of the disease, the fungus produces spores that serve as potent allergens or immunogens and give rise to both reaginic (IgE) and precipitating (IgG and IgM) antibodies in the patients.

Clinically, bronchopulmonary aspergillosis may present as adult-onset asthma or as an exacerbation of long-standing asthmatic disease. Wheezing, cough, increased sputum production, fever, and peripheral eosinophilia are common. Radiographically the specific findings of one or more nodular opacities, varying in size from 1.0 cm to almost the size of an entire lobe [30], may be seen in some patients, whereas others present pictures of recurrent pneumonitis or atelectasis of one or more segments of the lung [4]. Generally, radiologic findings resolve completely after about 6 wk and subsequent consolidations usually involve different lobes. However, depending on the severity of the tissue damage resulting from local immune responses and the extent of bronchial plugging by tenacious mucus, a variable pattern of both clinical and radiographic bronchiectasis may result.

When lung tissue from patients with asthmatic pulmonary eosinophilia is examined, the findings are generally the same as those of the prolonged pulmonary eosinophilias described above. But in addition, the walls of the distal air spaces may be markedly edematous and infiltrated with abundant mast cells and fibroblasts [2]. In these areas of local accumulations of mast cells, collections of eosinophils as well as mononuclear and plasma cells are prominant. Also distinctive in the pathology of the asthmatics in Liebow's series [2] was the finding of polyploid masses of granulation tissue containing very large numbers of eosinophils protruding into bronchioles and resembling the nasal polyps found in patients with allergic rhinitis.

E. Pulmonary Eosinophilia with Periarteritis Nodosa

In their classification scheme, Crofton *et al.* [1] recognized periarteritis nodosa as an entity sometimes associated with eosinophilic lung disease or peripheral blood eosinophilia. During subsequent years, it became clear that this condition is only one of a number of similar disease states characterized by pulmonary vasculitis, which may be associated with eosinophilia. These conditions have been reviewed in Chapter 13 of this volume and include serum sickness, systemic lupus erythematosus, rheumatoid arthritis, other collagen-vascular diseases, eosinophilic granuloma, Wegener's granulomatosis, allergic granulomatosis, lymphoid granulomatosis, and potentially any other disorder in which disseminated vasculitis occurs.

Each of these conditions has pathology extending beyond the confines of the lung and, as a result, presenting symptoms include generalized systemic complaints. The affected lung tissue itself is characterized by inflammation of blood vessels, most often the small arterioles, or by both vascular inflammation and concomitant granuloma formation. The eosinophils, when present, accumulate in the patterns described for prolonged pulmonary eosinophilic states (Section II B above). Peripheral blood eosinophilia may develop as well. Although the specific etiologies of these conditions are generally unknown, the mechanisms thought to be responsible for the vasculitic state and those felt to be involved in generating the accompanying eosinophilia have been investigated in some detail and will be discussed in Section V below.

F. Other Hypereosinophilic States with Pulmonary Eosinophilia

Pulmonary eosinophilia may also occur as one aspect of a generally severe and poorly characterized syndrome marked by profound peripheral blood eosinophilia and widespread tissue infiltration by these cells. These patients constitute the more severe categories of the spectrum of conditions grouped as the *hypereosinophilia syndromes* [31,32]. They usually present in middle age with systemic complaints of malaise, fatigue, weight loss, and symptoms of cardiopulmonary decompensation. Cardiac pathology is a regular feature in almost all instances—primarily mural thrombi, endocardial fibrosis, and valvular damage. Heptosplenomegaly is also common, occurring in more than 80% of cases and presumably the result of eosinophilic infiltrates in the periportal regions of the liver. Neurologic and pulmonary abnormalities each may be found in about 40% of reported cases [32]. Not all cases with pulmonary abnormalities, however, have eosinophilic infiltrates in the lung; many of the pulmonary changes are probably secondary to cardiac pathology. Still, autopsy results from this group of patients give evidence of definite eosinophilic pulmonary pathology in at least 24% of the cases. Hence, this syndrome also must be included among the groups of disease states that give rise to a picture of pulmonary eosinophilia.

Pulmonary eosinophilia, then, appears to represent a final common pathway for a wide variety of clinical states (Table 1), with an even greater diversity of etiologic agents. Before attempting to relate these clinical and pathologic states causally to recently delineated mechanisms of eosinophilia, one should like first to review present understandings of the eosinophil leukocyte itself and then to discuss laboratory observations leading to these current formulations of the mechanisms underlying an eosinophilic response.

III. The Eosinophil

A. Structure

Morphologically, characteristic acidophilic granules most strikingly distinguish the eosinophil from other types of polymorphonuclear leukocytes in man and most other species. Though many similarities between the eosinophil and other granulocytes have been noted [33], recent work has served to emphasize not only these similarities but also a number of significant differences among these cell types.

The eosinophil tends to have fewer lobulations of its nucleus (average, 2.3 lobes), more numerous mitochondria, a more well–developed Golgi apparatus, and distinct differences both in granular structure and in granular contents [34]. Like the neutrophil, the eosinophil has granules that are unit-membrane-bound vacuoles containing both enzymes and other types of molecules still functionally undefined. Archer and Hirsch [35], following the work of others [36], found that both rat and horse eosinophils contain a wide range of hydrolytic enzymes, including cathepsin, ribonuclease, arylsulfatase, β–glucuronidase, acid phosphatase, and peroxidase; a profibrinolysin (plasminogen) also has been described [37]. Major differences between the granule contents of eosinophils and neutrophils lie in the eosinophil's lack of the enzymes lysozyme, phagocytin, and alkaline phosphatase, and in its very high content of peroxidase. In fact, not only is eosinophil peroxidase quantitatively much greater than the corresponding neutrophil enzyme, myeloperoxidase, but it also is qualitatively and antigenically distinct [38,39].

Structurally the mature eosinophil granule is composed of a dense, osmophilic crystalloid core surrounded by a less dense homogeneous matrix [40] (Fig. 1). Recent studies by a number of investigators [41,42] localized zinc ions

TABLE 1 Pulmonary Eosinophilia

Classification	Clinical Data
1. Simple pulmonary eosinophilia (Loeffler's Syndrome)	Minimal symptoms; peripheral blood eosinophilia; spontaneous resolution within 1 mo.
2. Prolonged pulmonary eosinophilia	Symptoms may be severe: fever, weight loss, cough, dyspnea; duration greater than 1 mo or may be fatal; diminished pulmonary function; responses to steroids but may relapse.
3. Tropical eosinophilia	Persistent pulmonary symptoms including cough, dyspnea, asthma; malaise, fever, weight loss; marked blood eosinophilia; high levels of antifilarial antibody and very high levels of serum IgE; improvement after antifilarial chemotherapy (e.g., diethyl-carbamazine).
4. Pulmonary eosinophilia with asthma	Most commonly allergic bronchopulmonary aspergillosis either as complication of long–standing asthma or as a cause of adult–onset asthma; elevations of both specific reaginic and precipitating antibodies.
5. Pulmonary eosinophilia with periarteritis nodosa, and variants	Severe symptoms: pulmonary, systemic, and multisystem.

(presumably cofactors), as well as the enzyme activity of acid phosphatase and peroxidase, to the matrix of these granules, the "enzymatic storehouse" [43], while the dense central core has been implicated as the locus of an arginine–rich, low molecular-weight (6000–12,000 dalton) "major band protein" [44], the biologic function of which is yet to be defined. This single basic protein, moreover, accounts for greater than 50% of the total protein in the granular pool [35,44], an observation that becomes all the more remarkable when one considers that half the total cellular protein of the eosinophil is localized in these granules.

Radiologic Features	Pathologic Findings
Migratory, patchy "infiltrates" with a predominantly peripheral distribution.	Not well characterized.
Dense, progressive infiltrates primarily at periphery and nonsegmental.	Variable, but may include eosinophilic and mononuclear cell collections in alveoli and interstitium; occasional granuloma formation and even microangiitis.
Diffuse finely nodular infiltrates; increased interstitial markings.	Granulomatous nodules often surrounding degenerate microfilaria or with necrotic centers; alveolar and interstitial infiltrates composed of eosinophils and mononuclear cells.
Nodular opacities of varying size; recurrent pneumonia; atelectasis; occasional bronchiectasis.	Eosinophilic and mononuclear cell infiltrates of alveoli and interstitium; increased numbers of mast cells in walls of the air spaces.
Variable: interstitial markings, peripheral infiltrates, consolidations, nodules, and sometimes cavitations.	Variable, but characterized by vasculitis and granuloma formation, both sometimes associated with eosinophils.

B. Function

The quest for a specific function for the eosinophil leukocyte has stimulated much investigation and generated numerous hypotheses concerning the cell's role in host defense. As yet, however, the nature of this function remains elusive. As a result of these studies, however, a partial profile of the functional capabilities of the eosinophil can be defined.

Phagocytic activity of the eosinophil has been appreciated for many years [45] and, recently, newer techniques have permitted quantitative comparison of

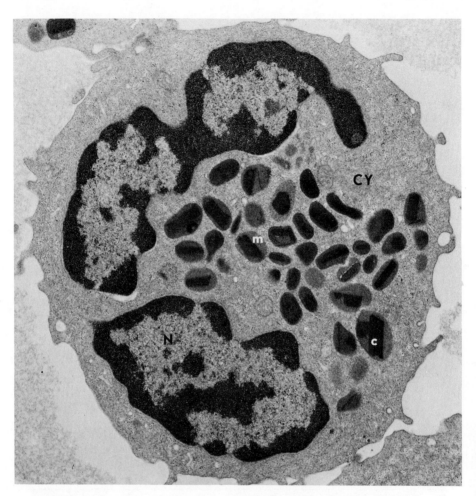

FIGURE 1 Electron micrograph of human eosinophil showing nucleus (N), cytoplasm (Cy), and characteristic granules composed of dense crystalloid core (c) and less dense homogeneous matrix (m). Photography available through the courtesy of K. U. Cehrs and A. S. Rosenthal. (16300X).

this activity with that of various other cell types. The eosinophil has been shown to be capable of ingesting bacteria [46], mycoplasma [47], candida [48], and other types of particles [49,50] in a manner qualitatively similar to, but quantitatively less efficient than, neutrophils.

Studying the metabolism of human leukocytes from patients with marked eosinophilia and comparing it to that of leukocytes from normal volunteers, Baehner and Johnston [51] and Mickenberg, Root, and Wolff [33] noted both relative elevations in resting levels of the eosinophil's oxidative metabolic pathways and a further relative enhancement of these enzyme activities after the cells had been stimulated to phagocytosis. Observations of these high levels of enzyme activity in these cells in the presence of their decreased microbial killing capacity led these investigators to attribute this less efficient killing to the relative deficiency in phagocytic activity already described. Subsequently, however, Cline [52], using a DNA-radiolabeling technique to study the intracellular viability of ingested bacteria, found that, compared to neutrophils and monocytes, eosinophil leukocytes were severely limited in their ability to inhibit the intracellular replication of several common species of bacteria. Thus, it appears that eosinophils not only phagocytose, but also kill, ingested microorganisms less efficiently than do neutrophils.

Interest in the eosinophil's capacity for phagocytosis, however, has not been limited to the ingestion of microorganisms and other particulate matter. In fact, early observations suggesting the importance of antigen and antibody union in inducing eosinophilia [53], led Sabesin [54] to use antigen–antibody complexes (ferritin–antiferritin) to demonstrate, by electron microscopy, the ability of eosinophils to ingest these complexes. Subsequently, others have confirmed his observations in a number of species and with a variety of experimental models [55-57]. Whether or not this ability of eosinophils to ingest antigen–antibody complexes is an important aspect of the cell's function, however, remains moot; it should be remembered that neutrophils, too, have this capability and may even perform it with equal or greater efficiency than do eosinophils [58].

The modulation of anaphylactic response by the "detoxification" of biologically active small molecules also has been proposed as a potential function of eosinophils. A number of different observations support this suggestion. Mast cell granules, which contain many of these active small molecules, have been shown repeatedly [59,60] to be ingested and subsequently broken down by eosinophils. Although when studied in vitro, both macrophages [60] and, probably, neutrophils share this ability with the eosinophil, it is not unlikely that the specific eosinophil-attracting properties of these mast–cell granules (see Section IV,B below) confer, on the eosinophil, distinct and qualitative advantages when performing this function in vivo. In addition, for years Archer (see Section IV,A below) advanced the notion that eosinophils (or soluble extracts derived from them) are effective in diminishing or blocking entirely the formation of intradermal edema normally generated by injection of inflammatory mediators (histamine, 5-hydroxytryptamine, and bradykinin) into the skin [61]. His experiments were performed on horses and demonstrated that not only were the eosinophils and eosinophil extracts effective against the edema stimulated directly by these mediators, but they were also effective against the edema generated indirectly following intradermal injection of horse erythrocytes into ponies having alloantibodies (isoagglutinins) to these red cells. More recently, Hubscher and Eisen [62], also studying extracts prepared from eosinophils, described an "eosinophil-derived inhibitor" that can block the *release* of histamine from sensitized target cells. Characterization of the material is incomplete, but their approach emphasizes, at least, continued interest in finding, for the eosinophil, a potential role in modulating allergic inflammatory reactions.

C. Kinetics

Only a limited number of studies of the kinetics of human eosinopoiesis and eosinophilia have been carried out [63-68], but a great deal of work on this subject has been performed with laboratory animals, primarily the guinea pig and rat. Though differences in detail exist among the various models, it is clear that certain strong generalizations do emerge from these studies.

The kinetics of the eosinophil can be divided into three descriptive phases: (a) production, (b) mobilization, and (c) redistribution; any of these may be modified by exogenous stimuli. When regarding the total eosinophil population in normal animals, it can readily be seen that, in fact, the eosinophil is not primarily a blood element. Rather, in the guinea pig, for example, it has been estimated that for every one eosinophil found in the blood, there are 400 such cells in marrow and another 300 in tissues [69]. For the rat, an estimated 200 marrow eosinophils and another 200 tissue cells exist for each one found in blood [70], and for man, a tissue:blood eosinophil ratio of 100:1 has been proposed [63].

Within the marrow space three general eosinophil "compartments" may be distinguished: (a) a dividing pool consisting of the youngest distinguishable cells, the promyelocytes and myelocytes; (b) a second compartment which contains cells that are more mature but still capable of dividing, the metamyelocytes; and (c) a compartment made up of maturing, nondividing eosinophils generally indistinguishable morphologically from the blood eosinophil. These last cells constitute the "marrow reserve" of eosinophils. About 50% to 75% of all developing eosinophils in the normal animal appear to be in the mature, eosinophil reserve population [71,72], and it is from this pool that the blood and, subsequently, tissue eosinophils are drawn.

In the rat the normal cell-cycle time for eosinophils within the marrow has been found to be about 30 hr and the transit time for cells to develop fully and peripheralize averages 5.5 days [72]. If one radiolabels eosinophils in vivo by pulsing techniques, the first cohort of labeled cells to appear peripherally marks the end of the maturational development of these cells following their last marrow mitosis and defines the "emergence time" or "marrow reserve transit time"; in man and guinea pigs this time has been estimated to be about 60 hr [69] and in rats, 41 hr [73].

Once the eosinophil has reached the blood stream, there is evidence that in the rat the removal of labeled eosinophils is exponential and that the blood half life of these cells is 6.7 hr [73]. In man, however, where the removal of [^{51}Cr]-labelled eosinophils from the blood of hypereosinophilic patients has been studied in considerable detail [64,74,75], the kinetics of eosinophil removal are complex and wholly different from the simple exponential decline described both for the rat eosinophil and for other human granulocytes [73,76,77]. Rather there first appears to be a marked exponential fall in the number of labeled eosinophils within the first 4 to 8 hr, followed by a rise or plateau in the number of labeled cells recovered throughout the second day, and finally a more gradual exponential or even arithmetic decline in labeled cells for several days thereafter. This complex, biphasic kinetic pattern suggests that there may be tissue sequestration of eosinophils with subsequent reentry of the cells into the blood stream, but details of the mechanisms underlying these observations remain obscure. Also, it is unclear whether or not this interesting cell–kinetics pattern observed in hypereosinophilic patients does, in fact, reflect that functioning in the normal individual.

Finally, after the eosinophils have left the peripheral blood in normal animals, they distribute themselves within the tissues in characteristic patterns [70]. However, once in these tissues, it is fair to generalize, their function, fate, and life span remain unknown.

Following eosinophilogenic stimuli, the overall kinetics of eosinophilopoiesis and eosinophil distribution must change. Spry [72,73] studied these changes with elegant detail in rats injected intravenously with muscle–stage larvae of *Trichinella spiralis,* a potent stimulus to eosinophilia [78]. In all three phases of eosinophil kinetics, he has been able to record alterations in these stimulated animals.

Production of eosinophils is seen to increase by the enhanced proliferation of marrow precursor cells. Cell cycle time decreases from 30 to 9 hr and this results in an increase of up to six additional divisions per precursor cell despite a reduction in average marrow transit time from 5.5 to 3.6 days.

Mobilization, too, is enhanced, as the emergence time is seen to fall from 41 to 18 hr, an observation that corresponds well to those of Hudson [69] in the foreign protein–stimulated guinea pig model. There, a decreased emergence time, from the normal 60 hr to less than 29 hr was demonstrated along with significant morphologic depletion of the guinea pig's eosinophil marrow reserve.

Finally, a short-term redistribution of eosinophils presumably from a "marginating pool" [77], could be shown by Spry [73] in response to *eosinophil releasing factor,* an activity found in the plasma of rats stimulated 12 to 24 hr previously, which induced significant eosinophilia in normal rats within 3 to 6 hr after its injection.

Another aspect of the kinetics of the eosinophil is found in the group of observations relating to the stimuli to eosinopenia. Both stress reactions [79] and the administration of corticosteroids [80] have long been known to depress the number of circulating eosinophils. Mechanisms underlying this eosinopenia are unknown, but recent evidence suggests that the steroids induce a reversible margination or sequestration of eosinophils and also decrease their release from the bone marrow [80]. Acute infection, too, will induce eosinopenia and probably by a mechanism distinct from that of the stress reaction alone [81]. Furthermore, there appears to be a link between the state of the autonomic nervous system and the level of blood eosinophilia. β-Adrenergic catecholamines are effective in producing prompt eosinopenia, and this effect can be reversed completely and specifically by β-blocking agents, such as propanolol [82]. Hence, the level of circulating eosinophils at any given time may reflect, in part, the functional state of an individual's autonomic nervous system [43].

In any case, it is clear that the kinetics of the eosinophil response are multifaceted and complex. Though the general outlines of the process of eosinophil maturation have been described in the work cited above, much of the detail of specific mechanisms and specific cellular interactions involved in these processes remains to be elucidated. Furthermore, a major problem that has yet to be approached successfully centers around the question of just what initiates the marrow's eosinophil response in the first place. A number of substances with the property of stimulating eosinophil chemotaxis has been described recently (see Section IV,B below), but their effects on the kinetics of eosinophilopoiesis and eosinophil distribution remain subjects for future investigation.

IV. Mechanisms of Eosinophilia

The study of eosinophil chemotaxis and the mechanisms mediating an eosinophilic response have progressed most rapidly in recent years. For the past 20 yr a number of laboratories have been actively engaged in studying the mechanisms of eosinophilia in a variety of animal models, and the results of their investigations have provided the foundations for both of the recent major advances in the field, i. e., an appreciation of the dependent link between the eosinophil response and the lymphoid immune system and the identification of at least four distinct molecular types of eosinophilotactic substances. These latter have been designated the *eosinophil chemotactic factor of anaphylaxis* (ECF-A), a mast cell product [83]; the eosinophil chemotactic factor produced by complement activation (ECF-C) [84]; and two lymphocyte-derived eosinophil chemotactic factors, one of which (ECF$_p$) requires the presence of specific antigen-antibody complexes before showing activity [85], and the other, termed *eosinophil stimulation promoter* (ESP), which is active even in the absence of such complexes [86].

Before describing each of these substances more fully and detailing the evidence functionally relating the eosinophil and the lymphocyte, one should like first to discuss the various model systems used in studying the mechanisms of eosinophilia and then to detail the results of investigations with these models, which have led to our present understandings of the subject.

A. Model Systems for the In Vivo Study of the Mechanisms of Eosinophilia

Peritoneal Eosinophilia

As described above (Section III,C), the eosinophil is not primarily a blood element but, in fact, a cell whose major role appears to be carried out in the tissues themselves. Accordingly, interest in the "tissue accumulation" of eosinophils has led a number of investigators to employ models in a number of species, using antigen introduced into the peritoneal cavity, to study the fluid exudate induced as a measure of "tissue" eosinophilia.

Speirs and his coworkers [87-89] first used this approach quantitatively to study eosinophilia in mice that received intraperitoneal injections of bovine serum albumin, ragweed extract, or toxoid preparations of tetanus and diphtheria after prior sensitization with one or another of these proteins. They were able to demonstrate two phases of the eosinophilic response in the peritoneal wash-out cells: an early phase that began in the first 6 to 12 hr, terminated by 24 hr, and was paralleled by a neutrophilic response; and a later phase that peaked at 4 days, was completed by 8 to 10 days, and generally was accompanied by mononuclear cells. The early eosinophilia was found to be part of the non-specific inflammatory reaction to foreign material, but the late response was shown to be antigen-specific. Furthermore, this late peak could be abolished by pretreating the animals with specific antibody to the challenging antigen [90] or by irradiating them [91]. The route of sensitization, too, appeared to affect the level of the eosinophil response; maximum late eosinophilia was found after subcutaneous immunization followed by intraperitoneal challenge, whereas immunization and challenge both by the intraperitoneal route resulted in only minimal eosinophilia [92]. Interestingly, the antibody responses (assessed by levels of tetanus antitoxin and presumably reflecting the immunoglobulin G class of antibodies) to the different immunization regimens varied inversely with the number of peritoneal eosinophils elicited.

Later, morphologic and antigen-radiolabeling studies allowed these workers to describe both the uptake of labeled antigen by peritoneal eosinophils (albeit along with similar uptake by other phagocytes) and the presence of intimate contacts between eosinophils and macrophages—observations that led them to suggest a possible role for the eosinophil in the antigen-processing phase of the immune response [93,94]. Furthermore, in recent studies by this group [95-97], this same model has been used to study the effects of immunologic manipulation and reconstitution on the generation of peritoneal eosinophilia. Their interesting observations, reviewed below in Section IV,C, have contributed significantly to the emerging appreciation of the dependent relationship between eosinophilia and certain aspects of the immune system.

Litt, too, in his early work [98] studied peritoneal eosinophilia, but in his system the guinea pig was used. He found that with repeated intraperitoneal sensitization to normal horse serum, human serum albumin, or hemocyanin, he could induce peritoneal eosinophilia in the guinea pig, with a maximum number of eosinophils seen 1 to 2 days after challenge. If several weeks were allowed to elapse after a period of sensitization, specific antigen rechallenge would lead to an accelerated and enhanced eosinophil response in the peritoneal cavity. Significant quantitative variation existed among animals, but the qualitative aspects of the response were consistent.

After demonstrating this biologic response to foreign protein sensitization, Litt turned to using the peritoneal cavity of primed guinea pigs (animals sensitized by repeated intraperitoneal injection of heterologous, noncross-reacting antigen) as in vivo reaction vessels in which to study the eosinophilotactic properties of a number of substances [53,99,100]. With this system, he showed that transfer of blood, serum, peritoneal lining, or lung tissue from sensitized animals into the peritoneal cavities of normal or primed guinea pigs, induced a subsequent peritoneal eosinophilia in recipients. Extracts of both the lung and peritoneal lining were also capable of transferring the eosinophilotactic activity. Further studies indicated that antibody had to be present in these preparations to transfer this reactivity. But antibody alone could not induce eosinophilia; antigen, too, was required. Then when the introduction of preformed antigen-antibody complexes into the peritoneal cavity resulted in eosinophilia, Litt postulated that these complexes were of primary importance in eliciting extravascular eosinophilia.

More recently, Parish [101] also turned to this same model in guinea pigs for further study. Using bovine plasma albumin as antigen, he confirmed the peritoneal eosinophilic response described by Litt but emphasized that the numbers of lymphocytes and other mononuclear cells in the peritoneal washout fluid also rise dramatically along with that of the eosinophils and that these cells may, in fact, play a role in mediating the eosinophilia.

Using this model further, Parish studied the relationship between homocytotropic antibodies (IgG_1 in the guinea pig) and the induction of eosinophilia. Primed animals were passively sensitized to a second antigen, by infusion of serum or serum fractions from hyperimmunized animals, and were then challenged with that antigen intraperitoneally. Eosinophilia resulted only when the infused antibody was of the homocytropic class IgG_1. Similarly, when antigen-antibody complexes of different classes were introduced into the peritoneal cavities of primed animals, again only complexes containing IgG_1 homocytotropic antibody were effective in inducing eosinophilia. However, though these experiments indicate the importance of homocytotropic antibody in generating the eosinophilia of this model, serum levels of this antibody, when induced by a number of different immunizing regimens, did not correspond at all with levels of peritoneal eosinophilia generated at the same time. Thus, Parish suggests that even in this single model more than one mechanism may be responsible for the generation and modulation of the eosinophilic response.

Finally, S. G. Cohen studied peritoneal eosinophilia in some of his more recent work on the mechanism of eosinophilia [102,103]. Using the mouse model, his group initially confirmed the observations by Speirs *et al.* [93] that there was both early and late eosinophilia in the peritoneal cavities of immunized and intraperitoneally challenged animals. Then, they showed that *Bordetella pertussis* vaccine, despite its profound effects in enhancing histamine sensitivity and anaphylactic responsiveness of the immune system [104], has no significant effect on the development of peritoneal eosinophilia. His group also extended to the mouse, observations made previously in guinea pigs, that it is only the homocytotropic antibody classes (IgE and IgG_1) that can induce peritoneal eosinophilia when injected intraperitoneally 24 hr prior to the injection of specific antigen [103]. Further, when specific antibodies of the nonhomocytotropic antibody class, IgG_2, were injected intraperitoneally, after the reaginic antibody but before antigenic challenge, the expected eosinophil response was aborted—an observation suggesting that blocking antibodies may be effective in regulating or terminating a homocytotropic antibody response. And, most recently, these investigators studied the eosinophilic response in this model using activators of the complement cascade (cobra venom factor and fumaropimaric acid) to demonstrate that complement plays no role in the homocytotropic–antibody–mediated generation of eosinophilia [103].

Lymph Node Eosinophilia

A second in vivo model of major importance in studies of the mechanisms of
eosinophilia was developed by S. G. Cohen, Kanter, and Gatto [105] when they
noted regional lymph node eosinophilia in rabbits 4 hr after a number of different substances were injected into the footpad. Initially, they observed that
neither antigen (bovine serum albumin) nor antibody alone would induce node
eosinophilia, but that when the two were administered sequentially, 30-min
apart, a marked regional node eosinophilia would result. Footpad injections of
preformed antigen–antibody precipitates or soluble complexes could not reproduce this response in the rabbit, and the administration of antihistamine or anti-
serotonin agents could not depress it. Further studies in the rabbit also demonstrated eosinophilic responses in the draining nodes after footpad injections of
glycogen, starch, insulin, and high molecular-weight dextran but not with simple
sugars or low molecular-weight dextran.

　　Later, however, when the same techniques were applied to the guinea pig,
first by Litt [106] and then by Cohen *et al.* [49,107], in contrast to findings in
the rabbit, draining nodes of the guinea pig developed local eosinophilia after
even single injections of heterologous protein (bovine serum albumin, hemocyanin, and others), homologous or heterologous gamma globulins in aggregated
or denatured states, soluble antigen–antibody complexes, and even a series of
polystyrene latex particles of varying size. Thus, these findings, taken together
with those in the rabbit, indicated that though certain types of stimuli (e.g.,
antigen–antibody complexes) may play a special role in inducing eosinophilia;
still, the physicochemical configuration of the stimulus, rather than the foreign
nature of the material itself, may be the major contributing factor to the eosinophilia of this model system.

　　In describing the kinetics of lymph node eosinophilia, Litt [108,109]
noted that the accumulation of eosinophils in response to a single footpad injection of heterologus protein was both very rapid (within minutes) and sensitive to
stimulation by even minute quantities of antigen (10^{-6} to $10^{-9}\mu g$ of protein).
Multiple injections of antigen (hemocyanin) over several weeks led to massive
local node eosinophilia after challenge, but treatment of the guinea pigs with
puromycin within 4 hr of specific-antigen challenge blocked this stimulated
eosinophil response [110]. These and other observations led him to conclude
that the capacity for active protein synthesis at the time of challenge was a necessary prerequisite for the development of eosinophilia in this model. He suggested that the protein being synthesized was, in fact, specific antibody and that
the induction of the eosinophilia, again, was mediated by specific antigen–antibody complexes [106,110]. Others [90,111], however, even taking these observations into consideration, have felt that while antigen–antibody complexes

do induce an accumulation of eosinophils, they may do so by more general mechanisms than Litt had envisioned; namely, by activating the complement cascade and generating chemotactic factors from these proteins (see Section IV,B below).

Cutaneous Eosinophilia

Again in an effort to study "tissue eosinophilia," several investigators used the skin as a reaction site at which local stimuli are relatively easy to effect and where eosinophils can readily accumulate and be studied by tissue biopsy.

Archer, in looking at the interactions between eosinophils and certain of the inflammatory mediators [61,112-114], injected large doses of histamine intradermally into ponies and found local edema formation, the appearance of eosinophils within 4 hr and a persistance of these cells for about 4 days. Superinjection of mepyramine, an antihistamine, into the sites shortly after the histamine, abolished both the local eosinophilia and edema. Moreover, if the initial injection of histamine was placed in an area with a high local concentration of eosinophils, no edema developed, although the cells themselves remained histologically unchanged. These observations suggested to Archer that the eosinophils might act as an antagonist to histamine and other inflammatory mediators (Section III,B above) and that histamine was a potent eosinophil chemotactic agent. Efforts to confirm this eosinophilotactic activity of histamine, however, both in vivo with other species and in vitro in Boyden chambers, have been unsuccessful [58,83,100] until recently [154].

S. G. Cohen [115] also used the model of cutaneous eosinophilia in the guinea pig to show that local eosinophilia in the skin could result from the same stimuli that induced an eosinophilic response in regional lymph nodes; namely, heterologus gamma globulin in native or aggregated states, preformed antigen–antibody complexes, or the sequential administration of antigen and antibody intradermally. He also noted that any local changes in the number of eosinophils were not reflected in the peripheral blood and that histamine had no effect on cutaneous eosinophilia in the guinea pig.

Subsequently, first Kay [116], and then Parish [101,117] also used this model in guinea pigs to study the effects of various classes of antibody on the production and mechanisms of production of local eosinophilia. They both demonstrated that passive sensitization of guinea pig skin with the homocytotropic antibody IgG_1 but not IgG_2, when followed by intravenous specific antigen resulted in positive passive cutaneous anaphylactic (PCA) reactions and the local accumulation of eosinophils. With preformed antigen–antibody complexes of both the IgG_1 and IgG_2 classes, however, intradermal injections regularly resulted in local eosinophilia, though these complexes appeared to elicit a local neutrophilia as well. Further observations with this model, by Kay [118], some in complement-depleted guinea pigs, were crucial to establishing the basic differences between the activities of ECF-A and ECF-C, as discussed more fully below in Section IV,B.

Blood Eosinophilia

Peripheral blood eosinophilia has fascinated many investigators, but because of difficulties with its experimental reproducibility and because major stimuli to eosinophilia are predominently extravascular, it has not been pursued extensively as a model system for studying the mechanisms of eosinophilia. Initially, Samter [119] used this aspect of the eosinophilic response in guinea pigs to make the intriguing observation that anaphylactically challenged lung tissue elicited blood eosinophilia when placed intraperitoneally in normal animals, However, the most extensive use of this model in studying the mechanisms of eosinophilia has more recently been in the work of Basten, Boyer, and Beeson [78,120,121], and later others of their coworkers [122-125,72,73] who have developed a model in the rat in which peripheral blood eosinophilia can be regularly induced by the intravenous injection of muscle-phase larvae of the parasitic nematode, *Trichinella spiralis.* In the natural infection of the rat with *Trichinella,* these same larvae normally would be ingested, mature in the intestine to adults, and then shed second-generation larvae to the muscle. The natural infection itself induces an eosinophilia [78], but the development of this eosinophilia is not so rapid and its reproducibility is not so great as that induced by the artificial route of sensitization.

With this model, these investigators have been able to study the hitherto unappreciated role of lymphoid cells in the generation of an eosinophilic response (Section IV,C below) along with numerous aspects of the kinetics of blood eosinophilia (Section III,C above). In addition, their observations emphasized the importance of the form or manner in which the antigen is presented to the animal on the subsequent development of eosinophilia. Particulate antigen (larvae or dextran), given intravenously, will induce a marked local inflammatory response in the lung and subsequent blood eosinophilia, whereas intravenous soluble *Trichinella* antigen alone will cause neither inflammation nor eosinophilia. However, if the soluble antigen is incorporated into complete Freund's adjuvant and injected subcutaneously, again there will be local inflammation in proximity to antigen and, again, peripheral blood eosinophilia develops.

Other In Vivo Models for the Study of Eosinophilia

A number of other models also have been employed in studying the mechanisms of eosinophilia in vivo. None has been used to the same extent as those already described, but several deserve mention because of the interesting work being done with them.

Speirs and his coworkers extended their investigations on immunologically altered and reconstituted mice (Sections IV,A and IV,C) to include studies of the eosinophil-containing "colony-forming units" in bone marrow and elsewhere [96]. Some of the observations they made with this model, in seeking to define factors important at the earliest stages of eosinophilopoeisis and the generation of an eosinophilic response, will be reviewed below (Section IV,C). Another interesting model has been proposed by Samter [126] for studying local, antigenically-induced eosinophilia in lung tissue following the administration of stimulating materials directly into lung parenchyma. In this model early and late peaks of eosinophilia developed after antigen stimulation, but mechanisms underlying these responses have yet to be characterized.

Though other interesting and potentially useful in vivo models have been formulated to study the mechanisms of eosinophilia [e.g., 127], experience with them is more limited than with those already described. Instead of pursuing these further here, I wish to turn now to some of the recent work in this area performed with a number of in vitro model systems. For, from these studies, initially stimulated by observations from the in vivo models, at least four effector agents capable of inducing local eosinophilia have been identified. After each has been described, it should be clear that they all, no doubt, play important roles in generating the eosinophilia observed both in the clinical states of pulmonary eosinophilia already outlined and in the in vivo experimental models described above.

B. Mediators

Eosinophil Chemotactic Factor of Anaphylaxis (ECF-A)

The observation by Kay ([116] and Section IV,A above) that in guinea pig skin only the homocytotropic antibody class IgG_1 was effective in producing positive PCA (passive cutaneous anaphylactic) reactions with local accumulation of eosinophils led Kay, Stechschulte, and Austen [83] to seek a factor released from anaphylactically-triggered mast cells, which was specifically chemotactic for eosinophils. By passively sensitizing fragments of guinea pig lung in vitro with specific IgG_1 antibody and then challenging this preparation with homologous antigen, or by challenging in vitro lung tissues taken from animals actively sensitized with homologous antigen previously, they were able to collect material that had been anaphylactically released from mast cells. In addition to finding the expected histamine and slow reacting substance of anaphylaxis (SRS-A) in these reaction mixtures, they were able to demonstrate another distinct entity, termed ECF-A, which manifested selective attraction for eosinophils when tested in the standard chemotactic–assay Boyden chamber.

Generation of this ECF-A showed a time course, divalent cation requirement, antigen–dose dependence, and complement independence that exactly paralleled that for histamine and SRS-A, the well-recognized products of mast-cell liberation. But it was separable from these other moieties not only functionally but also by Sephadex chromatography, susceptibility to boiling, and resistance to lyophilization. It has been shown to be a preformed short–chain peptide with a molecular weight between 500 and 600 daltons.

Subsequently, Kay and Austen [128] demonstrated the release of this same substance from human mast cells. In their experiments they passively sensitized human lung fragments with reaginic antibody, IgE, and then challenged these fragments with homologous antigen, finding the activity in the incubating medium. Subsequently, Parish [129] showed that the same activity can be released anaphylactically from human basophils. And, most recently, Wasserman *et al.* [130] isolated this same ECF-A material from a large–cell anaplastic tumor of human lung. Interestingly, the patient from whom this tumor was removed had both peripheral blood eosinophilia and local tumor eosinophilia. It is felt that this eosinophilotactic peptide was produced by the tumor in a manner analogous to that of the well–recognized, ectopically produced, peptide hormones.

Thus, in ECF-A a unique peptide has been described, which is markedly chemotactic for eosinophils and is released from tissue mast cells and circulating basophils concomitantly with other mediators of anaphylaxis. Since eosinophilia often is associated with an allergic state, this mechanism for the rapid generation of local eosinophilia no doubt is of major importance in accounting for many instances of eosinophilia seen clinically and in the experimental models described above.

Eosinophil Chemotactic Factor Derived From Complement (ECF-C)

The complement cascade of proteins provides three major chemotactic byproducts of its activation: C3a, C5a, and the trimolecular complex $\overline{C567}$ (Chapter 8 of this volume). These three moieties all had been shown to be chemotactic for neutrophilic leukocytes [131] prior to the demonstration by Ward [111]; Keller and Sorkin [132]; and Lachmann, Kay, and Thompson [133] that they were chemotactic for eosinophils as well. Further, Kay [84] showed that incubation of normal guinea pig serum with antigen–antibody complexes of either the IgG_1 or IgG_2 class generated a heat–stable product that was found to attract eosinophils selectively when tested in vitro against a mixed cell population. Characterization of this substance led to its identification as C5a, and the suggestion was advanced that this substance is biologically the most important eosinophil chemotactic factor derived from complement.

Just as the discovery of ECF-A provided a potential mechanistic explanation for the local eosinophilia found in many allergic states, so an appreciation of the activity of ECF-C offers a further possible explanation for the eosinophilia seen in other conditions in which the allergic state plays no part but in which the complement system may be assumed to be activated. Those determinants, which are known to activate this cascade either through the classic or alternate pathways [134], include antigen–antibody reactions of many types, immune complexes of all classes, aggregated proteins, certain polysaccharides of critical macromolecular character, and some bacterial products. Thus, it is clear that many different types of agents, in many different situations, may trigger the complement system and thereby generate factors chemotactic for eosinophils. Surely this mechanism, too, must play an important role in determining the eosinophilia seen in certain of the clinical eosinophilic syndromes and in a number of the in vivo models of eosinophilia already described above.

Eosinophil Chemotactic Factors Derived From Lymphocytes

A Chemotactic Lymphokine Requiring Activation by Antigen–Antibody Complexes (ECF_p)

Stimulated by the early observations of Arnason and Waksman [135] that reinjection of homologous antigen into the site of a previously positive, delayed hypersensitivity skin test in rats resulted in local eosinophilia, the "retest reaction," and by the observations of Basten, Boyer, and Beeson [120] linking the lymphoid immune system to the generation of eosinophilia (Section IV,C below), Cohen and Ward [85] sought to define an eosinophil chemotactic factor derived from lymphocytes. Lymph node lymphocytes were taken from guinea pigs sensitized previously to o-chlorobenzoyl–bovine gamma globulin (OCB–BGG) and cultured either in the presence or absence of this antigen. All studies were performed in the absence of complement. The fluid supernates from these cultures were then incubated in a complement-free environment either with homologous or heterologous antigen–antibody complexes or with no complexes at all. Finally, the material was tested for eosinophilotactic properties in a standard Boyden-chamber in vitro assay. The responding cell population in these chambers was the peritoneal exudate derived from guinea pigs that had received repeated intraperitoneal sensitization to heterologous antigen, in the manner of Litt [98], and consisted of 20% to 35% eosinophils along with other granulocytes and mononuclear cells.

With this system, Cohen and Ward [85] were able to demonstrate a factor in these antigen-stimulated lymphocyte culture fluids which, when reacted with species-specific, homologous antigen-antibody complexes, was found to be chemotactic for eosinophils. Neutrophils, too, were responsive to this substance but to a much lesser degree than were the eosinophils. These in vitro observations were then extended to the in vivo situation by injecting these cell-culture supernates, freed of antigen-antibody complexes, intradermally into normal guinea pigs and biopsying these sites 18 hr later. When supernates from antigen-stimulated lymphocyte cultures were used, significant eosinophilia developed, as in the case of in vitro studies, only if these supernates had been incubated previously with homologous antigen-antibody complexes. However, in contrast to in vitro findings, the injection of "unstimulated" supernates was also found to generate a significant (though lesser) degree of eosinophilia, but only if they, too, had been preincubated with homologous antigen-antibody complexes. Cohen and Ward interpreted this latter observation as evidence for some minimal spontaneous activation of cultured lymphocytes, even in the absence of antigen, that resulted in the production of small amounts of chemotactic factor, undetectable in the chamber assay but still recognizable by the presumably more sensitive in vivo cutaneous technique.

Subsequent efforts to characterize this lymphocyte-derived factor [136] led these authors to describe their material as a precursor substance (ECF_p) that requires activation by homologous immune complexes before evolving into a functional eosinophil chemotactic factor (ECF). The activating complexes must be of the IgG_2 class in the guinea pig model, with specificity directed against the antigen used both initially in sensitizing the animal and then in stimulating the lymphocytes in vitro. Actually this specificity is carrier-, not hapten-, dependent when tested with complex antigens, and in this regard ECF is similar to the well-described lymphokine MIF (migration inhibition factor). In fact, efforts to separate the activities of ECF_p and MIF by the physiochemical methods of Sephadex chromatography and agarose block electrophoresis were unsuccessful. However, separation could be achieved when the stimulated culture supernates were passed over specific antigen or antibody columns; MIF activity was unaffected by either column, but ECF_p activity was abolished after passage through the specific antibody-coated column. From these observations, the investigators suggested that ECF_p contains a fragment of specific antigen which is cleaved by coprecipitation with the homologous antigen-antibody complex in the course of being "activated" to a functional eosinophil chemotactic factor.

Thus, Torisu and his colleagues [136] were able to demonstrate for the first time that lymphocytes may account for still another mechanism of eosinophilia. In the appropriate situation (i.e., in states where delayed hypersensitivity and antibody production coexist with the presence of antigen), lymphocytes can be stimulated to produce a lymphokine that subsequently may be activated by specific antigen-antibody complexes and evolve into a molecule specifically chemoattractive to eosinophils.

Eosinophil Stimulation Promoter (ESP)

A second lymphokine with activity stimulatory to eosinophils has recently been described by Colley [86]. His model was the *Schistosoma mansoni* infected or immunized mouse, and his assay for eosinophil stimulation was the migration of eosinophils out of a peritoneal-exudate-agarose droplet maintained in cell culture either in the presence or absence of antigens or mitogens. In his experiments he noted that activation of lymphocytes, both by mitogen phytohemagglutinin and by specific antigens to which the donor animals were previously sensitized, resulted in the elaboration of a product into the cell-culture medium, which could stimulate eosinophils to migrate. This product, ESP, is neither complement-dependent nor immune-complex-dependent for its activity. It is heat-stable at $80°C$ for 30 min, resistant to ribonuclease, but sensitive to chymotrypsin; Sephadex chromatography yields a uniform peak of activity, with a molecular weight in the range of 31,000 daltons [137].

Though further characterization of this moiety and indications of both its biologic activity and chemotactic properties await additional studies, it appears that this factor is another unique eosinophil chemotactic agent. It is derived in an operationally different manner from the factor of Cohen and Ward [85], has no relation to the mast cell product ECF-A, and appears independent of complement as well. Being a lymphocyte product, moreover, it shares with ECF_p the potential of being the agent mechanistically responsible for the production of eosinophilia in those situations in which cell-mediated immunity may be etiologically involved in the development of the eosinophilic state.

C. The Role of the Lymphoid Immune System in the Eosinophilic Response

A link between eosinophilia and the immune response has long been postulated, but until recently the nature of the link was entirely unclear. Some investigators [58-61] felt that modulation of the anaphylactic immune response by mediator deactivation or other means was a role that belonged to the eosinophil. Others [135,138] argued that modulation of the entire immune response through effects on antigen, antibody, immune complexes, or lymphoid cells more readily defined the role of the eosinophil. Still others [87,93] speculated that through its phagocytic capabilities and intimate relations with the macrophage, the eosinophil may have a role in antigen processing or even antibody production. The definitive evidence necessary to prove the validity of any of these hypotheses, however, simply was not available.

Then Basten, Boyer, Beeson [78,120-125], and their colleagues developed a reproducible experimental model of peripheral blood eosinophilia in the rat (Section IV,A,4 above) which they were able to use in studying the effects of an altered immune system on the development of the eosinophilic response. Their model, it will be recalled, generated peripheral blood eosinophilia in rats sensitized to *Trichinella spiralis,* either naturally during the course of infection or artificially following injection of *Trichinella* larvae intravenously.

In a series of elegant experiments they made the following observations: (a) rechallenge of a previously sensitized animal led to an augmented and accelerated eosinophilic response, a "secondary response" resembling that of classic immune reactions; (b) the development of eosinophilia was independent of the humoral immune response; (c) the transfer of eosinophilia from a sensitized animal to a nonsensitized recipient could be achieved not by transfer of serum but only by infusion of syngeneic lymphocytes taken from the thoracic duct lymph 3 to 5 days after natural infection or from the peripheral blood 1 day after intravenous exposure to larvae; (d) depletion of lymphocytes by a number of means, including neonatal thymectomy, treatment with antilymphocyte serum, and thoracic duct drainage in appropriate settings depressed or abolished the eosinophil response; (e) reconstitution of irradiated rats required syngeneic cells from both normal bone marrow and thoracic duct lymph to restore the animals capacity to generate a normal eosinophil response after the intravenous injection of *Trichinella* larvae and if the donors of the bone marrow and thoracic duct cells had previously been sensitized to *Trichinella,* an accelerated eosinophilic response was seen in recipients challenged intravenously with larvae; and (f) findings in rats treated with a number of different immunosuppressive agents at various points in time relative to primary or secondary challenge with intravenous larvae were consistent with the known effects of the agents in altering the development of classic immune responses, suggesting the presence of inductive and proliferative phases in the generation of eosinophilia. Their findings, then, demonstrate very clearly that the eosinophilia generated in this model (and presumably in other situations as well) is a response intimately associated with a functional immune system.

Further support for this contention, moreover, has come from the results of studies by Speirs and his colleagues [95,97]. At the same time that the *Trichinella* model was evolving, these investigators were pursuing the potential interrelation between eosinophilia and the immune response by a somewhat different approach. Previously, they had characterized the peritoneal eosinophilic response in mice repeatedly sensitized intraperitoneally with tetanus toxoid (Section IV, A above). With this background, they used the same model to study the effects of immunologic manipulation and reconstitution on the ability of mice to develop peritoneal eosinophilia in response to the same challenging stimulus. Their recipient "experimental" mice, before being challenged by antigen, were lethally irradiated and then reconstituted with syngeneic tissue taken either from normal mice or from mice primed to the challenging antigen by prior immunization with tetanus toxoid. McGarry *et al.* [95] found that the absolute requirement for any reconstitution of the eosinophilic response was a source of eosinophil precursor stem cells, either from bone marrow or from fetal liver. But, more specifically, they noted that although the same moderate levels of eosinophilia could be achieved by the mice when reconstituted with primed bone marrow cells alone or with normal bone marrow cells in addition to thymus or spleen cells taken from either normal or primed donors, responsiveness was markedly augmented when both pools of reconstituting cells (bone marrow plus either thymus or spleen cells) were derived from primed animals. Thus, there appeared to be a cooperative interaction between two cell populations (presumably, bone-marrow–derived B cells and thymus–derived T cells) resulting in enhanced eosinophil responsiveness in these reconstituted mice.

Additional evidence for cellular cooperation among lymphoid elements in the induction of eosinophilia was subsequently presented by this group in their studies of the generation of eosionophil–containing hematopoeitic colony forming units (CFU) in mice lethally irradiated, bone marrow reconstituted, and then challenged with tetanus toxoid antigen [96]. In this experimental model, priming bone marrow donors alone by prior immunization with the antigen had no effect on the number of eosinophil–containing CFUs that developed after recipients were stimulated with antigen, as compared to the response of animals reconstituted with normal marrow. However, priming both marrow donors and recipients some weeks before irradiation and reconstitution led to markedly increased numbers of eosinophil–containing CFUs in both the marrow and spleen of recipient animals. Intermediate numbers of such CFUs were obtained in this system if the recipients alone were primed. Thus, it appeared that there was a population of immunologically–committed bone marrow cells in donor animals which were able to cooperate with similarly committed radioresistant elements in recipient animals to produce enhanced eosinophilopoeisis.

Then, most recently, in further reconstitution experiments seeking to define this cellular cooperative interaction more precisely, Ponzio and Speirs [97] were able to demonstrate that the transferable stimulus to eosinophilia, the "memory function" required for enhanced eosinophil responsiveness, is a property of thymus–derived (T cell) lymphocytes. And, moreover, when they operationally compared this population of "memory cells" for eosinophil responsiveness to the population of memory cells responsible for transferring secondary tetanus antitoxin antibody responsiveness to the reconstituted mice, they found that these two cell populations were separable and distinct. The implication here, of course, is that while the memory cells of both eosinophilia and antibody production appear to be lymphocytes, they are still distinct cell types and belong to different classes or subclasses of the total lymphoid cell pool.

Thus, the work from these two laboratories, as well as that from the laboratories involved in characterizing the lymphocyte–derived eosinophil chemotactic factors (Section IV,B above), has served to link firmly the lymphoid immune system with the generation of an eosinophil response. The details of this link, including its molecular mediators, are still unclear; what feedback effects the eosinophils themselves may have on lymphocyte function and what modulators may exist to regulate these cell to cell interactions are totally unknown. Clearly, however, findings of the past several years have greatly advanced our understandings of the eosinophil response and, indeed, have demonstrated with certainty its dependence, in many instances, on an intact lymphoid immune system.

V. Pulmonary Eosinophilia Reconsidered

Until recently, studies on the mechanisms of eosinophilia had concentrated both on phenomenologic observations directed towards defining the types of conditions and stimuli necessary for the induction of an eosinophilic response and on determining the functional role of these cells once they had localized to a particular site. Then, in the past few years a number of investigators, stimulated by these earlier observations, succeeded in isolating and partially characterizing at least four different effector moieties chemoattractive for eosinophils. Interestingly enough, each of these agents is characteristic of a specific type of immune injury or allergic response [139], and thus, each may have an important role in determining the eosinophilia seen in the broad and diverse spectrum of pulmonary disease discussed in Section II above.

ECF-A, the preformed mast–cell product, is released from these cells concomitantly with other mediators of Type I (immediate hypersensitivity) responses. And the local eosinophilia, which commonly accompanies these reactions, doubtless results primarily from the eosinophilotactic properties of released ECF-A.

ECF-C, on the other hand, is the complement–derived eosinophil chemotactic factor, which may be generated by any of the activators of the complement cascade. Although these activators include such substances as complex polysaccharides, molecular aggregates of proteins, endotoxin, and other bacterial products, from an immunologic or allergic point of view the most important activators are the direct interactions of antigen with antibody and the presence of discrete antigen-antibody complexes. Thus, it appears likely that while the effects of ECF-C in generating eosinophilia in vivo may be a response to numerous complement activators, its role in eliciting the eosinophilia accompanying allergic reactions may be restricted to those conditions marked by Type II (cytotoxic) and Type III (immune complex) responses, both being situations in which the activation of complement is a characteristic feature.

Both of the other effector agents are lymphocyte-derived products, or lymphokines. One of them (ECF$_p$) requires activation by homologous antigen-antibody complexes before it is chemotactic for eosinophils, whereas the other (ESP) is active in stimulating eosinophils without further modification. Since both are the products of specifically activated immune lymphocytes, their contributions to the generation of eosinophilia are probably limited to those situations in which Type IV allergic reactions (cell-mediated immunity) are etiologically important.

Initially (Section II above), one presented and described briefly the clinical conditions characterized by pulmonary eosinophilia. Now, having considered some of the experimental work on the mechanisms of eosinophilia, one shall turn again to clinical situations in an effort to relate these experimental findings to the pathogenesis of the disease states.

A. Simple Pulmonary Eosinophilia

The characteristic features of simple pulmonary eosinophilia or Loeffler pneumonia, it will be recalled, are peripheral blood eosinophilia, minimal symptoms that are self-limited and of short duration, and migratory pulmonary infiltrates found, on x-ray studies, to be generally patchy and pleural-based in distribution. Although direct evidence is lacking, these features are generally compatible with a Type I allergic reaction in which the allergen is reacting with specific mast-cell bound reaginic (IgE) antibody to elicit the release, from these cells, of biologically active mediator substances, including histamine, SRS-A, and ECF-A. The mediators may then act to increase the local concentration of cells and fluid and thereby contribute to the increased densities seen as the "infiltrates" in chest radiographs.

The patchy and peripheral distribution of these densities, moreover, corresponds in a general way to the distribution of mast cells in the lung [140], both being found primarily along the pleural surface linings and, to a lesser extent, scattered throughout the parenchyma as well. Since these cells serve as the nucleus for the reactions generated in a Type-I response, it is quite reasonable that their distribution should determine that of the infiltrates in Loeffler pneumonia. The transient and migratory nature of the infiltrates, furthermore, may result from any of a number of aspects of these Type I responses. For example, the naturally limited time-course of localized anaphylactic reactions, the potential effects of the attracted eosinophils in modulating mediator release from the mast cells [62] or in modulating the effects of the mediators themselves [61], or the physical migration of the antigenic stimulus itself in cases where the Loeffler picture is related to the presence of migrating larval forms of parasitic helminths. Finally, even though this localized reaction of allergen with cell-bound antibody should be expected to result in peripheral blood eosinophilia [98,126] as one observes, still it is an allergic reaction essentially confined to the pulmonary parenchyma. As such, in a patient who is not hyper-reactive to the effects of anaphylactic mediators, it may be expected to generate few systemic, and, perhaps, even minimal local symptoms.

Simple pulmonary eosinophilia, then, appears to manifest many of the aspects of Type I immune injury. However, it is unlikely that the entire pathologic picture can be accounted for by these immediate hypersensitivity responses, for it should be recalled that uncomplicated, extrinsic asthma—surely a model of immediate hypersensitivity disease—is rarely associated with eosinophilic pulmonary infiltrates. Furthermore, others have suggested that the pulmonary accumulations of eosinophils in the Loeffler syndrome may be primarily a result of the lung's "filtering" capabilities—either by (a) direct filtration of excessive numbers of circulating eosinophils responding to stimuli elsewhere, thereby providing a physiologic route of elimination for these cells [141] or by (b) trapping antigenic material or immune complexes, which may lead to multiple types of local immune injury and subsequent attraction or eosinophils, as already described. In any case, basic mechanisms underlying these pulmonary accumulations of eosinophils in the Loeffler syndrome remain unresolved at this time and, thus, so do the specific effector molecules responsible for attracting these cells.

B. Prolonged Pulmonary Eosinophilia

The prolonged eosinophilic pneumonias form a more heterogeneous group of syndromes than do the simple pulmonary eosinophilias. Their etiologies are diverse and in some cases unknown, and their pathologic characteristics extend from simple mast-cell hyperplasia to complex collections of multiple cell types often accompanied by granuloma formation and sometimes even with vasculitis. Clearly, then, there is no single category in the Coombs and Gell [139] classification of immunologic injury which can accomodate all features of this group of diseases. Though aspects of Type I responses are noted in some instances, both clinical and pathologic evidence suggests the predominant importance of immune complex reactions (Type III response) and cell–mediated immune responses (Type IV reaction) in the pathogenesis of most of these conditions. Moreover, even the dramatic effects of steroids seen in these diseases does little to distinguish among the different types of immune response involved, since it is well known that steroids are effective in altering responsiveness at multiple points in each of these immune reactions [142]. Hence, as it is likely that most, if not all, of the four types of immune response are involved in the pathogenesis of prolonged eosinophilic pneumonias, it is also likely that most, if not all, of the described effectors of eosinophilia play a role in localizing this cell type to the affected pulmonary parenchyma.

C. Tropical Eosinophilia

As described earlier, tropical eosinophilia is a condition resulting from filarial infection but bearing an unclear relation to classic filariasis. The pathogenesis of this disease state has yet to be defined, but certain of the clinical features suggest that at least some elements of immediate hypersensitivity, or Type I responsiveness, are involved. Supporting this notion, moreover, are the recent findings of Ezeoke *et al.* [143] and Kaplan and his coworkers [144] that while serum IgE levels in patients with classic filariasis are significantly elevated, the IgE values of patients with the tropical eosinophilia syndrome are increased to levels even 6 to 12 times higher than those in both classic filariasis and other helminth infections. Furthermore, this hyper–responsiveness of humoral immunity seen in tropical eosinophilia is not limited to the IgE class of antibodies alone; rather, in all antibody classes studied, markedly enhanced elevations of specific antifilarial antibody have been found [145].

In light of this latter observation and other clinical and radiologic features of the syndrome which suggest a disease state of greater severity than that resulting from simple Type I reactions alone, it is not unreasonable to suggest that Type III (antigen–antibody complex) reactions, too, may play a role in the pathogenesis of this disease. Cooperation between Type III and Type I reactions in producing severe asthmatic states has clearly been well-documented in other diseases, such as allergic bronchopulmonary aspergillosis, as described below. If, then, the pathology of tropical eosinophilia reflects the immune injury from Type I and Type III allergic responses, either independently or in concert, likely mediators for the eosinophilia seen in this condition are the mast–cell product ECF-A and the complement moiety ECF-C. Whether or not the lymphocyte-derived eosinophil chemotactic factors also contribute to the generation of the eosinophilia is still unknown, as the potential role of cellular immunity in the pathogenesis of this disease has yet to be explored.

D. Pulmonary Eosinophilia With Asthma

When asthma is associated with certain of the pulmonary eosinophilias, it is generally the consequence of allergy to extrinsic agents. Pure Type I responses induce a form of asthma characterized by paroxysmal onset, short duration, and ready reversibility by bronchodilator drugs. Systemic symptoms are minimal and the accompanying eosinophilia may well derive from the actions of ECF-A, the eosinophil chemotactic factor of anaphylaxis. Type III asthma [29], on the other hand, though dependent on the presence of some form of Type I reaction, is characterized by a gradual onset, prolonged duration, greater severity, poor reversibility, systemic fever, and leukocytosis. It is the product of the interaction of antigen and specific precipitating antibody which leads to an Arthus-type reaction, the inflammatory effects of which produce partial obstruction of the small airways. Since this inflammation is mediated by the activation of complement, the presence of eosinophilia in these instances probably reflects the activity of the complement-derived eosinophil chemotactic factor ECF-C.

In allergic bronchopulmonary aspergillosis, a prominent cause of pulmonary eosinophilia with asthma [29], both types of allergic responsiveness are evident [30,146]. Reagins and precipitins to aspergillus extracts may be demonstrated in serum, and skin testing with this material first yields a wheal and flare response and then Arthus-like reactivity. Clinical manifestations also exhibit features of both Type I and Type III reactivity. And interestingly, when the pathogenesis of the syndrome was studied experimentally [147,148], evidence accumulated that these two types of immune response do not simply coexist; rather, the Type I reaction appears to be required for the Type III response to proceed and for the full clinical syndrome to develop. Thus, this syndrome, which clearly forms a large proportion of the cases of pulmonary eosinophilia with asthma, has been shown conclusively to result from both Type I and Type III immune responses. The eosinophilia generated by these responses, therefore, presumably arises from the effects of both anaphylactic- and complement-derived eosinophil chemotactic factors; namely ECF-A and ECF-C. Whether or not Type IV reactions also contribute to the pathogenesis of bronchopulmonary aspergillosis is still unresolved.

E. Pulmonary Eosinophilia with Periarteritis Nodosa

This form of pulmonary eosinophilia is representative of that associated with a class of disease states (Section II,E above) in which the most characteristic pathologic feature is vasculitis, either with or without associated granuloma formation. Although the exact pathogenesis of these conditions is not understood, it is generally believed that the immune injury is generated by Type III (antigen-antibody) reactions, Type IV (cell-mediated) immune responses, or by a combination of both types of allergic reaction [149]. The interesting studies of the mechanisms involved in the dynamics of these vasculitic states have been reviewed elsewhere [149]; again, it is reasonable to propose that the mechanisms that generate the eosinophilia often accompanying these conditions reflect those that determine the vasculitis itself. When Type III reactions cause vasculitis, the associated eosinophilia probably arises from the effects of the complement–derived eosinophil chemotactic factor ECF-C. When evidence of Type IV immune injury is associated with the vasculitis, the accompanying eosinophilia may well be a response to lymphokine eosinophil chemotactic factors ECF_p and ESP.

F. Other Hypereosinophilic States with Pulmonary Eosinophilia

Finally, with regard to that collection of clinical entities manifesting generalized, infiltrative eosinophilia, which may often involve the lungs along with other tissues, little specific mechanistic information is available. Not only are the types of agents that cause the syndrome unknown, but even points in the life span of the eosinophil at which these agents operate is unclear. Thus, though one could speculate that the infiltrative nature of these severe forms of hypereosinophilic syndrome is related more to defects in cellular control mechanisms than to responses of normal cells to exaggerated but normal stimuli (as is presumed to be the case in other states of pulmonary eosinophilia described above), so little evidence is available that such speculation would be hazardous indeed. Definition of the mechanisms determining this systemic eosinophilia must await further investigation of this group of enigmatic conditions.

Finally, one must cite briefly, at least, a number of other clinical conditions that may sometimes be accompanied by pulmonary eosinophilia but which have not been discussed in the classification scheme described above. These include certain types of tumors [150], some forms of radiation therapy [151], and the results of treatment with a variety of cytotoxic agents [152]. In each of these instances, it is again unclear as to what underlying mechanisms are involved in generating the local eosinophilia observed. Perhaps, in some instances, direct trauma or tissue damage leads to nonspecific mast–cell discharge and results in the subsequent accumulation of eosinophilic infiltrates. Or, as has been suggested [153], perhaps in other instances new antigenic material ("tumor antigens" or altered host material) is generated in these abnormal clinical states. These new antigens, when presented to the host, may then initiate a variety of immune responses, the ultimate outcome of which may include the local accumulation of eosinophils via any of the specific effector mechanisms described above. In any case, further understanding of the pulmonary eosinophilia seen in these conditions will likely be achieved only after the basic immunologic and pathologic parameters involved have been defined more explicitly than they are at present.

VI. Summary

In summary, then, the pulmonary eosinophilias are a markedly heterogenous collection of clinical entities; until recently the few common denominators one could appreciate among them were generally of a descriptive nature only. Now, however, in light of a number of very basic and intriguing observations concerning the mechanisms underlying the induction of an eosinophilic response—observations made in several different laboratories over the years—certain similarities in the pathogenesis of these various clinical syndromes have become evident.

Thus far, four different effector moieties, specifically attractive or stimulatory for eosinophils, have been delineated (Fig. 2). Though one would anticipate that further such agents will be described, even these four are sufficient now to provide explanations for the mechanisms underlying the eosinophilia that accompanies diseases resulting from all four types of immune injury [139]. Thus, in conditions in which anaphylactic reactivity is the hallmark of the immune response, ECF-A probably mediates the eosinophilic response; in pathologic processes in which complement is activated, ECF-C most likely serves this function; and in disease states where a cellular immune response is involved in pathogenesis, the lymphokines ECF_p and ESP are likely responsible for generating the accompanying eosinophilia. In other words, mechanisms that lead to eosinophilia appear to parallel closely mechanisms of immune injury.

However, despite these recently acquired understandings of mechanisms responsible for the pulmonary eosinophilic response, it is evident that one has thus far successfully approached only the problems of eosinophil localization and, to some extent, mobilization. The earliest steps in the generation of eosinophilia, at the level of the bone marrow, are still poorly understood and, even more basically, the very significance of eosinophilia itself remains a mystery. Clearly, before pulmonary eosinophilia, or any other form of eosinophilia can be thoroughly appreciated, both of these problems will need to be approached again, hopefully with fresh ideas and new techniques that can be combined to yield a more revealing account of the eosinophil's life history and functional specificities than has heretofore been possible.

Acknowledgment

The author wishes to express his sincere appreciation to the following for their critical reviews of the manuscript: Drs. C. H. Kirkpatrick, S. G. Cohen, F. A. Neva,

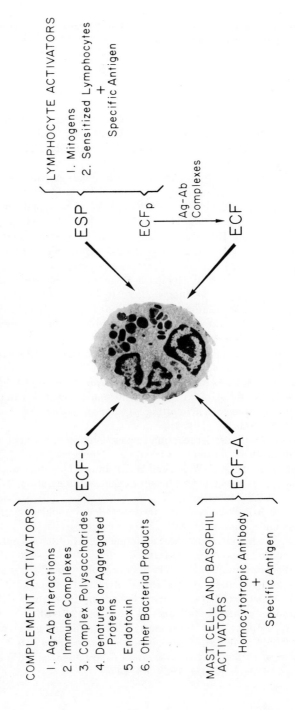

EOSINOPHIL CHEMOTACTIC FACTORS

LYMPHOCYTE ACTIVATORS

1. Mitogens
2. Sensitized Lymphocytes
   +
   Specific Antigen

ESP

ECFp → Ag-Ab Complexes → ECF

COMPLEMENT ACTIVATORS

1. Ag-Ab Interactions
2. Immune Complexes
3. Complex Polysaccharides
4. Denatured or Aggregated Proteins
5. Endotoxin
6. Other Bacterial Products

ECF-C

MAST CELL AND BASOPHIL ACTIVATORS

Homocytotropic Antibody
+
Specific Antigen

ECF-A

D. C. Dale, D. L. Hurley, and A. P. Kaplan; and to Ms. L. Johnson for her help
in preparing the manuscript.

References

1.   J. W. Crofton, J. L. Livingstone, N. C. Oswald, and T. M. Roberts, Pulmo-
     nary eosinophilia, *Thorax*, 7:1–35 (1952).
2.   A. A. Liebow and C. B. Carrington, The eosinophilic pneumonias, *Medi-
     cine*, 48:251–285 (1969).
3.   T. Hjorth, Pulmonary lesions with eosinophilia, *Scand. J. Respir. Dis.,
     Suppl.*, 72:132–138 (1970).
4.   L. A. Citro, M. E. Gordon, and W. T. Miller, Eosinophilic lung disease,
     Am. J. Roentgenol., Radium Ther. Nucl. Med., 117:787–797 (1973).
5.   W. Löffler, Zur Differential–Diagnose der Lungen Infiltrierungen: Über
     flüchtige Succedan–Infiltrate (mit Eosinophilia) Beitr, *Klin. Tuberk.*, 79:
     368–392 (1932).
6.   W. H. Reeder and B. E. Goodrich, Pulmonary infiltration with eosinophilia
     (PIE Syndrome), *Ann. Intern. Med.*, 36:1217–1240 (1952).
7.   H. Vogel and W. Minning, Contributions to clinical knowledge of lung
     ascariasis and to the question of transient eosinophilic lung infiltrates,
     Beitr. Klin. Tuberk., 98:620–654 (1942).
8.   J. E. Berk, Transitory pulmonary infiltrations, Correspondence *J.A.M.A.*,
     127:354–355 (1945).
9.   P. C. Beaver, Larva migrans, *Exp. Parasitol.*, 5:587–621 (1956).
10. D. Wright and E. Gold, Löffler's syndrome associated with creeping
     eruption (cutaneous helminthiasis). Report of 26 cases, *Arch. Intern.
     Med.*, 78:303–312 (1946).
11. H. Tuchman, Loeffler reaction to para–aminosalicylic acid, *Am. Rev.
     Tuberc.*, 70:171–175 (1954).
12. D. S. Feigenberg, H. Weiss, and H. Kirshman, Migratory pneumonia with
     eosinophilia associated with sulfonamide administration, *Arch. Intern.
     Med.*, 120:85–89 (1967).
13. R. J. M. Bell, Pulmonary infiltration with eosinophils caused by chlor-
     propamide, *Lancet*, 1:1249–1250 (1964).
14. F. W. Sunderman and F. W. Sunderman, Jr., Löffler's syndrome associated
     with nickel sensitivity, *Arch. Intern. Med.*, 107:405–408 (1961).
15. G. Diaconita and G. Goldis, Pathomorphology and pathogenesis of pulmo-
     nary paragonimiasis, *Acta Morphol. Acad. Sci. Hung.*, 12:315–331 (1964).
16. F. M. Willett and E. Oppenheim, Pulmonary infiltration with associated
     eosinophilia, *Am. J. Med. Sci.*, 212:608–612 (1946).
17. K. A. Elsom and F. J. Ingelfinger, Eosinophilia and pneumonitis in chronic
     brucellosis; A report of two cases, *Ann. Intern. Med.*, 16:995–1002 (1942).
18. J. Pepys. *Hypersensitivity Diseases of the Lungs Due to Fungi and Organic
     Dusts.* Basle, S. Karger, 1969, pp. 147.

19. W. G. Strauss and L. M. Griffin, Nitrofurantoin pneumonia, *J.A.M.A.*, **199**: 765–766 (1967).
20. C. B. Carrington, W. W. Addington, A. M. Goff, I. M. Madoff, A. Marks, J. R. Schwaber, and E. A. Gaensler, Chronic eosinophilic pneumonia, *N. Engl. J. Med.*, **280**:787–798 (1969).
21. C. Frimodt–Möller and R. M. Barton, Pseudo–Tuberculous condition associated with eosinophilia, *Indian Med. Gaz.*, **75**:607–613 (1940).
22. R. J. Weingarten, Tropical eosinophilia, *Lancet*, **1**:103–105 (1943).
23. D. L. Donohugh, Tropical eosinophilia. An Etiologic inquiry, *N. Engl. J. Med.*, **269**:1357–1364 (1963).
24. J. K. G. Webb, C. K. Job, and E. W. Gault, Tropical eosinophilia: Demonstration of microfilariae in lung, liver, and lymph–nodes, *Lancet*, **1**:835–842 (1960).
25. T. J. Danaraj, G. Pacheco, K. Shanmugaratnam, and P. C. Beaver, The etiology and pathology of eosinophilic lung (tropical eosinophilia), *Am. J. Trop. Med. Hyg.*, **15**:183–189 (1966).
26. P. C. Beaver, Filariasis without microfilaremia, *Am. J. Trop. Med. Hyg.*, **19**:181–189 (1970).
27. J. J. Buckley, Occult filarial infections of animal origin as a cause of tropical pulmonary eosinophilia (1958), *East Afr. Med. J.*, **35**:492–500 (1958).
28. W. S. V. Leeuwer, Z. Bien, W. Kremer, and H. Varekamp, On the significance of small–spored types of aspergilli (type of *Aspergillus fumigatus*) in the etiology of bronchial asthma, *Z. Immunitaetsforsch*, **44**:1–26 (1925).
•29. J. Pepys and G. Simon, Asthma, pulmonary eosinophilia, and allergic alveolitis, *Med. Clin. North Am.*, **57**:573–591 (1973).
•30. D. S. McCarthy and J. Pepys, Allergic broncho–pulmonary aspergillosis. Clinical Immunology: (1) Clinical Features, *Clin. Allergy*, **1**:261–286 (1971).
31. W. R. Hardy and R. E. Anderson, The hypereosinophilic syndromes, *Ann. Intern. Med.*, **68**:1220–1229 (1968).
32. M. J. Chusid, D. C. Dale, B. C. West, and S. M. Wolff, The idiopathic hypereosinophilic syndromes, *Medicine*, **54**:1–27 (1975).
33. I. D. Mickenberg, R. K. Root, and S. M. Wolff, Bactericidal and metabolic properties of human eosinophils, *Blood*, **39**:67–80 (1972).
34. D. Zucker–Franklin, Electron microscopic studies of human granulocytes: Structural variations related to function, *Semin. Hematol.*, **5**:109–133 (1968).
35. G. T. Archer and J. G. Hirsch, Isolation of granules from eosinophil leukocytes and study of their enzyme content, *J. Exp. Med.*, **118**:277–285 (1963).
36. R. Vercauteren, The properties of the isolated granules from blood eosinophiles, *Enzymologia*, **16**:1–13 (1953).
37. M. I. Barnhart and J. M. Riddle, Cellular localization of profibrinolysin (plasminogen), *Blood*, **21**:306–321 (1963).

38. T. Rytömaa, Relationship between tissue eosinophils and peroxidase activity, *Nature*, **192**:271–272 (1961).

39. R. J. Lehrer and M. J. Cline, Leukocyte myeloperoxidase deficiency and disseminated candidiasis: The role of myeloperoxidase in resistance to *Candida* infection, *J. Clin. Invest.*, **48**:1478–1488 (1969).

40. J. H. Hardin and S. S. Spicer, An ultrastructural study of human eosinophil granules: Maturational stages and pyroantimonate reactive cation, *Am. J. Anat.*, **128**:283–310 (1970).

41. E. Pihl, G. T. Gustafson, and B. Josefsson, Heavy metals in the granules of eosinophilic granulocytes, *Scand. J. Haematol.*, **4**:371–379 (1967).

42. P. M. Seeman and G. E. Palade, Acid phosphatase localization in rabbit eosinophils, *J. Cell. Biol.*, **34**:745–756 (1967).

43. R. W. Honsinger, Jr., D. Silverstein, and P. P. VanArsdel, The eosinophil and allergy: Why?, *J. Allergy and Clin. Immunol.*, **49**:142–155 (1972).

44. G. J. Gleich, D. A. Loegering, and J. E. Maldonado, Identification of a major basic protein in guinea pig eosinophil granules, *J. Exp. Med.*, **137**: 1459–1471 (1973).

45. L. Nattan-Larrier and M. Parvu, Rechershes sur le pouvoir phagocytaire des polynucléaires éosinophiles, *C. R. Soc. Biol.*, **66**:574–576 (1909).

46. M. J. Cline, J. Hanifin, and R. I. Lehrer, Phagocytosis by human eosinophils, *Blood*, **32**:922–934 (1968).

47. D. Zucker-Franklin, M. Davidson, and L. Thomas, The interaction of mycoplasmas with mammalian cells. I. Hela cells, neutrophils, and eosinophils, *J. Exp. Med.*, **124**:521–532 (1966).

48. T. Ishikawa, A. C. Dalton, and C. E. Arbesman, Phagocytosis of *Candida albicans* by eosinophilic leukocytes, *J. Allergy Clin. Immunol.*, **49**:311–315 (1972).

49. S. T. Kostage, A. P. Rizzo, and S. G. Cohen, Experimental eosinophilia XI. Cell responses to particles of delineated size, *Proc. Soc. Exp. Biol. Med.*, **125**:413–416 (1967).

50. G. T. Archer and J. G. Hirsch, Motion picture studies on degranulation of horse eosinophils during phagocytosis, *J. Exp. Med.*, **118**:287–294 (1963).

51. R. L. Baehner and R. B. Johnston, Jr., Metabolic and bactericidal activities of human eosinophils, *Br. J. Haematol.*, **20**:277–285 (1971).

52. M. J. Cline, Microbicidal activity of human eosinophils, *J. Reticuloendothel. Soc.*, **12**:332–339 (1972).

53. M. Litt, Studies in experimental eosinophilia III. The induction of peritoneal eosinophilia by the passive transfer of serum antibody, *J. Immunol.*, **87**:522–529 (1961).

54. S. M. Sabesin, A function of the eosinophil: Phagocytosis of antigen-antibody complexes, *Proc. Soc. Exp. Biol. Med.*, **112**:667–670 (1963).

55. M. Litt, Studies in experimental eosinophilia VI. Uptake of immune complexes by eosinophils, *J. Cell. Biol.*, **23**:355–361 (1964).

56. G. T. Archer, M. Nelson, and J. Johnston, Eosinophil granule lysis *in vitro* induced by soluble antigen–antibody complexes, *Immunology*, **17**:777–787 (1969).

57. T. Ishikawa, K. Wicher, and C. E. Arbesman, In vitro and in vivo studies on uptake of antigen–antibody complexes by eosinophils, *Int. Arch. Allergy Appl. Immunol.*, **46**:230–248 (1974).
58. W. E. Parish, Investigations on eosinophilia. The influence of histamine, antigen–antibody complexes containing gamma–1 or gamma–2 globulins, foreign bodies (phagocytosis) and disrupted mast cells, *Br. J. Dermatol.*, **82**:42–64 (1970).
59. R. A. Welsh and J. C. Geer, Phagocytosis of mast cell granule by the eosinophilic leukocyte in the rat, *Am. J. Pathol.*, **35**:103–112 (1959).
60. P. R. Mann, An electron–microscope study of the relations between mast cells and eosinophil leukocytes, *J. Pathol.*, **98**:183–186 (1969).
61. R. K. Archer. *The Eosinophil Leukocytes.* Oxford, Blackwell Scientific Publications, 1963.
62. T. Hubscher and A. H. Eisen, An eosinophil derived inhibitor (EDI) of histamine release, *J. Allergy Clin. Immunol.*, **51**:83–84 (1973) (abstr.).
63. P. A. Stryckmans, E. P. Cronkite, M. L. Greenberg, and L. M. Schiffer, Kinetics of eosinophil leukocyte proliferation in man. In *Proceedings 12th Congress, International Society Haematology,* New York, 1968.
64. J. C. Herion, R. M. Glasser, and J. G. Palmer, Eosinophil kinetics in two patients with eosinophilia, *Blood*, **36**:361–370 (1970).
65. S. N. Wickramasinghe and B. Moffatt, DNA synthesis during human eosinopoiesis, *Acta Haematol.*, **48**:158–163 (1972).
66. E. E. Osgood, A. J. Seaman, H. Tivey, and D. A. Rigas, Duration of life and of different stages of maturation of normal and leukemic leukocytes, *Rev. Hematol.*, **9**:543 (1954).
67. R. Gross, The eosinophils. In *The Physiology and Pathology of Leukocytes.* Edited by H. Braunsteiner and D. Zucker–Franklin. New York, Grune and Stratton, 1962, pp. 1–45.
68. D. Eidinger, M. Raff, and B. Rose, Tissue eosinophilia in hypersensitivity reactions as revealed by the human skin window, *Nature*, **196**:683–684 (1962).
69. G. Hudson, Quantitative study of the eosinophil granulocytes, *Semin. Hematol.*, **5**:166–186 (1968).
70. T. Rytömaa, Organ distribution and histochemical properties of eosinophil granulocytes in the rat, *Acta Pathol. Microbiol. Scand., Suppl.*, **140**:1–118 (1960).
71. G. Hudson, Changes in the marrow reserve of eosinophils following re-exposure to foreign protein, *Br. J. Haematol.*, **9**:446–455 (1963).
72. C. J. F. Spry, Mechanism of eosinophilia V. Kinetics of normal and accelerated eosionopoiesis, *Cell Tissue Kinet.*, **4**:351–364 (1971).
73. C. J. Spry, Mechanism of eosinophilia VI. Eosinophil mobilization, *Cell Tissue Kinet.*, **4**:365–374 (1971).
74. M. L. Greenberg and G. Chikkappa, Eosinophil production and survival in a patient with eosinophilia (Leukemia?), *Blood*, **38**:826 (1971) (abstr.).
75. D. C. Dale and S. M. Wolff, Personal communication. Unpublished observations.

76.   T. M. Fliedner, E. P. Cronkite, and J. S. Robertson, Granulocytopoiesis I. Senescence and random loss of neutrophilic granulocytes in human beings, *Blood*, **24**:402–414 (1964).

77.   J. W. Athens, O. P. Haab, S. O. Raab, A. M. Maner, H. Ashenbruker, G. E. Cartwright, and M. M. Wintrobe, Leukokinetic studies IV. The total blood, circulating and marginal granulocyte pools and the granulocyte turnover rate in normal subjects, *J. Clin. Invest.*, **40**:989–995 (1961).

78.   A. Basten, M. H. Boyer, and P. B. Beeson, Mechanism of eosinophilia I. Factors affecting the eosinophil response of rats to *Trichinella spiralis*, *J. Exp. Med.*, **131**:1271–1287 (1970).

79.   A. E. Renold, T. B. Quigley, H. E. Kennard, and G. W. Thorn, Reaction of the adrenal cortex to physical and emotional stress in college oarsmen, *N. Engl. J. Med.*, **244**:754–757 (1951).

80.   V. Andersen, F. Bro–Rasmussen, and K. Hougard, Autoradiographic studies of eosinophil kinetics: Effect of cortisol. In *Proceedings of the Twelfth Congress of the International Society of Hematology*, New York, 1968.

81.   J. E. Morgan and P. B. Beeson, Experimental observations on the eosinopenia induced by acute infection, *Br. J. Exp. Pathol.*, **52**:214–220 (1971).

82.   J. Koch–weser, Beta adrenergic blockade and circulating eosinophils, *Arch. Intern. Med.*, **121**:255–258 (1968).

83.   A. B. Kay, D. J. Stechschulte, and K. F. Austen, An eosinophil leukocyte chemotactic factor of anaphylaxis, *J. Exp. Med.*, **133**:602–619 (1971).

84.   A. B. Kay, Studies on eosinophil leukocyte migration II. Factors specifically chemotactic for eosinophils and neutrophils generated from guinea pig serum by antigen–antibody complexes, *Clin. Exp. Immunol.*, **7**:723–737 (1970).

85.   S. Cohen and P. A. Ward, In vitro and in vivo activity of a lymphocyte and immune complex–dependent chemotactic factor for eosinophils, *J. Exp. Med.*, **133**:133–146 (1971).

86.   D. G. Colley, Eosinophils and immune mechanisms I. Eosinophil stimulation promoter (ESP): A lymphokine induced by specific antigen or phytohemagglutinin, *J. Immunol.*, **110**:1419–1423 (1973).

87.   R. S. Speirs and U. Wenck, Eosinophil response to toxoids in actively and passively immunized mice, *Proc. Soc. Exp. Biol. Med.*, **90**:571–574 (1955).

88.   R. S. Speirs and M. E. Driesbach, Quantitative studies of the cellular responses to antigen injections in normal mice, *Blood*, **11**:44–55 (1956).

89.   R. S. Speirs, E. E. Speirs, and V. Jansen, A quantitative approach to the study of inflammatory cells, *Proc. Soc. Exp. Biol. Med.*, **106**:248–251 (1961).

90.   R. S. Speirs and M. X. Turner, The eosinophil response to toxoids and its inhibition by antitoxin, *Blood*, **34**:320–330 (1969).

91.   R. S. Speirs, Effect of x–irradiation on the cellular and humoral responses to antigen, *Ann. N. Y. Acad. Sci.*, **114**:424–441 (1964).

92.   M. X. Turner, R. S. Speirs, and J. A. McLaughlin, Effect of primary injection site upon cellular and antitoxin responses to subsequent challenging injection, *Proc. Soc. Exp. Biol. Med.*, **129**:738–743 (1968).

93.   R. S. Speirs and Y. Osada, Chemotactic activity and phagocytosis of eosinophils, *Proc. Soc. Exp. Biol. Med.,* **109**:929–932 (1961).
94.   R. S. Speirs and E. E. Speirs, Cellular localization of radioactive antigen in immunized and nonimmunized mice, *J. Immunol.,* **90**:561–575 (1963).
95.   M. P. McGarry, R. S. Speirs, V. K. Jenkins, and J. J. Trentin, Lymphoid cell dependence of eosinophil response to antigen, *J. Exp. Med.,* **134**: 801–814 (1971).
96.   V. K. Jenkins, J. J. Trentin, R. S. Speirs, and M. P. McGarry, Hematopoietic colony studies VI. Increased eosinophil–containing colonies obtained by antigen pretreatment of irradiated mice reconstituted with bone marrow cells, *J. Cell. Physiol.,* **79**:413–422 (1972).
97.   N. M. Ponzio and R. S. Speirs, Lymphoid cell dependence of eosinophil response to antigen III. Comparison of the rate of appearance of two types of memory cells in various lymphoid tissues at different times after priming, *J. Immunol.,* **110**:1363–1370 (1973).
98.   M. Litt, Studies in experimental eosinophilia. I. Repeated quantitation of peritoneal eosinophilia in guinea pigs by a method of peritoneal lavage, *Blood,* **16**:1318–1329 (1960).
99.   M. Litt, Studies in experimental eosinophilia. II. Induction of peritoneal eosinophilia by the transfer of tissues and tissue extracts, *Blood,* **16**:1330–1337 (1960).
100. M. Litt, Studies in experimental eosinophilia IV. Determinants of eosinophil localization, *J. Allergy,* **33**:532–543 (1962).
101. W. E. Parish, Eosinophilia I. Eosinophilia in guinea pigs mediated by passive anaphylaxis and by antigen–antibody complexes containing homologous IgGla and IgGlb, *Immunology,* **22**:1087–1098 (1972).
102. S. G. Cohen, T. M. Sapp, and P. N. Chiampi, Eosinophil leukocyte responses and hypersensitivity reactions in the *Bordetella pertussis*-treated mouse, *J. Allergy,* **46**:205–215 (1970).
103. S. G. Cohen, T. M. Sapp, and D. L. Reese, Homocytotropic antibody function in the mouse. Eosinophil responses, complement altering agents and eosinophilia, anaphylactic sensitization, *J. Allergy Clin. Immunol.,* **54**:263–273 (1974).
104. J. Munoz and R. K. Bergman, Histamine–sensitizing factors from microbial agents, with special reference to *Bordetella pertusis, Bacteriol. Rev.,* **32**:103–126 (1968).
105. S. G. Cohen, M. Kantor, and L. Gatto, Experimental eosinophilia III. Regional lymph node responses to reactions of tissue sensitization, *J. Allergy,* **32**:214–222 (1961).
106. M. Litt, Studies in experimental eosinophilia V. Eosinophils in lymph nodes of guinea pigs following primary antigenic stimulation, *Am. J. Pathol.,* **42**:529–549 (1963).
107. S. G. Cohen, T. M. Sapp, A. P. Rizzo, and S. T. Kostage, Experimental eosinophilia. VII. Lymph node responses to altered gamma globulins, *J. Allergy,* **35**:346–355 (1964).
108. M. Litt, Studies in experimental eosinophilia VII. Eosinophils in lymph

nodes during the first 24 hr following primary antigenic stimulation, *J. Immunol.,* **93**:807–813 (1964).

109. M. Litt, Studies in experimental eosinophilia VIII. Induction of eosino-
      philia by homologous 7Sγ1 antibody and by extremely minute doses of
      antigen. In *Proceedings 6th Congress of the International Association of
      Allergology,* 1967, pp. 38–53.

110. M. Litt, Studies of experimental eosinophilia IX. Inhibition by puro-
      mycin of the eosinophil response which hemocyanin elicits in guinea pig
      lymph nodes, *J. Immunol.,* **109**:222–226 (1972).

111. P. A. Ward, Chemotaxis of human eosinophils, *Am. J. Pathol.,* **54**:121–128
      (1969).

112. R. K. Archer, Eosinophil leukocytes and their reactions to histamine and
      5–hydroxytryptamine, *J. Pathol. Bacteriol.,* **78**:95–103 (1959).

113. R. K. Archer and J. Broome, Bradykinin and eosinophils, *Nature,* **198**:
      893–894 (1963).

114. R. K. Archer, On the functions of eosinophils in the antigen–antibody
      reaction, *Br. J. Haematol.,* **11**:123–129 (1965).

115. S. G. Cohen and T. M. Sapp, Experimental eosinophilia VIII. Cellular
      responses to altered globulins within cutaneous tissue, *J. Allergy,* **36**:
      415–422 (1965).

116. A. B. Kay, Studies on eosinophil migration. I. Eosinophil and neutrophil
      accumulation following antigen–antibody reactions in guinea pig skin,
      Clin. Exp. Immunol., **6**:75–86 (1970).

117. W. E. Parish, Eosinophilia II. Cutaneous eosinophilia in guinea pigs medi-
      ated by passive anaphylaxis with IgGl or reagin, and antigen–antibody
      complexes; Its relation to neutrophils and to mast cells, *Immunology,* **23**:
      19–34 (1972).

118. A. B. Kay and K. F. Austen, Antigen–antibody induced cutaneous eosin-
      ophilia in complement deficient guinea pigs, *Clin. Exp. Immunol.,* **11**:
      37–42 (1972).

119. M. Samter, M. A. Kofoed, and W. Pieper, A factor in lungs of anaphylac-
      tically shocked guinea pigs which can induce eosinophilia in normal ani-
      mals, *Blood,* **8**:1078–1090 (1953).

120. A. Basten and P. B. Beeson, Mechanism of eosinophilia II. Role of the
      lymphocyte, *J. Exp. Med.,* **131**:1288–1305 (1970).

121. M. H. Boyer, A. Basten, and P. B. Beeson, Mechanism of eosinophilia.
      III. Suppression of eosinophilia by agents known to modify immune
      responses, *Blood,* **36**:458–469 (1970).

122. M. H. Boyer, C. J. F. Spry, P. B. Beeson, and W. H. Sheldon, Mechanism
      of eosinophilia IV. The pulmonary lesion resulting from intravenous
      injection of *Trichinella spiralis, Yale J. Biol. Med.,* **43**:351–357 (1971).

123. R. S. Walls, A. Basten, E. Leuchars, and A. J. S. Davies, Mechanisms for
      eosinophilic and neutrophilic leucocytoses, *Br. Med. J.,* **3**:157–159
      (1971).

124. R. S. Walls and P. B. Beeson, Mechanism of eosinophilia VIII. Impor-
      tance of local cellular reactions in stimulating eosinophil production,
      Clin. Exp. Immunol., **12**:111–119 (1972).

125. R. S. Walls and P. B. Beeson, Mechanism of eosinophilia IX. Induction of eosinophilia in rats by certain forms of dextran, *Proc. Soc. Exp. Biol. Med.*, **140**:689–693 (1972).

126. M. Samter, Early eosinophilia induced in guinea pigs by intrapulmonary injection of antigenic determinants and antigens, *J. Allergy*, **45**:234–247 (1970).

127. R. Patterson, C. H. Talbot, and B. H. Booth, Bronchial eosinophilia in rhesus monkeys with IgE–mediated respiratory responses, *Int. Arch. Allergy*, **40**:361–371 (1971).

128. A. B. Kay and K. F. Austen, The IgE–mediated release of an eosinophil leukocyte chemotactic factor from human lung, *J. Immunol.*, **107**:899–902 (1971).

129. W. E. Parish, Eosinophilia III. The anaphylactic release from isolated human basophils of a substance that selectively attracts eosinophils, *Clin. Allergy*, **2**:381–390 (1972).

130. S. I. Wasserman, E. J. Goetzl, L. Ellman, and K. F. Austen, Tumor-associated eosinophilotactic factor, *N. Engl. J. Med.*, **290**:420–424 (1974).

131. P. A. Ward, C. G. Cochrane, and H. J. Müller–Eberhard, The role of serum complement in chemotaxis of leukocytes in vitro, *J. Exp. Med.*, **122**:327–346 (1965).

132. H. U. Keller and E. Sorkin, Studies on chemotaxis XIII. Differences in the chemotactic response of neutrophil and eosinophil polymorphonuclear leucocytes, *Int. Arch. Allergy*, **35**:279–287 (1969).

133. P. J. Lachmann, A. B. Kay, and R. A. Thompson, The chemotactic activity for neutrophil and eosinophil leucocytes of the trimolecular complex of the fifth, sixth and seventh components of human complement ($C\overline{567}$) prepared in free solution by the "reactive lysis" procedure, *Immunology*, **19**:895–899 (1970).

134. S. Ruddy, I. Gigli, and K. F. Austen, The complement system of man, *N. Engl. J. Med.*, **287**:489–495, 545–549, 592–596, and 642–646 (1972).

135. B. G. Arnason and B. H. Waksman, The retest reaction in delayed sensitivity, *Lab. Invest.*, **12**:737–747 (1963).

136. M. Torisu, T. Yoshida, P. A. Ward, and S. Cohen, Lymphocyte–derived eosinophil chemotactic factor II. Studies on the mechanism of activation of the precursor substance by immune complexes, *J. Immunol.*, **111**:1450–1458 (1973).

137. B. M. Greene and D. G. Colley, Partial characterization of a lymphokine: Eosinophil stimulation promoter (ESP), *Fed. Proc.*, **33**:746 (1974) (abstr.).

138. M. Litt, Eosinophils and antigen–antibody reactions, *Ann. N. Y. Acad. Sci.*, **116**:964–985 (1964).

139. R. R. A. Coombs and P. G. H. Gell, Classification of allergic reactions responsible for clinical hypersensitivity and disease. In *Clinical Aspects of Immunology*. Edited by P. G. H. Gell and R. R. A. Coombs. Philadelphia, F. A. Davis, 1968, pp. 575–596.

140. J. F. Riley. *The Mast Cells*. Edinburg and London, E & S Livingstone, Ltd., 1959, p. 182.

141.   S. G. Cohen, The eosinophil and eosinophilia, *N. Engl. J. Med.,* **290**:457–459 (1973).
142.   C. H. Kirkpatrick, Steroid therapy of allergic diseases, *Med. Clin. North Am.,* **57**:1309–1320 (1973).
143.   A. Ezeoke, A. B. Perera, and J. R. Hobbs, Serum IgE elevation with tropical eosinophilia, *Clin. Allergy,* **3**:33–35 (1973).
144.   A. P. Kaplan, F. A. Neva, and G. Pacheco. Unpublished observations.
145.   R. Viswanathan, Immunoglobulins in pulmonary eosinophilosis (Tropical eosinophilia), *Acta Med. Scand.,* **193**:219–222 (1973).
· 146.   D. S. McCarthy and J. Pepys, Allergic bronchopulmonary Aspergillosis. Clinical Immunology. II. Skin, nasal, and bronchial tests, *Clin. Allergy,* 1:415–432 (1971).
·147.   T. M. Golbert and R. Patterson, Pulmonary allergic aspergillosis, *Ann. Intern. Med.,* **72**:395–403 (1970).
148.   C. G. Cochrane, Mechanisms involved in the deposition of immune complexes in tissues, *J. Exp. Med.,* **134**:75s–89s (1971).
149.   A. S. Fauci, Pulmonary Vasculitis, this volume.
150.   M. V. Viola, E. Chung, and M. G. Mukhopadhyay, Eosinophilia and metastatic carcinoma, *Med. Ann. D.C.,* **41**:1–3 (1972).
151.   F. M. Muggia, N. A. Ghossein, and H. Wohl, Eosinophilia following radiation therapy, *Oncology,* **27**:118–127 (1973).
152.   A. M. Clarysse, W. J. Cathey, G. E. Cartwright, and M. M. Wintrobe, Pulmonary disease complicating intermittent therapy with methotrexate, *J.A.M.A.,* **209**:1861–1864 (1969).
153.   S. G. Cohen, Personal communication.
154.   R. A. Clark, J. I. Gallin, and A. P. Kaplan, The selective eosinophil chemotactic activity of histamine, *J. Exp. Med.,* (1975) in press.

Part III

DISEASES THAT ARE CONSEQUENCES OF ABERRANT OR DEFICIENT IMMUNOLOGIC REACTIONS IN THE LUNG

16

Replacement Therapy for Prevention and Treatment of Pulmonary Infections

REBECCA H. BUCKLEY

Duke University School of Medicine
Durham, North Carolina

I. Introduction

In those conditions characterized by deficiencies in specific humoral immunity, the systemic replacement of IgG antibodies with whole plasma or immunoglobulin concentrates is undoubtedly of benefit. This is most apparent in the significant prevention of serious or life-threatening systemic infections, but it is also seen in a reduced frequency and severity of pulmonary infections. Since neither of these therapies replaces the major form of antibody in external secretions, their effectiveness is actually somewhat surprising. New information on pulmonary host–defenses, derived from animal studies, suggests possible reasons for this benefit, however [1,2]. Rabbits immunized either parenterally or intranasally with killed *Pseudomonas* organisms were found to have IgG antibodies to these organisms in their bronchial secretions [1]. These antibodies were shown not only to be capable of agglutinating the organisms but to have superior opsonizing properties in alveolar macrophage-killing studies when compared to IgA antibodies [2]. Since no IgM or complement was detected in these secretions [1], IgG antibodies appeared to be the principal opsonin in rabbit respiratory secretions. If the same proves to be true for man, there would be a rational basis for humoral replacement therapy in the prevention and treatment of pulmonary infections, in addition to the clinical grounds cited above.

The successes noted following humoral replacement therapy for the first host defect found to predispose to chronic and recurrent pulmonary infection [3] led, for a time, to the rather widespread and indiscriminate use of gamma globulin injections in patients with recurrent lower respiratory infections [4]. Further misuse of this form of therapy has been fostered by the use of improper diagnostic tests and inappropriate normal laboratory values in evaluating pediatric-age patients with this problem. This has led to frequent erroneous diagnoses of humoral immunodeficiency and often to years of unnecessary injections of gamma globulin to children. From the wealth of information now accumulated in the world's literature about various immunodeficiency diseases and therapies presently available for them, two important points emerge relevant to the subject of this chapter. The first is that well-defined immunodeficiency is rare [5], and the second is that currently available forms of therapy for such defects leave much to be desired [6,7]. The latter is particularly true with respect to the prevention and treatment of infections of the respiratory and gastrointestinal systems in patients with these disorders, primarily because there is no effective way of replacing secretory IgA antibodies at mucous membrane surfaces, except by complete immunologic reconstitution through transplantation of immunocompetent tissue. Unfortunately, the latter therapy is available to only a select few with particular forms of immunodeficiency [6].

II. Indications and Contraindications

The only presently acceptable indication for either humoral or cellular replacement therapy for the control of pulmonary infections is the clear demonstration of a host deficit in one or both of these components.

A. Defects in Humoral Immunity

Passive antibody therapy is indicated in all immunodeficiency states in which antibody formation has been shown to be severely impaired [8,9]. These include especially those primary immunodeficiency diseases characterized by low or undetectable quantities of all five serum immunoglobulins, e.g., the a- or hypogammaglobulinemias. In addition, humoral replacement therapy is indicated for patients with X-linked immunodeficiency with hyper-IgM and even for normogammaglobulinemic immunodeficient patients whose ability to produce specific antibodies following immunization has been shown to be markedly impaired. Deficits in humoral immunity in which replacement therapy with gamma globulin or plasma is not indicated, however, include transient hypogammaglobulinemia of infancy and selective IgA deficiency. In the former situation, these infants usually have the capacity to make specific antibodies normally following immunization, despite low concentrations of all or some of the immunoglobulins during the first 15 to 18 months of life. Administration of passive antibody could conceivably suppress this ability and do more harm than good. In the case of selective IgA deficiency, the lack of appropriate replacement therapy is unfortunate, since it is, in all probability, the most common of the well-defined immunodeficiency disorders and a high percentage of individuals with this defect are subject to chronic and recurrent respiratory infection [10]. Patients with selective IgA deficiency usually have the ability to produce antibodies of the other immunoglobulin classes normally, however. Indeed a significant proportion of such individuals produce antibodies to IgA [11], and these have been implicated as the cause of anaphylactic transfusion reactions in some of these patients [12,13]. For this reason, humoral replacement therapy is contraindicated in this form of immunodeficiency. Moreover, even if products containing IgA could be given safely to patients with selective IgA deficiency, they still could not effect replacement of that immunoglobulin at mucous membrane surfaces, as mentioned above. This is due to the fact that secretory IgA in normal individuals derives from paragut and pararespiratory lymphoid tissue and is not transported from the intravascular compartment to external secretions, as originally thought. Indeed, even after intravenous infusions of large volumes of IgA-containing plasma into one agammaglobulinemic patient, an increase in IgA could not be detected in his external secretions; radiolabeled IgA infused into normal subjects could not be demonstrated in saliva or breast milk [14].

B. Defects in Cellular Immunity

Humoral replacement therapy has been of limited or no value in the treatment of patients with defects in cellular immunity, although it seems reasonable to use it in patients with combined humoral and cellular immunodeficiencies. The only certain effective replacement therapy for cellular immunodeficiency at present is successful immunologic reconstitution by transplanting suitable immunocompetent tissue [6,15]. There are only two immunodeficiency disorders that have been successfully treated in this manner. These are (a) severe combined immunodeficiency disease and (b) thymic hypoplasia, or the Di George syndrome. In the first condition, immunologic reconstitution has been achieved in a relatively large number of patients (estimated to be approximately 25 from reports collected at the Second International Workshop on Human Immunodeficiency Diseases in 1973) by transplants of histocompatible bone marrow [15]. In addition, it has been estimated that an approximately equal number of unsuccessful attempts have been made to achieve immunologic reconstitution by bone marrow transplants in infants with this disorder. In the Di George syndrome, the basic abnormality lies in the failure of structures derived from the third and fourth branchial pouches, including the thymus and parathyroid glands, to develop. Immunologic improvement has been noted in three infants with this syndrome given either transplants of fetal thymus [15] or a thymus gland implanted in a millipore diffusion chamber [16]. In all other immunodeficiency disorders characterized by combined deficits in humoral and cellular immunity, the impairment in cellular immunity is only partial, and even grafts compatible at the major human histocompatibility complex are eventually rejected, unless the patient's cellular immunity is further suppressed by sublethal doses of cyclophosphamide or total body irradiation [6,15]. Since knowledge of the proper tissues to transplant in these forms of immunodeficiency is incomplete at the present time, and since such immunosuppression creates a grave risk in these patients, it seems most inadvisable to attempt reconstitution in them at the present state of knowledge.

C. Other Genetically Determined Defects

In addition to its use in the treatment of antibody deficiency states, it is possible that humoral replacement therapy may be extended in the future to other types of genetically determined defects in protein synthesis or function, which may relate to chronic and recurrent pulmonary infection or disease. Such conditions include (a) inherited deficiencies or abnormalities in function of components of the complement system and (b) a_1-antitrypsin deficiency. Fresh plasma infusions have been employed successfully in the treatment of patients with C5 dysfunction [17] and in a patient who lacked an inhibitor of an enzyme, GBC-ase, which acts on properdin factor B (glycine–rich β-glycoprotein, or GBG) and who exhibited a resultant hypercatabolism of C3 [18]. Patients of both types are subject to recurrent severe infections, which diminish greatly following plasma therapy. Plasma infusions have also been used in the treatment of attacks of angioedema in patients with an hereditary deficiency of the inhibitor of C1 esterase. The use of such infusions in this condition is highly controversial, however, since their value to date has not been convincing, and there is the potential danger that symptoms may increase since more substrate for the uninhibited C1 esterase is provided. There are no published reports on the use of plasma infusions for persons deficient in a_1-antitrypsin. It is possible that such therapy may be precluded in immunocompetent a_1-antitrypsin deficient patients if antibodies to genetically different forms of the enzyme are induced by such infusions.

D. Risks in Subjects with Normal Immunocompetence

While undoubtedly many persons with normal humoral immunity have received injections of immune serum globulin (ISG, gamma globulin) without apparent adverse effects, several reports of putative allergic reactions following such injections have been made, and there are a number of theoretic dangers to this usually unnecessary practice. Plasma infusions and ISG injections have been shown to commonly induce antibodies to immunoglobulin alloantigens genetically different from those of the recipient [19,20]. Moreover, reactions to plasma infusions have been noted in at least two persons known to have such antibodies in their serum prior to the infusions [21,22]. In experimental animals, antiallotype antibodies have been found to suppress antibody formation in fetuses having immunoglobulins of the particular allotype [23]. From these observations it has been postulated that maternal antibodies to human fetal immunoglobulin allotypes could have a role in the production of transient immunodeficiency disease of infancy; no firm evidence for this has been forthcoming, however. Heiner [24] reported that ISG preparations derived from placentas also contain nonimmunoglobulin proteins that appear to represent placenta-specific antigens. Heterologous antisera prepared against placental ISG produced arcs on immunoelectrophoresis against placentally derived ISG that were not seen with anti-whole human serum antisera. These arcs were still produced after absorption of the antiplacental ISG antisera with normal human serum but not after absorption with minced placental tissues. It is not known whether administration of such preparations to female children or to women in the childbearing age has resulted in any of the theoretically possible adverse consequences of immunization against placental antigens. Finally, in addition to the above considerations, it is also possible that passive antibody, in the form of gamma globulin injections or plasma infusions given to normal individuals, may suppress endogenous antibody formation to antigens they have not previously encountered. There is ample evidence for this phenomenon in experimental studies in animals, and it was on this rationale that the administration of anti-Rh (D) gamma globulin preparations to Rh (D) negative women at delivery was begun to prevent the formation of antibodies to fetal red cell Rh (D) antigens. While the success of the latter form of passive immunotherapy is unquestioned, the extent to which antibodies to other antigens have been suppressed by such therapy has not been examined in man.

III. Types of Therapy

Replacement therapy for the prevention and treatment of pulmonary infections in immunodeficient patients consists of either (a) passive therapy in the form of immune serum globulin (ISG) or plasma infusions to correct deficits in humoral immunity or (b) active replacement in the form of immunocompetent tissue transplants for cellular or combined immunodeficiency disorders.

A. Passive or Humoral Immunotherapy

Immune Serum Globulin (ISG) for Intramuscular Use

This material is ordinarily prepared from outdated blood bank plasma or from placentas by the alcohol-salt fractionation method of Cohn *et al.* [25] and is supplied commercially in solutions containing 14.5 to 16.5 g/100 ml of IgG [24]. Although these preparations consist principally of IgG, they have also been shown to contain varying quantities of IgA, IgM, IgD, albumin, $\beta_1 C$, transferrin and placenta-specific proteins. The content of these latter proteins depends primarily upon whether the material is derived from plasma or placental sources and upon technical variations in their preparation [24]. Gamma globulin derived from placentas usually contains more IgA, IgM, and IgD than does that prepared from plasma [24], but the quantities of these proteins present even in the placentally derived preparations (less than 5% of the total protein for any one of the immunoglobulins A, M, or D) are probably inconsequential from a clinical standpoint in view of the very short half lives of these immunoglobulins [26]. The one exception to this statement is that patients with selective IgA deficiency may have life-threatening anaphylactic reactions to the small amount of IgA present in ISG preparations [12]. Gamma globulin prepared by the alcohol-salt fractionation method has been found to be remarkably stable, showing little change in concentrations of gamma migrating protein or clinical effectiveness when stored at $4°C$ for as long as 4 yr [27]. Such preparations have been shown to aggregate and fragment, however, as well as to demonstrate anticomplementary activity to varying degrees upon storage. These changes occur more often in preparations from which ethanol is not completely removed by dialysis and in those contaminated to a greater degree by endogenous plasmin [27]. This anticomplementary activity is due to the formation of aggregates that have the ability to activate the complement system [28]; it is to this property that clinical reactions to gamma globulin injections have often been attributed [29]. The half life of IgG in such preparations has been shown to vary from 17.5 to 22.1 days, with a mean of 19.8 days in normal subjects [30]. It is likely to be even longer in agammaglobulinemic patients, since the mean half life of IgG given in plasma or isolated from it by ion-exchange chromatography was shown to be 32 days in five such patients studied by Stiehm and Fudenberg [20]. The half life is also likely to be affected by the clinical state of the patient, since other studies also showed a shortened survival for IgG in these patients during episodes of infection [20].

The recommended dose of ISG for the treatment of primary humoral immunodeficiency is 0.1 g/kg-month (0.6 to 0.7 ml/kg-month) after a loading dose of two to three times that amount. These doses, of necessity, require the administration of large volumes by the intramuscular route, resulting in great discomfort to the recipient. It is generally considered inadvisable to give more than 20 to 30 ml at a time, or 40 ml per month, and no more than 5 ml per injection site because of this and other reasons discussed below. Many physicians who treat older patients with severe humoral deficiency recommend giving 10 ml of ISG per week to avoid giving too large a dose at any one time. The preferred injection sites are the buttocks, but the anterior thighs and deltoids may also be used. It is well to point out that the dose recommended above has been arrived at empirically from arbitrary clinical trials [5,31] but that, in practice, it has seemed to be nearly as effective as twice that amount [5]. Since half the above recommended dose was ineffective in one large study [5], and since there is considerable variability in immunoglobulin and antibody content from lot to lot of commercially available preparations, further investigation of optimal dosage is needed. Furthermore, there would appear to be a need for establishing routine objective parameters for use in following the efficacy of therapy in such patients in addition to the subjective evaluations of clinical effectiveness.

As mentioned above, there are several theoretically possible adverse effects from the administration of homologous antibody globulins. In addition, there are well-documented adverse reactions to ISG because of problems unique to its fractionation and administration. The repeated large volumes administered intramuscularly to patients with immunodeficiency not only cause a great deal of pain but are a source of considerable psychologic difficulty in some children with these defects. Adverse local reactions that have been encountered include sterile abscesses, fibrosis, and sciatic or other nerve injuries. Infrequent, but sometimes serious, systemic reactions were also reported by the British Medical Research Council Working Party on Hypogammaglobulinemia to have affected 32 of 175 (18%) patients treated over an 11-yr period with ISG, and one death occurred [5]. It became necessary to discontinue therapy in five of these patients, in part, because of such reactions. As noted above, systemic reactions in agammaglobulinemic patients are believed to be due to entry of aggregated immunoglobulin molecules into the intravascular compartment during administration of large intramuscular volumes. This is thought to result in activation of the complement system and generation of anaphylotoxin and other vasoactive substances [29]. In one agammaglobulinemic patient, however, the reaction was thought to be due to an antibody to aggregated gamma globulin in the recipient's serum, which could be demonstrated by agar gel diffusion [32]. Systemic reactions to ISG injections have also been noted in patients with selective IgA deficiency who have antibodies to IgA [12]. Symptoms of such reactions may appear from seconds to minutes to several hours after the injections and include flushing and facial swelling, dyspnea, cyanosis, anxiety, nausea, vomiting, malaise, hypotension, and even loss of consciousness. The treatment should be the immediate administration of epinephrine and antihistamines. In the Medical Research Council Working Party on Hypogammaglobulinemia study, it was noted that agammaglobulinemic boys with affected male relatives were significantly spared from systemic reactions and that the frequency of such reactions did not appear to correlate with the degree of anticomplementary activity of the batches of gamma globulin employed [5]. Indeed, the distribution of reactions among the 40 different batches used was random. These observations led members of the Working Party to suggest that the mechanism of the reaction may be related to the underlying disease of the recipient. It was also noted that such reactions could start at any stage of treatment and that the incidence did not change with length of therapy, arguing against a mechanism involving some form of immunization. In any case, until more is known about their nature, patients with a history of such reactions should be given a small test dose of ISG from a different supplier before such therapy is resumed. The test dose should be given in an extremity so that a tourniquet may be applied in the event of any sign of an adverse reaction. Skin testing with ISG preparations was found to be of no help in guiding the course of future therapy in such patients [5,33].

Intravenous Gamma Globulin Preparations

These ISG preparations have all been treated in some way to render them aggregate-free and to eliminate anticomplementary activity. While several have undergone testing or are being tested in carefully supervised clinical trials, they are not available commercially, since none has been licensed for general use in the United States. There are several advantages to the administration of ISG by the intravenous route: (a) much larger doses can be given than would be possible by the intramuscular route, (b) the action is more rapid, (c) there is no loss due to local proteolysis, and (d) the therapy is far less painful. Unfortunately, reactions to intravenous infusions of unmodified ISG are more frequent and more severe in patients who stand to benefit most from them—e.g., patients with antibody deficiency—than in normal individuals, for reasons that are poorly understood [33]. The symptoms and signs of such reactions are similar to those that occur with intramuscular ISG injections but may also include chills, fever, pallor, and fatigue beginning 1 to 2 hr after the infusion. There has been considerable interest for over a decade now in the development of ISG preparations that would be safe for intravenous use, and several approaches have been tried [33]. These include

(a) physical removal of high molecular-weight aggregates by ultracentrifugation or gel filtration, (b) treatment of the preparations with proteolytic enzymes, (c) treatment with certain chemicals that affect specific sites on the gamma globulin molecule or with sulfhydryl bond reducing agents, and (d) incubation of these preparations at a low pH for varying periods of time. Successful removal of aggregates by ultracentrifugation requires an extremely high centrifugal force and does not appear to be practical for the large-scale production of ISG for intravenous use. Treatment of such preparations with proteolytic enzymes, such as trypsin, pepsin, or plasmin, eliminates anticomplementary activity quite effectively and renders them safe for intravenous use [30,34,35]. Unfortunately, however, immunoglobulin molecules subjected to enzymatic treatment fragment into low molecular-weight subunits that are more rapidly cleared from the circulation than is the intact molecule, thereby compromising the duration of passive immunity rendered. Plasmin-treated gamma globulin preparations appear to be far superior to those treated with other proteolytic enzymes, since a considerable proportion of the plasmin-treated material retains a sedimentation coefficient of 6.5 S and a half life of 18 days, both just slightly less than those of intact IgG [30]. Most promising, however, are preparations that have been rendered free of anticomplementary activity by treatment with sulfhydryl bond reducing agents followed by alkylation with iodoacetamide. The immunoglobulins in these preparations reportedly retain the sedimentation characteristics and antibody potency of those in the untreated material and no low molecular-weight fragments are generated. Apparently the IgG molecules remain held together by noncovalent bonds; it is not clear why anticomplementary activity is lost by this treatment. Some of these preparations are currently undergoing initial clinical trials, and the doses being given are roughly those recommended for the intramuscular preparations.

Plasma Infusions

There are several obvious advantages to the use of plasma infusions in the treatment of severe humoral immunodeficiencies: (a) antibodies of all five immunoglobulin classes can be provided in significant quantities, (b) such intravenous infusions are far less painful than intramuscular ISG injections and thus have greater patient acceptability, (c) adverse reactions are few, and (d) higher serum immunoglobulin concentrations can be effected than with intramuscular ISG injections. In addition, the donor can be immunized to provide higher titers of some antibodies than can be achieved with pooled gamma globulin. The disadvantages include: (a) the potential danger of transmitting homologous serum hepatitis, (b) the risk of graft-versus-host (GVH) disease in infants with severe combined immunodeficiency disease from residual immunocompetent cells contained in most plasma preparations, and (c) the inconvenience or impracticality of performing plasmaphereses on a regular basis in some clinical settings. The risk of homologous hepatitis can be greatly reduced by careful donor selection, using guidelines described below. The danger of GVH can be avoided either by carefully removing all cellular elements, by irradiating the plasma sufficiently to destroy the GVH potential of the immunocompetent cells, or both. Finally, enlisting the aid of regional blood banks in conducting donor plasmaphereses helps to reduce the impracticality of this form of therapy.

We first became impressed with the potential usefulness of plasma infusions for the treatment of immunodeficiency while using them as a sustaining measure in infants with severe combined immunodeficiency who were awaiting transplantation [7]. For use in those patients, we either removed all cellular elements from the plasmas by high–speed centrifugation or irradiated them with 3000 rads prior to their administration. Graft versus host reactions did not occur in any of the patients as a consequence of the infusion of plasma so treated, and we found that we achieved nearly adult levels of each of the three major immunoglobulins and normal antibody titers to a number of antigens. Following our experience in those patients, we became interested in the use of plasma therapy in patients whose defects involved mainly the humoral limb of the immunologic system. Stimulating this interest was the fact that several patients with infantile X-linked agammaglobulinemia, whom we were following, required chronic antibiotic therapy, in addition to injections of gamma globulin at doses of 100 mg/kg every 3 wk, in order to remain free of overt lower respiratory infection. A review of the literature on the use of plasma therapy in immunodeficiency revealed that it had been employed on only a very limited basis, the experience of Stiehm et al. [14] being the most extensive. Because of the potential advantages of this form of replacement, however, we began, 5½ yr ago, to evaluate periodic plasma infusions in the treatment of immunodeficiency and have used them to treat 15 patients with severe humoral immunodeficiency followed at this institution during this period. The group includes 4 patients with infantile X-linked agammaglobulinemia, 7 with B-lymphocyte agammaglobulinemia, 2 with unclassified agammaglobulinemia, and 2 with X-linked immunodeficiency with hyper-IgM. All plasma donors have been carefully screened for a history of hepatitis and by testing their sera for hepatitis-B antigen by counterelectrophoresis and, more recently, by radioimmunoassay. In most cases a "buddy" system is used whereby the same donor, usually a parent, is used repeatedly. This minimizes the risk of hepatitis since once a donor is established as being safe, the danger of his transmitting hepatitis in the future is negligible. For 2 patients, their husbands serve as donors and for 1, a brother. One patient has no relatives suitable for periodic plasma donations and he is currently receiving plasma from a group of professional blood donors whose blood has been used repeatedly for other recipients in whom there has been no subsequent development of homologous hepatitis. In most instances, the donors are of the same ABO and Rh blood types as the recipient but, in 2 cases, there are minor mismatches, e.g., the donor plasmas contain antibodies in low titer against recipient red cell antigens. In these cases, appropriate soluble blood group substances are added to the plasmas to neutralize the antibodies prior to infusion into the patients. The dose of plasma employed varies according to the donor's serum IgG concentration but is usually selected to provide the recipient with 100 mg/kg IgG every 3 wk and, in most cases, is approximately 10 ml/kg. As with ISG therapy, the dose for the first treatment is usually twice that amount. The results of serum immunoglobulin measurements 3 wk after plasma infusions in the first four patients begun on this form of therapy are presented in Table 1 and compared with results of similar measurements in six other agammaglobulinemic patients 3 wk after they had received 0.6 ml/kg of ISG intramuscularly [7]. Serum IgG concentrations averaged 113 mg/100 ml higher in the plasma-treated group than in the gamma globulin-treated group and low, but higher, than baseline concentrations of IgA and IgM could be detected after 3 wk in the plasma-treated but not in the ISG-treated patients. In addition, as shown in Table 2, only one gamma globulin-treated patient had detectable anti-B antibodies, none had antibodies to A cells or diphtheria toxoid, and all had low to absent antitetanus antibody titers. All plasma-treated patients, on the other hand, had normal antibody titers to tetanus toxoid and low titers to diphtheria toxoid. One Type O recipient of Type O plasma had near normal isohemagglutinin titers. One possible reason for the lower antibody titers in the group treated with gamma globulin is the fact that samples of three different commercial sources of ISG showed marked variability in their content of antitetanus antibody and each had very low titers of antidiphtheria antibody (Table 2). Another possible cause of both the lower immunoglobulin concentrations and lower antibody titers in the ISG treated patients 3 wk post-treatment is that denaturation of gamma globulin takes place during the alcohol-salt fractionation procedure and more rapid catabolism of this preparation is caused by proteolysis by local tissue enzymes in the intramuscular injection sites.

The results of our experience with plasma therapy in the other 11 patients are in keeping with those described above for the first 4, except that we are unable to maintain serum immunoglobulin concentrations of that magnitude in our larger teen-age and adult patients because it is difficult to obtain the volumes of plasma required to achieve the dosage given above. In addition, we observed evidence of more rapid catabolism of the infused immunoglobulins in 2 patients who experienced acute episodes of infection. In general, however, the clinical status of each of these patients has improved considerably since plasma therapy was initiated. Only 1 experienced a serious infection, and this was

TABLE 1 Comparison of Serum Immunoglobulin Concentrations in Patients with Deficits in Humoral Immunity 3 Wk after Plasma Infusions or Gamma Globulin Injections

Patient	Treatment status	IgG[a]	IgA[a]	IgM[a]
1	Pre–plasma	125	0	0
	Post–plasma[b]	256	9	4
2	Pre–plasma	50	0	0
	Post–plasma[b]	262	9	4
3	Pre–plasma	56	13	11
	Post–plasma[c]	249	18	15
4	Pre–plasma	205	5	6
	Post–plasma[d]	231	7	5
5	Pre–gamma globulin	125	0	0
	Post–gamma globulin	148	0	0
6	Pre–gamma globulin	65	0	15
	Post–gamma globulin	155	0	9
7	Pre–gamma globulin	47	0	9
	Post–gamma globulin	103	0	9
8	Pre–gamma globulin	130	0	0
	Post–gamma globulin	170	0	0
9	Pre–gamma globulin	25	0	11
	Post–gamma globulin	145	0	18
10	Pre–gamma globulin	60	0	0
	Post–gamma globulin	102	0	0

[a] Concentrations expressed in mg/100 ml.
[b] Average values from twenty–three 3–wk post–treatment sera.
[c] Average values from five 3–wk post–treatment sera.
[d] Average values from two 3–wk post–treatment sera.

TABLE 2 Comparison of Antibody Titers[a] in Immunodeficiency Patients 3 Wk after Treatment with Plasma or Gamma Globulin

Patient	Treatment status	Blood type	Anti–A	Anti–B	Tetanus	Diphtheria
1[c]	Donor	A+	0	256	5×10^5	81
	Pre–plasma	O+	0	0	243	0
	Post–plasma	-	0	0[b]	2×10^4	81
2[c]	Donor	A+	0	256	5×10^5	81
	Pre–plasma	AB+	0	0[b]	0	0
	Post–plasma	-	0	0[b]	2×10^4	27
3[d]	Donor	O+	256	256	12.9×10^7	0
	Pre–plasma	O+	0	0	0	0
	Post–plasma	-	16	4	4.3×10^7	0
Commercial globulin	Co.A	-	0	0	1.6×10^6	81
	Co.B	-	0	0	6×10^4	9
	Co.C	-	0	0	3.5×10^9	243
4[c]	3 wk–Post–gamma globulin	-	0	0	243	0
5[c]	3 wk–Post–gamma globulin	-	0	0	81	0
6[c]	3 wk–Post–gamma globulin	-	0	0	243	0
7[c]	3 wk–Post–gamma globulin	-	0	4	0	0
8[c]	3 wk–Post–gamma globulin	-	0	0	243	0

[a]Expressed as reciprocal of highest dilution giving positive reaction.
[b]A and B blood group substances added to donor plasma before infusions.
[c]Infantile X-linked agammaglobulinemia.
[d]Acquired hypogammaglobulinemia.

meningitis due to an enterovirus. That patient subsequently recovered, without sequelae. A number of patients formerly requiring chronic antibiotic therapy in addition to ISG have been able to discontinue it and the frequency of required courses of antibiotics has been reduced in all.

In contrast to our initial experience in which there were no adverse effects from plasma therapy in any of the patients during the first 2½ yr of evaluation, we subsequently encountered adverse reactions in 3 patients, 1 of whom is not included in the above group of 15 since therapy could not be started because of the adverse effect. In keeping with the observation by the British Medical Council Working Party on Hypogammaglobulinemia that boys with affected lateral male relatives were significantly spared from adverse reactions to ISG [5], there were no reactions in any of our patients with infantile X–linked agammaglobulinemia. Each of the 3 patients in whom untoward reactions were observed had normal percentages of peripheral blood B lymphocytes bearing surface immunoglobulins of all three major classes and were diagnosed as having B–lymphocyte agamma-globulinemia. In 1 patient, the reaction occurred only when he received plasma from his mother and not when he received it from his brothers. The reaction began approximately 1 hr after the infusion was started, after he had received one full unit of plasma, and was characterized by chills, fever, and a drop in his peripheral blood leukocyte count. The mother's plasma was later found to contain cytotoxic antibodies to HL–A antigens present on the patient's leukocytes. In another patient with B–lymphocyte agammaglobulinemia, a reaction characterized by chills, but no fever or chest oppression, began 1 to 2 hr after the infusion began on two occasions, followed by prolonged lethargy. Although the etiologies of those reactions remain undefined, the possibility exists that they could have been due to the minor red cell antigen mismatch between donor and recipient. Against that, however, are the facts that there was no sign of a hemolytic transfusion reaction, direct Coombs tests were negative following both, and the patient received plasma from the same donor on other occasions with no untoward effects. This patient is now receiving plasma from a pool of professional donors matched for the same blood type, without adverse effects.

The third patient's reaction was very different from the aforementioned. This occurred in a girl who had a serum IgG concentration of 280 mg/100 ml, no detectable IgA by single radial diffusion, an IgM concentration of 14 mg/100 ml, and impaired antibody formation to a number of antigens. Since she had normal percentages of immunoglobulin–bearing B lymphocytes, her findings were considered to be most consistent with a diagnosis of B–lymphocyte hypogamma-globulinemia. She has no history of ever having received blood transfusions or ISG. Within seconds after an ABO and Rh–compatible paternal plasma infusion the patient experienced a sensation of tightness of the skin of her face, intense dyspnea, moderate cyanosis, vomiting, defecation, mild hypertension, and subsequent somnolence. The plasma was discontinued immediately; only a total of 15 ml was given. There were no changes in her vital signs other than the transient blood pressure rise, and she did not require treatment with emergency medications. All signs of the reaction subsided within 1 hr except for the somnolence, which lasted several hours. There was no evidence of a hemolytic transfusion reaction, and a direct Coombs test shortly after the reaction was negative. Her serum β_1 C concentration, in a sample collected 15 min following the reaction, was slightly higher than that in a sample obtained immediately before the infusion began. Subsequent analysis of the patient's pretreatment serum in the laboratory of Dr. H. H. Fudenberg revealed that it contained a titer greater than 1:1024 of anti–IgA antibodies, as detected by the chromic chloride passive hemagglutination method. Moreover, the antibodies reacted with all of several different IgA myeloma protein coats, indicating that they did not have isospecificity. The reaction experienced by this patient is similar to the anaphylactic transfusion reactions reported in patients with selective IgA deficiency who had anti–IgA antibodies [12,13]. The unusual feature of this patient, however, is that although she had no detectable serum IgA, she did not have normal or elevated concentrations of IgG and IgM, as is usually seen in patients with selective IgA deficiency. This experience indicates that anti–IgA antibodies may exist in patients other than those with typical selective IgA deficiency. We feel that it is imperative that this possibility be investigated before replacement therapy is started in other patients with absent serum IgA who have significant quantities of immunoglobulins of the other two major classes, even though the concentrations may be abnormally low.

B. Active or Cellular Immunotherapy

Bone Marrow Transplantation

As noted in the early part of this chapter, bone marrow transplantation has been employed successfully in the immunologic reconstitution of a number of infants with severe combined immunodeficiency disease. In all instances where success was achieved, the donor and recipient were shown to be histocompatible in mixed leukocyte culture but not necessarily for the serologically defined HL-A antigens [36,37]. The donor, in most cases, was a histocompatible sibling, but in a few instances was another relative who, because of consanguinity or recombinational events within the major histocompatibility complex, was compatible with the patient at the MLR locus [36-38]. All incompatible marrow grafts given infants with severe combined immunodeficiency disease either led to fatal GVH reaction or were unsuccessful because the infant died of complications of the primary disease without evidence of adequate immunologic reconstitution [15]. Bone marrow transplantation has been attempted in 3 patients with infantile X-linked agammaglobulinemia, in 1 with the Wiskott-Aldrich syndrome, and in 1 with ataxia telangiectasia [15]. Only in the case of the Wiskott-Aldrich patient was chimerism achieved; immunologic improvement was not seen except for minimal changes in the patient with Wiskott-Aldrich syndrome and in the one with ataxia telangiectasia.

Fetal Thymus and Liver Transplants

Fetal thymus transplants have been used in the treatment of patients with the Di George syndrome, as mentioned earlier, and immunologic improvement occurred [6,15]. The mechanism of the improvement is unclear, however. Fetal thymus transplants into infants with severe combined immunodeficiency disease have been unsuccessful in all but a few cases in which partial immunologic reconstitution was achieved [39]. Interest in the use of fetal tissues to correct the defect in infants with severe combined immunodeficiency who have no histocompatible donors has been rekindled by the latter report as well as by the recent success in reconstituting three of these infants with an infusion of fetal liver cells [40,41].

Transfer Factor

The potential usefulness of transfer factor therapy for cellular immunodeficiency is discussed elsewhere in this section (see Chapter 24).

References

1. H. Y. Reynolds and R. E. Thompson, Pulmonary host defenses. I. Analysis of protein and lipids in bronchial secretions and antibody responses after vaccination with Pseudomonas aeruginosa, *J. Immunol.,* **111**:358–368 (1973).
2. H. Y. Reynolds and R. E. Thompson, Pulmonary host defenses. II. Interaction of respiratory antibodies with Pseudomonas aeruginosa and alveolar macrophages, *J. Immunol.,* **111**:369–380 (1973).
3. O. C. Bruton, Agammaglobulinemia, *Pediatrics,* **9**:722–727 (1952).
4. M. E. Miller, Uses and abuses of gammaglobulin, *Hosp. Pract.,* **4**:38–43 (1969).
5. Medical Research Council Working Party on Hypogammaglobulinemia, Hypogammaglobulinemia in the United Kingdom, *Medical Research Council Special Report Series,* No. 310, 1971, pp. 1–319.
6. R. H. Buckley, Reconstitution: Grafting of bone marrow and thymus. In *Progress in Immunology.* Edited by D. B. Amos. New York and London, Academic Press, Inc., 1971, pp. 1061–1080.

7. R. H. Buckley, Plasma therapy in immunodeficiency diseases, *Am. J. Dis. Child.,* **124**:376–381 (1972).

8. H. H. Fudenberg, R. A. Good, H. C. Goodman, W. Hitzig, H. G. Kunkel, I. M. Roitt, F. S. Rosen, D. S. Rowe, M. Seligmann, and J. R. Soothill, Primary immunodeficiencies: Report of a World Health Organization committee, *Pediatrics,* **47**:927–946 (1971).

9. M. D. Cooper, W. P. Faulk, H. H. Fudenberg, R. A. Good, W. Hitzig, H. G. Kunkel, F. S. Rosen, M. Seligmann, J. F. Soothill, and R. J. Wedgwood, Classification of primary immunodeficiencies, *N. Engl. J. Med.,* **288**:966–967 (1973).

10. R. H. Buckley, Clinical and immunologic features of selective IgA deficiency. In *Immunodeficiency Diseases in Man and Animals.* Edited by D. Bergsma, R. A. Good, J. Finsted, and N. W. Paul. Stanford, Conn., Sinauer Associates, Inc., 1975, pp. 134–141.

11. G. N. Vyas, A. S. Levin, and H. H. Fudenberg, Intrauterine isoimmunization caused by maternal IgA crossing the placenta, *Nature,* **225**:275–276 (1970).

12. G. N. Vyas, H. A. Perkins, and H. H. Fudenberg, Anaphylactoid transfusion reactions associated with anti–IgA, *Lancet,* **2**:3–12 (1968).

13. A. P. Schmidt, H. F. Taswell, and G. J. Gleich, Anaphylactic transfusion reactions associated with anti–IgA antibody, *N. Engl. J. Med.,* **280**:188–193 (1969).

14. E. R. Stiehm, J.-P. Vaerman, and H. H. Fudenberg, Plasma infusions in immunologic deficiency states: Metabolic and therapeutic studies, *Blood,* **28**:918–937 (1966).

15. R. H. Buckley, Transplantation. In *Immunologic Disorders in Infants and Children.* Edited by E. R. Stiehm and V. A. Fulginiti. Philadelphia, W. B. Saunders Co., 1973, pp. 591–623.

16. R. W. Steele, C. Limas, G. B. Thurman, M. Scheulein, H. Bauer, and J. A. Bellanti, Familial thymic aplasia. Attempted reconstitution with fetal thymus in a Millipore diffusion chamber, *N. Engl. J. Med.,* **287**:787–791 (1972).

17. J. C. Jacobs and M. E. Miller, Fatal familial Leiner's disease: A deficiency of the opsonic activity of serum complement, *Pediatrics,* **49**:225–232 (1972).

18. C. A. Alper, N. Abramson, R. B. Johnston, Jr., J. H. Jandl, and F. S. Rosen, Increased susceptibility to infection associated with abnormalities of complement–mediated functions and of the third component of complement (C3), *N. Engl. J. Med.,* **282**:349–354 (1970).

19. J. C. Allen and H. G. Kunkel, Antibodies against γ–globulin after repeated blood transfusions in man, *J. Clin. Invest.,* **45**:29–39 (1969).

20. E. R. Stiehm and H. H. Fudenberg, Antibodies to gamma–globulin in infants and children exposed to isologous gamma–globulin, *Pediatrics,* **35**:229–235 (1965).

21. H. H. Fudenberg and B. R. Fudenberg, Antibody to hereditary gamma-globulin (Gm) factor resulting from maternal–fetal incompatibility, *Science,* **145**:170–171 (1964).

22. K. Fischer, Immunohämatologische und klinische Befunde bei einem trans-
     fusionszwrischenfall infolge Gm(a)–antikorperbildung, *Bibl. Haematol.*,
     23:434–440 (1965).
23. L. A. Herzenberg, L. A. Herzenberg, R. C. Goodlin, and E. C. Rivera,
     Immunoglobulin synthesis in mice. Suppression by anti–allotype antibody,
     J. Exp. Med., **126**:701–713 (1967).
24. D. C. Heiner and L. Evans, Immunoglobulins and other proteins in com-
     mercial preparations of gamma globulin, *J. Pediatr.*, **70**:820–827 (1967).
25. E. S. Cohn, F. R. N. Gard, D. M. Surgenor, B. D. Barnes, R. K. Brown,
     G. Derouaux, J. M. Gillespie, F. W. Kahnt, W. F. Lener, C. H. Liu, D. Mittel-
     man, R. F. Mouton, K. Schmid, and E. Uroma, A system for the separation
     of the components of human blood: Quantitative procedures for the sepa-
     ration of the protein components of human plasma, *J. Am. Chem. Soc.*,
     72:465–474 (1950).
26. T. A. Waldmann and W. Strober, Metabolism of immunoglobulins, *Prog.
     Allergy*, **13**:1–110 (1969).
27. M. MacKay, L. Vallet, and B. S. Cambridge, The characterization and
     stability during storage of human immunoglobulin prepared for clinical use,
     Vox Sang., **25**:124–140 (1973).
28. C. L. Christian, Studies of aggregated γ–globulin. I. Sedimentation, electro-
     phoretic, and anticomplementary properties, *J. Immunol.*, **84**:112–121
     (1960).
29. H. B. Richerson and P. M. Seebohm, Anaphylactoid reaction to human
     gamma globulin, *Arch. Intern. Med.*, **117**:568–572 (1966).
30. C. A. Janeway, E. Merler, F. S. Rosen, S. Salmon, and J. D. Crain, Intra-
     venous gamma globulin. Metabolism of gamma globulin fragments in
     normal and agammaglobulinemic persons, *N. Engl. J. Med.*, **278**:919–923
     (1968).
31. C. A. Janeway, F. S. Rosen, E. Merler, and C. A. Alper. *The Gamma
     Globulins.* Boston, Little, Brown, 1967.
32. E. F. Ellis and C. S. Henney, Adverse reactions following administration
     of human gamma globulin, *J. Allergy*, **43**:45–54 (1969).
33. S. Barandun, P. Kistler, F. Jeunet, and H. Isliker, Intravenous administra-
     tion of human γ–globulin, *Vox Sang.*, **7**:157–174 (1962).
34. B. V. Jager, Intravenous administration of modified gamma globulin, *Arch.
     Intern. Med.*, **119**:60–64 (1967).
35. M. J. Simons, M. J. Schumacher, and R. Fowler, Intravenous gamma
     globulin therapy of immunoglobulin deficiency diseases, *Aust. Paediatr. J.*
     4:127–133 (1968).
36. R. A. Gatti, H. J. Meuwissen, H. D. Allen, R. Hong, and R. A. Good,
     Immunological reconstitution of sex–linked lymphopenic immunological
     deficiency, *Lancet*, **2**:1366–1369 (1968).
37. B. Dupont, V. Andersen, V. Faber, R. A. Good, K. Henriksen, F. Juhl,
     C. Koch, N. M. Berat, B. Park, A. Svegaard, and A. Wiik, Immunological

reconstitution in severe combined immunodeficiency with HL–A incompatible bone marrow graft. Donor selection by mixed lymphocyte culture, *Transplant, Proc.,* 5:905–908 (1973).

38. J. M. Vossen, J. de Koning, D. W. Van Bekkum, K. A. Dicke, V. P. Eijsvoogel, W. Hijmans, E. Van Loghem, J. Radl, J. J. Van Rood, D. Van der Waaij, and L. J. Dooren, Successful treatment of an infant with severe combined immunodeficiency by transplantation of bone marrow cells from an uncle, *Clin. Exp. Immunol.,* 13:9–20 (1973).

39. A. J. Ammann, D. W. Wara, S. Salmon, and H. Perkins, Thymus transplantation. Permanent reconstitution of cellular immunity in a patient with sex–linked combined immunodeficiency, *N. Engl. J. Med.,* 289:5–9 (1973).

40. R. Keightley, A. R. Lawton, L. Y. F. Wu, E. J. Yunis, and M. D. Cooper, Lymphoid differentiation of allogeneic fetal liver cells in a child with severe combined immunodeficiency (SCID), *Clin. Res.,* 22:86 (1974) (abstr.).

41. R. H. Buckley and W. Hitzig, unpublished data.

17

Kinetics of Penetration and Clearance of Antibiotics in Respiratory Secretions

JAMES E. PENNINGTON

National Institute of Allergy and Infectious Diseases
National Institutes of Health
Bethesda, Maryland

I. Introduction

The use of antimicrobial agents in the treatment of bacterial pulmonary infections has not been uniformly successful. The spectrum of pulmonary infectious diseases includes certain pathologic conditions notably resistant to antibiotic therapy. Chronic bronchitis, bronchiectasis, certain forms of pulmonary abscess, and cystic fibrosis with bronchitis, are extremely difficult conditions to treat; despite long and intensive antibiotic treatment, pathogenic bacteria often persist. In contrast, acute bronchopneumonia and lobar pneumonia caused by penicillin sensitive, gram-positive organisms, are often quite amenable to antibiotic treatment in the patient with otherwise normal host–defense mechanisms.

Factors that determine success or failure in treating pulmonary bacterial infection include the immune state of the host and the virulence of the infecting organism, including the sensitivity of the organism to available antibiotics. One of the most important factors is the ability to achieve at the site of infection concentrations of appropriate antibiotic agents that will exceed the minimal inhibitory concentration of the infecting organism. Except for highly protein bound drugs, serum antibiotic concentrations may be used as a guide to the concentrations achieved in interstitial spaces [1-3]. However, in chronic bronchitis,

pulmonary abscess, and bronchiectasis, the ability of antibiotic agents to penetrate areas of purulence, stasis, fibrosis, and anatomic destruction may be far less
than the ability of these agents to reach interstitial and alveolar pulmonary infections. Therefore, an adequate concentration of antibiotics in blood does not
assure an adequate concentration of antibiotic in the bronchial lumen [4].

This chapter will examine the factors critical for antibiotic penetration
into, and clearance from, bronchial secretions. This will be followed by a discussion of clinical and animal studies, which address the problem of achieving adequate intrabronchial antibiotic concentrations. Finally, alternative means of
achieving therapeutic antibiotic levels in bronchial secretions will be discussed.

II. Pharmacokinetics of Antibiotics in Bronchial Secretions

The pharmacologic concept of drug penetration across biologic membrane barriers is well-documented [2]. In some instances, such as with basement membranes and most capillary endothial cells, free drug passage is the rule [2]. However, in passing from blood to bronchial lumen, an antibiotic must pass through
a complex series of plasma–cellular membranes, intralumenal mucus, bacterial
debris, and various other protein accumulations. This series of organic barriers
is known as the blood–bronchus barrier. Once the antibiotic reaches the bronchial compartment, the rate at which it accumulates and clears will determine
the net effective concentration achieved for the degree of penetration.

A. Penetration

Two major factors influence the penetration of an antibiotic from blood to bronchus. These are, permeability of and the mode of transport across bronchial tissues, which might be passive diffusion or active transport.

Tissue permeability to antibiotics depends upon drug and host factors.
Drug factors include molecular size and structure [5-7]. Antibiotics of large
molecular weight have been shown to enter bronchial secretions more readily
than do those of smaller molecular weight in most instances [6,7]. Antibiotics
that contain benzene rings (erythromycin) penetrate bronchial secretions well
[6], whereas those derived from sugars (aminoglycosides) penetrate with more
difficulty, probably due to their hydrophilic nature [5,6]. Relative lipid solubil-
ity of the antibiotic is another important factor in tissue penetration [2,5,8,9].
In general, lipophilic molecules diffuse across membranes more easily; however,
some exceptions to this may occur for antibiotics [5,6]. Antibiotics in ionized

form are relatively lipid insoluble; therefore, the pKa of an antibiotic in relation to the pH of bronchial tissues and fluids (usually in the pH range 6-8 [10,11]) is also of concern [2,5].

The degree of antibiotic binding to serum and tissue proteins has been shown to influence their diffusability across membranes and to affect their antibacterial activity [1,9,12-14], with unbound, free drug being the active antimicrobial fraction. Therefore, such highly protein-bound antibiotics as cloxacillin and oxacillin are less able to pass from blood into the interstitial spaces. Intravascular protein-bound antibiotic acts as a reservoir in supplying free drug to replace that which diffuses to extravascular spaces [15]. Once the antibiotic reaches bronchial secretions, most of it will be in a free, unbound state, since protein concentrations in bronchial secretions are much lower than in serum [11,16]. Mucus binding and penetration through mucus has been studied in vitro, and the capability of antibiotics to penetrate respiratory tract mucus may be another important variable in achieving adequate intrabronchial antibiotic concentrations at the site of infection [6].

Host factors also seem to be an important determinant for tissue permeability to antibiotics. The integrity of the blood–bronchus barrier may be damaged by such factors as bronchial inflammation or bronchial injuries, causing anatomic alterations in tissue barriers. In states of bronchitis and bronchial pneumonia, the increased local inflammation may enhance permeability to antibiotic molecules. In this pathologic state, both free and protein-bound antibiotics might gain access to bronchial secretions by leakage across inflamed tissues. When inflammation subsides, coincident with improvement of the clinical status of the patient, bronchial penetration of antibiotics might then be much more difficult. Also, anatomic damage to bronchial walls from excessive coughing, bronchoscopy, or other causes, can induce intrabronchial bleeding. This in turn may allow blood-borne antibiotics to pass freely into the bronchus. Direct evidence of this phenomenon has been found for gentamicin [17]; blood-tinged bronchial secretions obtained by bronchoscopy contained higher concentrations of antibiotic than did specimens that were free of blood.

Besides the permeability of bronchial tissues to antibiotics, the mode of drug transport from blood to bronchial lumen influences the net penetration. Passive (free) diffusion of antibiotic from the blood in capillaries of the bronchial wall to the bronchial lumen may be the sole means of transport [2]. Higher serum concentrations of antibiotic would be expected to create larger concentration gradients from blood to bronchus and, therefore, lead to higher concentrations in sputum [15]. Over the short distances involved in normal tissues, passive diffusion could provide an efficient means of antibiotic transport. However, in pathologic states, such as pulmonary abscess and bronchiectasis, the antibiotic must diffuse across distances of several millimeters or more. This has been shown to be a highly inefficient process [1].

An active transport mechanism might also account for antibiotic transport across the blood–bronchus barrier [2]. This energy–consuming process could allow the drug to pass against concentration gradients [5]. However, a maximum capacity for the active transport of the drug must exist. Thus, serum antibiotic concentrations above a certain critical level would be ineffective in causing further elevations in bronchial concentrations of antibiotic. Antibiotic transport could occur by a combination of passive diffusion assisted by an active process, thus a selectivity of transport mechanisms for various drugs might exist.

B. Accumulation and Clearance

After an antibiotic has penetrated the blood–bronchus barrier, it may accumulate in bronchial secretions. Accumulation of antibiotics in extravascular spaces has been demonstrated [3]. Patients with chronic bronchitis seem especially prone to slow clearance of intrabronchial antibiotics [18]. If antibiotics are collected in pooled intrabronchial secretions, the net local concentration might rise, if selective absorption or evaporation of water occurs. In some situations, local intrabronchial antibiotic might persist for periods of time after the antibiotic has been cleared from serum. Thus, in certain situations, bronchial antibiotic concentrations could exceed serum concentrations.

Clearance of antibiotics from the bronchial lumen may occur by reabsorption across the blood–bronchus barrier. This would be maximal as serum concentrations drop below those in the bronchus and could be minimized if serum antibiotic levels are kept consistently higher than the bronchial concentration. Respiratory cleansing mechanisms, such as mucociliary movement and cough, undoubtedly are important in clearing antibiotics from the respiratory tract. Finally, intrabronchial metabolism and degradation of antibiotic molecules could occur. Penicillinase producing bacterial organisms have been shown to cause ampicillin inactivation in bronchial secretions [19].

III. Clinical Studies

Clinical studies have shown that sterilization of sputum is critical to the effective treatment of pulmonary infections [4,10,20,21]. In many forms of bacterial infection, the concentration of antibiotic in serum is used to guide effective therapy. However, in planning the most efficacious regimen of antibiotic therapy for pulmonary infections, antibiotic concentrations in infected human sputum and bronchial secretions seem more relevant [4,10,20]. Although antibiotic concentrations in sputum may not be equivalent to local tissue levels at the site of infection, the correlation seems closer than that between serum and bronchial tissues [4,22]. For this reason, a number of investigators have examined the ability of various antibiotics to enter human bronchial secretions and sputum. Certain problems, questions, and controversies have been encountered.

A. General Topics

Assay System

Because of the bacteria in infected sputum, a diffusion method rather than titration must be used for antibiotic assay [22]. This implies that standard curves must be made with known concentrations of antibiotics in various dilutions. It may be important to construct standard curves for the sputum antibiotic assay, using pooled bronchial secretions as diluent [23,24]; however, for ampicillin, gentamicin, and carbenicillin this seems unimportant [10,11].

Specimens

Specimens of bronchial secretions for antibiotic analysis may be obtained directly from the lower respiratory tract by a bronchoscope, endotracheal tube, or by tracheostomy. These secretions are preferable to expectorated material, which could be contaminated by saliva. Since expectorated sputum is often easier to obtain, however, this material is frequently used for clinical studies. The concentration of antibiotic in saliva has been measured and found to vary considerably for penicillin [25], ampicillin [10,20], and cephalexin [26], but usually is much lower than concentrations in sputum. Thus, some dilutional error in antibiotic concentration in sputum might exist when the specimen is contaminated with saliva. This appears to be of minimal practical importance, however, when adequate methods are used to collect sputum [26].

Whether sputum is collected at specific times and correlated with concomitant serum specimens [10,25,26], or whether sputum specimens are pooled over 6-, 12-, or 24-hr periods [7,20] may be more important. Both systems have been used, but pooling sputa over long periods may give misleading data when attempts are made to correlate antibiotic concentrations of the pooled sputa to individual serum antibiotic concentrations [26]. The lack of correlation between serum and sputum antibiotic concentrations, found by some investigators [7,20], may be explained on this basis. One study, however, comparing pooled 24-hr sputum ampicillin concentrations to concentrations in specimens obtained 6 hr after a single dose, showed little differences [22].

Clinical Entity

The type of pathologic process involving pulmonary tissue may affect the bronchial penetration of antibiotics. However, in a study involving patients with pneumonia and bronchitis, as well as patients with infectious complications of pneumothorax, bronchial neoplasm, and pulmonary infarction, there was no significant difference in the sputum penicillin levels achieved in the various groups of patients [25].

Bronchial Inflammation

Inflammation of infected bronchial tissues is an expected finding. When adequate antibacterial therapy is instituted, the inflammation regresses and sputum production is reduced concomitantly [20,21,26]. Increased penetration of ampicillin and cephalexin into bronchial secretions during inflammatory conditions, with significantly decreased penetration as the inflammation subsides, has been well-documented [10,20,26]. This phenomenon did not occur with gentamicin, however [17].

Since the ability to achieve bactericidal levels of ampicillin or cephalexin in sputum seems to depend on the presence of bronchial inflammation, early, high–dose, intensive antibiotic therapy for bronchial infection has been proposed [20,21,26]. By achieving bactericidal bronchial concentrations of antibiotic quickly, complete sterilization of bronchial tissues may occur. As therapy continues and inflammation subsides, the bronchial antibiotic concentrations will fall into the bacteriostatic (or lower) range, and by then, the hope of preventing a relapse of bronchitis is probably lost. One study with ampicillin in patients with chronic bronchitis has shown that doses of 1 g or more every 6 hr are needed to achieve bactericidal sputum concentrations in most patients [22].

Correlation with Serum Levels

That serum and sputum antibiotic concentrations are often markedly different has been well-documented [4,6,10,20,25,26], however, controversy exists concerning the exact relationship between serum and sputum concentrations. If antibiotic is transported from blood to bronchus by simple diffusion, a direct correlation between serum and sputum concentrations would be found. Therefore, raising the dose of antibiotic administered would be expected to increase the sputum antibiotic level, if increased serum levels were produced. This direct relationship has been found by most investigators [10,25-27]. However, a few studies implied a somewhat independent relationship between serum and bronchial concentrations of antibiotic [7,20]. In one clinical trial [20], ampicillin was given in variable doses, including 250 mg, 500 mg, and 1 g orally, and 1 g intramuscularly. The serum concentration of antibiotic rose concomitantly with dose, whereas sputum concentrations ranged from 0.3 to 0.8µg/ml, correlating poorly with serum levels. The conclusion was that an active process governs ampicillin transport from blood to bronchus and that above a maximum serum concentration, further increases in serum antibiotic levels would be ineffective in raising sputum levels due to saturation of an active transport system. Exceptional cases in which higher doses of ampicillin consistently led to higher sputum concentrations were explained by break-down of the normal blood-bronchus barrier, with antibiotic leakage.

In general, almost all studies show that higher doses of antibiotics produce higher sputum levels. Although a rate-limiting active process may exist, this seems to be of little practical importance in planning drug therapy. Although great individual variation in sputum antibiotic concentrations between patients is the rule, much of this discrepancy may be eliminated if closer attention is given to the precise timing of sputum and serum specimen collection.

The mode of antibiotic administration (e.g., oral, intramuscular, intravenous infusion) may well be an important factor influencing sputum antibiotic concentration. Since the magnitude and duration of serum antibiotic concentrations are directly related to the route of administration, it seems likely that effective sputum concentrations might be achieved more reliably by one route of administration than by another. This has, in fact, been demonstrated for ampicillin [20].

Penicillinase Producing Organisms

Colonization of the bronchial tree with penicillinase-producing gram-negative bacteria has been reported in certain patients with chronic bronchitis [19]. Although these organisms may have little direct pathogenic effect, their ability to cause penicillinase-mediated inactivation of ampicillin in sputum has been shown [19]. Since the effective treatment of *Hemophilus influenzae* depends upon adequate sputum ampicillin levels, an indirect pathogenicity for these organisms seems likely. The addition of cloxacillin to the ampicillin regimen has been clinically effective in inhibiting this penicillinase effect [19]. Other investigators have found penicillinase producing organisms to be a less impressive problem [10,25].

Miscellaneous

The effects of exogenously administered adrenal corticosteroids and ACTH upon sputum ampicillin concentrations in patients with chronic bronchitis was examined in one study [10]. In the same study, patients taking diuretic medications were compared to those who were not in their ability to obtain adequate levels of ampicillin in sputum. The concentrations of ampicillin achieved in sputum were not affected by corticosteroid and ACTH, or by the diuretic drugs.

B.   Sputum Concentrations of
Various Antibiotics

When judging the clinical efficacy of a given antibiotic in treating respiratory tract infections, clearing of pus and bacteria from sputum suggests a successful regimen. Unfortunately, the high rate of relapse or frank failure in treating bronchitis and bronchiectasis has led to concern that concentrations of antibiotics in sputum may be lower than the bactericidal or even bacteriostatic concentration for the pathogenic bacteria being treated. For example an ampicillin concentration of $0.3\mu g/ml$ will inhibit 50% of *H. influenzae* isolates. A concentration of $0.6\mu g/ml$, however, is required to kill 50% of the isolates, while 97% of the isolates will be inhibited at this level [22]. If killing is crucial to successful antimicrobial therapy, it is obvious that higher doses of ampicillin would be needed.

The effectiveness of any given antibiotic dose schedule in treating a respiratory tract infection may be judged more precisely, therefore, if both the minimal inhibitory concentration (MIC) and minimal bactericidal concentration (MBC) for the pathogenic organism as well as the exact concentration of drug achieved in the sputum with a given dose of antibiotic are known. If, for example, an isolate of *H. influenzae* has an MBC of $0.6\mu g/ml$, 1 g (or more) of ampicillin by mouth every 6 hr will be required to achieve a sputum concentration greater than the MBC of this organism [22].

The results of clinical studies in which concentrations of antibiotics in bronchial secretions or sputum were measured are summarized in Table 1. Mean peak values are given, although great individual variation in sputum antibiotic levels was the rule rather than the exception. Based upon bacteriologic data, including MICs and MBCs, Table 1 might be used for more effective antibiotic treatment of respiratory infections.

IV.   Animal Model

Beyond the ability to measure antibiotic concentration in individual bronchial secretion and sputum specimens for a given drug and dose, the kinetics of antibiotic penetration into, and its clearance from bronchial secretions, seem important. It may be that different drugs are transported into sputum by different mechanisms. Some drugs may accumulate in the bronchus, whereas others might be cleared quickly. Certain drugs may be much more dependent on concomitant serum levels for adequate blood–bronchus penetration than do other drugs. Finally, the route of antibiotic administration might be a critical factor in achieving effective sputum levels.

One drug might best diffuse into sputum after a large blood–bronchus concentration gradient is established by rapid intravenous injection, whereas the transport of another drug might be more dependent on the prolonged, albeit lower, serum concentrations after intramuscular administration. The total time interval during which the sputum antibiotic concentration exceeds the MIC or MBC of the infecting organism may be a crucial factor in effective treatment of respiratory tract infections.

Attempts are usually made in human clinical studies to gather sputum and serum specimens at specific times after a dose of antibiotic. However, problems in obtaining sputum specimens upon demand in some patients, and the changing clinical setting from day to day in a given patient, make precise sputum-kinetic studies in humans difficult. For this reason, very few good clinical studies describing the appearance and disappearance curves for various antibiotics in human bronchial secretions have appeared in the literature. To date no study has appeared outlining the pharmacokinetic effect of antibiotics in sputum that various methods and routes of drug administration might have.

To allow a reproducible, readily available, and precise system for monitoring antibiotic concentrations in bronchial secretions over given periods of time, a dog model was developed [11,24]. It is now possible to compare different antibiotic drugs as well as different doses and routes of administration.

In this dog model, American foxhounds (or any available large dog) are anesthetized and intubated with an indwelling rubber endotracheal tube. Anesthesia does not seem to seriously alter antibiotic concentrations [24]. Bronchial secretion specimens may be obtained through this tube by a small-bore, plastic catheter, with a syringe attached for suction. These specimens may be collected at precise time intervals before and after antibiotic administration, and concomitant serum specimens can easily be obtained. This model eliminates the problem of bronchial secretion contamination by saliva.

Since the normal canine respiratory tract is relatively dry, subcutaneous doses of pilocarpine may be administered to stimulate bronchial secretion. The dose of pilocarpine used is small so that quantities of secretion are small enough (0.5 to 1.0 ml/hr) to avoid serious dilutional errors. One study has shown that pilocarpine probably does not greatly alter the constituents of bronchial secretions [11].

TABLE 1 Concentration of Antibiotics in Sputum and Bronchial Secretions

Antibiotic	Dose (mg) and route of administration[a]	Mean peak sputum concentration (µg/ml)	Type of infection[b]	Reference
Penicillin G[c]				
Procaine	600,000 qd IM	≤0.05	B,Bs	4
	600,000 bid IM	≤0.05		
Crystalline	1,000,000 qid IM	0.5		
Penicillin G				
Benzyl	1,000,000 bid IM	0.25	P,B,O	25
	2,000,000 bid IM	0.31		
	3,000,000 bid IM	1.20		
Ampicillin	250 qid po	0.08	B	22
	500 qid po	0.24		
	1,000 qid po	0.33		
Ampicillin	1,000 qid IM	0.3–0.8	B	20
Ampicillin	250 qid po	0.3	CF	7
Ampicillin	250 qid po	0.3	P,B,Bs,A,O	10
	500 qid po	0.26		
	1,000 qid po	0.65		
Cloxacillin	250 qid po	0.55	CF	7
Methicillin	250 qid po	0.22	CF	7

Carbenicillin	200/kg IV	0	CF	27
	600/kg IV	78		
Amoxycillin	500 qid po	0.40	B	47
Erythromycin	250 qid po	0.55	CF	7
Sulphadiazine	500–1500 qid po	0.1–3.76	CF	7
Sulphadimidine	500–1500 qid po	0.1–3.76	CF	7
Cephaloridine	250 qid IM	0.04	CF	7
Cephalexin	500 qid po	0.32	P,B	26
Clindamycin	300 po	2.7	CF	Unpublished[d]
Lincomycin	250 qid po	0.43	CF	7
Tetracycline HCl	250 qid po	0.80	CF	7
Doxycycline	100 po	1.5	B,O	48
Gentamicin	80 IM	1.85	P,B,O	17
Gentamicin	1/kg/qd IM	0.04	CF	7
	2/kg/qd IM	0.20		
Gentamicin	4–5 kg/qd IV	1.5	CF	27
Gentamicin	80 tid IM	<0.5	P,B	31
Gentamicin	80–120 tid IM	0.1–6.0	B,Bs	33

[a] po = by mouth; IM = intramuscular; IV = intravenous; qd = each day; bid = twice daily; tid = three times daily; qid = four times daily.
[b] P = pneumonia; B = bronchitis; Bs = bronchiectasis; A = pulmonary abscess; CF = cystic fibrosis, with bronchitis; O = other.
[c] For penicillin, dose in units rather than milligrams and concentration is expressed as units per milliliter. 1 unit Penicillin G = 0.6μg.
[d] Personal communication, J. A. Raeburn, Department of Human Genetics, Western General Hospital, Edinburgh, Scotland.

The lack of bronchial inflammation in this dog model makes it difficult to correlate precisely antibiotic concentrations of certain drugs, such as ampicillin and cephalexin, in infected human and normal dog bronchial secretions. However, human studies have shown that for gentamicin, mucoid and purulent bronchial secretions have comparable concentrations [17]. Studies for gentamicin also show a good correlation between dog and human bronchial secretion levels at comparable milligram per kilogram doses [11,17]. For these reasons, aminoglycoside antibiotics seem especially well-suited for study in this model. A dog model of *Pseudomonas* pneumonia has recently been described [28]. This refinement of the present model may allow study of antibiotic kinetics in the inflamed canine bronchus.

Figure 1 depicts the typical types of curves that can be constructed, using this model to compare two aminoglycosides. The relatively slow disappearance of

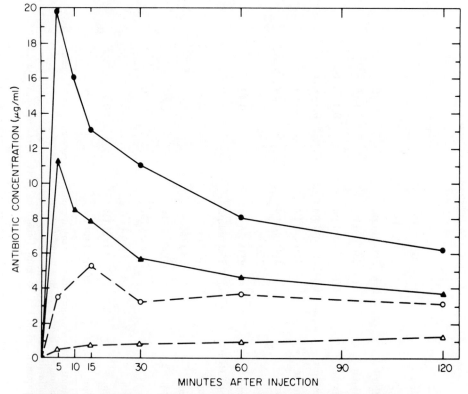

FIGURE 1 Comparison of serum and bronchial secretion concentrations of gentamicin to tobramycin, after 1.7 mg/kg intravenous injection. Gentamicin: serum ●——●; bronchial secretions ○– – –○. Tobramycin: serum ▲——▲; bronchial secretions △– – –△.

both antibiotics in bronchial secretions, when compared to serum, could be accounted for by a cumulative effect. The later peak concentration, shown by tobramycin in bronchial secretions, implies the presence of an active concentrating mechanism that continues to transport antibiotic into the bronchus despite a rapid fall in serum levels. Figure 2 illustrates the use of this model in studying the effect of different routes of administration of the same drug. The intramuscular route appears to create a lower, but more sustained, bronchial concentration of gentamicin than does the intravenous route. Thus, intrabronchial gentamicin appears to exceed the MIC of many bacteria for a longer total time when given by the intramuscular route of administration.

Carbenicillin has been studied with this model [11]. With this drug bronchial concentrations about 20% of those in serum were achieved. Amphotericin B and 5-fluorocytosine also have been studied [29]. Amphotericin B was absent from bronchial secretions, even after maximum intravenous dosage. 5-Fluorocytosine, however, showed good penetration of the blood—bronchus barrier. Early studies with clindamycin indicate that this drug penetrates into bronchial secretions quite well.

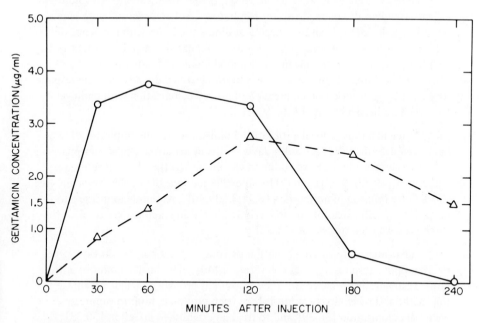

FIGURE 2 Comparison of bronchial secretion concentration of gentamicin after 1.7 mg/kg intravenous, ○——○, and after 1.7 mg/kg intramuscular injection, △- - -△.

V. Antibiotic Aerosols and Tracheobronchial Instillations

Since parenterally administered antibiotics penetrate the blood–bronchus barrier unpredictably and often inadequately, antibiotic aerosols and local antibiotic instillation in the infected tracheobronchial tree have been proposed. Enthusiasm for local antibiotic therapy of respiratory tract infection has varied, but some investigators reported encouraging results and have vigorously advocated this mode of therapy [18,30,31]. Other investigators, however, reported disappointing results with this therapeutic modality [32,33]. The local use of polymyxins and aminoglycoside antibiotics for gram–negative respiratory infections has been especially popular, due to the high incidence of systemic toxicity when these drugs are used parenterally and their relatively low degree of systemic absorption from the tracheobronchial tree [34].

An increasing number of patients, hospitalized for antibiotic treatment of primary bacterial pneumonia, are developing nosocomial pulmonary colonization and occasionally fatal superinfection with new bacterial strains, often *Staphylococcus aureus* or gram–negative bacilli [35]. Hospitalized patients with non-infectious illness also seem at risk for respiratory tract colonization with gram–negative bacilli [36,37], and the degree of illness correlates with incidence of colonization [37]. The same organisms that colonize the respiratory tract will lead to nosocomial pneumonia in a substantial number of patients [36,38]. Therefore, aerosolized antibiotics or antibiotics instilled directly into the respiratory tract for prevention or suppression of airway colonization with pathogenic bacteria have been advocated [36,39,40].

Three methods of local antibiotic administration to the respiratory tract have been described: (a) aerosol–spray into the upper airway (posterior pharynx) [40]; (b) aerosol administered to the tracheobronchial tree through respiratory equipment [30,33,36,39], and (c) local instillation into the tracheobronchial tree via catheter infusion of antibiotic [18,31,32,39,40]. Attempts to infuse antibiotic into specific areas of pulmonary infection, using radiography to place the catheter, have been successful [18,32].

Advocates of upper airway antibiotic spray suggest polymyxin B to effectively suppress respiratory tract colonization [40]. The small amount of antibiotic systemically absorbed from the pharynx is probably a major advantage of this method. Lower airway aerosols have been proposed, both to suppress bacterial colonization [36,39] and to treat an established infection [30,33]. Promising results with this technique for prophylaxis against airway colonization have been reported [36,39]; however, treatment of actual infection has met with mixed results [30,33]. Some impressive clinical results have been reported using local instillation of gentamicin into the respiratory tract of tracheostomized patients with gram–negative bacillus pneumonia [31].

Distribution and deposition of aerosols in the tracheobronchial tree depend upon particle size, electrical charge, and physical properties [41]. It has been shown that large amounts of aerosolized material collect in midline pulmonary structures, and very little may reach peripheral lung parenchyma [42]. Pathologic anatomy and alterations in breathing patterns may also affect the pulmonary distribution of aerosols [43]. One investigator demonstrated excellent peripheral distribution of aerosolized kanamycin [30], using an animal model. In another study, a pulmonary scan technique was used to detect radioactive material instilled by direct infusion into the tracheobronchial tree [18]. In this later study, excellent bronchial distribution was demonstrated using segmental infusions, and the local infusion method was recommended as superior to aerosols.

The addition of a mucolytic agent with antibiotic aerosols and instillation has been suggested as a means of increasing antibiotic penetration into thick purulent sputum. Acetylcysteine [18], pancreatic dornase [44], trypsin [36], streptokinase–streptodornase [36], and NaI [32] have all been used for this purpose. Acetylcysteine should not be used with carbenicillin as they are incompatible [34].

Any antibiotic aerosol or instillation produces some local bronchial irritation, and the threat of bronchial constriction always exists [34]. Although this has been of minor importance in some clinical series [30,39,40], there has been a report of airway obstruction in 2 patients following inhalation of 10 to 15 mg of aerosolized polymyxin B [45]. In another series, inhaled colistin was poorly tolerated in three of 17 patients [33].

The local use of antibiotics in tracheobronchial infection has been advocated to avoid the systemic side effects that accompany parenteral antibiotic therapy. This implies that very little antibiotic is absorbed systemically from the tracheobronchial tree. One study has shown that penicillin can reach therapeutic levels in the blood either after tracheal instillation or aerosol inhalation [46]. Table 2 reviews the findings in several studies involving antibiotics with known serious side effects. Except for one study [31], very little antibiotic was detected in serum. Systemic side effects were absent in all studies when local antibiotic administration was used alone.

The emergence of highly resistant strains of bacteria during systemic antibiotic therapy of primary pulmonary infection has been documented [35]. One concern with aerosols or other local forms of antibiotic administration has been that bacterial pathogens more resistant to antimicrobial drugs might emerge in the respiratory tract. This has, in fact, now been documented for colistin [39].

TABLE 2 Serum and Sputum Concentrations of Antibiotics Administered to the Tracheobronchial Tree

Drug	Dose administered to tracheobronchial tree (mg)[a]	Serum concentration (µg/ml)	Sputum concentration (µg/ml)	Reference
Kanamycin	250 bid or tid	0	ND[b]	30
Gentamicin	20 qid	0.2–2.0	0.1–20.0	33
Gentamicin	40 q 4 hour	1.3–6.8	7.5–>20	31
		(mean = 2.6)	(mean = >20)	
Polymyxin B	0.1 tid	0–0.1	0.2–1.5	18
	0.3 tid	0–0.15	0.9–1.4	
	1.0 tid	ND	1.8–3.1	
Colistin	50 tid	<0.25	–	39
	100 tid	<0.25	–	
Amphotericin B	5 qd	0	ND	32

[a]qd = each day; bid = twice daily; tid = three times daily; qid = four times daily.
[b]ND = None detected.

Polymyxin B, when used locally in the respiratory tract, seems to lead to gram-positive bacterial colonization [36], but not to colonization with polymyxin B resistant organisms [18]. One group of investigators has suggested that polymyxin B may favorably alter the flora of the tracheobronchial tree so that more antibiotic susceptible gram–positive organisms would replace the gram–negative bacilli [40].

Currently, antibiotic aerosols or instillations seem best reserved for seriously ill patients who require assisted ventilation, or who have a tracheostomy, or both. In these patients, vigorous attempts at preventing nosocomial pneumonia is warranted. Also, in progressive, life-threatening gram–negative bacillary pneumonia, which is unresponsive to parenteral antibiotics, the local instillation or aerosolization of antibiotics into the tracheobronchial tree may produce dramatic results in some patients [30,31].

VI. Summary

The penetration of antibiotics across the blood–bronchus barrier is crucial for adequate sterilization of the infected tracheobronchial tree. Unfortunately, this penetration is unpredictable, and for many antibiotics a therapeutic concentration in bronchial secretions and sputum is not achieved. Increased bronchial inflammation seems to help certain antibiotics pass into bronchial secretions, and higher serum levels of antibiotics tend to produce higher sputum concentrations. In certain situations the use of antibiotic aerosols or instillation of antibiotic directly into the respiratory tract may be of clinical benefit.

References

1. W. F. Verwey, H. R. Williams, Jr., and C. Kalsow, Penetration of chemotherapeutic agents into tissues, *Antimicrob. Agents Chemother.*, **1965**: 1016–1024 (1966).
2. C. A. Hogben, Biological membranes and their passage by drugs. In *Handbook of Experimental Pharmacology. Concepts in Biochemical Pharmacology.* Edited by B. B. Brodie and J. R. Gillette. Part I, Vol. 28. New York, Springer–Verlay, 1971, pp. 1–8.
3. M. Barza and L. Weinstein, Penetration of antibiotics into fibrin loci in vivo. I. Comparison of penetration of ampicillin into fibrin clots, abscesses, and "interstitial fluid", *J. Infect. Dis.*, **129**:59–65 (1974).
4. J. R. May, The laboratory background to the use of penicillin in chronic bronchitis and bronchiectasis, *Br. J. Tuberc.*, **49**:166–173 (1955).
5. R. A. Fishman, Blood–brain and CSF barriers to penicillin and related organic acids, *Arch. Neurol.*, **15**:113–124 (1966).

6.   B. A. Saggers and D. Lawson, Some observations on the penetration of antibiotics through mucus in vitro, *J. Clin. Pathol.,* **19**:313–317 (1966).

7.   B. A. Saggers and D. Lawson, In vivo penetration of antibiotics into sputum in cystic fibrosis, *Arch. Dis. Child.,* **43**:404–409 (1968).

8.   G. L. Biagi, M. C. Guerra, A. M. Barbaro, and M. F. Gamba, Influence of lipophilic character on the antibacterial activity of cephalosporins and penicillins, *J. Med. Chem.,* **13**:511–516 (1970).

9.   M. Barza, T. Samuelson, and L. Weinstein, Penetration of antibiotics into fibrin loci in vivo. II. Comparison of nine antibiotics: Effect of dose and degree of protein binding, *J. Infect. Dis.,* **129**:66–72 (1974).

10. S. M. Stewart, M. Fisher, J. E. Young, and W. Lutz, Ampicillin levels in sputum, serum, and saliva, *Thorax,* **25**:304–311 (1970).

11. J. E. Pennington and H. Y. Reynolds, Concentrations of gentamicin and carbenicillin in bronchial secretions, *J. Infect. Dis.,* **128**:63–68 (1973).

12. W. F. Verwey and H. R. Williams, Jr., Relationships between the concentrations of various penicillins in plasma and peripheral lymph, *Antimicrob. Agents Chemother.,* **1961**:476–483 (1962).

13. C. M. Kunin, Clinical significance of protein binding of the penicillins, *Ann. N. Y. Acad. Sci.,* **145**:282–290 (1967).

14. M. Barza, J. Brusch, M. G. Bergeron, and L. Weinstein, Penetration of antibiotics into fibrin loci in vivo. III. Intermittent vs. continuous infusion and the effect of probenecid, *J. Infect. Dis.,* **129**:73–78 (1974).

15. J. Crofton, Some principles in the chemotherapy of bacterial infections—II, *Br. Med. J.,* **2**:209–212 (1969).

16. H. Y. Reynolds and H. H. Newball, Analysis of proteins and respiratory cells obtained from human lungs by bronchial lavage, *J. Lab. Clin. Med.,* **84**:559–573 (1974).

17. O. Wieser, H. Regula, and W. Wundt, Die ausscheidung von gentamicin über den bronchialbaum, *Dtsch. Med. Wochenschr.,* **96**:870–972 (1971).

18. R. J. Ramirez and E. F. O'Neill, Endobronchial polymyxin B: Experimental observations in chronic bronchitis, *Chest,* **58**:352–357 (1970).

19. J. L. Maddocks and J. R. May, "Indirect pathogenicity" of penicillinase-producing enterobacteria in chronic bronchial infections, *Lancet,* **1**:793–795 (1969).

20. J. R. May and D. M. Delves, Treatment of chronic bronchitis with ampicillin. Some pharmacological observations, *Lancet,* **1**:929–933 (1965).

21. J. R. May, The bacteriology and chemotherapy of chronic bronchitis, *Br. J. Dis. Chest,* **59**:57–65 (1965).

22. J. R. May, Ampicillin in the therapy of chronic bronchitis, *Postgrad. Med. J., Suppl.,* **40**:193–197 (1964).

23. J. M. Kaplan, G. H. McCracken, Jr., and E. Snyder, Influence of methodology upon apparent concentrations of antibiotics in tissue, *Antimicrob. Agents Chemother.,* **3**:143–146 (1973).

24. J. E. Pennington and H. Y. Reynolds, Tobramycin in bronchial secretions, *Antimicrob. Agents Chemother.,* **4**:299–301 (1973).

25. F. F. Hafez, S. M. Stewart, and M. E. Burnet, Penicillin levels in sputum, *Thorax,* **20**:219–225 (1965).

26. G. M. Halprin and S. M. McMahon, Cephalexin concentrations in sputum during acute respiratory infections, *Antimicrob. Agents Chemother.,* **3**: 703–707 (1973).

27. M. I. Marks, R. Prentice, R. Swarson, E. K. Cotton, and T. C. Eickhoff, Carbenicillin and gentamicin: Pharmacologic studies in patients with cystic fibrosis and pseudomonas pulmonary infections, *J. Pediatr.,* **79**:822–828 (1971).

28. D. C. Dale, H. Y. Reynolds, J. E. Pennington, R. J. Elin, T. W. Pitts, and R. G. Graw, Granulocyte transfusion therapy of experimental pseudomonas pneumonia, *J. Clin. Invest.,* **54**:664–671 (1974).

29. J. E. Pennington, E. R. Block, and H. Y. Reynolds, Five–fluorocytosine and amphotericin B in bronchial secretions, *Antimicrob. Agents. Chemother.,* **61**:324–326 (1973).

30. M. Bilodeau, J. C. Roy, and M. Giroux, Studies of absorption of kanamycin by aerosolization, *Ann. N. Y. Acad. Med.,* **132**:870–878 (1966).

31. J. Klastersky, C. Geuning, E. Mouawad, and D. Daneau, Endotracheal gentamicin in bronchial infections in patients with tracheostomy, *Chest,* **61**:117–120 (1972).

32. R. J. Ramirez, Pulmonary aspergilloma. Endobronchial treatment, *N. Engl. J. Med.,* **271**:1281–1285 (1964).

33. A. Pines, H. Raafat, and K. Plucinski, Gentamicin and colistin in chronic purulent bronchial infections, *Br. Med. J.,* **2**:543–545 (1967).

34. W. F. Miller, Aerosol therapy in acute and chronic respiratory disease, *Arch. Intern. Med.,* **131**:148–155 (1973).

35. J. R. Tillotson and M. Finland, Bacterial colonization and clinical super-infection of the respiratory tract complicating antibiotic treatment of pneumonia, *J. Infect. Dis.,* **119**:597–624 (1969).

36. M. H. Lepper, S. Kofman, N. Blatt, H. F. Dowling, and G. G. Jackson, Effect of eight antibiotics used singly and in combinations on the tracheal flora following tracheotomy in poliomyelitis, *Antibiot. and Chemother.,* **4**:829–843 (1954).

37. W. G. Johanson, A. K. Pierce, and J. P. Sanford, Changing pharyngeal bacterial flora of hospitalized patients. Emergence of gram–negative bacilli, *N. Engl. J. Med.,* **281**:1137–1140 (1969).

38. W. G. Johanson, A. K. Pierce, J. P. Sanford, and G. D. Thomas, Nosocomial respiratory infections with gram–negative bacilli. The significance of colonization of the respiratory tract, *Ann. Intern. Med.,* **77**:701–706 (1972).

39. H. D. Rose, M. B. Pendharker, G. S. Snider, and R. C. Kory, Evaluation of sodium colistimethate aerosol in gram–negative infections of the respiratory tract, *J. Clin. Pharmacol.,* **10**:274–281 (1970).

40. S. Greenfield, D. Teres, L. S. Bushnell, J. Hedley-Whyte, and D. S. Feingold, Prevention of gram–negative bacillary pneumonia using aerosol

polymyxin as prophylaxis. I. Effect on the colonization patterns of the upper respiratory tract of seriously ill patients, *J. Clin. Invest.*, **52**:2935–2940 (1973).

41. L. T. Greene, Aerosols. In *Handbook of Experimental Pharmacology. Concepts in Biochemical Pharmacology*. Edited by B. B. Brodie and J. R. Gillette. Part I, Vol. 28. New York, Springer–Verlag, 1971, pp. 88–102.

42. G. D. Patterson and G. H. Kamp, Retention of liquid aerosols in the lung, *Am. Rev. Respir. Dis.*, **95**:443–446 (1967).

43. I. S. Goldberg and R. V. Lourenco, Deposition of aerosols in pulmonary disease, *Arch. Intern. Med.*, **131**:88–91 (1973).

44. R. Spier, E. Witebsky, and J. R. Paine, Aerosolized pancreatic dornase and antibiotics in pulmonary infections: Use in patients with postoperative and nonoperative infections, *J.A.M.A.*, **178**:878–886 (1961).

45. G. Marschke and A. Sarauw, Danger of polymyxin B inhalation, *Ann. Intern. Med.*, **74**:296–297 (1971).

46. E. A. Gaensler, J. R. Beakey, and M. S. Segal, Pharmacodynamics of pulmonary absorption in man. I. Aerosol and intratracheal penicillin, *Ann. Intern. Med.*, **31**:582–594 (1949).

47. J. R. May and A. Ingold, Amoxycillin in the treatment of chronic nontuberculous bronchial infections, *Br. J. Dis. Chest.*, **66**:185–191 (1972).

48. J. Gartmann, Doxyzyklinkonzentrationen im lungengewebe, in der bronchialwand und im bronchialsekret, *Schweiz. Med. Wochenschr.*, **102**:1484–1486 (1972).

18

Vaccines for Nonbacterial Disease of the Lower Respiratory Tract

ROBERT M. CHANOCK

National Institute of Allergy and Infectious Diseases
National Institutes of Health
Bethesda, Maryland

I. Viruses and Mycoplasmas of Sufficient Importance in Lower Respiratory Tract Disease to Warrant Attempts at Immunoprophylaxis

At least 120 viruses and one mycoplasma have been shown to cause acute respiratory tract disease in man [1]. Although it would be desirable to provide protection against each of these agents, such an approach is clearly impractical at this time because of a number of constraints to be described subsequently. For this reason a system of priorities is needed so that the most important pathogens are given first consideration. Fortunately, the relative importance of various viral and mycoplasmal respiratory pathogens is well-understood and this understanding provides a secure base for ordering priorities in the development and use of vaccines. It should be emphasized that the importance of the different lower respiratory tract pathogens varies considerably with age, epidemiologic setting, and underlying pulmonary pathology. Accordingly, the formulation of vaccines must vary to reflect the specific needs of individuals in these different categories.

A. Agents that are Primary Causes of Lower Respiratory Tract Disease

Influenza A and B Viruses

These viruses are most important in adults, although their impact in young children should not be discounted. It is now clear that influenza A virus and, to a lesser extent, influenza B virus are important causes of croup in infants and young children. In adults influenza A virus is the most important primary viral pathogen of the lower respiratory tract in terms of disability and serious disease [2]. Influenza A virus can cause a fatal pneumonia without the participation of pathogenic bacteria, and a significant number of influenza fatalities occur in this manner [2-4].

Respiratory Syncytial Virus (RSV)

This virus is the most important lower respiratory tract pathogen of early life [5]. For example, RSV is responsible for most bronchiolitis illnesses of infancy. Furthermore, this virus is a major cause of pneumonia during infancy and early childhood.

Parainfluenza Viruses

These viruses, especially Types I, II, and III, are the major etiologic agents of acute laryngotracheobronchitis (croup) of infancy and childhood [5].

Adenoviruses

Viruses of this group rank next in importance as primary respiratory viral pathogens. Types I, II, III, V, and VII are relatively important causes of pneumonia and less severe respiratory disease in infants and young children [6]. In addition, Type IV and Type VII viruses and, to a lesser extent, Type III virus are the most common causes of acute febrile respiratory tract disease in populations of military recruits [7,8].

M. pneumoniae

This organism is the single most important cause of nonbacterial pneumonia in older children and young adults [8,9]. In special groups, such as military recruits and college students, *M. pneumoniae* assumes an even greater significance than in the general population [10-12].

B. Agents that Provoke Acute Bacterial Pneumonia

Influenza A virus causes more fatal illness by initiating a sequence of events that lead to bacterial pneumonia than by acting as a primary, self-sufficient pathogen [2-4]. During the years when influenza A virus has been epidemic in the United States, 20,000 to 40,000 excess deaths from respiratory disease occurred and the terminal event in most of these fatal illnesses was bacterial pneumonia [2-4,13, 14]. Clearly, influenza A virus is the most frequent virus responsible for initiating fatal respiratory disease.

It is suspected that mild viral respiratory disease caused by viruses other than influenza may often provoke the development of severe or fatal bacterial pneumonia. Many patients progress from what appears to have been a mild viral upper respiratory illness to bacterial pneumonia. However, it is usually not possible to document such a viral infection by recovering the virus and/or demonstrating a serologic response [15]. In this situation, specimens for laboratory detection of viral infection, of necessity, are collected when the diagnosis of bacterial pneumonia is established, and it may be too late, at this time, to recover virus that has disappeared from the respiratory tract.

C. Agents that Cause an Exacerbation of Chronic Lung Disease

There is convincing evidence that rhinovirus infection is frequently associated with exacerbation of chronic lung disease, such as chronic bronchitis and emphysema [16]. Although rhinoviruses act infrequently as primary pathogens of the lower respiratory tract, their effect upon lungs with underlying chronic damage is both dramatic and important in terms of respiratory disease morbidity and ultimately, mortality. It has been suggested that RSV may play a role similar to that of the rhinoviruses, but evidence to support this view is not particularly convincing.

II. Obstacles to Successful Immunoprophylaxis

A. Antigenic Shift in Influenza A Viruses

A major shift in one or both surface glycoproteins of influenza A virus occurs approximately each decade. Between major shifts, significant antigenic drift occurs. The major shifts are thought to result from recombination (or gene reassortment) between influenza A viruses of man and animals or birds [17]. It is postulated that the genes which code for the surface glycoproteins, i.e., the hemagglutinin and neuraminidase enzyme, are transferred from the animal or avian influenza A virus to the human virus during an infection in which a host is dually infected with a human virus and an animal or avian virus. Antigenic drift on the other hand is thought to represent the phenotypic expression of point mutation in genes that code for the two surface glycoprotein antigens [17].

Major antigenic shift from reassortment of influenza virus genes poses a special problem in the development and production of an influenza virus vaccine designed to meet the threat of a recently emerged pandemic strain of virus with novel surface antigen (hemagglutinin) or antigens (hemagglutinin and neuraminidase). For example, when a major shift in one or both surface glycoproteins occurred in 1957 and again in 1968, it was not possible to develop, prepare, and distribute vaccine containing the new virus in time to affect the course of pandemic or epidemic disease [18].

Fortunately the noninfluenzal respiratory pathogens do not undergo rapid, significant shifts in surface antigenic determinants.

B. Large Multiplicity of Distinct Rhinovirus Serotypes

One hundred distinct rhinovirus serotypes are now recognized, and it is unlikely that the magnitude of antigenic diversity is completely understood at this time [19]. This multiplicity of rhinovirus serotypes constitutes a serious impediment to any attempt at specific immunoprophylaxis, whether it involves inactivated virus antigen or live attenuated virus.

C. Transient Nature of Resistance to Certain Lower Respiratory Tract Pathogens

Reinfection occurs with high frequency with certain viruses, such as RSV and Type III parainfluenza virus [20-22]. Disease affecting the lower respiratory tract may occur during such reinfection, but generally the severity of illness is less than that associated with primary infection [21-23]. Nonetheless, a considerable amount of illness and dissemination of virus can occur during reinfection with RSV and Type III parainfluenza virus. Since primary, symptomatic infection does not provide complete or long-lasting protection, it is unlikely that immunization with inactivated antigen or live attenuated virus will be successful in preventing reinfection or irradicating these viruses from the community. For the present, the aim of vaccines for viruses, such as RSV and the parainfluenza viruses, must, of necessity, be limited to preventing serious disease during primary infection.

It is not known how long the host remains resistant to an influenza A virus that has not undergone significant antigenic variation. This type of important information has been difficult to obtain, in part, because of the frequency with which influenza A virus changes antigenic structure. Influenza B virus undergoes antigenic change more slowly than does Type A virus, and this has made it possible to assess the duration of resistance to Type B virus. It appears that significant resistance to influenza B virus disease does not persist more than 3 yr [24].

Resistance to viruses of the adenovirus group and to *M. pneumoniae* appears to be relatively long-lasting, as suggested by the age-distribution of illness caused by these pathogens. The adenovirus serotypes, which cause disease in infants and young children (Types 1, 2, 3, 5, and 7) and which infect most individuals by the time they are adults, rarely initiate illness in adults [8]. Similarly, *M. pneumoniae* produces its major impact as a lower respiratory tract pathogen during childhood and adolescence, while illness in older adults is uncommon [9,10].

D. Need in Certain Circumstances to Immunize Early in Life

There is a need to immunize against several important pediatric respiratory pathogens early in life. The extreme case is RSV, which produces its major impact on the lower respiratory tract during the first 3 months [25]. If an RSV vaccine is to be useful, it must be effective in inducing resistance to disease when administered during the first month of life. Unfortunately, this is a difficult period in which to attempt immunization since the host's immunologic processes are not fully responsive to antigenic stimulation. In addition, antibody in serum, which is passively acquired from the mother, may act to suppress the infant's immunologic response.

III. Nature of Resistance to Respiratory Tract Viruses and Mycoplasmas

Critical to the development of effective vaccines for the control of acute disease of the respiratory tract is an understanding of the immunologic factors that provide protection against important respiratory pathogens.

A. Systemic Immunity

Serum Antibody

In a number of situations, serum antibody has been found to be ineffective in protecting the host against infection or disease caused by respiratory viruses and mycoplasma. There is evidence from observations made during natural infection with RS virus as well as experimental infection with parainfluenza Type I virus and Type XIII rhinovirus that serum antibody does not correlate closely with resistance. Similar evidence has been obtained recently for experimental infection with *M. pneumoniae* in the hamster.

Respiratory syncytial virus produces its major impact during the first few months of life. Bronchiolitis and pneumonia caused by RS virus occur most often during the second month of life, and there is a decrease in incidence thereafter with increasing age [25]. Young infants uniformly possess a moderate to high level of serum antibody passively acquired from the mother [25]. Despite the presence of passive serum antibody, RS virus is the major respiratory tract pathogen of early infancy. This constitutes the most dramatic evidence for the ineffectiveness of serum antibody in viral disease of the lower respiratory tract.

Observations made during a series of volunteer studies strongly suggested that serum antibody did not provide protection against upper respiratory tract disease caused by parainfluenza Type I virus or rhinovirus Type XIII [26,27]. It should be emphasized that there have been no serious attempts to evaluate the role of serum antibody in resistance to lower tract disease caused by the parainfluenza viruses. Resolution of this question will require careful prospective study of young children, with the collection of appropriate serum and respiratory secretion specimens.

During recent studies in hamsters, the intramuscular and intranasal routes of administration of inactivated *M. pneumoniae* vaccine were shown to be equally effective in stimulating the development of serum antibody [28,41]. However, only the latter route of administration induced demonstrable resistance to the development of lung lesions produced by challenge with virulent organisms. In this situation it appeared that immune defenses other than serum antibody were responsible for resistance.

For one group of viruses, serum antibody appears to play a significant role in resistance to lower respiratory tract disease. Resistance to adenovirus infection differs from the situation for myxoviruses, paramyxoviruses, and rhinoviruses. With the latter viruses, it appears that local immunologic defense mechanisms in the respiratory tract are of major importance in host resistance. Recent experience with a live Type IV adenovirus vaccine administered in an enteric-coated capsule of tablet suggested that serum antibody provided definite protection against adenovirus infection and illness [1,29]. When Type IV adenovirus was given in this way, the virus produced a silent infection limited to the lower intestinal tract. Individuals infected by this method developed moderately high levels of serum neutralizing antibody, but nasal secretion antibody was not induced [30,31]. Miliary recruits who received Type IV adenovirus vaccine in an enteric-coated capsule or tablet prior to an epidemic exhibited significant resistance to infection and almost complete resistance against disease caused by this virus. In this setting, in which a dissociation of serum antibody and local respiratory tract antibody was achieved, it appeared that serum antibody by itself was sufficient to provide protection against adenovirus and its effects. This finding suggests that Type IV adenovirus produces a type of infection different from that produced by the myxoviruses, paramyxoviruses, or rhinoviruses. It may be that adenovirus infection penetrates to a deeper level than the more superficial myxoviruses and rhinoviruses. Certain features of adenovirus infection, such as latency, prolonged shedding, and lymph node involvement, are consistent with this view.

Cell-mediated Immunity

Systemic cell-mediated immune responses have been observed following experimental infection of guinea pigs with influenza A and parainfluenza Type III viruses [32]. It was of some interest that the cell-mediated immune response to Type III parainfluenza virus appeared to develop more rapidly than did serum antibody. Systemic cell-mediated immune response to *M. pneumoniae* has also been detected in the experimentally infected hamster [33]. The significance of this type of response in bringing about resolution of infection or protecting the host against subsequent infection with the homologous agent is not understood at this time.

B. Local Immunity

That a local antibody system exists within the respiratory tract has been well-established during the past decade [34]. Plasma cells located beneath the respiratory mucosa produce immunoglobulins, predominantly IgA, which are secreted into the respiratory secretions. Most of the antiviral activity in respiratory secretions is associated with secretory (or dimeric) 11 S IgA. Recently, evidence has been presented for the existence of a local cell-mediated immune system in the respiratory tract, which is separate from that of systemic cell-mediated immunity [35].

There is increasing evidence that local immunologic mechanisms in the respiratory tract play a major role in protecting the host against disease caused by a number of viral and mycoplasmal pathogens. It is not clear, however, whether local antibody or cell-mediated immunity is of greater importance or whether both are of equal importance. Possibly the situation varies for different agents.

Evidence that local immunity is often a prime determinant of resistance is both direct and indirect. The latter evidence may be summarized in the following manner. Successive reinfections with RS virus lead to significant partial resistance so that adults generally develop a mild illness in response to the virus. In contrast, initial infection in early life usually is associated with febrile respiratory disease. Relatively high levels of serum neutralizing antibody do not protect the young infant against serious lower respiratory tract disease caused by RS virus [25]. Furthermore, infants who developed both serum antibody and a systemic cell-mediated immune response following administration of an inactivated RS virus vaccine were not protected against this virus [36–38]. Since a series of sequential infections appear to confer partial resistance upon the host, it is likely that local rather than systemic immunity is of prime importance.

Direct evidence for the protective effect of local immunity comes from experimental studies in man and animals. Over 20 years ago, it was shown that resistance to influenza A virus in the mouse correlated well with antibody in respiratory tract secretions, while antibody in serum did not appear to be effective [39]. This finding should not be surprising when one considers the superficial nature of this myxovirus infection in the lung. Local defense mechanisms (antibodies in secretions?) are strategically located to intercept virus when it attacks the respiratory epithelium.

Similarly, in hamsters *M. pneumoniae* produces a very superficial infection in which the organism is localized to the surface of the respiratory epithelium [40]. This mycoplasma does not appear to grow in the respiratory epithelial cells or to penetrate the basement membrane of the respiratory epithelium. In several experiments the effectiveness of immunization by the parenteral and intranasal routes was compared, and it was found that the latter procedure induced greater resistance in the lungs despite the fact that the former type of immunization stimulated a slightly higher level of serum antibody [28,41]. Thus, in experimental *M. pneumoniae* infection in the hamster local immunologic defenses appear to be of prime importance.

In man, studies in volunteers provided evidence for a major role of local respiratory tract immunity in certain viral infections involving the upper respiratory tract. Unfortunately, there is no direct evidence that bears upon the possible role of local immunity in lower respiratory tract disease, although the natural history of RS virus infection (described above) strongly suggests that local immunologic mechanisms may be of major importance in protecting the host. In volunteers, resistance to upper respiratory tract infection or disease produced by Type I parainfluenza virus, RS virus or rhinovirus Type XIII correlated better with level of antibody in respiratory tract secretions than with that of antibody in serum [26,27,42]. Recently a similar correlation was observed for 11 S, IgA, local secretory antibody for *M. pneumoniae,* and resistance to mild respiratory disease produced by this organism [43]. Since some of the illnesses in this study involved the lower respiratory tract, the correlation just described may constitute the first preliminary evidence that local immunity has a role in lower respiratory tract disease in man.

In the studies just described, local respiratory tract antibody appeared to be a relatively reliable index of immunity. However, it should not be considered as any more than that at this time since secretory antibody may only correlate with another local immune mechanism (such as cell–mediated immunity), which is the true determinant of resistance. In any case, local respiratory antibody provides a reliable indication of host resistance and, as such, it can serve a valuable function in assessing the immunogenicity of respiratory vaccines.

IV. Vaccines Licensed for Prevention of Viral Respiratory Disease

A. Influenza—Inactivated

The only formulation currently licensed for prophylaxis of human viral respiratory disease is influenza vaccine. There has been considerable dispute concerning the protective efficacy of inactivated influenza virus (Type A and B) vaccine administered parenterally. In large part, the poor performance of inactivated influenza vaccine can be ascribed to the use of preparations containing an inadequate quantity of antigen. When vaccine preparations containing sufficient antigenic mass have been used, impressive protection has been provided against influenzal disease. In these circumstances the level of protection has approached 70% to 90% [44]. For example, in the military routine yearly immunization with potent vaccine has affected a dramatic and almost complete suppression of epidemic influenza during interpandemic periods [45].

Recent advances in virus purification and concentration have been applied to large scale processing of inactivated influenza antigens, and this has made it possible to prepare, on a regular basis, vaccine of high potency. In addition, recent vaccines have been relatively free of much of the toxic reactivity associated with older, less pure vaccines.

If local respiratory tract immunity plays such a decisive role in resistance, why have parenterally administered inactivated influenza vaccines provided significant protection? The answer may lie in the observation that the local respiratory antibody system can be stimulated by parenterally administered antigen. This has been seen with influenza A virus, rhinovirus Type XIII and parainfluenza virus Type I [27,46–48]. However, the local antibody mechanisms can be stimulated more efficiently and more frequently by direct administration of either live or inactivated antigen into the nasopharynx. The superiority of local administration of antigen applies only to material in aqueous form. If antigen is mixed with mineral or peanut oil adjuvant and inoculated parenterally, it will stimulate a local antibody response which often equals that produced by infection or local instillation of antigen [49,50]. Questions concerning the long-term safety of mineral and peanut oil adjuvants have been raised, but the available evidence does not confirm these fears [49,51]. In any case, an oil adjuvant cannot be considered for use with inactivated respiratory viral vaccines until the issue of long-term safety has been resolved with finality.

Influenza A virus is unique among the 120 viruses that cause respiratory tract disease in man in that it periodically undergoes an abrupt change in the structure of its coat antigens. This type of abrupt shift, which occurs approximately every 10 years, poses a special problem for control of influenzal disease through vaccination. Abrupt change in the outer structure of the virus renders the entire population susceptible to infection and illness, since immunity produced against influenza viruses, which had infected in the past, does not affect the new altered virus and thus does not protect against it. At such a time, when vaccine is most needed, it is generally in shortest supply. For example, at the crest of the 1957 Asian and 1968 Hong Kong epidemics the quantity of inactivated vaccine produced for the new variants was insufficient to affect the course of epidemic influenza in the United States [18]. Approximately 20,000 to 40,000 persons died in the United States in each of these epidemics. Furthermore, the economic loss to the nation caused by the Hong Kong epidemic has been estimated conservatively at 4 billion dollars [52]. There was not enough time between the isolation and characterization of the new virus and the beginning of the epidemic to prepare sufficient inactivated vaccine. Clearly what is needed is a method for the rapid production of vaccine when the threat of pandemic disease arises.

Recently, a new technique was introduced for shortening the time required for the development and production of a new inactivated influenza virus vaccine. Ordinarily, a newly isolated strain of influenza virus grows poorly in eggs, and a period of several months is usually required to select a mutant that replicates to high titer in eggs. Recently, it was shown that strains of virus that grow well in eggs can be produced rapidly through the mechanism of genetic recombination (or reassortment). The high growth potential in eggs of a well-adapted laboratory strain can be transferred to a newly isolated strain via genetic recombination [53]. In essence, the gene (or genes) that controls growth in eggs is transferred from the old egg-adapted strain to the newly isolated virus. This results in a virus that has the outer antigenic coat of the new virus and the growth potential in eggs of the egg-adapted virus. Whether this application of the principles of virus genetics will close the time gap sufficiently to effect the course of future epidemics remains to be seen.

Rapid development, production, and widespread use of inactivated influenza virus vaccine will not solve the influenza problem for all segments of the population. If inactivated vaccine for a new strain could be produced with sufficient speed and in sufficient quantity, it should be possible to protect that portion of the population most at risk of developing fatal disease following influenza virus infection, namely individuals over 60 yr of age. Unfortunately, little benefit can be expected for the other segment of the population at greatest risk, i.e., infants and young children. Although mortality is not high in this age group, the young have an increased risk of developing serious lower respiratory tract disease during an influenza epidemic. The most extreme manifestation of this predilection is obstructive croup, which is often serious and life-threatening [54]. The impact of influenza A and B viruses in the pediatric population has been almost completely overlooked by those charged with the responsibility for preventing influenza. Unfortunately, the current purified inactivated vaccines cannot be recommended for routine use in infants and young children because of the unacceptably high frequency of local and systemic reactions produced by such preparations. Clearly, another approach to immunoprophylaxis in this age group is indicated.

B. Adenovirus—Inactivated

In the past, inactivated adenovirus vaccine containing Serotypes III, IV, and VII was licensed for use in man. The vaccine was used primarily in the military where the majority of acute febrile respiratory tract illnesses was caused by Type IV virus and to a lesser extent Type VII and Type III viruses [7,55,56]. The use of inactivated adenovirus vaccine was justified in terms of high respiratory tract disease morbidity, hospitalization, and costly disruption of military training. The first experimental, inactivated vaccines prepared from viruses grown in monkey, kidney tissue culture were extremely effective in preventing adenovirus disease. However, subsequent production lots of licensed vaccine exhibited a variable degree of potency. In some instances, very little protection was conferred [56].

Monkey, kidney grown, adenovirus vaccines were withdrawn from distribution when it was found that a portion of, or the whole, SV-40 genome was integrated into the genome of each of the adenovirus vaccine strains [57–59]. The use of vaccines containing adenovirus SV-40 hybrid viruses was suspended, since it was known that SV-40 virus induced tumors in suckling hamsters and transformation of human cells in tissue culture [60]. Attempts to develop vaccine strains free of SV-40 genetic material and capable of growing in monkey kidney cells failed. It soon became clear that the SV-40 genetic material in the adenovirus SV-40 hybrid virus provided an essential helper function for the growth of adenovirus in monkey kidney cells [59]. In numerous experiments it was shown that Type III, Type IV, and Type VII adenoviruses were unable to grow in simian cells in the absence of the helper function provided by SV-40.

V. Experimental Inactivated Vaccines

A. Respiratory Syncytial Virus (RS Virus)

RS virus is the most important respiratory tract pathogen of early life, and for this reason it has been given one of the highest priorities in vaccine development. After several early, relatively unconcentrated inactivated vaccines were found to be weakly antigenic, a 100 times concentrated vaccine containing alum adjuvant was prepared from virus grown in vervet monkey kidney tissue culture in an effort to determine whether resistance could be induced to RS virus. The concentrated vaccine was quite antigenic and stimulated high levels of serum antibody and systemic cell-mediated immunity in seronegative infants [36-38]. It came as a surprise, therefore, that the vaccine did not induce resistance to RS virus infection. More striking than failure of the vaccine to protect against infection was the unexpected response of vaccinees to RS virus infection. These individuals developed serious obstructive lower respiratory tract disease (bronchiolitis) with an unusually high frequency [36-38]. Clearly the vaccine had induced an altered and exaggerated state of reactivity to infection and this effect was limited to the younger vaccinees who had not been infected with RS virus previously [38]. Presumably these individuals lacked protective local respiratory tract immunity. The exaggerated response to infection in individuals who received the inactivated RS virus vaccine could have resulted from a cytotoxic or Arthus reaction produced in the lung by interaction of vaccine-induced serum antibody and RS virus antigen. It is also possible that vaccine-induced cell-mediated immunity could have been responsible, acting alone or in concert with serum antibody.

B. Parainfluenza

Antigenic inactivated vaccines have been prepared for the parainfluenza viruses, which are second in importance only to RS virus as pediatric respiratory viral pathogens. Although a trivalent vaccine containing egg grown viruses induced appreciable levels of serum antibody in infants and children, the preparation did not induce resistance to naturally occurring parainfluenza virus disease [61,62].

C. Rhinoviruses

Intranasal instillation of an unconcentrated, inactivated Type XIII rhinovirus vaccine stimulated antibodies in both serum and nasal secretions and induced significant resistance to experimental illness [27]. In contrast, the same vaccine, given by the intramuscular route, stimulated antibody primarily in serum; volunteers so vaccinated were not protected against experimentally induced illness. Since intranasal instillation of vaccine represents a simple method for administering antigen, conceivably this approach could be used to provide protection against rhinoviruses in individuals with chronic lung disease who are at-risk of developing an exacerbation of their pulmonary disease during rhinovirus infection. Unfortunately, the large multitude of rhinovirus serotypes (over 100) constitutes a major obstacle to the success of this approach. Also, methods for producing higher yields of rhinovirus from tissue culture and techniques for enhancing and prolonging the local secretory antibody response must be developed if this type of immunization is to be practical.

D. Adenovirus

A promising approach to adenovirus immunoprophylaxis involves the use of DNA-free, virus capsid subunits. Partially purified protein capsid subunits have been shown to stimulate the development of serum neutralizing antibody. Recently, highly purified, DNA-free, Type V hexon and fiber antigens were found to be antigenic in adults who lacked preexisting serum neutralizing antibody [63]. Further, vaccinees were shown to be resistant to the effects of a challenge with virulent, Type V virus [63]. There was a suggestion, however, that the seronegative adults involved in the vaccine trial may have been infected with Type V virus previously, so that the antibody responses observed may have been secondary rather than primary in nature. Nonetheless, this is an exciting approach to the use of highly purified, nucleic acid-free, protein subunits for vaccination.

E. *M. pneumoniae*

The need for an effective vaccine for *M. pneumoniae,* an organism that very rarely produces fatal disease, is indicated by (a) the high incidence of *M. pneumoniae* disease in children and young adults, especially military recruits and college students, (b) the frequent prolonged course of disease prior to diagnosis, and (c) the failure of effective chemotherapeutic compounds, such as tetracycline or erythrocycin, to eradicate the organism from the respiratory tract [64]. Formalin-inactivated vaccines have been developed which stimulate serum antibody in volunteers lacking preexisting metabolism-inhibiting antibody. Vaccines prepared from organisms grown in a chemically defined medium supplemented with chloroform extract of egg yolk, or in a serum-free medium of unidentified composition, were moderately antigenic and provided approximately 50% protection against pneumonia resulting from naturally occurring infection [65,66].

Vaccine preparations containing a high concentration of antigen were prepared recently using a new technique for cultivating and purifying organisms.

M. pneumoniae grows luxuriantly on glass and remains tenaciously attached to the glass surface despite repeated washings with saline or water [67]. This property makes it possible to remove constituents of the medium from the organisms, which then can be scraped from the glass surface to yield a highly concentrated, purified suspension of mycoplasmas suitable for use in an inactivated vaccine. Conditions necessary to retain the antigenicity of the organisms growing on glass, such as maintaining a neutral pH, have been defined and incorporated into the protocol for vaccine production [68].

Although older vaccines of moderate antigenic potency have provided approximately 50% protection in field trials, several experiences have raised questions that must be resolved before further large-scale use of inactivated vaccine can be recommended.

In one volunteer study, men who failed to develop serum antibody in response to inactivated vaccine developed more severe disease following challenge with virulent organisms than did unvaccinated controls [69]. The basis for this apparent sensitization is not understood completely, but the possibility that this phenomenon will occur must be taken into account when inactivated *Mycoplasma* vaccine is used. Since volunteers who developed a serologic response to inactivated vaccine in the above-mentioned study exhibited significant resistance to challenge with wild type organisms, it is possible that a vaccine which is 100% immunogenic and stimulates a long-lived serologic response could be recommended for the prophylaxis of *M. pneumoniae* disease.

Recently, an experience with a more potent inactivated vaccine than was used in the adult volunteer study cast an additional pall over the prospects for an inactivated vaccine. Children who were inoculated parenterally with vaccine developed evidence of cell-mediated immunity to *M. pneumoniae,* but in most instances a serum antibody response was not detected [70]. This type of split immunologic response raises a number of questions concerning the safety of inactivated *M. pneumoniae* vaccine in individuals who have not been infected with the organism previously.

VI. Experimental Live Vaccines

The development of experimental live vaccines has taken two directions. With the adenoviruses, an attempt was made to produce a selective infection in an area of the body where disease manifestations rarely occur. On the other hand, efforts to develop live vaccines for influenza and respiratory syncytial viruses and *M. pneumoniae* have been directed toward producing attenuated mutants that could be administered directly into the respiratory tract. The latter approach was taken for influenza, RS virus and *M. pneumoniae* because the major importance of local respiratory tract immunity in resistance to these respiratory pathogens, has recently been recognized.

A. Adenovirus

The development of live vaccines for the prevention of adenovirus illness has proceeded slowly because of the possible oncogenic effects associated with this group of viruses. A number of the adenovirus serotypes have been shown to induce tumor formation when injected into suckling hamsters. However, vigorous attempts to link these viruses to tumors in man have been uniformly unsuccessful [71,72].

Although effective vaccines are needed for at least eight adenovirus serotypes (Types I, II, III, IV, V, VII, XIV, and XXI), initial efforts involving live virus were restricted to the development and evaluation of a vaccine for Type IV virus [30]. This virus causes large-scale epidemics of acute respiratory disease in military recruits, and this epidemiologic situation offers an ideal setting in which to evaluate the efficacy of a vaccine. Furthermore, Type IV virus lacks oncogenic potential for newborn hamsters [30].

Type IV virus was used as a model, with the expectation that the enteric approach to vaccination could be applied to other adenovirus serotypes of importance in human disease when the specter of oncogenesis has been completely dispelled. Type IV virus was administered by an atypical route so as to bypass the region of the body, i.e., the respiratory tract, in which disease manifestations usually develop. When Type IV virus was placed in an enteric–coated capsule or tablet and fed to adult volunteers, a selective infection of the lower intestinal tract occurred. In this manner the upper respiratory tract was bypassed and infection was confined to the lower intestinal tract, an area in which manifestations of disease do not develop during natural infection. This type of experimental infection was asymptomatic and stimulated the development of moderately high levels of serum neutralizing antibody [30]. Finally, infection did not spread from enterically infected volunteers or military recruits to susceptible contacts, despite close and prolonged exposure [29,30].

In subsequent studies it was found that enteric infection was transmitted in some instances from husband to wife or vice versa; however, secondary infection did not result in respiratory tract disease [73]. Although, on occasion, transmission may occur between marital partners, it seems clear that contact infection is not a risk in closely associated groups of military recruits.

To date, enteric–coated Type IV virus, grown in human diploid fibroblast culture, has been given to several hundred thousand mulitary recruits without evidence of untoward effect. The vaccine has been highly effective in preventing acute respiratory tract disease caused by Type IV virus. If vaccine is given prior to an epidemic, essentially complete protection against febrile disease caused by Type IV is provided [29].

In several military recruit centers, suppression of Type IV virus by vaccination has led to the emergence of Type VII virus as a cause of epidemic disease [74]. Currently an experimental Type VII enteric virus formulation for use in preventing resurgent Type VII disease in military recruits is being evaluated and the results are most encouraging [75]. Type VII virus behaves like Type IV virus; enteric administration of Type VII virus leads to a silent, selective intestinal infection that does not spread to individuals in close contact with the infected subject [75]. In addition, Type IV and Type VII viruses can be administered simultaneoulsy by the enteric route, without interference occurring [75,76].

Whether the live enteric vaccine or purified subunit vaccine approach will be favored ultimately is difficult to predict at this time. It is likely, however, that the balance will shift toward enteric live vaccines as concern regarding the danger of oncogenesis recedes.

B. Influenza

During the past few years interest and effort in the development of techniques for the attenuation of influenza viruses has increased anew, with the expectation that the most promising strains might be useful for the prevention of influenzal disease. Live influenza virus vaccine offers a potential advantage over inactivated vaccine in that its stimulation of local respiratory tract immunologic defenses may be more effective. Further, 100 to 1000 times more live vaccine can be prepared from an egg than is the case with inactivated vaccine. Finally, it may be possible to respond to a pandemic or epidemic challenge, posed by a new virus, more rapidly using defined genetic techniques to achieve attenuation.

Four separate techniques by which attenuation can be achieved have been described by workers in the field: (a) recombination of a pathogenic variant with an antigenically distinct virus strain known to be attenuated for man; (b) serial passage at low temperature to derive a "cold" mutant and the transfer of this property to pathogenic strains by recombination; (c) use of a chemical mutagen to induce temperature sensitive (TS) mutants and the transfer of the TS property by recombination to pathogenic strains; and (d) selection of inhibitor resistant mutants.

In early studies, methods used to achieve attenuation were based upon prolonged serial passage of virus in eggs [77,78]. This essentially blind approach was time-consuming, and to some extent the outcome was unpredictable as there were no in vitro markers that indicated the desired attenuated mutant had been recovered and selectively favored during passage. During the past few years, attenuated influenza A viruses have been derived through genetic recombination, and this has considerably shortened the time required to obtain potentially suitable vaccine strains [79,80]. When two different influenza A viruses infect the same cell, genetic recombinants are produced with high efficiency [81]. The basis for this unusual property is thought to be the segmented state of the influenza A virus genome, which is postulated to facilitate reassortment of genes, i.e., RNA segments, into maturing virus particles [82].

During a recent study in the United Kingdom genetic recombinants were obtained from a mixed infection involving the pathogenic influenza A/Hong Kong/1968 (H3N2) virus and the completely attenuated influenza A/PR-8/1934 (H0N1) virus [79,80]. Recombinants possessing the surface hemagglutinin and neuraminidase antigens (H3N2) of the Hong Kong virus, and the high growth yield of the older PR-8 (H0N1) strain, exhibited independent assortment of virulence for man and for the mouse. Two of the four recombinants studied in detail were attenuated for man to a degree thought suitable for a live vaccine strain [79]. One of the two suitably attenuated recombinants, 64D, was studied further in several hundred volunteers, and no clinical reactions were detected against the background of normal intercurrent respiratory disease [83]. In a closed population, infection did not spread from infected vaccinees to close contacts. Further, alternating passage of the 64D virus in eggs and in man was performed, and there was no evidence that the virus acquired increased virulence during successive infections in man. This was interpreted as evidence for genetic stability of the property of attenuation.

Since the PR-8 strain has a clouded passage history, workers in Britain explored the possibility of using another donor of avirulence. The Okuda strain of influenza A (H2N2) was selected for this purpose [84]. This virus had been passaged over 200 times in eggs and had been shown, in Japan, to be attenuated for children as well as for adults [84]. The Okuda strain produces distinct plaques in chick embryo kidney culture monolayers and this means that virus clones can now be selected by picking plaques rather than by terminal dilution methods.

It appears that virulence is the result of the efficient functioning of a number of different steps in the replicative cycle. Interference with any of these can lead to a reduction in virulence. Thus, attenuated strains produced by genetic recombination presumably contain one or more genes derived from the attenuated parent, and this gene, or these genes, limit replication of the recombinant virus in man. There is considerable experimental evidence which supports the polygenic nature of virulence of influenza virus [85]. Accordingly, attenuation of influenza virus by recombination is thought to result from a redistribution of avirulent and virulent genes from the two parental viruses.

Attempts to find markers that correlate with the degree of attenuation exhibited by recombinant viruses have had some success. Preliminary results in one study suggested that there was a correlation between virulence for man and the ability of a virus to stop ciliary activity in organ cultures of human trachea [86]. Also, attenuated strains were found to replicate less well in such cultures. These characteristics of one attenuated recombinant strain were found to be stable on serial passage in man.

Another approach to attenuation of influenza A and B viruses made use of the technique of "cold adaptation." This approach represents an extension of previous findings reported from the USSR [87]. In the recent studies, "cold" mutants were initially selected by step-wise "adaptation" of virus to growth at 25°C, a temperature at which naturally occurring virus grows very poorly [88]. This adaptation procedure generally required 5 to 8 months. By abruptly shifting the temperature for growth of virus to 25°C and picking plaques that developed at the low temperature, it has been possible to select stable "cold" mutants within 4 months [88]. Mutants evaluated for attenuation in man were selected by this method. More recently, it was shown that the property of growth at low temperature could be transferred by recombination to new antigenic variants; this procedure took only 5 to 7 wk [89].

In the laboratory cold mutants suitably attenuated for man were found to share six properties: (a) high level of growth at 25°C in primary chick kidney tissue culture (PCKTC) and embryonated eggs; (b) high efficiency of plaque formation in PCKTC at 25°C; (c) uniform, round 3-mm plaques at 25°C and 33°C and small irregular plaques at 37°C; (d) temperature sensitivity manifest by restriction of growth in eggs at 40°C and failure to produce plaques at 40°C; (e) acid lability; and (f) avirulence for ferrets which nevertheless developed high levels of serum antibody following infection [88]. In certain instances, strains that were over-attenuated for ferrets were produced by "cold adaptation"; these strains characteristically produced small irregular plaques at 25°C and had a labile hemagglutinin. Such strains were poorly immunogenic in ferrets.

The clinical response of volunteers to "cold" mutants of influenza A/1968 (H3N2) and influenza B/1969, which had been grown in avian leukosis virus-free eggs was evaluated recently [80,90]. Initially, the influenza A mutant was shown to be safe and immunogenic. Similar results were observed when the influenza B mutant was studied. Further, the influenza A and B mutants could be administered simultaneously to man without encountering interference in antibody production. Although vaccinees frequently shed virus, transmission of "cold" mutants did not occur under conditions highly favorable for contact infection. These observations were extended and confirmed in a series of studies performed in Naval recruits [91]. Thus, it appears that influenza viruses adapted to growth at lower temperature were suitably attenuated for man. Since cold mutants are likely to possess multiple genetic defects, including one or more temperature-sensitive lesions, it is not clear what constitutes the genetic basis for attenuation. This situation undoubtedly will be clarified when future recombinants of cold mutants and wild-type viruses bearing new surface antigens are evaluated in man.

The third approach to attenuation involves the production of TS mutants of influenza A virus. TS mutants were prepared, with the expectation that their temperature-sensitive defects would restrict virus growth in vivo, at the temperature of the lower respiratory tract ($37°C$), whereas replication should not be completely impaired in the cooler environment of the upper respiratory passages ($32°$ to $34°C$) [92,93]. TS mutants of a 1965 influenza A (H2N2) virus were produced by growing the virus in the presence of a chemical mutagen, 5-fluorouracil, and the TS lesions were then transferred to Hong Kong influenza A (H3N2) virus by genetic recombination [92,93]. Four such genetically distinct influenza A (H3N2) TS recombinants, grown in bovine kidney (BK) tissue culture, were evaluated for in vitro properties in tissue culture and for in vivo properties in the hamster and in man. The four TS recombinants exhibited a spectrum of temperature sensitivity; one recombinant had a shut-off temperature for plaque formation of $37°C$, another shut-off at $38°C$, while the remaining two recombinants had a shut-off temperature of $39°C$ [92]. The $37°C$ shut-off recombinant did not infect seronegative volunteers. The $39°C$ shut-off recombinants infected each of the seronegative volunteers tested and appeared to be attenuated; however, attenuation was not complete since most of the volunteers developed respiratory tract symptoms, in some instances, associated with low-grade fever [92, 94]. The TS recombinant, with intermediate temperature sensitivity, infected almost all seronegative volunteers and appeared to be satisfactorily attenuated, even for young children who lacked serum antibody [92,95]. Thus, there appeared to be a direct relationship between degree of temperature sensitivity in vitro and level of attenuation for man. In the initial volunteer studies it was shown that the $38°C$ recombinant, TS-1[E], induced moderate levels of serum and nasal wash neutralizing antibodies and stimulated complete protection to experimental challenge with a virulent wild-type suspension of Hong Kong virus [92]. Furthermore, it was found that the TS-1[E] virus did not spread from infected vaccinees who were shedding virus to close susceptible contacts.

In addition, $10^6 TCID_{50}$ of the TS-1[E] recombinant grown in avian leukosis virus-free eggs were given to seronegative volunteers, and their response was compared to that of men given BK culture grown virus. The egg-grown recombinant was found to be attenuated, antigenic, genetically stable, and did not differ perceptibly in its effect on seronegative volunteers from the BK grown virus [96]. Thus the important properties of the TS-1[E] recombinant appeared to be genetically determined and not influenced by the host in which the virus was grown.

Attenuation of the virus was further confirmed in a recent study by the finding that $10^7 TCID_{50}$ of egg-grown virus produced a similar, benign clinical response, although virus replication was extensive enough to induce an immunologic response in serum and nasal secretions, which approached that stimulated by the wild-type, virulent virus [96].

Evidence that the lower respiratory tract was not involved during TS-1[E] infection was provided in a study in which seven young adults who had low or undetectable serum HI antibody for the Hong Kong virus were investigated [97]. Each of the volunteers was infected following administration of 10^6 $TCID_{50}$ of TS-1[E] virus, but none of them developed any alteration in pulmonary function over a 60-day period.

The TS-1[E] vaccinees, as a group, shed approximately 3000-fold less virus from the nasopharynx than did volunteers infected with wild-type virus, indicating that the recombinant was also attenuated for the upper respiratory tract. To date, virus isolates from 48 volunteers to whom the TS-1[E] virus was administered have been examined for their temperature sensitivity, and each isolate was shown to retain the TS phenotype, thus documenting the genetic stability of this virus in man. The inability of the TS-1[E] virus to produce contact infection is probably due, in part, to its failure to induce cough or extensive sneezing and also to its high human infectious $dose_{50}$ (HID_{50}) which appears to be approximately 10^5 $TCID_{50}$/ml [96]. The high HID_{50} of the TS-1[E] virus may be of particular importance, since the quantity of virus produced in the nasopharynx is relatively small.

The ease with which the TS-1[E] lesion could be transferred from the Hong Kong TS-1[E] mutant to other influenza A viruses by recombination suggests that it should be possible to effect a rapid transfer of this genetic lesion to new viruses that assume pandemic or epidemic importance. Presumably, transfer of the TS-1[E] lesion will confer attenuation on the recipient virus. Fortunately, this type of transfer can be made to new strains, since the TS-1[E] lesion does not involve genes that code for the surface glycoprotein antigens—the hemagglutinin and the neuraminidase enzyme [92].

The fourth approach used to attenuate influenza virus is based on observations made in the USSR a number of years ago. Inhibitor resistant mutants of influenza viruses were derived in several laboratories in the USSR [77]. Later, similar strains were produced in Britain by the serial passage of virus in the presence of horse serum that contained a potent inhibitor of hemagglutination activity [98]. Such mutants were frequently, but not always, found to be attenuated for man. Recently, Belgian workers derived a mutant of influenza A/1969 (H3N2) virus completely resistant to inhibitors of viral hemagglutination in the serum of guinea pigs and horses [99]. This in vitro marker was found to be stable after passage of the mutant in eggs, experimental animals, and man.

Inhibitor resistant influenza A (H3N2) virus has been given to approximately 1000 individuals, 16 to 75 years of age, without evidence of any untoward reaction. Lower respiratory tract symptoms were not observed [99]. It appeared that approximately 10^7 EID_{50}, given in two doses, were required to induce a serum hemagglutination-inhibition (HI) antibody response in 80% to 95% of individuals with a prevaccine serum HI titer of 1:32 or less. This dose of virus was also effective in stimulating a local nasal antibody response in the same proportion of vaccinees. Vaccine virus could be recovered from 25% of vaccinees, but the amount of virus excreted appeared to be low. Virus recovered from infected vaccinees retained its inhibitor resistance. In three separate closed populations infection did not spread from infected vaccinees to close contacts.

The biologic basis for attenuation of serum inhibitor-resistant influenza A viruses is not fully understood. Presumably, inhibitor-resistant viruses undergo a mutation in the gene that codes for the surface glycoprotein responsible for hemagglutination. If this type of change in the structure of hemagglutinin is responsible for attenuation, then it will not be possible to transfer attenuation to new influenza viruses of public health importance. Each new influenza virus will have to be approached as a new situation, and inhibitor-resistant mutants will need to be derived and evaluated de novo.

It is of interest that each of the four different approaches to attenuation of influenza virus yielded avirulent virus several orders of magnitude less infectious for man than the parent, wild-type virus. Each of the attenuated viruses grew considerably less well in the respiratory tract of man than did the parental, wild-type virus and this was associated with a benign clinical response to infection. Further, contact infection did not appear to occur with any of the candidate vaccine strains; presumably this was a manifestation of the small quantity of virus produced during infection and the low infectivity of each of these viruses for man. However, each of the candidate strains appeared to be moderately antigenic, stimulating antibody against both hemagglutinin and neuraminidase antigens. Although the immunologic response to infection with attenuated viruses did not equal that induced by natural infection, there was evidence that the level of response was sufficient to protect the host from virulent virus. For example, prior infection with the TS-1[E] recombinant induced complete resistance to experimental challenge with virulent virus [92]. Similarly, there was evidence that the inhibitor-resistant mutant of a 1969 (H3N2) virus provided protection against natural challenge with homologous virus and, more recently, the heterologous 1972 London (H3N2) virus [100]. There is no information available concerning the duration of vaccine immunity. Finally, it should be noted that the need to match antigens of a live vaccine virus to those of the epidemic strain appears to be as great as that previously recognized for inactivated influenza vaccines.

C. Respiratory Syncytial Virus (RS Virus)

As mentioned earlier, consideration of the epidemiology of RS virus infection strongly suggested that local defense mechanisms in the respiratory tract played a major role in resistance to illness caused by this virus. For this reason, a high priority was given to the development of an attenuated strain of RS virus that would induce resistance to the virus in young infants without producing significant illness. In the early phase of this effort, a cold mutant of RS virus was evaluated in infants and children [101]. This mutant produced a silent infection in individuals previously infected with RS virus. However, mild lower respiratory disease developed in one of three seronegative infants given the candidate vaccine strain. These observations indicated that a considerable degree of attenuation had been achieved, but the residual virulence of the low–temperature adapted strain made it unacceptable for use in young infants, the group for whom an RS virus vaccine is most urgently needed.

Encouraged by the partial success of the low–temperature adapted RS virus strain, efforts were directed at the development of other candidate RS viruses, which might offer the possibility of greater attenuation. One such strain was a TS mutant induced by the chemical mutagen 5-fluorouridine [102]. This strain, designated TS-1, was chosen for clinical evaluation on the basis of its behavior in vitro in tissue culture and in vivo in the hamster host. This mutant did not produce plaques, i.e., did not initiate foci of infection, at $37°C$ or above in tissue culture, unlike wild–type virus, which produced plaques without restriction at $39°C$. In the hamster, infection with the mutant was limited to the cooler upper respiratory tract ($32°$ to $34°C$), and virus did not grow in the lungs where the temperature was $37°C$. The mutant appeared to be stable genetically in the hamster. In later studies adult volunteers, all of whom were seropositive, underwent a silent infection following nasopharyngeal administration of the mutant, and they were resistant to subsequent challenge with virulent, wild–type virus [103,104]. Finally, the TS-1 mutant appeared to be stable genetically in adults in that the isolates obtained from the volunteers retained the TS property.

Encouraged by the response of adult volunteers, studies were extended into younger individuals. Each of the 32 infants and children studied were infected when the mutant was administered by the nasopharyngeal route [105]. Twenty-five of the children had been infected with natural RS virus previously, whereas the remaining seven infants were thought to have escaped prior infection. Following infection with the mutant, individuals in the former group failed to develop symptoms or developed at most mild rhinorrhea. In contrast, the seven infants without prior RS virus experience developed moderate rhinorrhea and one of these individuals subsequently developed otitis media. Mild to moderate rhinitis may be an acceptable price to pay for protection against serious RS virus disease of the lower respiratory tract in early life. However, the occurrence of secondary otitis media is probably not acceptable, and for this reason efforts have been initiated to produce a mutant slightly more attenuated than TS-1.

Also, genetic instability has been a problem with the TS-1 mutant. A small proportion of the virus recovered from the young vaccinees exhibited evidence of genetic alteration, as indicated by a partial or complete loss of the TS property [106]. Although genetic alteration of the TS-1 mutant in vivo in children was not associated with any untoward clinical reaction, this type of genetic lability is not desirable. For this reason, attempts are now underway to introduce multiple TS mutations into candidate vaccine strains slated for clinical evaluation in infants. Hopefully, this will minimize the possibility of reversion from the TS phenotype as well as effect a greater reduction in virulence than was seen with the TS-1 mutant.

D. *Mycoplasma pneumoniae*

Infection with this organism appears to be quite superficial, involving only the respiratory epithelium. Further, local, immune defense mechanisms in the respiratory tract seem to be more effective in protecting the host than is systemic immunity. When considered together, these observations provide a basis for pursuing the development of an attenuated mutant that could be administered locally into the respiratory tract and that would stimulate local immune processes in this area.

Initially, a series of temperature sensitive mutants of *M. pneumoniae* were produced by exposing the organism to N-methyl-N'-nitro-N-nitrosoguanidine (NTG) [107]. Mutants were recovered which were restricted in growth in vitro at $37°C$ or $38°C$. At $37°C$ and $38°C$ the wild-type organism grew without restriction. Missence mutants of the TS class were sought, with the expectation that their temperature-sensitive defects would restrict growth in vivo at the temperature of the lower respiratory tract ($37°C$), whereas replication should not be seriously impaired in the cooler environment of the upper respiratory passages ($32°C$ to $34°C$). It was shown that TS mutants, as a group, were attenuated for the Syrian hamster, and prior infection with the mutants induced resistance to subsequent challenge with wild-type organisms [108].

Five of the most genetically stable mutants were subjected to more detailed analysis [64]. These mutants exhibited a gradient of temperature sensitivity; however, each of the mutants was completely stable genetically in vivo as well as in vitro.

The mutant with intermediate temperature sensitivity (TS 640) was the first to be evaluated in man [64]. In the laboratory, mutant TS 640 was found to be partially restricted in growth on agar at $37°C$ and completely restricted at $38°C$. The mutant was studied in 11 volunteers who lacked preexisting serum metabolism–inhibiting (MI) antibody. Each of the volunteers was infected and nine of the men underwent a silent infection. However, two of the volunteers developed bronchitis, which indicated that this mutant possessed sufficient residual virulence to disqualify it as a candidate vaccine strain. Nonetheless, the results of the study were encouraging, since the TS 640 mutant exhibited significant loss of virulence and the mutant was genetically stable in man, i.e., each of the isolates recovered from the volunteers retained the TS property.

The next mutant after TS 640 in the temperature–sensitivity gradient was TS H43, and this organism was completely restricted in growth on agar at 37°C. In a second volunteer trial, TS H43 was given by the nasopharyngeal route to 16 volunteers who lacked serum MI antibody, with the expectation that it would be more attenuated than the TS 640 mutant. Each of the volunteers became infected and developed a significant immunologic response, however, none of the men became ill [28]. Furthermore, in each instance the organisms recovered from the infected volunteers retained the TS phenotype of the mutant. Thus, the TS H43 mutant appeared to be suitably attenuated and genetically stable in man. At this point, expanded study of the TS H43 mutant appears indicated, since the organism possesses many of the properties desired of a strain to be used for prevention of *M. pneumoniae* disease.

References

1. R. M. Chanock, Control of acute mycoplasmal and viral respiratory tract disease, *Science*, **169**:248–256 (1970).
2. T. Francis, Jr. and H. F. Maassab, Influenza viruses. *Viral and Rickettsial Infections of Man*. Fourth edition. Philadelphis, L. B. Lippincott, 1965, pp. 689–740.
3. C. H. Stuart–Harris, Clinical characteristics, Twenty years of influenza epidemics, *Am. Rev. Respir. Dis.*, **83**:54–61 (1961).
4. D. E. Rogers, General discussion, *Am. Rev. Respir. Dis.*, **83**:61–67 (1961).
5. R. M. Chanock and R. H. Parrott, Acute respiratory disease in infancy and childhood: Present understanding and prospects for prevention, *Pediatrics*, **36**:21–39 (1965).
6. C. D. Brandt, H. W. Kim, A. J. Vargosko, B. C. Jeffries, J. O. Arrobio, B. Rindge, R. H. Parrott, and R. M. Chanock, Infections in 18,000 infants and children in a controlled study of respiratory tract disease. I. Adenovirus pathogenicity in relation to serologic type and illness syndrome, *Am. J. Epidemiol.*, **90**:484–500 (1969).
7. R. J. Huebner, W. P. Rowe, and R. M. Chanock, Newly recognized respiratory tract viruses. In *Annual Review of Microbiology*. Vol. 12. Edited by C. E. Clifton, S. Raffel, and M. P. Starr. Palo Alto, Annual Reviews Inc., 1958, pp. 49–76.

8. J. Van der Veen, The role of adenoviruses in respiratory disease, *Am. Rev. Respir. Dis.,* Suppl., **88**:167–180 (1963).
9. H. M. Foy, G. E. Kenny, R. McMahan, A. M. Mansy, and J. T. Grayston, Mycoplasma pneumoniae. Pneumonia in an urban area, *J.A.M.A.,* **214**: 1666–1672 (1970).
10. R. M. Chanock, Mycoplasma infections of man, *N. Engl. J. Med.,* **273**: 1199–1206 (1965).
11. R. M. Chanock, H. H. Fox, W. D. James, R. R. Gutekunst, R. J. White, and L. B. Senterfit, Epidemiology of M. pneumoniae infection in military recruits, *Ann. N. Y. Acad. Sci.,* **143**:484–496 (1967).
12. A. S. Evans and M. Brobst, Bronchitis, pneumonitis, and pneumonia in University of Wisconsin students, *N. Engl. J. Med.,* **265**:401–409 (1961).
13. C. D. Dauer and R. E. Serfling, Mortality from influenza, *Am. Rev. Respir. Dis.,* **83**:15–28 (1961).
14. A. D. Langmuir and J. Housworth, A critical evaluation of influenza surveillance, *Bull. W. H. O.,* **41**:393–398 (1969).
15. M. A. Mufson, Y. Chang, V. Gill, S. C. Wood, M. J. Romansky, and R. M. Chanock, The role of viruses, mycoplasmas, and bacteria in acute pneumonia in civilian adults, *Am. J. Epidemiol.,* **86**:526–544 (1967).
16. A. C. Stenhouse, Rhinovirus infection in acute exacerbations of chronic bronchitis: A controlled prospective study, *Br. Med. J.,* **3**:461–463 (1967).
17. R. G. Webster, On the origin of pandemic influenza viruses, *Curr. Top. Microbiol.,* **59**:76–105 (1972).
18. R. Murray, Production and testing in the USA of influenza virus vaccine made from the Hong Kong variant in 1968–69, *Bull. W. H. O.,* **41**:495–496 (1969).
19. A. Z. Kapikian, R. M. Conant, V. V. Hamparian, R. M. Chanock, E. C. Dick, J. M. Gwaltney, Jr., D. Hamre, W. S. Jordan, Jr., G. E. Kenny, E. H. Lennette, J. L. Melnick, W. J. Mogabgab, C. A. Phillips, J. H. Schieble, E. J. Stott, and D. A. J. Tyrrell, A collaborative report: Rhinoviruses—extension of the numbering system, *Virology,* **43**:524–526 (1971).
20. H. H. Bloom, K. M. Johnson, R. Jacobsen, and R. M. Chanock, Recovery of parainfluenza viruses from adults with upper respiratory illness, *Am. J. Hyg.,* **74**:50–59 (1961).
21. R. M. Chanock, R. H. Parrott, K. M. Johnson, A. Z. Kapikian, and J. A. Bell, Myxoviruses: Parainfluenza, *Am. Rev. Respir. Dis.,* **88**:152–166 (1963).
22. M. Beem, Repeated infections with respiratory syncytial virus, *J. Immunol.,* **98**:1115–1122 (1967).
23. H. V. Coates and R. M. Chanock, Clinical significance of respiratory syncytial virus, *Postgrad. Med.,* **35**:460–465 (1964).
24. C. E. Hall, M. K. Cooney, and J. P. Fox, The Seattle Virus Watch. III. Comparative epidemiologic observations of infections with influenza A and B viruses, 1965–1969, in families with young children, *Am. J. Epidemiol.,* **98**:365–380 (1973).
25. R. H. Parrott, H. W. Kim, J. O. Arrobio, D. S. Hodes, B. R. Murphy, C. D. Brandt, E. Camargo, and R. M. Chanock, Epidemiology of respiratory

syncytial virus infection in Washington, D.C.: II. Infection and disease
with respect to age, immunologic status, race, and sex, *Am. J. Epidemiol.,*
98:289–300 (1973).

26. C. B. Smith, R. H. Purcell, J. A. Bellanti, and R. M. Chanock, Protective
     effect of antibody to parainfluenza type 1 virus, *N. Engl. J. Med.,* **275**:
     1145–1152 (1966).

27. J. C. Perkins, D. N. Tucker, H. L. S. Knopf, R. P. Wenzel, A. Z. Kapikian,
     and R. M. Chanock, Comparison of protective effect of neutralizing anti-
     body in serum and nasal secretions in experimental rhinovirus type 13
     illness, *Am. J. Epidemiol.,* **90**:519–526 (1969).

28. H. Greenberg, C. Helms, and R. M. Chanock, Asymptomatic infection of
     adult volunteers with a temperature sensitive mutant of mycoplasma
     pneumoniae, *Proc. Natl. Acad. Sci. U.S.A.,* **71**:4015–4019 (1974).

29. W. P. Edmondson, R. H. Purcell, B. F. Gundelfinger, J. W. P. Love, W.
     Ludwig, and R. M. Chanock, Immunization by selective infection with
     type 4 adenovirus growth in humans diploid culture. II. Specific protec-
     tive effect against epidemic disease, *J.A.M.A.,* **195**:453–459 (1966).

30. R. M. Chanock, W. Ludwig, R. J. Huebner, T. R. Cate, and L. W. Chu,
     Immunization by selective infection with type 4 adenovirus grown in
     human diploid tissue culture. I. Safety and lack of oncogenicity and
     tests for potency in volunteers, *J.A.M.A.,* **195**:445–452 (1966).

31. T. J. Smith, E. L. Buescher, F. H. Top, Jr., W. A. Altermeier, and J. M.
     McCowan, Experimental respiratory infection with type 4 adenovirus
     vaccine in volunteers: Clinical and immunological responses, *J. Infect.
     Dis.,* **122**:239–248 (1970).

32. R. E. Wetherbee, Induction of systemic delayed hypersensitivity during
     experimental viral infection of the respiratory tract with a myxovirus of
     paramyxovirus, *J. Immunol.,* **111**:157–163 (1973).

33. G. Biberfeld, Communications. Macrophage Migration inhibition in
     response to experimental mycoplasma pneumoniae infection in the
     hamster, *J. Immunol.,* **110**:1146–1150 (1973).

34. T. B. Tomasi and J. Bienenstock, Secretory immunoglobulins, *Adv.
     Immunol.,* **9**:1–96 (1968).

35. R. H. Waldman and C. S. Henney, Cell–mediated immunity and antibody
     responses in the respiratory tract after local and systemic immunization,
     J. Exp. Med., **134**:482–494 (1971).

36. R. M. Chanock, R. H. Parrott, A. Z. Kapikian, H. W. Kim, and C. D.
     Brandt, Possible role of immunologic factors in pathogenesis of RS virus
     lower respiratory tract disease. In *Perspectives in Virology VI.* Edited by
     M. Pollard. New York, Academic Press, Inc., 1968, pp. 125–139.

37. H. W. Kim, J. G. Canchola, C. D. Brandt, G. Pyles, R. M. Chanock, K.
     Jensen, and R. H. Parrott, Respiratory syncytial virus disease in infants
     despite prior administration of antigenic inactivated vaccine, *Am. J. Epide-
     miol.,* **89**:422–434 (1969).

38. A. Z. Kapikian, R. H. Mitchell, and R. M. Chanock, An epidemiologic

study of altered clinical reactivity to respiratory syncytial (RS) virus infection in children previously vaccinated with an inactivated RS virus vaccine, *Am. J. Epidemiol.,* **89**:405–421 (1969).

39. S. Fazekas de St. Growth and M. Donnelley, Studies in experimental immunology of influenza: IV. The protective value of active immunization, *Aust. J. Exp. Biol. Med. Sci.,* **28**:61–75 (1950).

40. A. M. Collier, Pathogenesis of mycoplasma pneumoniae infection as studied in human fetal trachea in organ culture. In *Pathogenic Mycoplasmas.* New York, Associated Scientific, 1972, pp. 307–327.

41. G. W. Fernald and W. A. Clyde, Jr., Protective effect of vaccines in experimental mycoplasma pneumoniae disease, *Infect. Immunol.,* **1**:559–565 (1970).

42. J. Mills, H. L. S. Knopf, J. E. Van Kirk, and R. M. Chanock, Significance of local respiratory tract antibody to respiratory syncytial virus. In *The Secretory Immunologic System.* Edited by D. H. Dayton, Jr., P. A. Small, R. M. Chanock, H. E. Kaufman, and T. B. Tomasi, Jr. Washington, D.C., Govt. Printing Off., 1971, pp. 149–165.

43. H. Brunner, H. B. Greenberg, W. D. James, R. L. Horswood, R. B. Couch, and R. M. Chanock, Antibody to mycoplasma pneumoniae in nasal secretions and sputa of experimentally infected human volunteers, *Infect. Immunol.,* **8**:612–620 (1973).

44. F. M. Davenport, Killed influenza virus vaccines: Present status suggested use, desirable developments. International Conference on the Application of Vaccines Against Viral, Rickettsial, and Bacterial Diseases of Man. Washington, D.C., 1970, pp. 89–95.

45. F. M. Davenport, Present status of inactivated influenza virus vaccines. First International Conference on Vaccines Against Viral and Rickettsial Diseases of Man. Washington, D.C., Pan American Health Organization, 1967, pp. 3–8.

46. R. H. Waldman, J. A. Kasel, R. V. Fulk, Y. Togo, R. B. Hornick, G. G. Heiner, A. T. Dawkins, and J. J. Mann, Influenza antibody in human respiratory secretions after subcutaneous or respiratory immunization with inactivated virus, *Nature,* **218**:594–595 (1968).

47. J. A. Kasel, E. B. Hume, R. V. Fulk, Y. Togo, M. Huber, and R. B. Hornick, Antibody responses in nasal secretions and serum of elderly persons following local or parenteral administration of inactivated influenza virus vaccine, *J. Immunol.,* **102**:555–562 (1969).

48. C. B. Smith, J. A. Bellanti, and R. M. Chanock, Immunoglobulins in serum and nasal secretions following infection with type 1 parainfluenza virus and injection of inactivated vaccines, *J. Immunol.,* **99**:133–141 (1967).

49. A. F. Woodhour, A. Friedman, R. E. Wiebel, and M. R. Hilleman, Clinical and laboratory studies of improved adjuvant 65 influenza vaccines. Internal Symposium on Influenza Vaccines for Man and Horses, London. *Symp. Ser. Immunobiol. Stand.,* **20**:125–132 (1972).

50. D. S. Freestone, S. Hamilton–Smith, G. C. Schild, R. Buckland, S. Chinn,

and D. A. J. Tyrrell, Antibody response and resistance to challenge in volunteers vaccinated with live attenuated detergent split and oil adjuvant A2/Hong Kong/68 (H3N2) influenza vaccines, *J. Hyg.*, **70**:531–543 (1972).

51. G. W. Beebe, A. H. Simon, and S. Vivona, Long–term mortality follow up of army recruits who received adjuvant influenza virus vaccine in 1951–1953, *Am. J. Epidemiol.*, **95**:337–346 (1972).

52. J. Kavets, ScD Thesis. Influenza and public policy. Boston, Massachusetts, Harvard School of Public Health, 1972.

53. E. D. Kilbourne, Future influenza vaccines and the use of genetic recombinants, *Bull. W. H. O.*, **41**:643–645 (1969).

54. A. Vargosko, R. M. Chanock, R. J. Huebner, A. H. Luckey, H. W. Kim, C. Cumming, and R. H. Parrott, Association of type 2 hemadsorption (parainfluenza 1) virus and asian influenza A virus with infectious coup, *N. Engl. J. Med.*, **261**:1–9 (1959).

55. M. R. Hilleman, R. A. Stallones, R. L. Gauld, M. S. Warfield, and S. A. Anderson, Prevention of acute respiratory illness in recruits by adenovirus (R1–APC–ARD) vaccine, *Proc. Soc. Exp. Biol. Med.*, **92**:337–383 (1956).

56. R. W. Sherwood, E. L. Buescher, R. E. Nitz, and J. W. Cooch, Effects of adenovirus vaccine on acute respiratory disease in U.S. army recruits, *J. Am. Med. Assoc.*, **178**:1125–1127 (1961).

57. R. J. Huebner, R. M. Chanock, B. A. Rubin, and M. J. Casey, Induction by adenovirus type 7 of tumors in hamsters having the antigenic characteristics of SV40 virus, *Proc. Natl. Acad. Sci.*, **52**:1333–1340 (1964).

58. W. P. Rowe and S. G. Baum, Evidence for a possible genetic hybrid between adenovirus type 7 and SV40 viruses, *Proc. Natl. Acad. Sci.*, **52**: 1340–1347 (1964).

59. W. P. Rowe and S. G. Baum, Studies of adenovirus SV40 hybrid viruses. II. Defectiveness of the hybrid particles, *J. Exp. Med.*, **122**:955–966 (1965.

60. B. E. Eddy, G. S. Borman, G. E. Grubbs, and R. D. Young, Identification of the oncogenic substance in rhesus monkey kidney cell cultures as simian virus 40, *Virology*, **17**:65–75 (1962).

61. J. Chin, R. L. Magoffin, L. A. Shearer, J. H. Schieble, and E. H. Lennette, Field evaluation of a respiratory syncytial virus vaccine and a trivalent parainfluenza virus vaccine in a pediatric population, *Am. J. Epidemiol.*, **89**:449–463 (1969).

62. V. A. Fulginiti, J. J. Eller, O. F. Sieber, J. W. Joyner, M. Minamitani, and G. Meiklejohn, Respiratory virus immunization, *Am. J. Epidemiol.*, **89**: 435–448 (1969).

63. R. B. Couch, J. A. Kasel, H. G. Pereira, A. T. Haase, and V. Knight, Induction of immunity in man by crystalline adenovirus type 5 capsid antigens, *Proc. Soc. Exp. Biol. Med.*, **143**:905–910 (1973).

64. H. Brunner, H. Greenberg, W. D. James, R. L. Horswood, and R. M. Chanock, Decreased virulence and protective effect of genetically stable

temperature–sensitive mutants of mycoplasma pneumoniae, *Ann. N. Y. Acad. Sci.,* **225**:436–454 (1973).

65. R. M. Chanock, C. B. Smith, W. T. Friedewald, R. R. Gutenkunst, P. Steinberg, S. Fuld, K. E. Jensen, L. B. Senterfit, and B. Prescott, Mycoplasma pneumoniae infection—prospects for live and inactivated vaccines. First International Conference on Vaccines Against Viral and Rickettsial Diseases of Man. Pan American Health Organization, Washington, D.C. *Science,* **147**:132–140 (1967).

66. W. J. Mogabgab, Mycoplasma pneumoniae vaccines. International Conference on the Application of Vaccines Against Viral, Rickettsial, and Bacterial Diseases of Man. Washington, D.C., 1970, pp. 117–126.

67. N. L. Somerson, W. D. James, B. E. Walls, and R. M. Chanock, Growth of mycoplasma pneumoniae on a glass surface, *Ann. N. Y. Acad. Sci.,* **143**: 384–389 (1967).

68. J. D. Pollack, N. L. Somerson, and L. B. Senterfit, Effect of pH on the immunogenicity of mycoplasma pneumoniae, *J. Bacteriol.,* **97**:612–619 (1969).

69. C. B. Smith, W. T. Friedewald, R. H. Alford, and R. M. Chanock, Mycoplasma pneumoniae infections in volunteers, *Ann. N. Y. Acad. Sci.,* **143**: 471–483 (1967).

70. G. W. Fernald and P. Glezen, Humoral and cellular immune responses to an inactivated mycoplasma pneumoniae vaccine in children, *J. Infect. Dis.,* **127**:498–504 (1973).

71. R. J. Huebner, The problem of oncogenicity of adenoviruses. First International Conference on Vaccines Against Viral and Rickettsial Diseases of Man. Washington, D.C., Pan American Health Organization, 1967, pp. 73–80.

72. R. V. Gilden, J. Kern, Y. K. Lee, F. Rapp, J. L. Melnick, J. L. Riggs, E. H. Lennette, B. Zbar, H. J. Rapp, H. C. Turner, and R. J. Huebner, Serologic surveys of human cancer patients for antibody to adenovirus T antigens, *Am. J. Epidemiol.,* **91**:500–509 (1970).

73. E. D. Stanley and G. G. Jackson, Spread of enteric live adenovirus type 4 vaccine in married couples, *J. Infect. Dis.,* **119**:51–59 (1969).

74. E. L. Buescher, Respiratory disease and the adenoviruses, *Med. Clin. North. Am.,* **51**:769–779 (1967).

75. F. H. Top, Jr., B. A. Dudding, P. K. Russell, and E. L. Buescher, Control of respiratory disease in recruits with types 4 and 7 adenovirus vaccines, *Am. J. Epidemiol.,* **94**:142–146 (1971).

76. R. B. Couch, R. M. Chanock, T. R. Cate, D. J. Long, and V. Knight, Immunization with types 4 and 7 adenovirus by selective infection of the intestinal tract, *Am. Rev. Respir. Dis.,* **88**:394–403 (1963).

77. V. M. Zhdanov, Present status of live influenza virus vaccines. First International Conference on Vaccines Against Viral and Rickettsial Diseases of Man. Washington, D.C., Pan American Health Organization, 1967, pp. 9–15.

78. A. S. Beare, M. L. Bynoe, and D. A. J. Tyrrell, Investigation into the attenuation of influenza viruses by serial passage, *Br. Med. J.*, 4:482–484 (1968).

79. A. S. Beare and T. S. Hall, Recombinant influenza-A viruses as live vaccines for man, *Lancet*, 2:1271–1273 (1971).

80. A. S. Beare, H. F. Maassab, D. A. J. Tyrrell, A. N. Slepushkin, and T. S. Hall, A comparative study of attenuated influenza viruses, *Bull. W. H. O.*, 44:593–598 (1971).

81. R. W. Simpson and G. K. Hirst, Temperature–sensitive mutants of influenza A virus: Isolation of mutants and preliminary observations on genetic recombination and complementation, *Virology*, 35:41–49 (1968).

82. G. K. Hirst, Mechanism of influenza recombination, *Virology*, 55:81–93 (1973).

83. A. S. Beare and D. A. J. Tyrrell. Unpublished data.

84. Y. Okuno and K Nakamura, Prophylactic effectiveness of live influenza vaccine, *Biken, J.*, 9:89–95 (1966).

85. E. D. Kilbourne, Influenza virus genetics, *Prog. Med. Virol.*, 5:79–126 (1963).

86. S. R. Mostow and D. A. J. Tyrrell, Detection of attenuation of recombinant influenza viruses in vitro, *Lancet*, 2:116–117 (1972).

87. A. A. Smorodincev, The efficacy of live influenza vaccines, *Bull. W. H. O.*, 41:585–588 (1969).

88. H. F. Maassab, T. Francis, Jr., F. M. Davenport, A. V. Hennessy, E. Minuse, and G. Anderson, Laboratory and clinical characteristics of attenuated strains of influenza virus, *Bull. W. H. O.*, 41:589–594 (1969).

89. H. Maassab, A. P. Kendal, and F. M. Davenport, Hybrid formation of influenza virus at 25° (35234), *Proc. Soc. Exp. Biol. Med.*, 139:768–773 (1972).

90. F. M. Davenport, A. V. Hennessy, E. Minuse, H. F. Maassab, G. R. Anderson, J. R. Mitchell, J. C. Heffelfinger, and C. D. Barret, Jr., Pilot studies on mono and bivalent live attenuated influenza virus vaccines. Proceedings of the Symposium on Live Influenza Vaccine. Zagreb, Yugoslav Academy of Sciences, 1971, pp. 105–113.

91. E. A. Edwards, R. E. Mammen, M. J. Rosenbaum, R. O. Peckinpaugh, J. R. Mitchell, H. F. Maassab, E. Minuse, A. V. Hennessy, and F. M. Davenport, Live influenza vaccine studies in human volunteers. International Symposium on Influenza Vaccines for Men and Horses. Edited by F. T. Perkins and R. H. Regamey. *Series Immunobiol. Standard*, 20:289–294 (1973).

92. B. R. Murphy, E. G. Chalhub, S. R. Nusinoff, and R. M. Chanock, Temperature sensitive mutants of influenza virus. II. Attenuation of ts recombinants for man, *J. Infect. Dis.*, 126:170–178 (1972).

93. J. Mills and R. M. Chanock, Temperature–sensitive mutants of influenza virus. I. Behavior in tissue culture and in experimental animals, *J. Infect. Dis.*, 123:145–157 (1971).

94. B. R. Murphy, D. S. Hodes, S. R. Nusinoff, S. Spring–Stewart, E. L. Tierney, and R. M. Chanock, Temperature sensitive mutants of influenza virus. V. Evaluation in man of an additional ts recombinant virus with a 39°C shutoff temperature, *J. Infect. Dis.*, **130**:144–149 (1974).

95. R. H. Parrott and H. W. Kim. Unpublished data.

96. B. R. Murphy, E. G. Chalhub, S. R. Nusinoff, J. Kasel, and R. M. Chanock, Temperature–sensitive mutants of influenza virus. III. Further characterization of the ts–1[E] influenza A recombinant (H3N2) virus in man, *J. Infect. Dis.*, **128**:479–487 (1973).

97. W. H. Hall, R. G. Douglas, Jr., D. A. Zaky, R. W. Hyde, D. Richman, and B. R. Murphy, Evaluation of an attenuated virus in normal adults (The role of pulmonary function studies in vaccine trials), *J. Clin. Invest.*, (1975). In press.

98. A. S. Beare, Laboratory characteristics of attenuated influenza virus, *Bull. W. H. O.*, **41**:595–598 (1969).

99. C. Huygelen, J. Peetermans, E. Vascoboinic, E. Berge, and G. Colinet, Live attenuated influenza virus vaccine in vitro and in vivo properties. International Symposium on Influenza Vaccines for Men and Horses. London, *Series Immunobiol. Standard*, **20**:152–157 (1973).

100. C. Huygelen. Unpublished data.

101. H. W. Kim, J. O. Arrobio, G. Pyles, C. D. Brandt, E. Camargo, R. M. Chanock, and R. H. Parrott, Clinical and immunological response of infants and children to administration of low–temperature adapted respiratory syncytial virus, *Pediatrics*, **48**:745–755 (1971).

102. M. A. Gharpure, P. F. Wright, and R. M. Chanock, Temperature–sensitive mutants of respiratory syncytial virus, *J. Virol.*, **3**:414–421 (1969).

103. P. F. Wright, W. G. Woodend, and R. M. Chanock, Temperature–sensitive mutants of respiratory syncytial virus: In vivo studies in hamsters, *J. Infect. Dis.*, **122**:501–512 (1970).

104. P. F. Wright, J. Mills, V. Chanock, and R. M. Chanock, Evaluation of a temperature–sensitive mutant of respiratory syncytial virus in adults, *J. Infect. Dis.*, **124**:505–511 (1971).

105. H. W. Kim, J. O. Arrobio, C. D. Brandt, P. Wright, D. Hodes, R. M. Chanock, and R. H. Parrott, Safety and antigenicity of temperature sensitime (TS) mutant respiratory syncytial virus (RSV) in infants and children, *Pediatrics*, **52**:56–63 (1973).

106. D. S. Hodes, H. W. Kim, R. H. Parrott, and R. M. Chanock, Genetic alteration in a temperature–sensitive mutant of respiratory syncytial virus after replication in vivo, *Proc. Soc. Exp. Biol. Med.*, **145**:1158–1164 (1974).

107. P. Steinberg, R. L. Horswood, and R. M. Chanock, Temperature sensitive mutants of mycoplasma pneumoniae. I. In vitro biologic properties, *J. Infect. Dis.*, **120**:217–224 (1969).

108. P. Steinberg, R. L. Horswood, H. Brunner, and R. M. Chanock, Temperature–sensitive mutants of mycoplasma pneumoniae. II. Response of hamsters, *J. Infect. Dis.*, **123**:179–187 (1971).

19

Antibacterial Vaccines for Lower Lung Infections

MALCOLM S. ARTENSTEIN

Walter Reed Army Institute of Research
Washington, D.C.

I. Introduction

Vaccines against bacterial infections have been prepared by a variety of techniques, which have at least one major feature in common—the bacteria or purified products extracted from them are administered to the subject in a fashion that will stimulate the development of specific immunity mechanisms. All bacteria contain a variety of antigens to which the host responds immunologically, but not all of these responses enhance host–resistance to infection. Thus, group A β–hemolytic streptococcus infection induces humoral antibodies to certain antigens, such as streptolysin O and the group A carbohydrate, yet these have no effect on resistance to subsequent infection; rather, the M protein of the streptococcal cell wall is the virulence antigen to which antibodies confer type–specific immunity. In developing a vaccine, then, it is imperative that the product contain the relevant antigen in an immunogenic form. This can often be accomplished by using a vaccine consisting of the whole bacterial cell inactivated by one means or another. But such vaccines containing millions of dead bacteria are usually quite toxic to the host. Therefore, some type of detoxification must be accomplished.

Killed whole cell vaccines do not always contain the important antigen(s) in sufficient concentration to stimulate immunity, and multiple injections may be required. The use of live attenuated vaccines can circumvent some of these problems, since the viable strain multiplies in the host presenting the significant antigen(s) in higher concentration or in a more natural form. Yet live vaccines present a series of problems related to safety and potency, which must be solved prior to large-scale use. Another approach to the development of vaccines, which has been spurred by recent advances in the field of chemistry, is to extract and purify the relevant antigen from bacterial cultures. In this way the antigen can be concentrated, if necessary, and administered free from toxic materials. In the subsequent sections of this chapter examples of these approaches to bacterial vaccines will be presented.

Very few vaccines against bacterial pulmonary pathogens are currently available for general medical use. However, a somewhat larger number are in the experimental stage. Both categories are listed in Table 1.

II. Pertussis

Whooping cough (pertussis), once a highly prevalent, highly feared childhood disease, has become a medical rarity in the United States. The declining incidence of whooping cough has been directly related to the widespread use of effective pertussis vaccines, which began in the 1940s [1]. The success of these vaccines may also be responsible for the fact that little new has been learned about pertussis during the past decade, despite advances in knowledge of the immunology of many other infectious diseases during this period.

Bordetella pertussis is the etiologic agent in the great majority of cases, although certain respiratory viruses, especially adenoviruses, and related bacteria (*B. parapertussis*) occasionally provoke similar illnesses [2,3]. The pathogenesis of the clinical manifestations is unclear even today. The infection is undoubtedly transmitted from person to person by respiratory droplets. The bacteria initially proliferate on the mucosal surface of the bronchial tree. Masses of bacteria are found on the surface of the bronchial epithelium in close apposition to cilia. The exudate is purulent, and necrosis of the mucous membrane develops. In man, bronchiolitis, bronchopneumonia, atelectasis, and even lobar pneumonia develop in the first few weeks of the infection. Much of this pathology may be due to secondary invading pyogenic organisms, since *B. pertussis* is, itself, not an invasive bacterium.

The organism produces a number of toxic substances (heat-stable endotoxin, and heat-labile toxin, lymphocytosis promoting factor, histamine sensitizing factor), the roles of which in pathogenesis are not clear. Furthermore, the

TABLE 1 Bacterial Vaccines Against Pulmonary Pathogens

Type of vaccine	Stage of development
Whole Cell Killed	
Pertussis	Licensed
Plague	Licensed
Viable Attenuated	
Tuberculosis	Licensed
Tularemia	Experimental
Purified (or Partially Purified)	
Anthrax	Licensed
Pneumococcus	Experimental
Hemophilus influenzae	Experimental
Pseudomonas	Experimental
Streptococcus	Experimental

nature of the protective antigen is also not clearly established. The lymphocytosis promoting factor (LPF) has been studied by Morse [4,5], where work has shown that, in mice, injection of *B. pertussis* causes the number of normal small lymphocytes in the circulation to increase. The lymphocytosis is not the result of increased production of lymphocytes but is due to the entry into the circulation of mature lymphocytes derived from tissue pools such as lymph nodes and spleen. Lymphocyte promoting factor appeared to be associated with extracts of the cell surface that have a filamentous morphology [6]. These same fractions have histamine–sensitizing activity.

The histamine sensitizing factor (HSF) is of considerable interest because microgram quantities markedly sensitize mice to histamine, serotonin, and anaphylaxis. This factor apparently does this by blocking certain β–adrenergic receptors needed for the activities of epinephrine. The subject has recently been reviewed by Munoz and Bergman [7]. Chemically, HSF appears to contain protein and lipid. In addition, highly purified preparations of HSF induce protection of mice against challenge with *B. pertussis*. Histamine sensitizing factor is thought, to also play a role in some of the neurologic complications of both pertussis infection and vaccination [8]. Antigenic analysis of *B. pertussis* based on surface agglutinins has been defined by Eldering *et al.* [9]. In these studies, all species of *Bordetella* appeared to contain a similar heat–stable agglutinin (O antigen). Heat–labile agglutinins analogous to *E. coli* K antigens were also found and were called *factors*. Factors 1 through 6 were found in *B. pertussis* only; factor 7 was found in all cultures of *Bordetella*. Subsequent workers indicated that these factors are not the protective antigen, although most vaccines induce agglutinin formation.

The mechanism of both natural and vaccine–induced immunity is unknown. Although a number of humoral antibodies are formed after immunization or infection (agglutinins, hemagglutinins, opsonins), they do not appear to be the significant immunity factors. There is some natural resistance in the early postnatal period, suggesting passively transferred immunity (IgG) from the mother. Yet, young women of childbearing age appear to lack circulating protective antibodies. Immunity induced by vaccine does not appear to be durable. Lambert, *et al.* [10] have shown that the attack rate of pertussis was 21% in individuals immunized within the 4 yr preceding exposure, whereas the attack rate among individuals immunized more than 12 yr before an outbreak was 95%. The suggestion has been raised [11] that pertussis in adults may be quite prevalent but may not be diagnosed because of its atypical symptomatology and because appropriate culture procedures are not used. Many of the features of pertussis immunity suggest that local respiratory tract antibodies may be important; however, studies of secretory IgA activity have not been published.

Pertussis vaccine is a whole–cell vaccine detoxified with 0.02% merthiolate and stored at 4°C for several months. Adsorption with aluminum salts provides better and longer protection. The most frequently used vaccine preparation is the combination with diphtheria and tetanus toxoids (DPT). Efficacy of vaccines in field trials has been correlated with results of intracerebal inoculation tests in mice and, therefore, this assay has become the standard method for determining potency [8]. With current vaccines, primary immunization is recommended to begin at age 6 to 8 wk and to consist of three injections given at 4- to 6-wk intervals, with a fourth dose administered 1 yr later [12]. A booster dose should be given at the time the child enters school (age 3 to 6 yr).

III. Tuberculosis

Tuberculosis, although no longer the scourge it once was, is still a formidable clinical problem, even in developed countries. Knowledge of immunity to tuberculosis has advanced markedly in recent years as the field of cellular immunology has begun to be unravelled. Yet even now this knowledge is incomplete.

Mycobacterium tuberculosis is probably one of the most successful of what are called *intracellular* parasites. Following primary infection most people develop an enhanced resistance to infection with *Mycobacterium tuberculosis* and only a minority show progressive illness. Concomitant with their acquired resistance, infected, nonill persons develop a delayed-type hypersensitivity to tuberculin, a protein antigen of the organism. Considerable evidence exists to show that humoral antibodies against various antigens of *Mycobacterium tuberculosis* play no role in immunity to the disease. Delayed hypersensitivity, defined as the dermal response to tuberculin, is probably only an accompanying facet of immunity, since immunization with purified tuberculin in animals does not induce immunity to challenge with virulent organisms, although hypersensitivity develops [13,14].

BCG vaccination is an attempt to replace the natural primary virulent TB infection, with all of its attendant risks, with an avirulent organism that is also capable of inducing immunity.

BCG is an attenuated live bacterial vaccine derived originally by Drs. Calmette and Guerin in France, in 1908, from a virulent strain of *Mycobacterium tuberculosis* var. bovis. Although most studies have shown a significant reduction in new cases of tuberculosis in vaccinated as compared to control groups [15], use of the vaccine is still rather controversial in the United States. Among the reasons for the controversy is the disrepute engendered by the Lubeck disaster in Germany in 1930 in which 72 children died of tuberculosis after accidentally receiving a vaccine containing a virulent strain of *Mycobacterium tuberculosis*. The fear that the BCG vaccine might revert to virulence is unfounded, as documented by hundreds of millions of safe vaccinations during the past 40 yr.

Vaccination with BCG is performed by intradermal inoculation or by scarification or multiple puncture. The concentration of BCG in the vaccine must be sufficient to convert 80% to 90% of tuberculin-negative recipients to positive in 6 to 8 wk [16]. Tuberculin skin-test negative subjects ordinarily develop a painless papule (3 to 7 mm in diameter) within 48 hr. This progresses so that by 1 month a sharply defined ulcer (4 to 8 mm in diameter and 1 to 2 mm in depth) covered with a dry scab is noted. By 3 months, the ulcer usually is healed, leaving a small red depressed scar [17]. Regional lymph node enlargement may develop in a varying proportion of vaccinated individuals, the incidence varying with different lots of liquid vaccine [18]. However, this complication was not noted in several thousand vaccinations with lyophilized vaccine [19]. Adenitis, when it occurred, progressed to suppuration in almost half of the cases. Nonsuppurative "BCGitis" regressed in a few weeks or months, whereas suppurative adenitis required up to 8 months to heal. Antituberculous therapy does not appear to influence the course of this complication. Aronson *et al.* [17] showed that INH therapy administered for 2 months after BCG vaccination did not increase the rate at which local BCG ulcers healed.

A. Development of Tuberculin Hypersensitivity

In one study [20], a positive skin test (≥6 mm induration to 0.1 ml of 1:100 or 1:500 old tuberculin) developed in 99% of vaccinated individuals, with only a slight falling-off in the percentage of reactors after 2 yr. By 5 yr, 87% were still positive and at 9 yr, 80%. However, in the control population in this same study, positive skin tests were observed at 2 yr in 20% and at 9 yr in 52%. In another study [21], conversion rates to 5TU of PPD (intermediate) at 8 wk and 1 yr after BCG vaccination were 97% and 60%, respectively. Six percent to 7% of nonvaccinated controls were PPD positive at 1 yr.

BCG vaccination in the United States has been recommended only for tuberculin skin-test negative persons at high risk of exposure. Such groups would include: (a) medical personnel who deal with patients or laboratory workers exposed to TB in specimens or animals; (b) individuals who are unavoidably exposed to infectious TB in the home; (c) patients and employees of mental hospitals, prisons, and other such institutions in which the incidence of TB is known to be high; (d) children and certain adults living in communities in which the mortality from TB is unusually high [15,18,20,22]. For persons who are immunized with BCG but who may remain exposed to TB for the 2 to 3 months before immunity develops, INH prophylaxis can be administered for 2 months without a significant reduction in BCG efficiency [21,23], although a positive skin test may not develop in a significant proportion of those who received INH.

A number of long-term field studies have shown BCG to be from 60% to 80% effective in preventing new cases of tuberculosis [15,18,20]. One particular study has shown very little effectiveness, but this result has been criticized in several major respects [15,18]. The major problems associated with BCG vaccine are those related to standardization and stability of the product. Of great concern is the necessity to prevent mutation to virulence or introduction of a virulent mycobacterial contaminant. Production requirements quite clearly outline the techniques to be used [16]. With the advent of new uses of BCG as a nonspecific stimulant of immunity, such as in cancer and leukemia [24], it is anticipated that these technical problems will be resolved because of increased demands for products with reproducible characteristics.

IV. Vaccination Against Pneumococcal Pneumonia

Diplococcus pneumoniae infection is probably the most highly prevalent cause of bacterial pneumonia in man [25]. As such, it has received intensive study for many years and much of our knowledge of the organism and immunity to it has been known for a long time [26,27]. The capsular polysaccharide of the organism is believed to be responsible for the pathogenicity of the *Pneumococcus* and also represents the type-specific antigen. At present, over 82 distinct capsular serotypes are recognized, a fact which in itself indicates a serious problem in terms of vaccine development. The chemical composition of many of these capsular antigens is known [28]. All are polysaccharides, but the sugars comprising the polymers are different and, thus, each type is immunologically distinct. Actually, there is some degree of crossreactivity among some of the pneumococal polysaccharides, and also some crossing with polysaccharides of certain other bacteria and plants [29]. Typing of pneumococcal isolates has shown that certain types are more frequent human pathogens than others. A number of recent studies to determine the prevalence of pneumococcal types has been reviewed by Austrian [30] and are summarized in Table 2. It can be seen that 10 specific types account for about 75% of severe human pneumococcal infections. Clinical experience has shown that a number of nonspecific factors increase susceptibility to pneumococcal pneumonia. Among these are preceding viral respiratory infection, old age, chronic pulmonary disease, and congestive heart failure. Animal and human experience have shown that immunity to infection can be induced by previous infection or by active or passive immunization. (Prior human infection with *Pneumococcus* does not produce an absolute immunity to reinfection. Strauss and Finland [31] have shown that at least 3% of the patients with pneumonia developed a second attack within 2 yr, and in 25% the serotype was the same as that which caused the initial infection.) Both local and systemic factors appear to play a role in host resistance. Bull and Mc Kee [32] showed that rabbits can become immune to infection produced by nasal challenge with virulent pneumococci by prior nasal infection or prior intranasal immunization with killed organisms. Mac Leod *et al.* [33], in studies of pneumococcal vaccines in humans, showed type-specific protection against pneumonia, and also a 55% reduction in pharyngeal carriage rate in vaccinated subjects compared to controls. Local respiratory secretory antibodies against pneumococci have not been reported, but type-specific antipneumococcal IgA antibodies have been identified in human colostrum [34].

TABLE 2 Pneumococcal Types Causing Disease[a]

Types	Percent	Disease	Place
1, 3, 4, 7, 8, 12	60	Bacteremia	USA
1, 6, 7, 14, 19, 23	80	Middle ear	USA
1, 3, 4, 7, 8, 12	46	Bacteremia	Denmark
1, 3, 8	85	Bacteremia	Scotland
1, 3, 4, 8, 12	59	Blood, lung	England
1, 3, 7, 8	?	Pneumonia	New Guinea
1, 2, 3, 4, 7, 8, 12	82	Pneumonia	So. Africa

[a]From Austrian [30].

TABLE 3   Trial of Pneumococcal Polysaccharide Vaccine in Elderly Subjects 1937–1943[a]

A.

Vaccine group	Incidence/1000 of pneumonia (all etiologies)	Mortality/1000
Vaccinated Types I, II, and III	17.2	6.2
Control	44	19

B. Pneumococcal Serotypes Causing Pneumonia

Vaccine group	No. of cases with Types I, II, and III	(Rate/1000)	No. of cases of all other types	(Rate/1000)
Vaccinated 99 cases	3	30.3	31	313
Control 227 cases	33	145.3	63	277

[a]From Kaufman [16].

The classic studies of Wood [35] characterized the importance of phago-cytosis in host defense against pneumococcal infection. Phagocytosis and subse-quent intracellular killing of pneumococci occur in the absence of antibodies, a process he called *surface phagocytosis*. Only the highly encapsulated Type 3 organism was resistant to surface phagocytosis, a fact that may explain the con-siderable virulence of this serotype. Nevertheless, the presence of opsonic anti-bodies greatly accelerated the phagocytic events and speeded the recovery of the host. For some years before the advent of antibiotics, hyperimmune antiserum was used in therapy, with a significant lowering of case fatality rates [36].

The immune response to pneumococcal polysaccharides has a number of unique features that deserve comment. Immunologic paralysis following the injection of mice with doses of polysaccharide greater than those required for immunization was described by Felton and coworkers in 1955 [37]. The nature of the phenomenon is still under active investigation. There is some evidence that large doses of pneumococcal polysaccharides may result in suboptinal anti-body responses in humans [38]. According to current concepts, large molec-ular-weight bacterial polysaccharides stimulate B cells of the lymphoid system directly, there being no evidence for T-cell activation. There is some recent evi-dence, however, that T cells may have both a suppressor and an amplifier effect on the antibody response of polysaccharide stimulated B cells, at least in the mouse [39]. Attempts at vaccination against pneumococcal disease have a long history, which has been reviewed extensively [26,33,40]. Two definitive trials of purified multivalent polysaccharide vaccines have shown the efficacy of this procedure. Kaufman [40] immunized over 5000 elderly individuals in a chronic disease hospital over a 6-yr period and reported significant reductions in inci-dence and mortality from pneumonia as compared to a control nonvaccinated group. Table 3 shows a summary of his results. Mac Leod and others tested a polysaccharide vaccine containing four serotype antigens in an Army camp dur-ing World War II [33]. Vaccine was administered as a single injection containing 30 to 60μg of each antigen. Results (Table 4) showed a highly significant reduc-tion in cases of pneumonia caused by the specific serotypes included in the vaccine.

TABLE 4   Pneumococcal Vaccine Field Trial[a]

	Vaccine group	Controls
No. men	8586	8449
No. cases pneumonia		
Types I, II, V, VII	4	26
Other types	56	59

[a]From Mac Leod *et al.* [33].

Thus, vaccination with pneumococcal polysaccharides can be a highly effective means of preventing pneumococcal pneumonia in high risk groups. The problems to be overcome in reaching this goal are twofold: (a) technical aspects related to producing a vaccine with 10 specific polysaccharide antigens and (b) lack of motivation on the part of physicians and public health authorities that such a vaccine is needed. The data and logic provided by Austrian [30] have begun to make some inroads in both of these problem areas.

References

1. G. F. Brooks and T. M. Buchanan, Pertussis in the United States, *J. Infect. Dis.*, **122**:123–125 (1970).
2. J. D. Connor, Etiologic role of adenoviral infection in pertussis syndrome, *N. Engl. J. Med.*, **283**:390–394 (1970).
3. J. Wilkins and P. F. Wehrle, Pertussis. In *Communicable and Infectious Diseases.* Seventh Edition. Edited by F. H. Top and P. F. Wehrle. St. Louis, Mo., C. V. Mosby Co., 1972, pp. 440–449.
4. S. I. Morse and S. K. Riester, Studies on the leukocytosis and lymphocytosis induced by *Bordetella pertussis, J. Exp. Med.,* **125**:401–408 (1967).
5. S. I. Morse, Studies on the lymphocytosis induced in mice by *Bordetella pertussis, J. Exp. Med.,* **121**:49–68 (1965).
6. J. H. Morse and S. I. Morse, Studies on the ultrastructure of *Bordetella pertussis.* I. Morphology, origin, and biological activity of structures present in the extracellular fluid of liquid cultures of *Bordetella pertussis, J. Exp. Med.,* **131**:1342–1357 (1970).
7. J. Munoz and R. K. Bergman, Histamine–sensitizing factors from microbial agents, with special reference to *Bordetella pertussis, Bacteriol. Rev.,* **32**: 103–126 (1968).
8. M. Pittman, *Bordetella pertussis*–bacterial and host factors in the pathogenesis and prevention of whooping cough. In *Infectious Agents and Host Reactions.* Edited by S. Mudd. Philadelphia, W. B. Saunders Co., 1970, pp. 239–270.
9. G. Eldering, C. Hornbeck, and J. Baker, Serological study of *Bordetella pertussis* and related species, *J. Bacteriol.,* **74**:133–136 (1957).
10. H. J. Lambert, Epidemiology of a small pertussis outbreak in Kent County, Michigan, *Public Health Rep.,* **80**:365–369 (1965).
11. S. I. Morse, Pertussis in adults, *Ann. Intern. Med.,* **68**:953–954 (1968).
12. Report of the Committee on Infectious Diseases. Am. Acad. Pediatrics. Sixteenth edition, 1970, p. 5.
13. G. B. Mac Kaness, The immunology of antituberculous immunity, *Am. Rev. Respir. Dis.,* **97**:337–344 (1968).
14. G. P. Youmans and A. S. Youmans, Recent studies on acquired immunity in tuberculosis. In *Current Topics in Microbiology.* Berlin, Heidelberg, Springer–Verlag, **48**:130–178 (1969).

15. R. J. W. Rees, BCG vaccination in mycobacterial infections, *Br. Med. Bull.,* 25:183–188 (1969).

16. WHO Expert Committee on Biological Standardization, Requirements for Dried BCG Vaccine, *W. H. O. Tech. Rep. Series,* 329:25–49 (1966).

17. J. D. Aronson, H. C. Taylor, and D. L. Kirk, The effects of isoniazid treatment on the tuberculin reaction and on the healing of BCG–induced ulcers, *Am. Rev. Tuberc. Pulm. Dis.,* 74:7–14 (1956).

18. D. W. Smith, Why not vaccinate against tuberculosis, *Ann. Intern. Med.,* 72:419–422 (1970).

19. E. Chaves–Carballo and G. A. Sanchez, Regional lymphadenitis following BCG vaccination (BCGitis), *Clin. Pediatr.,* 11:693–697 (1972).

20. S. R. Rosenthal, E. Loewinsohn, M. L. Graham, D. Liveright, M. G. Thorne, and V. Johnson, BCG vaccination against tuberculosis in Chicago. A twenty–year study statistically analyzed, *Pediatrics,* 28:622–641 (1961).

21. H. M. Vandiviere, M. Dworski, I. G. Melvin, K. A. Watson, and J. Begley, Efficacy of bacillus calmette–guerin and isonizid–resistant bacillus calmette–guerin with and without isonizid chemoprophylaxis from day of vaccination. II. Field trial in man, *Am. Rev. Respir. Dis.,* 108:301–313 (1973).

22. E. L. Kendig, The place of BCG vaccine in the management of infants born of tuberculous mothers, *N. Engl. J. of Med.,* 281:520–523 (1969).

23. D. T. Smith, Which children in the United States should receive BCG vaccination?, *Clin. Pediatr.,* 9:632–634 (1970).

24. G. Mathé, Experimental doses and first clinical controlled trials of leukemia active immunotherapy. *Progress in Immunology–First International Congress of Immunology.* Edited by B. Amos. New York, Academic Press, 1971, pp. 959–969.

25. S. Rabinovich and I. M. Smith, Pneumonias, Bacterial. In *Communicable and Infectious Diseases.* Edited by F. H. Top and P. F. Wehrle. Seventh edition. St. Louis, C. V. Mosby Company, 1972, pp. 457–479.

26. R. Heffron, Pneumonia with special reference to pneumococcus lobar pneumonia. New York, Commonwealth Fund, 1939.

27. C. M. Mac Leod. *The Pneumococci in Bacterial and Mycotic Infections of Man.* Edited by R. J. Dubos. Third edition. Philadelphia, J. B. Lippincott Company, 1958, pp. 230–247.

28. E. A. Kabat and M. M. Mayer. *Kabat and Mayer's Experimental Immunochemistry.* Second edition. Illinois, Charles C. Thomas, 1971, p. 847.

29. *Ibid.,* p. 848.

30. R. Austrian, The current status of pneumococcal disease and the potential utility of polyvalent pneumococcal vaccine. In Proceedings, International Conference on the Application of Vaccines Against Viral Rickettsial, and Bacterial Diseases of Man, 14–18 December 1970. Scientific Publication Number 226. Washington, D.C., Pan American Health Organization, 1971, pp. 359–363.

31. E. Strauss and M. Finland, Further studies on recurrences in pneumococcic pneumonia with special reference to the effect of specific treatment, *Ann. Intern. Med.,* 16:17–32 (1942).

32. C. G. Bull and C. M. Mc Kee, Respiratory immunity in rabbits. VI. The effects of immunity on the carrier state of the pneumococcus and *Bacillus bronchisepticus, Am. J. Hyg.,* 8:723–729 (1928).

33. C. M. Mac Leod, R. G. Hodges, M. Heidelberger, and W. G. Bernhard, Prevention of pneumococcal pneumonia by immunization with specific capsular polysaccharides, *J. Exp. Med.,* 82:445–465 (1945).

34. R. P. Mouton, J. W. Stoop, R. E. Ballieis, and N. A. J. Muls, Pneumococcal antibodies in serum and external secretions, *Clin. Exp. Immunol.,* 7:201–210 (1970).

35. W. B. Wood, Studies on the cellular immunology of acute bacterial infections. In *The Harvey Lectures, 1951-1952.* New York, Academic Press, 47:72–98 (1953).

36. M. Finland, W. C. Spring, and F. C. Lowell, Specific treatment of the pneumococci pneumonias; an analysis of the results of serum therapy and chemotherapy at the Boston City Hospital from July 1938 through June 1939, *Ann. Intern. Med.,* 13;1567–1594 (1940).

37. L. D. Felton, G. Kauffman, B. Prescott, and B. Ottinger, Studies on the mechanism of the immunological paralysis induced in mice by pneumococcal polysaccharides, *J. Immunol.,* 74:17–26 (1955).

38. J. M. Ruegsegger and M. Finland, The influence of dosage and route of injection on the antibody response of human subjects to the specific carbohydrate of the type VIII pneumococcus, *J. Clin. Invest.,* 14:833–836 (1935).

39. P. J. Baker, N. D. Reed, P. W. Stashak, and D. F. Amsbaugh, Regulation of the antibody response to type III pneumococcal polysaccharide. I. Nature of regulatory cells, *J. Exp. Med.,* 137:1431–1441 (1973).

40. P. Kaufman, Pneumonia in old age, *Arch. Intern. Med.,* 79:518–531 (1947).

20

Genetic Factors in Atopic Allergic Disease

BERNARD B. LEVINE

New York University School of Medicine
New York, New York

I. Introduction

A. Background Information

The purpose of this paper is to review the literature pertaining to hereditary factors in atopic allergic diseases and recent experiments in our laboratory on the genetic control of reagin (IgE) production in the mouse and in man. The historic development of current concepts of human allergic diseases encompasses a time span of approximately 70 yr. During this time, we learned to recognize several groups of diseases mediated in part by specific antibodies, sensitized lymphoid cells, or both. These include IgE-mediated diseases, such as allergic rhinitis, allergic asthma, anaphylaxis, and urticaria; diseases mediated by antibodies, including serum sickness, certain types of arteritis, arthritis, and nephritis; some hematological disorders and autoimmune diseases; and diseases mediated by cellular hypersensitivity, including contact dermatitis, certain inflammatory aspects of infectious diseases, as well as some autoimmune diseases. This is by no means

---

This review was supported by a grant from the U.S. Army Medical Research and Development Command.

an all-inclusive list. Several mechanisms may play a role in a given disease, e.g., cellular hypersensitivity may be important in some cases of asthma or rhinitis and there are complexities in the mediation of immunologic tissue damage involving the interplay of sensitized cells and serum antibodies of different classes. Thus it is sometimes difficult to speak exclusively of Type I, II, or III allergic diseases, as several inter-related mechanisms may be involved in the generation of an immunologic disease. For example, the deposition of immune complexes in the kidney may be enhanced by the presence of IgE antibodies, prior reaction of which with antigen causes a local change in the permeability of glomerular membranes for antigen-antibody complexes [1]. Similarly, the killing action of sensitized lymphoid cells on target cells may be inhibited by IgG "blocking or enhancing" antibodies of the same specificity. Finally, the generation of immunologically mediated diseases involves additional factors that are not primarily immunologic, e.g., nervous, infectious, hormonal, and metabolic factors. This multitude of mechanisms makes for a complexity of genetic controls in a clinical allergic disease.

The clinical allergist deals mainly with only a few of these immunologic diseases, termed *allergic diseases.* These are hay fever and allergic rhinitis, vasomotor rhinitis, allergic and idiopathic asthma, food allergies, eczema (both atopic and allergic contact dermatitis), urticarias, anaphylaxis, drug allergy, and serum sickness.

B. Historic Aspects

In 1906 von Pirquet introduced the term *allergy* to cover reactions and diseases caused by the body's altered reactivity to foreign substances. Coca and Cooke [2] categorized allergic reactions into five groups: anaphylaxis, serum sickness, hypersensitivity to infection, allergic contact dermatitis, and a newly introduced category, the atopic diseases of man. They included hay fever, asthma, and food allergies under atopic diseases. The term *atopy* is a Greek word meaning strange or unusual. It means literally: a- (no), top- (place), y- (ness), i.e., having no place relative to current experience.

Why did Coca and Cooke consider these diseases strange? In the 20 years preceeding the introduction of the term atopy, anaphylaxis had been discovered by Portier and Richet [3] and by Smith [4] and it had been suggested that hay fever and asthma were similar in mechanism to anaphylaxis in experimental animals [5]. However, Coca and Cooke [2] were sufficiently impressed with the differences between experimental anaphylaxis in animals and hay fever and asthma in man that they introduced the term atopy. Among these differences were observations that large doses of strong antigens (which were really antigen mixtures, e.g., horse serum or crude toxins) sensitized more than 90% of test animals. By contrast, only 5% to 10% of the human population developed hay fever or asthma as a consequence of sensitivity to ambient allergens. In animal anaphylaxis, serum precipitating antibodies could be demonstrated readily and such sera could passively transfer anaphylactic sensitivity to nonsensitive recipients. Finally, pregnant sensitive mothers could transfer sensitivity to their offspring through the placenta or colostrum. In contrast, in human hay fever and asthma, serum precipitins were not found. Indeed, only a year or two before the term atopy was introduced, sensitivity was transferred successfully in allergic man [6,7]. Moreover, it was known that hay fever and asthma were not transferred placentally to newborn infants from sensitive mothers. Many authors had noted that asthma and hay fever frequently occurred in certain families, and Coca and Cooke [2] were strongly impressed with the importance of hereditary factors in the causation of these allergic diseases. In experimental anaphylaxis, hereditary factors controlling the development of sensitivity (and the elicitation of reactions) were not appreciated by these early investigators.

Because of these arguments, Coca and Cooke [2] felt that asthma and hay fever represented hypersensitivity mechanisms fundamentally different from anaphylaxis in experimental animals. Consequently they called asthma and hay fever *atopic diseases*. As I will discuss later, Coca and Cooke's arguments cannot now be considered valid. That is, when minute doses of antigen are used for sensitization, clear-cut heritable factors can be brought out in experimental anaphylaxis. Also, by using minute doses of antigen, IgE production with very little IgG production ensues, i.e., the sera will transfer sensitivity but does not contain precipitins, as is the situation in man (vide infra). However, there still appears to be some advantage in using the term atopy in clinical situations. This term communicates a compound notion that several diseases (allergic rhinitis, allergic and idiopathic asthma, infantile eczema, possibly vasomotor rhinitis, some food allergies and urticaria) are commonly associated in certain individuals and families, and that one or a few basic mechanistic factors (currently not understood) are common to these diseases and are heritable.

II. Clustering of Asthma, Eczema, and Hay Fever

There is considerable evidence for the association of these atopic diseases in certain individuals. First, there are numerous publications showing this association, although most do not offer unequivocal evidence. These studies have been summarized by Schwartz [8]. Basically they showed that asthmatics have a higher prevalence of eczema and hay fever and vice versa than does a nonallergic population. As Schwartz pointed out, these studies presented statistical difficulties in interpreting data due to differences in allergic and control populations and in the diagnostic methods used. A most carefully documented retrospective clinical study was published by Edgren [9]. Edgren's test series consisted of 331 persons seen at a Dermatology Clinic for infantile eczema 16 to 40 yr previously. His control series consisted of 298 patients seen for nonallergic skin lesions at the same clinic during the same time period. In the study the allergic diseases developed by the two populations during the 16 to 40 yr subsequent to the diagnosis of infantile eczema were determined by interview. In the eczema group, 23% developed asthma, 10% developed hay fever, and 27% developed urticaria. In the control group 2% developed asthma, 2% developed hay fever, and 6% developed urticaria. These differences are, of course, highly significant statistically. Stifler [10] studied, retrospectively, 40 patients diagnosed as having infantile eczema at a clinic at Johns Hopkins Medical School 21 yr previously. He found that in the 21-yr interval, 13 (32%) had developed hay fever, 3 (8%) had developed asthma alone, and 5 (13%) had developed hay fever and asthma. A control population was not included in the study. Reasonable prevalence figures for hay fever in that area, in that time period, would be 7% to 13% and about 3% to 6% for asthma. Thus the 45% figure for hay fever and 21% figure for asthma in the population with eczema is significantly higher than normal.

Two lines of evidence indicate that atopic dieases are heritable: (a) family studies in which the prevalence of atopic diseases in families of an atopic propositus is significantly higher than in families of nonatopic propositi or in the population at large; and (b) studies comparing monozygotic and dizygotic twins for concordance in atopic diseases.

The idea that hay fever is subject to inheritance appeared early in the literature, but the first real study on this issue was by Cooke and Vander Veer [11]. They studied individuals for hay fever, asthma, urticaria, and acute gastroenteritis following the ingestion of certain foods, such as strawberries and fish. Diagnosis of these diseases in antecedents (mother and father) was made by history alone. Of 504 patients studied, there was a positive family history of allergic disease in 48.4%. Of 63 nonallergic people, there was a positive family history of atopic disease in 9.5%. The authors did not include atopic eczema in this study, but stated that a history of eczema was commonly elicited in these patients. The results of this study were generally confirmed by another study from that laboratory published 8 yr later [12]. In this work, only hay fever and asthma were studied; urticaria and food allergy were not included. The clinical material consisted of 462 patients with hay fever, or asthma, or both "... in all of which a hypersensitive condition was demonstrated by a positive intradermal test which was in complete accord with this history." The control group consisted of 115 nonallergic individuals. In the atopic group, a positive antecedent history of atopic disease was obtained in 58% as compared to 7% for the control nonallergic population.

In another study on 400 patients with asthma, Adkinson [13] found that 48% had a positive family history of asthma. From these and other studies, it was widely agreed among allergists that genetic factors were of great importance in atopic diseases [14-16]. An extensively detailed and documented family study on 191 probands with asthma and 200 control probands was published in 1952 by Schwartz [8]. This investigator collected data on the occurrence of the following diseases in the families: asthma, hay fever, vasomotor rhinitis, Besnier's prurigo, eczema, urticaria, Quinke's edema, migraine, gastrointestinal allergy, epilepsy, ichthyosis, and psoriasis. The family members studied comprised individuals from four generations: children, siblings, parents, parents' siblings, and grandparents. Family members were interviewed personally wherever possible, rather than relying upon the memory of the proband. Some of Schwartz's results are shown in Table 1. Before discussing them, some comment on the diagnostic categories is in order.

By allergic asthma was meant clinical asthma due to clear-cut allergic factors. Nonallergic asthma was asthma in which no clear-cut allergenic precipitating factor was found. In the latter diagnostic group, nonspecific factors, such as respiratory infections or fumes, could precipitate asthma. Schwartz stated that this division was rough and was not meant to imply that the nonallergic group was truly nonallergic, but rather that in this group specific allergic factors were exceedingly difficult to document. In the allergic asthma group, allergenic incitants were readily found. Some of the other diagnostic categories Schwartz used are subject to argument; as vasomotor rhinitis, he included all cases of rhinitis (but not common cold) that lacked a seasonal factor. However, this category probably included cases of allergic rhinitis to perennial allergens, e.g., danders, feathers, dusts, and others. His cases of Besnier's prurigo appear to be virtually all atopic (infantile) eczema. This diagnosis was used when some trace of the disease still remained. However, where only a history of infantile eczema was obtained, then the case was placed in a category labeled *eczema,* and this category also included clear-cut allergic contact dermatitis. Because of this heterogeneity, I do not show his data on eczema in Table 1, but the reader should appreciate that the prevalence of Besnier's prurigo (or atopic eczema) in his study is artificially low. Table 1 shows that asthma, hay fever, vasomotor rhinitis (which included nonseasonal allergic rhinitis), and Besnier's prurigo occurred significantly more frequently in families of patients with asthma than in families of subjects that did not have asthma, whereas there were no differences in the occurrence of urticaria or migraine in the two kinds of families. However, when urticaria was further broken down, it appeared that among daughters and sisters of probands (but not among mothers), urticaria occurred more frequently in families of patients with asthma. This latter conclusion is unconfirmed.

TABLE 1 Prevalence of "Allergic" Diseases in Family Members of Patients with Asthma and in Nonallergic Controls[a]

	No. of probands	No. of relatives examined	Asthma		Hay fever		Vasomotor rhinitis		Besneir's prurigo		Urticaria		Migraine	
			n	%	n	%	n	%	n	%	n	%	n	%
Allergic asthma	74	631	51	8.1	8	1.3	40	6.3	3	0.4	60	9.5	33	5.2
Nonallergic asthma	117	1005	107	10.7	6	0.6	62	6.2	5	0.5	74	7.4	52	5.2
Total asthma	191	1636	158	9.7	14	0.9	102	6.2	8	0.5	134	8.2	85	5.2
Nonallergic controls	200	1790	24	1.3	6	0.3	25	1.4	0	0.0	129	7.2	74	4.1

[a]From Schwartz [8].

Thus the family studies indicate that the propensity to develop hay fever, asthma, atopic eczema, and perhaps urticaria, certain food allergies and vasomotor rhinitis runs in families, suggesting genetic control. Studies in twins support this idea. Many studies on single twin pairs (or small numbers) have been published (reviewed by Schwartz [8]). The data taken as a whole are not consistent, but, in general, among monozygotic twins, concordance in allergic disease was seen more commonly than was discordance. This subject was studied extensively by Spaich and Ostertag in 1936 [17]. They studied 71 pairs of twins in which one or both members had an allergic disease. Of the monozygotic twins, 2 of 7 pairs were concordant for asthma, i.e., in 2 pairs, both members had asthma and in 5 pairs, only one member had asthma. Of the dizygotic twins, only 1 of 14 pairs was concordant for asthma. For hay fever, 2 of 3 monozygotic twin pairs and 1 or 2 dizygotic twin pairs were concordant. Spaich and Ostertag also presented data on concordance in other allergic diseases, but these data cannot be interpreted clearly as they included migraine and food–related abdominal symptoms under *other allergic diseases.*

Studies on twins confirm, in a general way, the notion that atopic diseases are under a demonstrable genetic control. Although atopy appears to be familial, some workers suggested that the familial occurrence of a specific disease may be more striking than is the familial occurrence of atopy in general. For example, in studies by Clarke *et al.* [18] and by Spaich and Ostertag [17], asthma occurred more frequently than did hay fever in the families of patients with asthma, and hay fever occurred more frequently than did asthma in the families of patients with hay fever. Further work on this issue would be welcome. At present, it appears likely that both the general and the specific diseases may be under genetic control.

III. Genetic Factors in Atopy

Two questions arise in connection with the preceeding data: (a) what factors are shared in common by various atopic diseases, and (b) what is the nature of controlling genetic factors? Regarding the first question, atopic diseases are clearly diverse, e.g., reagin production involved in hay fever, eosinophilia and bronchial hypersensitivity in idiopathic asthma, and the dermal disease of atopic eczema. The factor(s) common to these diseases are not yet clearly known. It may be that one common factor is complex autonomic abnormality manifested as a partial diffuse β-adrenergic blockade [19-20], vagotonia, or both [21-22]. Salvaggio *et al.* [23] suggested that mucous membrane permeability to antigens differs for atopic and nonatopic subjects. Stember and Levine's [24] data point to an important role of mucous membrane permeability in the development of hay fever. As permeability is controlled in part by the autonomic nervous system, the two notions can be brought together. Other factors, e.g., local IgA antibody production, are also possible, and it will be important to determine these common factors as such information can be the basis for developing more effective preventatives and treatments for atopic diseases.

As to the second question, these diseases are based on many factors, both genetic and environmental. It is of relatively little value to discuss the mode of transmission of a multifactorial disease. It is more meaningful to study individual genetic factors and their transmission. The greatest progress will be made when genes on a single locus can be identified and their genetic transmission, function, and relationship to other factors and the disease are characterized.

IV. Genetic Studies on Reagin Production in Mice

With this approach in mind, we set out to study one aspect of the atopic spectrum, IgE antibody (reagin) formation. First animal models were established and then the information obtained from the animal models was applied to studies in atopic man. I will now review studies from our laboratory which led to the identification of two kinds of genetic controls of reagin production in the mouse and one genetic control of reagin production in man. The latter is an *Ir* gene that permits the recognition of ragweed antigen E in low concentrations as antigenic. It appears to be necessary (but not sufficient) for the generation of ragweed hay fever (due to antigen E) in man.

The initial experiments [25] yielded a model in mice for reagin production similar to that in man spontaneously allergic to aeroallergens. In our first experiments groups of mice of eight different inbred strains were immunized with antigens mixed with aluminum hydroxide gel adjuvant and injected intraperitoneally. Sera were drawn at intervals and assayed for $IgG_1(\gamma_1)$ and for reaginic antibodies by passive cutaneous anaphylaxis (PCA) in CFW mice. Both γ_1 and reaginic antibodies in mice are homocytotropic, i.e., capable of mediating homologous PCA reactions and in vitro histamine release from homologous peritoneal mast cells. Gamma-1 antibodies were assayed by PCA after a 2-hr sensitization period and reagin by PCA with a 49 to 72 hr sensitization period. Considerable data indicate that the two antibodies can be assayed quite well by this means. Mouse reagin is similar in many properties to IgE antibodies in man.

When mice were immunized with a single 100μg dose of antigen, all eight strains made clear-cut immune responses, although quantitative differences in antibody titers were seen. Figure 1 shows typical results with BPO_{25}-BGG

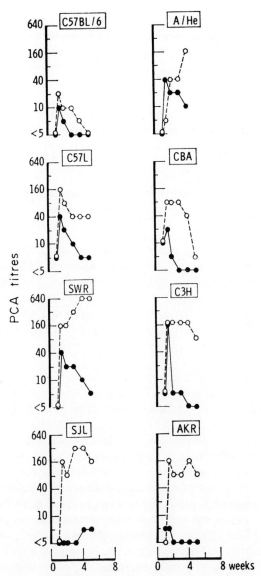

FIGURE 1 Immune responses to 100 g BPO$_{25}$–BGG plus 20 mg Al(OH)$_3$ gel injected intraperitoneally at 0 time. Reagin ●——●; IgG$_1$ ○– – –○. Reprinted by permission from *Int. Arch. Allergy* **39**:156–171 (1970).

(benzylpenicilloyl-bovine γ-globulin) as antigen. By contrast, when repeated minute doses (0.1μg) of antigen were used for immunization, clear-cut "all-or-none appearing" strain differences in immune responsiveness were brought out (Fig. 2). In most responding strains, the following characteristics of the immune response were noted:

1. Strain differences were in immune responsiveness in general rather than in reagin production uniquely.

2. In the low-antigen dose system, reagin production was a prominent part of the immune response in most strains.

3. Reagin production was persistent over long time periods and was subject to marked booster responses to repeated doses of antigen.

4. In other experiments, using antigen-antibody binding at limiting antigen concentrations, it was seen that the reagin induced by repeated low-antigen doses was of relatively high binding avidity to antigen. These similarities to reagin production in spontaneously sensitized man suggest that this mouse system may be a useful experimental model for reagin-mediated allergic diseases, such as ragweed hay fever.

The next studies established some of the immunologic and genetic properties of the low-antigen dose system in inbred mice. From immunization experiments of many inbred mouse strains with three different antigens, BPO_{25}-BGG, ovalbumin, and ovomucoid in low doses, it was seen that the responsiveness of a given mouse strain was antigen-specific, i.e., one strain was a good responder to one antigen but a poor responder to another antigen. Further, when good and poor responders to a given antigen were grouped, responsiveness correlated with *H-2* genotype [26,27]. Representative data are shown in Table 2. Breeding experiments and immunization of congenic strain pairs (at the *H-2* locus) established that genetic control was by a single autosomal locus closely linked to the *H-2* system. Data from breeding experiments, shown in Table 3, demonstrate that the F_1 generation are good responders, i.e., the responder trait is autosomal dominant. The (F_1 × poor responder) backcross yielded approximately 50% responders, consistent with control by a single gene. Responsiveness to ovomucoid was linked to the $H-2^a$ genotype in the backcross generation.

Previous studies in mice by McDevitt and Chinitz [28] had established an *H-2* linked single locus genetic control of immune responsiveness to synthetic branched chain polypeptides (T,G)-A--L and (H,G)-A--L. This has been called the *IR-1* gene. The unique properties of the present system were the

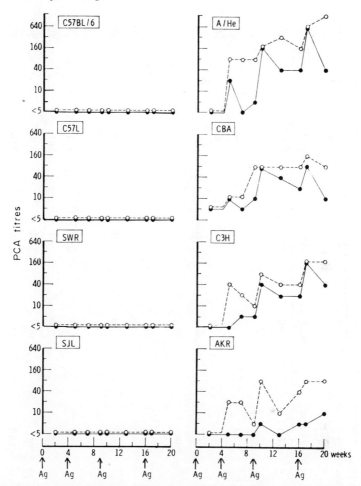

FIGURE 2 Immune responses to repeated 0.1 g doses of BPO_{25}–BGG plus 0.1 mg $Al(OH)_3$ gel injected intraperitoneally at times indicated by "Ag." Reagin ●——●; IgG_1 ○– – –○. Reprinted by permission from *Int. Arch. Allergy* **39**:156–171 (1970).

finding that for protein antigens minute doses were required for immunization to bring out strain differences, and in this system genetic control over immune responsiveness per se included control over reagin production. Also, where minute doses of antigen are used, reagin production (relative to production of IgG antibodies) was accentuated as compared with responses to high doses of antigen.

As to the genetic mapping of this locus, recent studies on recombinant strains place this locus between the *K* end of the *H–2* system and the *SS–Slp*

TABLE 2 BPO–Specific Antibody Responses of Inbred Strains of Mice Following Immunization with Either a Single High Dose or Repeated Small doses of BPO_{25}–BGG^a

H-2 type	Mouse strains[b]	Immunization with					
		(A)				(B)	
		HA[b]	IgG₁ 100μg once[c]	Reagin	HA	IgG₁ 1.0μg twice	Reagin
a	A/HeJ	8	160	40	128	320	160
b	C57BL/6J	1	20	10	2	0	0
b	C57L/J	4	160	40	4	0	0
b	LP/J	nt[d]	nt	nt	0	0	0
b	129/J	nt	nt	nt	0	0	0
d	BALB/cJ	16	40	10	0	0	0
d	DBA/2J	16	80	20	0	0	0
k	AKR/J	16	160	5	256	320	0
k	CBA/J	8	80	20	64	160	80
k	CE/J	nt	nt	nt	128	320	80
k	C3H/HeJ	64	160	160	128	320	80
k	C57BR/ckj	32	160	80	4	40	10

k C58/J	nt	nt	64	160	40
k MA/J	nt	nt	4	20	0
k RF/J	16	160	4	20	5
k ST/bJ	nt	nt	512	320	5
q BUB/BNJ	nt	nt	0	0	0
q DBA/1J	nt	nt	0	0	0
s SLJ/J	128	320	16	10	0
? SWR/J	32	640	0	0	0

a(A) columns: Antibody titers at 9 or 14 days after a single injection of 100µg of BPO$_{25}$–BGG plus 20 mg of Al(OH)$_3$ gel i.p.; serum pools of three mice. (B) columns: Antibody titers at 7 days after a secondary injection of 1.0µg of BPO$_{25}$–BGG plus 1.0 mg of Al(OH)$_3$ gel i.p.; serum pools of three mice.

bHemagglutination titers (reciprocal $\times\ 10^{-3}$); HA tests negative at 1:2000 are shown as zero.

cIgG$_1$ and reaginic antibody reciprocal titers, as measured by PCA tests in CRW recipient mice with sensitization periods of 2 or 48 hr, respectively; PCA reactions at 1:5 are shown as zero. All data from Vaz and Levine [26].

dnt = not tested.

TABLE 3   Immune Responses to Ovomucoid of C57BL × A/He Generations

Generation		Immune Response[a]		$H\text{-}2^a$ Antigen[b]
		IgG_1	Reagin	
Parental				
C57BL	(8F)	0	0	Absent
A/He	(6F)	80–320	160–640	Present
	(1F)	0	0	Present
F_1				
C57BL × A/He	(10M)	10–80	10–160	Present
	(7F)	40–640	80–640	Present
F_1 Backcross				
F_1 × C57BL				
Females	13	0	0	Absent
	14	10–160	10–80	Present
Males	11	0	0	10 absent, 1 present
	6	5–80	20–160	Present

[a]Ninth day after two 1.0μg doses of OM 4 wk apart.
[b]RBC typed with C57BL anti–A.

locus [29–31]. Lieberman and Humphrey's [30–31] studies indicate more than one immune response locus in the chromosome region between the K and $SS\text{-}Slp$ regions of the $H\text{-}2$ system, but further studies of this nature will be required to establish this point. The precise mode of action of the gene product, which is crucial for immune responsiveness, is not yet clear. Recent data support the view that the product is expressed in T–cell helper function [32], and it is not clear whether it also may be expressed in B cells. The product acts on "carrier" function of the immunogen, i.e., it permits recognition of immunogenic carriers, following which B cells may respond to various haptenic determinants on the carrier, with the production of antibodies of various classes. We speculate that the gene product may be a specific receptor (nonimmunoglobulin?) for the carrier present on T–cell surface membranes. Antigen–induced antibody synthesis is controlled by many genes. The Ir gene is only one of several classes of genes controlling immune responses, but these are apparently crucial for the multiclassed antibody response to antigen in minute doses.

An altogether different kind of genetic factor, which controls immune serum reagin titers uniquely, was found in mice. The experimental data may be summarized as follows: When a large number of mouse strains was immunized with multiple antigens (and in various doses) all strains produced IgG antibody to one or another antigen. However, with regard to serum reagin titers, some strains made high titers, some made moderate titers, and some had little or no serum reagin [33–34]. The most thoroughly studied strains are the RF ($H\text{-}2^k$) and SJL

($H\text{-}2^s$) strains. For example, in response to immunization with two 10-μg doses of ovalbumin given 4 wk apart, RF made antibody titers of 1:2560 (γ_1) and 1:640 (reagin), whereas SJL made titers of 1:2560 (γ_1) and less than 1:10 reagin. Similarly, poor reagin responses for SJL were seen for six other antigens. This system differs in properties from the first system described above:

1. There is no dose effect.

2. There is no antigen specificity.

3. The effect is on reagin uniquely.

4. Genetic control is by more than one locus and not linked to *H-2*.

As to the last point, breeding experiments showed the following: (RF $\times$ SJL)F_1 were all good reagin producers and the ($F_1 \times$ SJL) backcross segregated out 50% good serum reagin producers, 25% poor serum reagin producers, and 25% intermediate producers. The latter segregants bred true when crossed to SJL partners, thus indicating a true intermediate class. This kind of backcross result showed control by more than one locus, but is consistent with two loci. Our unpublished data indicated this genetic effect is upon reagin production rather than upon degradation. The properties of the system indicate the genetic expression in B-cell function, although the molecular details of what may be involved are not yet known.

Both these genetic controls were seen to operate in determining whether or not a given mouse strain will produce reagin to a given antigen. Thus, immunization of SJL to ovalbumin will yield γ_1 antibodies but not reagin. Immunization of DBA/1 with low doses of BPO-BGG will not yield antibody responses detectable by PCA, neither γ_1 nor reagin; asH-2^q do not respond to this antigen in minute doses. However, the (SJL $\times$ DBA/1)F_1 will respond with both reagin to ovalbumin and reagin to BPO-BGG, i.e., both genetic effects, reagin production and responsiveness to BPO-BGG, are dominant traits. Further studies in this field will be concerned with development of other kinds of genetic controls of reagin production in inbred mice and the dissection of cellular and molecular mechanisms involved in these controls. In addition to genetic controls, environmental factors are also important determinants of reagin production in the mouse.

V. Genetic Studies in Allergic Man

Returning to the problem of genetic control of reagin production in allergic man, my colleagues and I first sought to determine whether or not *Ir* genes would be

demonstrated in man and whether they play an important role in the generation
of allergic diseases. Ragweed hay fever was chosen as the disease in which to
look for *Ir* genes. It was felt that *Ir* genes could be most easily demonstrated
since ragweed pollenosis is a disease mediated by an immune response (reagin) to
minute doses of purified proteins (e.g., antigen E), and probably other antigens
contained in pollen, and it was sufficiently common to occur in several members
of a family. Family studies rather than population studies were deemed necessary
to directly demonstrate *Ir* genes. In our earliest family studies one family was
found in which ragweed pollenosis correlated with *HL-A* haplotype in three successive generations, suggesting the importance of *Ir* genes in ragweed hay fever
[35]. More recently, in collaboration with Dr. Rishon Stember and Dr. Madrilena
Fotino, we have been able to demonstrate *Ir* genes specific for antigen E and have
shown that these are necessary (but not sufficient) to permit ragweed hay fever
to occur. Seven families in which ragweed hay fever occurred in more than one
member were studied for clinical ragweed hay fever, IgE response to antigen E,
and HL-A haplotype. Details of experimental methods used are given in the
publication [36]. Figure 3 and Table 4 depict one of the seven families. In this
family, four of six (67%) family members that had the HL-A1, HL-A8 [1,8]

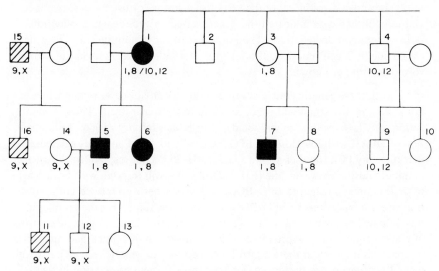

FIGURE 3 Representation of "R" family. Completely darkened circles or
squares represent patients with ragweed hay fever. Lined circles and squares
represent subjects with relatively weak skin reactivity to antigen E but no hay
fever. Lower numbers are haplotypes. Upper numbers represent subject number
for whom genetic and immunologic data are in Table 4. From B. B. Levine,
et al. [36].

TABLE 4 Clinical, Genetic, and Immunologic Features of Members of the "R" Family

Subject	Age (years)	HL-A Haplotype	Ragweed hay fever	Immediate wheal- and flare-skin reactivity			
				Ragweed extract (PNU/ml)		Antigen E (μg/ml)	
				100	1	10^{-3}	10^{-5}
1	60	1 8/10 12	Severe	−	4+	3+	1+
2	48	10 x /9 5	None	0	0	0	0
3	49	1 8/10 12	None	0	0	0	0
4	58	10 x /10 12	None	0	0	0	0
5	37	1 8/10 x	Severe	−	3+	2+	1+
6	35	1 8/10 x	Severe	−	ŗ+	4+	1+
7	24	1 8/5 x	Severe	−	4+	3+	1+
8	19	1 8/11R	None	0	0	0	0
9	25	2 7/10 12	None	0	0	0	0
10	26	2 7/10 x	None	0	0	0	0
11	12	9 x /10 x	None	−	2+	2+	0
12	16	9 x /10 4	None	0	0	0	0
13	14	10 x /1 Mapi	None	0	0	0	0
14	36	9 x /1 Mapi	None	0	0	0	0
15	59	9 x / x x	None	4+	2+	1+	0
16	24	9 x /1 Mapi	None	3+	1+	1+	0

aFrom B. B. Levine, *et al.* [36].

haplotype had intense immediate wheal-and-flare skin reactivity to antigen E in dilute solutions, indicating IgE antibody and severe ragweed hay fever. Neither of the two subjects with the other *HL-A* haplotype of the propositus (HL-A10, 12) had immediate skin reactivity to antigen E nor clinical ragweed hay fever. Of the blood relatives of the propositus who lacked the 1,8 haplotype, none of seven had ragweed hay fever. Six of the seven did not have reactivity to antigen E. One of the seven (subject 11, a grandson of the propositus) had a relatively weak skin reactivity to antigen E. In this exceptional case, another haplotype correlating with IgE antibody responsiveness to antigen E was inherited from the maternal side of the family. The figure shows that the maternal grandfather, a maternal uncle, the mother, and subject 11 all had the HL-A9, X haplotype and that subject 11 and his maternal grandfather and uncle all had weak skin reactivity to antigen E without clinical hay fever (Table 4).

Data for the seven families are totaled in Table 5. Twenty of 26 (77%) family members with the hay fever-associated haplotypes, had ragweed hay fever and intense skin reactivity to antigen E. By contrast, none of the 11 family members who had other haplotypes of the propositi (and lacked the hay fever-associated haplotype) had clinical ragweed hay fever. Ten of these 11 did not have skin reactivity to antigen E and one had relatively weak skin reactivity to antigen E. This difference in the frequency of IgE antibody responsiveness to antigen E (and clinical ragweed hay fever) between family members with the hay fever-associated haplotype and family members with the other haplotype of the propositus is highly significant statistically ($P<0.01$). The table also shows the frequency of IgE antibody responsiveness to antigen E and ragweed hay fever in blood relatives of the propositus who had neither of the haplotypes of the propositus. None of the 20 subjects in this group had clinical hay fever and three of 20 had relatively weak wheal-and-flare skin reactivity to antigen E. In one of these three subjects, a different ragweed hay fever-associated HL-A haplotype can be seen to have been introduced from the maternal side of the family (see Fig. 3).

These results show a highly significant statistical correlation between clinical ragweed hay fever and an intense IgE antibody immune response specific for antigen E with an HL-A haplotype in successive generations of the seven families studied. This linkage of intense IgE antibody responsiveness to antigen E (and ragweed hay fever) and HL-A haplotype through successive generations of the seven families implies a close genetic linkage between the HL-A system and a genetic locus controlling immune responsiveness to antigen E. If this immune responsiveness gene is similar to the *Ir* loci in the mouse, then it should also control the production of the IgG antibody specific for antigen E, and immune responsiveness should be antigen-specific. These two parameters were studied. First, serum IgG antibodies specific for antigen E were assayed by Dr. Kimishage

TABLE 5 Association of IgE Immune Response to Antigen E[a] and Ragweed Hay Fever with *HL–A* Haplotype in Successive Generations[b]

Family members[c]	Ratio (percentage) of family members having ragweed hay fever and intense wheal and flare reactivity to antigen E	Ratio (percentage) of family members having relatively weak wheal and flare reactivity to antigen E but without ragweed hay fever
Having the hay fever–associated haplotype	20/26 (77)	–
Having the other haplotype of the propositus[d]	0/11	1/11 (9)
Not having the hay fever–associated haplotype[e]	0/20	3/20 (15)

[a]As detected by intense direct wheal and flare skin reactivity to dilute solutions of allergens.
[b]Data for seven families are totaled.
[c]The propositus and blood relatives of the propositus are included.
[d]Excluding family members with both haplotypes of the propositus.
[e]This group of 20 includes the 11 family members with the other haplotype of the propositus. Data from Levine *et al.* [36].

Ishizaka in subjects from the family depicted in Figure 3. Three kinds of subjects were chosen. Subjects 1 and 6 who have the hay fever-associated haplotype and an intense IgE antibody responsiveness were found to have small amounts of IgG antibody to antigen E in their sera. Subjects 4 and 9 who have the other haplo-type of the propositus had no detectable IgG antibody for antigen E in their sera. Subjects 3 and 8 who have the hay fever-associated haplotype but no hay fever nor wheal-and-flare reactivity to antigen E, nevertheless had trace amounts of IgG antibody to antigen in their sera. Thus the gene controlling IgE immune responsiveness to antigen E also appears, according to these preliminary data, to control IgG responsiveness to antigen E.

As a preliminary study of antigenic specificity of the system, the 37 family members with either haplotype of the propositi were skin tested for wheal-and-flare reactivity with dilute (10 PNU/ml) solutions of timothy grass pollen extract and cat dander (hair) extract. Intense skin reactivity (3+ to 4+) to dilute solu-tions of cat dander extract was found in two of 26 (8%) family members with the other haplotype of the propositus. Thus the HL-A linked control of immune responsiveness to antigen E appears to show antigenic specificity, i.e., IgE anti-body responsiveness did not extend to two unrelated antigens.

The data presented above thus indicate the presence in human beings of a genetic locus, closely linked to the HL-A system, which controls IgE antibody responsiveness to antigen E and permits the development of ragweed hay fever. Preliminary data further indicate that this genetic factor controls immune respon-siveness in at least two antibody classes, IgE and IgG, and shows antigenic speci-ficity. This genetic factor is similar in immunologic properties to *H-2* linked *Ir* genes in mice. We tentatively refer to it as a human *Ir* gene and call this gene the *Ir-antigen E* gene. This appears to be the first demonstration of an *Ir* gene in man. More recently Marsh *et al.* [37] and Buckley *et al.* [38] have reported evi-dence indicating *Ir* genes in man specific for other antigens.

Several points merit brief discussion. First, in the seven families studied, the *Ir-antigen E* gene was linked to seven different *HL-A* haplotypes (*W-28, X; HL-A10, Da*(6); *HL-A3,* 7; *HL-A1,* 8; *HL-A2, W14; HL-A2, X;* and *HL-A2, W-14*). Whether one or more of these haplotypes will be frequently or always linked to an *Ir-antigen E* gene in this or in other populations remains to be deter-mined. In this regard, it is not known whether only one or several different *Ir-antigen E* genes exist. Further, we presume that *Ir* genes specific for other anti-gens exist in man and that these may be necessary for the development of immu-nologic diseases specific for other antigens. Second, a rough estimate of the frequency of *Ir-antigen E* genes in our local population can be given. In the seven families studied, 20 of 26 (77%) family members who possessed *Ir-antigen E* genes had intense IgE responsiveness to antigen E and clinical hay fever. These seven families were not selected at random, however, but were basically selected for expressivity of clinical hay fever; that is, an equal number of families were interviewed but not selected for study because clinical hay fever, while present in the propositus, did not appear in the other members of the family. Thus the 0.77 rate of expressivity of the *Ir-antigen E* genes (as an intense reagin response to antigen E) may be about twice as high as in the general population. To calculate the likely approximate prevalence of subjects possessing *Ir* genes in our local population, we use the following data [24] : 10% of our local population have intense wheal–and–flare reactivity to dilute solutions of antigen E, and 40% of ragweed hay fever patients also react intensely to timothy pollen allergens in dilute solution as compared with 4% of subjects who are not ragweed reactive. These data are consistent with a high (30% to 40%) prevalence of individuals with *Ir-antigen E* genes in our local population, with a rate of expression of the *Ir* genes as a reagin response of about 0.3.

The presence of an *Ir-antigen E* gene is viewed as necessary but not sufficient for the development of an intense IgE immune response to antigen E and clinical hay fever. The trait controlled by the *Ir* gene is inherited as a Mendelian dominant. For expression, i.e., for the individual to mount an IgE immune response to repeated minute doses of antigen E, additional factors, both genetic and environmental, are required. The nature of these additional factors are not clearly known. Among environmental factors sufficient for its expression is adequate exposure to airborne allergen and its diffusion through mucous membranes to lymphoid cells. An additional genetic factor might be one similar to a genetic control described in inbred mice, which permits a strong IgE antibody response to a variety of antigens. However, this factor may not frequently be limiting in outbred man. Nevertheless, Hamburger and Basaral [39] suggested a genetic control of basal IgE levels in man on the basis of statistical analysis of serum IgE levels in normal adults. Other factors not directly related to the function of lymphatic tissues have been suggested as influencing immune responsiveness to airborne allergens, i.e., permeability of mucous membrane [23,24] , and permeability factors may be limiting the expression of the *Ir-antigen E* gene in man. Other nonimmune factors are probably also operative in determining, in patients with intense IgE antibody responses to ragweed antigens, the nature of the clinical result (e.g., rhinitis vs. rhinitis plus asthma) and its severity [19]. It will be important to learn the nature of the various environmental and genetic factors which permit the expressivity of *Ir-antigen E* genes.

VI. Clinical Application of Genetic Studies

There is a potential clinical usefulness for these findings. Haplotyping families that have high incidences of antigen–specific allergic diseases might serve to identify those young family members at–risk for these diseases in which preventive measures might be instituted.

Currently my colleagues and I believe that in order for an individual to develop ragweed hay fever under conditions of natural exposure in the New York City area, that person must possess an *Ir*-gene specific for antigen E (or for another clinically important ragweed antigen). The nature of other genetic information needed to develop hay fever is not clearly known. Probably many separate genes are needed, some of which are possessed by the great majority of the population (e.g., structural genes for IgE synthesis), some of which are possessed by only a fraction of the population at–risk and are thus factors that limit the prevalence of hay fever. These genetic factors control both immunologic processes (e.g., related to production and secretion of high avidity IgE antibody, which is a complex process) and nonimmunologic processes (e.g., mucous membrane permeability to allergenic materials, mediator release, vascular response to mediators, neurohumoral and metabolic processes). Additionally, environmental factors that influence these processes also determine which of the individuals who possess the required genetic background will express the trait. Thus, it can be appreciated that individuals may possess a gene, such as an *Ir-antigen E* gene, and yet not express it as clinical hay fever if they lack other necessary genetic information, or if environmental factors, such as inadequate exposure, prevent phenotypic expression. Yet these individuals will pass the *Ir-antigen E* gene to some of their children and grandchildren who then might express it with clinical hay fever. This is one explanation for "skip generations." Thus in further genetic studies in atopic diseases, it will be important to have a marker for the gene under investigation, so that it can be detected in an individual even in the absence of the atopic disease.

In summary, certain of the allergic diseases appear to be associated in individuals and families. These are asthma (both allergic and idiopathic), allergic rhinitis, atopic eczema, and possibly vasomotor rhinitis, urticaria, and bonafide food allergy. Multiple factors, both genetic and environmental are involved in the generation of these diseases.

Recent studies have demonstrated two distinct kinds of genetic controls of IgE antibody formation in inbred mice. One of these has also been shown to exist in man and appears necessary but not sufficient for the generation of ragweed hay fever. This is the *Ir-antigen E* gene(s), which permits the individual to recognize as antigens, low concentrations of antigen E.

Atopic diseases are based on many genetic and environmental factors. Some factors are unique for individual diseases and some (one or a small number) are probably common to all. The latter are not clearly appreciated as yet, although mucosal permeability factors and β–adrenergic blockade factors have been suggested.

In depth understanding of the genetic controls of atopy will require studies on the many individual factors involved in atopy, their function, their genetic transmission, and their interplay to cause atopic diseases.

References

1. P. M. Henson and C. G. Cochrane, Immune complex disease in rabbits. The role of complement and of a leukocyte–dependent release of vasoactive amines from platelets, *J. Exp. Med., 133*:554–571 (1971).
2. A. F. Coca and R. A. Cooke, On the classification of the phenomenon of hypersensitiveness, *J. Immunol., 8*:163–182 (1923).
3. P. Portier and C. Richet, De l'action anaphylactique de certains venins, *C. R. Seances Soc. Biol., 54*:170–172 (1902).
4. T. Smith, Degrees of susceptibility to diptheria toxin among guinea pigs. Transmission from parent to offspring, *J. Med. Res., 8*:341–348 (1904).
5. S. J. Meltzer, Bronchial asthma as a phenomenon of anaphylaxis, *J. Am. Med. Assoc., 55*:1021–1024 (1910).
6. M. A. Ramirez, Horse asthma following blood transfusion: Report of a case, *J. Am. Med. Assoc., 73*:984–985 (1919).
7. C. Prausnitz and H. Kustner, Studien Über die Ueberempfindlichkeit, *Zbl. Bakt.* (Orig.), *86*:160 (1921).
8. M. Schwartz, Heredity in bronchial asthma, *Acta Allergol., 5*:Suppl. 2: 11–288 (1952).
9. G. Edgren, Prognose und erblichkeitsmomente bei ekzima infantum, *Acta Paediatr.,* Suppl. 30:1–204 (1943).
10. W. C. Stifler, Jr., A 21 year follow–up of infantile eczema, *J. Pediatr., 66*: 166–167 (1965).
11. R. A. Cooke and A. Vander Veer, Human sensitization, *J. Immunol., 1*: 201–305 (1916).
12. W. C. Spain and R. A. Cooke, Studies in specific hypersensitivity: II. The familial incidence of hay fever and bronchial asthma, *J. Immunol., 9*:521–569 (1924).
13. J. Adkinson, The behavior of bronchial asthma as an inherited characteristic, *Genetics, 5*:363–418 (1920).
14. F. M. Rackemann. *Clinical Allergy. Asthma and Hay fever.* New York, The Macmillan Company, 1931, pp. 1–607.
15. W. T. Vaughan and J. H. Black. *Practice of Allergy.* Second edition. St. Louis, Mosby, 1948, pp. 1–1145.
16. S. L. Feinberg. *Allergy in Practice.* Chicago, Year Book Publishers, 1944, pp. 1–819.
17. D. Spaich and M. Ostertag, Untersuchungen über allergische Erkrankungen bei Zwillingen, *Z. Menschl. Vererb. Konstitutions–lehre, 19*:731–752 (1936).

18. J. A. Clarke, Jr., H. H. Donalley, and A. F. Coca, On the influence of heredity in atopy, *J. Immunol.,* **15**:9–11 (1928).

19. A. Szentivanyi, The beta adrenergic theory of atopic abnormality in bronchial asthma, *J. Allergy,* **42**:203–232 (1968).

20. R. H. Carr, W. W. Busse, and C. E. Reed, Failure of catecholamines to inhibit epidermal mitosis in vitro, *J. Allergy Clin. Immunol.,* **51**:255–262 (1973).

21. H. Eppinger and L. Hess. *Die Vagotonie.* Berlin, 1910, pp. 1–99.

22. J. A. Waindorff, The response of sweat glands to acetylcholine in atopic subjects, *Br. J. Dermatol.,* **83**:306–311 (1970).

23. J. Salvaggio, H. Kayman, and S. Leskowitz, Immunologic responses of atopic and normal individuals to aerosolized destran, *J. Allergy,* **38**:31–40 (1966).

24. R. H. Stember and B. B. Levine, Prevalence of allergic diseases, penicillin hypersensitivity, and aeroallergen hypersensitivity in various populations, *J. Allergy Clin. Immunol.,* **51**:100 (1973) (abstr.).

25. B. B. Levine and N. M. Vaz, Effect of combinations of strain, antigen dose on reagin production in the mouse. A mouse model for human atopy, *Int. Arch. Allergy,* **39**:156–171 (1970).

26. N. M. Vaz and B. B. Levine, Immune responsiveness of inbred mice to low doses of antigen: Relationship to histocompatibility (H–2) type, *Science,* **168**:852–854 (1970).

27. N. M. Vaz, J. M. Phillips–Quagliata, B. B. Levine, and E. M. Vaz, H–2 linked genetic control of immune responsiveness to ovalbumin and ovomucoid, *J. Exp. Med.,* **134**:1335–1348 (1971).

28. H. O. McDevitt and H. Chinitz, Genetic control of antibody response: Relationship between immune response and histocompatability (H–2) type, *Science,* **163**:1207–1208 (1969).

29. H. O. McDevitt, B. D. Deak, D. C. Schreffler, J. Klein, J. H. Stimpfling, and G. D. Snell, Genetic control of the immune response. Mapping of the *Ir–1* locus, *J. Exp. Med.,* **135**:1259–1278 (1972).

30. R. Lieberman and W. Humphrey, Association of H–2 types with genetic control of immune responsiveness to IgA allotypes in the mouse, *Proc. Natl. Acad. Sci. USA,* **68**:2510–2513 (1971).

31. R. Lieberman and W. Humphrey, Separation of Ir genes for IgG and IgA allotypes in the mouse, *Fed. Proc.,* **31**:777 (1972).

32. G. F. Mitchell, F. C. Grumet, and H. O. McDevitt, The effect of thymectomy on the primary and secondary response of mice to poly–L(Tyr,Glu)–poly–D,L–Ala––poly–L–lys, *J. Exp. Med.,* **135**:126–135 (1972).

33. B. B. Levine and N. M. Vaz, Genetic control of reagin production in mice, *Fed. Proc.,* **30**:469 (1971) (abstr.).

34. B. B. Levine, Genetic factors in reagin production in mice. In *Biochemistry of the Acute Allergic Reactions.* Second International Symposium. Edited by K. F. Austen and E. L. Becker. Oxford Blackwell Scientific Publications, 1971, pp. 1–11.

35. B. B. Levine. The John Sheldon Memorial Lecture at the Annual Meeting of the American Academy of Allergy, Chicago, February, 1971.

36. B. B. Levine, R. H. Stember, R. H. Fotino, and M. Fotino, Ragweed hay fever: Genetic control and linkage to HL-A haplotypes, *Science,* **178**: 1201–1203 (1972).

37. D. G. Marsh, W. B. Bias, S. H. Hsu, and L. Goodfriend, Association of an HL-A7 crossreacting group with a specific reaginic antibody response in allergic man, *Science,* **179**:691–693 (1973).

38. C. E. Buckley, III, F. C. Dorsey, R. B. Corley, W. B. Rolph, M. A. Wordburg, and F. B. Amos, HL-A linked human immune response genes, *Proc. Natl. Acad. Sci. USA,* **70**:2157–2161 (1973).

39. R. N. Hamburger and M. Bazarel, IgE levels in twins confirm genetic control in human beings, *J. Allergy Clin. Immunol.,* **49**:91 (1972) (abstr.).

21

The Pharmacologic Modulation of Mediator Release from Human Basophils and Mast Cells

ALLEN P. KAPLAN

National Institute of Allergy and Infectious Diseases
National Institutes of Health
Bethesda, Maryland

I. Introduction

The treatment of asthma, regardless of type or etiology, frequently necessitates the use of many different types of drugs in order to relieve the patients respiratory distress. Thus one might utilize bronchodilators, such as isoproterenol, aminophylline, and epinephrine, to relieve bronchospasm, antibiotics to treat infection, expectorants to reduce mucus plugging of small bronchioles, antihistamines to antagonize the bronchoconstrictive and permeability effects of histamine, disodium cromoglycate to inhibit mediator release from tissue mast cells, and steroids to reverse an apparent β-receptor blockade. It has become clear, however, that many of these agents, such as the bronchodilators, also modulate the release of mediators from basophils or tissue mast cells. Observations such as these have provided new insights into the biochemical steps that lead to the release of mediators as well as the manner by which these therapeutic agents act. Most studies have been performed using IgE–dependent mediator release as the model; thus the observations made are directly pertinent to allergic or extrinsic asthma although the effects of drugs in "intrinsic" asthma may be the same, even though the underlying etiology is not known. It is the purpose of this review to describe the mechanisms of modulating mediator release from basophils and mast cells as they relate to the manifestations and therapy of asthma.

A. The Role of IgE in Mediator Release

Approximately 50 yr ago Prausnitz and Kustner first identified reaginic activity
in human sera and demonstrated that skin sensitizing activity could be passively
transferred from allergic to normal individuals, indicating that an antibody might
be involved. The immunoglobulin class to which this reaginic activity belonged
was not determined until 1966 when Ishizaka *et al.* [1] provided evidence that
the reaginic activity of sera from ragweed sensitive patients could not be removed
after absorption with myeloma proteins of the known IgG, IgM, IgD, or IgA
classes and suggested that reagin belonged to a unique class of immunoglobulin
tentatively designated γE (IgE). This globulin was inactivated by heating at $56°C$
for 2-4 hr [2] as originally described for human skin sensitizing antibodies [3]
and was later partially purified from ragweed sensitive serum and definitively
identified [4]. About this time, a heat-labile homocytotropic antibody in atopic
(allergic) serum was shown to be capable of passively sensitizing human leukocytes
[5] and monkey lung for antigen-induced histamine release [6] or human lung
for the antigen-dependent release of both histamine and slow-reacting substance
of anaphylaxis (SRS_A) [7,8], providing evidence that the passive transfer experiment could be performed in vitro and mediator release observed in a direct
fashion.

Studies of the role of IgE in mediator release were greatly facilitated by the
discovery of an atypical myeloma protein termed IgND, [9] which appeared to
be a new class of immunoglobulin [10] and was subsequently shown to have IgE
antigenic determinants in its Fc fragment [11]. This myeloma protein could
specifically inhibit the Prausnitz-Kustner reaction [12], a property shown to reside in binding sites of the Fc fragment of IgE for human skin [13].

The studies of Lichtenstein and Osler [14] indicated that leukocytes from
ragweed sensitive patients release histamine upon incubation with the appropriate antigen. Subsequently, antibody to IgE was shown to substitute for antigen
in this system and liberate histamine [15], indicating that cell-bound IgE is a
critical component of the release reaction. Utilizing [^{125}I] anti-IgE for histamine
release, it was shown that IgE was actually bound to basophil leukocytes through
its Fc fragment [15-17], thus identifying the critical cell in the leukocyte system
responsible for histamine release. In tissue systems, the critical cell appeared to
be the mast cell [18], and using the human lung model, IgE has also been shown
to be responsible for the observed mediator release upon antigenic challenge.
Experiments, which conclusively demonstrated this, are as follows: depletion of
IgE from the serum of a ragweed sensitive patient with monospecific antihuman
IgE to leave the concentrations of IgG, IgA, IgM, and IgD unchanged removed
the capacity of the serum to prepare monkey [19] or human [20] lung fragments
for the antigen-induced release of histamine and SRS_A. Conversely, antisera to

the other immunoglobulin classes had no effect. IgE myeloma protein was found to compete for the receptor sites and abolish the capacity of allergic serum to sensitize the lung fragments for antigen-induced mediator release [20,21]. Challenge with antihuman IgE of human lung [22] or of monkey lung fragments prepared with atopic serum, purified IgE myeloma [19], or the Fc fragment of IgE myeloma [23] also elicited mediator release, whereas challenge with antisera to other human immunoglobulin classes did not.

Studies by Ishizaka using human basophils have estimated that a minimum of two IgE molecules in proximity are required for antigen-induced mediator release and presented evidence for the likelihood of bridging of two IgE molecules by multivalent antigen. This antigen was capable of binding to one of the Fab fragments of each IgE, thereby bridging two molecules [24-26]. They have further estimated the number of IgE molecules per basophil in the order of 10,000-40,000, with a binding constant of approximately 10^8 to 10^{10} liters/mol, indicating very firm binding [27]. This is consistent with the inability of IgE to be washed off the cells. Nevertheless some exchange of cell bound IgE with fluid phase $[^{125}I]$ IgE can be demonstrated, indicating that the binding, although firm, is nevertheless reversible. A diagrammatic representation of antigen-induced mediator release from IgE sensitized cells is shown in Figure 1.

A second heat-stable immunoglobulin of the IgG class has also been shown to participate in mediator release in a variety of animals. These include IgG_1 of

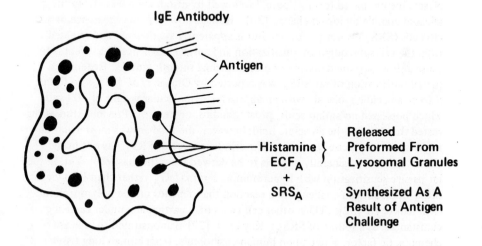

FIGURE 1 Drawing of mediator release from an IgE-sensitized basophil or mast cell after interaction with antigen.

the guinea pig, IgG_a of the rat, and IgG_1 of the mouse [28,29]. However, an IgG subclass having this function in man has not been identified. Periodically, reports of such an immunoglobulin in man have appeared but when assessed further have generally been confused with IgE. One can demonstrate IgG bound to human basophils, and mediator release can be observed with anti-IgG. However, the concentration of antiserum required is 100 to 1000 times as high as that of anti-IgE in order to yield comparable histamine release (Table 1). IgG does possess weak affinity for basophils; thus washed basophils contain only about 1% the quantity of bound IgG compared to IgE. Since immunization via the upper respiratory tract does not result in the production of high levels of IgG antibody (IgA and IgE predominate), a role for IgG in hay fever or asthma presently appears unlikely. This does not, however, preclude the possibility of an IgG reagin being present in man, which, under certain circumstances, can be of pathogenic significance.

B. Mediators of Immediate Hypersensitivity

The best characterized and most frequently assessed mediator released from basophils or mast cells is histamine, which is present in the lysosomal granules of the cell bound to cationic polypeptides and a heparin-like material. These granules appear to be extruded by fusion of the lysosomal membrane with the plasma membrane to form a "pore," followed by histamine release from the released granule by ion-exchange [30]. Human slow-reacting substance of anaphylaxis (SRS_A) is not preformed but is apparently synthesized and released from the cell subsequent to sensitization and antigen challenge. Its effect is to cause a slow, sustained contraction of bronchial smooth muscle. Recently, a partial purification of rat SRS_A was reported by Orange *et al.* [31] who found it to be an acidic molecule with an approximate molecular weight of 400 and which possessed no amino acids, prostaglandins, or steroids. Previous studies suggested that it might be an acidic lipid; however, the final answer must await determination of its precise structure. The cellular source of SRS_A has not been clearly defined; it generally appears to be derived from the mast cell. Yet, in the rat passive sensitization with hyperimmune serum (IgG_A rather than IgE) yields SRS_A upon antigen challenge in a reaction that depends on the polymorphonuclear leukocyte [32]. Thus, other cell types may participate, under certain circumstances, as a source of SRS_A. Kay *et al.* [22] demonstrated the release of a chemotactic factor, active upon human eosinophils, from human lung tissue sensitized with IgE antibody and challenged with antigen. This has been termed *Eosinophilic Chemotactic Factor of Anaphylaxis* (ECF_A) [33] and appears to be a preformed peptide with an approximate molecular weight 500 to 1000,

TABLE 1 Histamine Release[a] from Human Leukocytes by Anti-IgG vs. Anti-IgE[b]

					Dilution				
	1:32	1:64	1:128	1:256	1:512	1:1024	1:2048	1:4096	1:8192
Anti-IgG	90	150	30	–	–	–	–	–	–
Anti-IgE	–	–	15	37.5	90	135	180	150	90

[a]Values for histamine released in nanograms as determined by bioassay using the isolated guinea pig ileum [Clark and Kaplan, unpublished observations].

[b]IgG and IgE antibody studied at equivalent antibody nitrogen content.

apparently in the same granule fraction with histamine [34]. The release of other mediators from basophils or mast cells may occur directly as a consequence of antigen challenge or may be secondarily recruited from other cells. The release of histamine and serotonin from rabbit platelets, as a consequence of IgE-dependent release of mediators from rabbit basophils is an example of such a mechanism [35]. In an analogous fashion, kinins or prostaglandins may be recruited into the allergic reaction, but their source and mechanism of release have not been extensively studied.

C. The Mechanism of Mediator Release and Its Pharmacologic Control

Mediator release has been shown to be noncytotoxic and is considered to be analogous to secretory processes observed in other cells. An intact glycolytic pathway is essential, since mediator release is inhibited by the addition of iodoacetic acid or by incubation with 2-deoxyglucose when the glucose concentration is limited. The reaction also requires the presence of calcium ions [20,36]. The sequence of histamine release from IgE-sensitized human leukocytes has been divided into two stages, an initial stage dependent upon antigen but independent of calcium ions and a subsequent antigen–independent phase that then requires calcium ions [36]. This sequence has also been observed in the human lung system and, in addition, antigen–induced activation of an esterase appears to be a prerequisite for mediator release [20].

In 1968 Lichtenstein and Margolis [37] demonstrated that histamine release from human leukocytes could be inhibited by catecholamines, such as isoproteranol or epinephrine. These agents activate the enzyme adenyl cylcase, which catalyzes the formation of cyclic $3'5'$ AMP from ATP. Methylxanthines, such as theophylline or caffeine, also inhibit histamine release and elevate the cellular level of cyclic $3'5'$ AMP by inhibiting phosphodiesterase, the enzyme that destroys cyclic $3'5'$ AMP by converting it to $5'$ AMP. Both observations suggested that the inhibition of mediator release observed might be a consequence of elevated levels of cyclic $3'5'$ AMP. The ability of catecholamines plus methylxanthines to synergistically inhibit histamine release and of dibutryl cyclic AMP itself to inhibit release fulfilled the criteria considered critical for the demonstration of a role for cyclic AMP in a given system. The ability of propanolol, a β–adrenergic blocking agent, to inhibit the effect of catecholamines provided further evidence to suggest that the basophil possesses a β–receptor [38]. Studies with lung tissue provided evidence for the presence of receptors of the a– and β–adrenergic type as well as cholinergic receptors that modulate IgE-mediated reactions. Initially, it was found that IgE-mediated release of both histamine and SRS_A from human lung could be inhibited by β-adrenergic

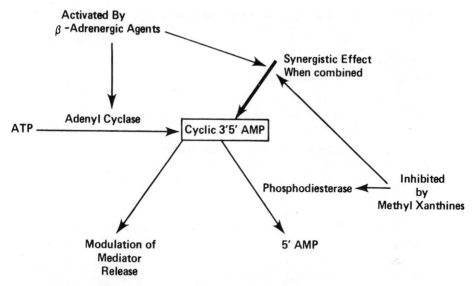

FIGURE 2   Affect of β–adrenergic agents and methylxanthines upon the formation of cyclic 3'5' AMP.

stimulators [21] and, subsequently, that a-adrenergic stimulation caused an increase in mediator release [20,39]. Thus a mixture of epinephrine, an agent that possesses both a and β effects plus propranolol, a β-blocker, yielded the predicted a enhancement. This effect could then be inhibited by the a antagonist, phenoxybenzamine. Direct measurement of cyclic AMP levels revealed an inverse relationship between tissue cyclic 3'5' AMP levels and mediator release [39]. Enhancement of the immunologic release of both histamine and SRS_A has also been shown to be demonstrable by addition of cholinergic agents, such as carbamylcholine chloride, the effect of which could be inhibited by atropine. However, no effect upon cyclic AMP levels was observed. Since cholinergic agents were known to act upon the cyclic GMP system, the effect of 8-bromo-cyclic GMP upon antigen–induced mediator release was investigated and a dose-dependent enhancement was found, providing further indirect evidence that the cholinergic enhancement depends upon the level of cyclic GMP [40]. A summary of the effects of adrenergic and cholinergic agents upon cyclic 3'5' AMP and mediator release is shown in Table 2.

Histamine, a product of the release reaction has been shown to inhibit the release process from human leukocytes and is associated with an increased level of cyclic AMP [41,42]. However, it is effective only during the first few minutes of the reaction, before much histamine is actually released. This effect, although apparently modulated by a rise in cyclic AMP, was not inhibited by propranolol,

TABLE 2 Pharmacologic Control of Mediator Release from Human Lung

Stimulus		C–AMP	Mediator release
β–Adrenergic Agent	Isoproterenol or Epinephrine	↑	↓
α–Adrenergic Agent	Phenylephrine or Norepinephrine + propranalol	↓	↑
Cholinergic Agent	Acetylcholine or Carbachol	No Change (? ↑ C–GMP)	↑
Prostaglandins E_1 and E_2 (low dose)		↓	↑
Prostaglandins E_1 and E_2 (high dose)		↑	↓
Histamine		↑	↓

indicating that histamine is not acting on the β–receptor [42]. Furthermore, its inhibitory effect was not inhibited by antihistamines, suggesting that it may act via the H_2 receptor [43], as is the case for histamine stimulation of gastric secretion, rather than by the H_1 receptor which causes smooth muscle contraction and increased vascular permeability.

Prostaglandins E_1 and E_2 were also shown to inhibit the immunologic release of histamine from human leukocytes by increasing the level of cyclic AMP through a separate prostaglandin receptor [42] distinct from the β–receptor. In the human lung system, high doses of prostaglandins E_1 and E_2 had essentially the same effect as in the leukocyte system. However, low doses depressed cyclic AMP levels and enhanced the release of mediators [44]. Recently, evidence for IgE–dependent release of prostaglandins E_1, E_2, and F_2a from human lung has been presented [45]. Thus, the release of prostaglandins may not only act directly upon bronchial muscle tone (F_2a is a potent bronchoconstrictor), but E_1 and E_2 may act as a regulator capable of increasing or depressing the release of mediators, depending upon its concentration.

Microtubules have been implicated in the terminal steps of the secretory process. Challenge with antigen appears to cause aggregation of microtubules, a process that depends upon calcium. Thus colchicine, an agent that binds to microtubules and inhibits aggregation, was found to inhibit IgE–dependent histamine release from leukocytes, whereas deuterium oxide (D_2O), which facilitates aggregation, blocks the action of colchicine and itself enhances the release of histamine [46,47]. It is possible that phosphorylation of microtubule protein by protein kinases activated by cyclic 3'5' AMP may be the mechanism by which its inhibitory action is manifested [48].

The sequence of biochemical events in the antigen-induced release of mediators from human lung has suggested a sequence of events in which the initial activation of a DFP activatable esterase requires calcium and is followed in sequence by a glucose-requiring, a second calcium requiring, and cyclic-AMP modulating steps [49]. This cannot be clearly related to the two-step sequence seen with human leukocytes in which an antigen-dependent, calcium-independent step occurs first at which point agents influencing cyclic AMP levels exert their effect before the calcium-dependent, glucose-requiring step. It is clear that details of the surface and intracellular chemistry of the basophil and mast cell will be required in order to further clarify individual steps leading to the release of mediators in each cell type.

D. Abnormalities of Mediator Release in Asthma and The Role of Drug Therapy

In 1968 Szentivanyi [50] proposed the theory of β-adrenergic blockade as the underlying cellular abnormality in bronchial asthma. There is considerable indirect evidence to support this theory; for example, a diminished adenyl cyclase response to isoproterenol has been observed when leukocytes from patients with asthma are compared to those from normal subjects [51-55]. Furthermore, patients with severe asthma fail to evoke a hyperglycemic response to the administration of epinephrine [56,57], a function known to be mediated by a β-receptor effect. Determination of urinary cyclic AMP in this population after epinephrine was administered revealed little increase compared to that observed in normal subjects [58]. Alternatively, these defects could be viewed as being caused by hyperactivity of a-receptors. In support of this possibility, phentolamine, a standard a-blocking agent was found to possess some β-agonist activity that could be blocked with propranolol, yet it acted synergistically with isoproteranol to correct the diminished response of leukocytes from patients with asthma to isoproteranol. Possibly its a-blocking effect allowed the full β effect of isoproteranol to be expresed [59].

Theoretically, any agent that acts to diminish the release of mediators should be efficacious in bronchial asthma. Thus, the effect of isoproteranol and aminophylline may be to diminish the release of mediators as well as to exert a direct dilating effect upon bronchial smooth musculature. Since the effect of both a-adrenergic and cholinergic stimulation is to enhance the release of mediators, a-blocking agents and atropine might be effective in asthma and are presently being evaluated. Symptoms of certain subpopulations of asthmatics may be related to cholinergic or a-adrenergic effects and may respond to these agents.

The new agent, disodium cromoglycate, has been shown to be beneficial in bronchial asthma, although somewhat more so in extrinsic asthma [60-69]. It is also effective in the treatment of asthma induced by exercise [70,71], by hyperventillation [72], and by certain chemical irritants [73]. This agent is taken by inhalation and acts upon the cell to block the release of mediators [74,75], although its site of action is unknown. Steroids undoubtedly affect the cell in many ways. However, there is evidence that they can reverse the diminished response of patients with asthma to β-adrenergic stimuli and may therefore act, in part, to normalize the function of the β-receptor [54,76]. Certainly a better understanding of the underlying cellular defect(s) in asthma will provide a more rational approach to the use of known agents. Hopefully it will lead to the development of drugs that act to block specific reactions or reverse defined biochemical abnormalities and thereby increase our ability to deal with patients who respond poorly to our present regimens.

References

1.   K. Ishizaka, T. Ishizaka, and M. M. Hornbrook, Physicochemical properties of reaginic antibody. IV. Presence of a unique immunoglobulin as a carrier of reaginic activity, *J. Immunol.*, **97**:75–85 (1966).
2.   K. Ishizaka, T. Ishizaka, and A. E. O. Menzel, Physicochemical properties of reaginic antibody. VI. Effect of heat on γE, γG and γA antibodies in the sera of ragweed sensitive patients, *J. Immunol.*, **99**:610–618 (1967).
3.   M. H. Loveless, Immunologic studies of Pollinosis. I. The presence of two antibodies related to the same pollen–antigen in the serum of treated hay–fever patients, *J. Immunol.*, **38**:25–50 (1940).
4.   K. Ishizaka and T. Ishizaka, Identification of IgE antibody as a carrier of reaginic activity, *J. Immunol.*, **99**:1187–1198 (1967).
5.   D. A. Levy and A. G. Osler, Studies on the mechanisms of hypersensitivity phenomena. XIV. Passive sensitization in vitro of human leucocytes to ragweed pollen, *J. Immunol.*, **97**:203–212 (1966).
6.   L. Goodfriend, B. A. Kovacs, and B. Rose, In vitro sensitization of monkey lung fragments with human ragweed atopic serum, *Int. Arch. Allergy*, **30**: 511–518 (1966).
7.   P. Sheard, P. G. Killingback, and A. M. J. N. Blair, Antigen–induced release of histamine and SRS–A from human lung passively sensitized with reaginic serum, *Nature* (London), **216**:283–284 (1967).
8.   W. E. Parish, Release of histamine and slow reacting substance with mast cell changes after challenge of human lung sensitized passively with reagin in vitro, *Nature*, **215**:738–739 (1967).
9.   S. G. O. Johansson and H. Bennich, Immunologic studies of an atypical (myeloma) immunoglobulin, *Immunology*, **13**:381–394 (1967).

10. S. G. O. Johansson, H. Bennich, and L. Wide, A new class of immunoglobulins in human serum, *Immunology*, 14:265–272 (1968).

11. H. Bennich, K. Ishizaka, T. Ishizaka, and S. G. O. Johansson, A comparative antigenic study of γE globulin and myeloma IgND, *J. Immunol.*, 102: 826–831 (1968).

12. D. R. Stanworth, J. H. Humphrey, H. Bennich, and S. G. O. Johansson, Specific inhibition of the Prausnitz–Kustner reaction by an atypical human myeloma protein, *Lancet*, 2:330–332 (1967).

13. D. R. Stanworth, J. H. Humphrey, H. Bennich, and S. G. O. Johansson, Inhibition of Prausnitz–Kustner reaction by proteolytic cleavage fragments of a human myeloma protein of immunoglobulin class E, *Lancet*, 2:17–18 (1968).

14. L. M. Lichtenstein and A. G. Osler, Studies in the mechanisms of hypersensitivity phenomena. IX. Histomine release from human leukocytes by ragweed pollen antigen, *J. Exp. Med.*, 120:507–530 (1964).

15. T. Ishizaka, K. Ishizaka, S. G. O. Johansson, and H. Bennich, Histamine release from human leukocytes by anti–γE antibodies, *J. Immunol.*, 102: 884–892 (1969).

16. K. Ishizaka, R. DeBernardo, H. Tomioka, L. M. Lichtenstein, and T. Ishizaka, Identification of basophil granulocytes as a site of allergic histamine release, *J. Immunol.*, 108:1000–1008 (1972).

17. A. L. Sullivan, P. Grimley, and H. Metzger, Electron microscopic localization of immunoglobulin E on the surface membrane of human basophils, *J. Exp. Med.*, 134:1402–1416 (1971).

18. H. Tomioka and K. Ishizaka, Mechanisms of passive sensitization. II. Presence of receptors for IgE in monkey mast cells, *J. Immunol.*, 107: 971–978 (1971).

19. T. Ishizaka, K. Ishizaka, R. P. Orange, and K. F. Austen, The capacity of human immunoglobulin E to mediate the release of histamine and slow reacting substance of anaphylaxis (SRS_A) from monkey lung, *J. Immunol.*, 104:335–343 (1970).

20. R. P. Orange, M. A. Kaliner, and K. F. Austen, The immunologic release of histamine and slow reacting substance of anaphylaxis from human lung. III. Biochemical control mechanisms involved in the immunologic release of the chemical mediators. In Second International Symposium on the Biochemistry of the Acute Allergic Reactions. Edited by K. F. Austen and E. L. Becker. Oxford, England, Blackwell Scientific, 1971, pp. 189–202.

21. R. P. Orange, W. G. Austen, and K. F. Austen, The immunological release of histamine and slow reacting substance of anaphylaxis from human lung. I. Modulation by agents influencing cellular levels of cyclic 3′,5′–adenosine monophosphate, *J. Exp. Med.*, Suppl., 134:136s–148s (1971).

22. A. B. Kay and K. F. Austen, The IgE–mediated release of an eosinophil leukocyte chemotactic factor from human lung, *J. Immunol.*, 107:889–902 (1971).

23.   K. Ishizaka, T. Ishizaka, and E. H. Lee, Biologic function of the Fc frag-
      ments of E myeloma protein, *Immunochemistry*, 7:687–702 (1970).
24.   K. Ishizaka and T. Ishizaka, Mechanisms of reaginic hypersensitivity, *Clin.
      Allergy*, 1:9–24 (1971).
25.   K. Ishizaka and T. Ishizaka, Immune mechanisms of reversed type reaginic
      hypersensitivity, *J. Immunol.*, 103:588–595 (1969).
26.   K. Ishizaka and T. Ishizaka, Induction of erythema wheal reactions by sol-
      uble antigen–γE antibody complexes in humans, *J. Immunol.*, 101:68–78
      (1968).
27.   T. Ishizaka, C. S. Soto, and K. Ishizaka, Mechanisms of passive sensitization.
      III. Number of IgE molecules and their receptor sites on human basophil
      granulocytes, *J. Immunol.*, 111:500–511 (1973).
28.   K. J. Block and J. L. Ohman, The stable homocytotropic antibodies of
      guinea pig, mouse, and rat; and some indirect evidence for the in vivo inter-
      action of homocytotropic antibodies of two different rat immunoglobulin
      classes at a common receptor on target cells. In Second International Sym-
      posium on the Biochemistry of the Acute Allergic Reactions. Edited by
      K. F. Austen and E. L. Becker. Oxford, England, Blackwell Scientific,
      1971, pp. 45–64.
29.   E. L. Becker and K. F. Austen, Anaphylaxis. In *Textbook of Immuno-
      pathology*. Vol. 1. Edited by P. A. Miescher and H. J. Muller–Ebechard.
      New York, Grune and Stratton, 1968, pp. 76–93.
30.   B. Uvnas, Quantitative correlation between degranulation and histamine
      release in mast cells. In Second International Symposium on the Biochem-
      istry of the Acute Allergic Reactions. Edited by K. F. Austen and E. L.
      Becker. Oxford, England, Blackwell Scientific, 1971, pp. 175–188.
31.   R. P. Orange, R. C. Murphy, M. L. Karnovsky, and K. F. Austen, The phys-
      icochemical characteristics and purification of slow–reacting substance of
      anaphylaxis, *J. Immunol.*, 110:760–770 (1973).
32.   R. P. Orange, M. D. Valentine, and K. F. Austen, Release of slow–reacting
      substance of anaphylaxis in the rat: Polymorphonuclear leukocyte,
      Science, 157:318–319 (1967).
33.   A. B. Kay, D. J. Stechschulte, and K. F. Austen, An eosinophil leukocyte
      chemotactic factor of anaphylaxis, *J. Exp. Med.*, 133:602–619 (1971).
34.   S. E. Wasserman, E. J. Goetzl, and K. F. Austen, Immunologic release of
      preformed eosinophil chemotactic factor of anaphylaxis (ECF–A) from
      isolated mast cells, *Fed. Proc.*, 32:819 (1973) (abstr.).
35.   J. Benveniste, P. M. Henson, and C. G. Cochrane, Leukocyte–dependent
      histamine release from rabbit platelets. The role of IgE, basophils, and a
      platelet–activating factor, *J. Exp. Med.*, 136:1356–1377 (1972).
36.   L. M. Lichtenstein and R. DeBernardo, The immediate allergic response:
      In vitro effect of cyclic AMP active and other drugs on the two stages of
      histamine release, *J. Immunol.*, 107:1131–1136 (1971).
37.   L. M. Lichtenstein and S. Margolis, Histamine release in vitro: Inhibition
      by catecholamines and methyxanthines, *Science*, 161:902–903 (1968).
38.   H. R. Bourne, L. M. Lichtenstein, and K. L. Melmon, Pharmacologic

control of allergic histamine release in vitro: Evidence for an inhibitory role of 3',5'-adenosine monophosphate in human leukocytes, *J. Immunol.*, **108**:695–705 (1972).

39. R. P. Orange, M. A. Kaliner, P. J. LaRaia, and K. F. Austen, The immunological release of histamine and slow–reacting substance of anaphylaxis from human lung. II. Correlation of changes in cellular levels of cyclic adenosine 3'5'–monophosphate with the release of chemical mediators, *Fed. Proc.*, **30**:1725–1729 (1971).

40. M. A. Kaliner, R. P. Orange, and K. F. Austen, Immunological release of histamine and slow–reacting substance of anaphylaxis from human lung. IV. Enhancement by cholinergic and alpha adrenergic stimulation, *J. Exp. Med.*, **136**:556–567 (1972).

41. H. R. Bourne, K. L. Melmon, and L. M. Lichtenstein, Histamine augments leukocyte adenosine 3'5'–monophosphate and blocks antigenic histamine release, *Science*, **173**:743–745 (1971).

42. L. M. Lichtenstein and H. R. Bourne, Inhibition of allergic histamine release by histamine and other agents which stimulate adenyl cyclase. In Second International Symposium on the Biochemistry of the Acute Allergic Reactions. Edited by K. F. Austen and E. L. Becker. Oxford, England, Blackwell Scientific, 1971, pp. 161–174.

43. J. W. Black, W. A. M. Duncan, C. J. Durant, C. R. Ganellin, and E. M. Parsons, Definition and antagonism of histamine H_2–receptors, *Nature*, **236**:385–390 (1972).

44. A. I. Tauber, M. A. Kaliner, D. J. Stechschulte, and K. F. Austen, Immunologic release of histamine and slow reacting substance of anaphylaxis from human lung. V. Effects of prostaglandins on release of histamine, *J. Immunol.*, **111**:27–32 (1973).

45. P. J. Piper and J. L. Walker, The release of spasmogenic substances from human chopped lung tissue and its inhibition, *Br. J. Pharmacol.*, **47**:291–304 (1973).

46. E. Gillespie and L. M. Lichtenstein, Heavy water enhances IgE mediated histamine release from human leukocytes: Evidence for microtubule involvement, *Proc. Soc. Exp. Biol. Med.*, **140**:1228–1230 (1972).

47. E. Gillespie and L. M. Lichtenstein, Histamine release from human leukocytes: Studies with deuterium oxide, colchicine, and cytochalasin B, *J. Clin. Invest.*, **51**:2941–2947 (1972).

48. D. M. P. Goodman, H. Rasmussen, F. Dibella, and C. G. Guthnow, Jr., Cyclic adenosine 3':5'–monophosphate–stimulated phosphorylation of isolated neurotubule subunits, *Proc. Natl. Acad. Sci.*, **67**:652–659 (1970).

49. M. A. Kaliner and K. F. Austen, A sequence of biochemical events in the antigen–induced release of chemical mediators from sensitized human lung tissue, *J. Exp. Med.*, **138**:1077–1094 (1973).

50. A. Szentivanyi, The beta–adrenergic theory of the atopic abnormality in bronchial asthma, *J. Allergy*, **42**:203–232 (1968).

51. J. W. Smith and C. W. Parker, The responsiveness of leukocyte cyclic

adenosine monophosphate to adrenergic agents in patients with asthma, *J. Lab. Clin. Med.,* **76**:993–994 (1970).

52.   P. J. Logsdon, E. Middleton, Jr., and R. G. Coffey, Stimulation of leukocyte adenyl cyclase by hydrocortisone and isoproterenol in asthmatic and nonasthmatic subjects, *J. Allergy Clin. Immunol.,* **50**:45–50 (1972).

53.   C. J. Falliers, R. R. deCardosa, H. N. Bane, R. G. Coffey, and E. Middleton, Jr., Discordant allergic manifestations in monozygotic twins: Genetic identity vs. clinical, physiologic, and biochemical differences, *J. Allergy,* **47**: 207–219 (1971).

54.   C. W. Parker and J. W. Smith, Alterations in cyclic adenosine monophosphate metabolism in human bronchial asthma. I. Leukocyte responsiveness to beta–adrenergic agents, *J. Clin. Invest.,* **52**:48–59 (1973).

55.   C. W. Parker, M. L. Baumann, and M. G. Huber, Alterations in cyclic adenosine monophosphate metabolism in human bronchial asthma. II. Leukocyte and lymphocyte responses to protaglandins, *J. Clin. Invest.,* **52**:1336–1341 (1973).

56.   S. D. Lockey, Jr., J. A. Glennon, and C. E. Reed, Comparison of some metabolic responses in normal and asthmatic subjects to epinephrine and glucagon, *J. Allergy,* **40**:349–354 (1967).

57.   E. Middleton, Jr. and S. R. Fonke, Metabolic response to epinephrine in bronchial asthma, *J. Allergy,* **42**:288–299 (1968).

58.   R. A. Bernstein, L. Linarelli, M. A. Facktor, G. A. Friday, A. L. Drash, and P. Fireman, Decreased urinary adenosine $3'5'$ monophosphate (cyclic AMP) in asthmatics, *J. Allergy,* **80**:772–779 (1972).

59.   P. J. Logsdon, D. V. Carnright, E. Middleton, Jr., and R. G. Coffey, The effect of phentolamine on adenylate cyclase and on isoproterenol stimulation in leukocytes from asthmatic and nonasthmatic subjects, *J. Allergy Clin. Immunol.,* **52**:148–157 (1973).

60.   I. W. B. Grant, S. Channell, and J. C. Drever, Disodium cromoglycate in asthma, *Lancet,* **2**:673 (1967).

61.   J. B. L. Howell and R. E. C. Altounyan, A double–blind trial of disodium cromoglycate in the treatment of allergic bronchial asthma, *Lancet,* **2**: 539–542 (1967).

62.   P. H. Kinder, P. Meisner, N. B. Pride, and R. S. B. Pearson, Disodium cromoglycate in the treatment of bronchial asthma, *Lancet,* **2**:655–657 (1968).

63.   F. Moran, J. D. H. Bankier, and G. Boyd, Disodium cromoglycate in the treatment of allergic bronchial asthma, *Lancet,* **2**:137–139 (1968).

64.   D. G. Robertson, S. W. Epstein, and D. A. Warrell, Trial of disodium cromoglycate in bronchial asthma, *Br. Med. J.,* **1**:552–554 (1969).

65.   J. L. Chen, N. Moore, P. S. Norman, and T. Van Melve, Disodium cromoglycate, a new compound for the prevention of exacerbations of asthma, *J. Allergy,* **43**:89–100 (1969).

66.   M. Lopez, F. C. Lowell, and W. Franklin, A controlled trial of disodium cromoglycate in the treatment of bronchial asthma, *J. Allergy,* **44**:118–121 (1969).

67. J. H. Toogood, N. M. Lefcoe, D. K. Rose, and D. R. McCourtie, A double-blind study of disodium cromoglycate for prophylaxis of bronchial asthma, *Am. Rev. Respir. Dis.,* **104**:323–330 (1971).

68. T. Gebbie, E. A. Harris, T. V. O'Donnell, and G. F. S. Spears, Multicentre, short–term therapeutic trial of disodium cromoglycate, with and without prednisone in adults with asthma, *Br. Med. J.,* **4**:576–580 (1972).

69. M. Silverman, N. M. Connioly, L. Balfour–Lynn, and S. Godfrey, Long-term trial of disodium cromoglycate and isoprenaline in children with asthma, *Br. Med. J.,* **2**:378–381 (1972).

70. S. E. Davies, Effect of single administration of disodium cromoglycate on exercise induced asthma. In *Disodium Cromoglycate in Allergic Airways Disease.* Edited by J. Pepys and A. W. Frankland. London, Butterworths, 1970, pp. 55–61.

71. P. A. Eggleston, C. W. Bierman, W. E. Pierson, S. J. Stamm, and P. P. van Arsdel, A double–blind trial of the effect of cromolyn sodium on exercise-induced bronchospasm, *J. Allergy Clin. Immunol.,* **50**:57–63 (1972).

72. P. S. Clarke, Effect of disodium cromoglycate on exacerbations of asthma produced by hyperventillation, *Brit. Med. J.,* **1**:317–319 (1971).

73. J. Pepys and C. A. C. Pikering, Asthma due to inhaled chemical fumes aminoethyl ethanolamine in aluminum soldering flux, *Clin. Allergy,* **2**: 197–204 (1972).

74. J. S. G. Cox, Disodium cromoglycate (TPL 670) ('intal'): A specific inhibitor of reaginic antibody–antigen mechanisms, *Nature* (London), **216**: 1328–1329 (1967).

75. J. S. G. Cox, Disodium cromoglycate—Mode of action and its possible relevance to the clinical use of the drug, *Brit. J. Chest Dis.,* **65**:189–204 (1971).

76. C. W. Parker, M. G. Huber, and M. C. Baumann, Alterations in cyclic AMP metabolism in human bronchial asthma. III. Leukocyte and lymphocyte responses to steroids, *J. Clin. Invest.,* **52**:1342–1348 (1973).

22

Immunotherapy (Desensitization) in Allergic Conditions of the Respiratory Tract

PHILIP S. NORMAN

The Johns Hopkins University School of Medicine
Baltimore, Maryland

I. Introduction

The therapeutic procedure known as desensitization or immunotherapy is widely established in the practice of medicine. In the United States approximately 3000 specialists in allergy build their practice around this technique, considering that it should be contemplated regularly when allergy is established and employed frequently if the particulars of the situation warrant. In addition, family physicians, pediatricians, and internists employ the same technique from time to time, although with less specialized training in the details of its use. Furthermore, many such physicians administer the many injections involved in the treatment after highly specific recommendations from a consultant specialist in allergy. A number of commercial companies concern themselves with the collection of various types of allergens, such as pollens, molds, animal danders, insects, and so forth, which may be used in the technique, and prepare sterile solutions for final

These investigations were supported by Grants AI 04866, AI 08270 and AI 10304 from the National Institute of Allergy and Infectious Diseases, National Institutes of Health, and Contract FDA-73-156 from the Food and Drug Administration. This is publication no. 149 of the O'Neill Memorial Research Laboratories.

compounding and prescription by physicians. This effort grew largely as a result of empirical observations that injections of allergen extracts will ameliorate a patient's symptoms.

Although a few investigators concerned themselves with the immunologic and physiologic consequences of taking such injections, the principal basis for their continued use has been the experience developed by a sizable number of physicians who repeatedly used the technique in practice. Although the value of such practical experience is not to be discounted, this review will concern itself largely with those systematic observations and controlled experiments that attempt to develop some of the basic principles underlying any therapeutic benefit that may be derived from such injections. The approach of the review will be principally historic but with exceptions in order to develop ideas fully in appropriate places. Since studies of the method and potential improvements are an ongoing process, this review must be considered a progress report rather than a final statement. Practical recommendations derived from organized experiments and that have withstood the test of repeated use are possible only to a very limited degree.

Credit for introducing "prophylactic inoculation against hay fever" is generally given to Noon [1], who seemed to be unaware of the hypersensitivity nature of disease due to the inhalation of pollen. Rather, it was his notion that pollens contained a specific toxin that incited symptoms in some people and that it might be appropriate to immunize such patients with a vaccine composed of extracts of the pollen. Pollens of several species of grass were extracted with distilled water, aided by freezing and thawing several times, and were then sterilized by boiling for 10 min after being sealed in glass tubes. Patients received subcutaneous injections of the pollen extract, starting with minute doses and increasing it every 3 or 4 days. Treatment was started some weeks before the expected season of pollination. Results were tested principally by instilling drops of the pollen extract into the eye and observing the reaction. This was done several times during the course of injection therapy. The first effect of the inoculation was to lower resistance for a few days, after which resistance was increased so that larger amounts of a pollen extract could be instilled before a reaction was observed. Approximately a 100-fold increase in the amount required for a reaction was observed after a number of such injections, and the patients were considered to be improved during the natural exposure to grass pollen.

This work was taken up by Freeman [2] who continued to give such injections to a larger number of patients. Although he noted that some patients with hay fever were not improved, a number were noticeably less reactive during pollen exposure, and the success of the method seemed established. Other physicians quickly took up the technique of preparing extracts of allergens and giving repeated subcutaneous injections in gradually larger doses.

At the same time, the theory of "allergy" was developing rapidly, and it became generally accepted that allergic reactions to inhaled protein materials were mediated by antibody mechanisms similar to those responsible for anaphylaxis in animals. Hence the condition was not the result of any toxic reaction of materials contained in pollens and other allergens. The process of inoculation, therefore, became known as *desensitization* to fit with this improved knowledge of the pathogenesis of allergic disease.

By 1918 Cooke [3] was able to write an extensive review of his experience with desensitization in both rhinitis and asthma, employing extracts of pollen, sachets, animal danders, and foods. Subsequently, it has been more or less customary to prepare extracts of almost any suspected allergen and, if positive tests can be obtained either by direct skin tests, the Prausnitz–Küstner reaction, or mucosal test, to employ a desensitization regimen in an attempt to alleviate symptoms. As already noted, the evaluation of results has been largely by direct observation and therefore empirical. Attempts to evolve techniques for more objective observation of the protection achieved or to conduct controlled experiments lagged considerably behind the introduction of the method.

Feinberg, Stier, and Grater [4] extended Noon's original observations concerning protection against the instillation of extracts of allergens applied directly to mucous membranes. Twenty patients who had undergone desensitization were compared with 20 who had not received treatment. In the desensitized patients the amount of extract required to elicit a reaction was higher than it was in the untreated patients. There was, however, no independent method of matching the two groups to be sure that in the absence of treatment they would have had equal sensitivity.

II. Controlled Efficacy Studies in Pollen Allergy

Frankland [5] carried out an organized trial of four different types of grass pollen extract in 200 cases of seasonal hay fever, assigning patients at random to (a) timothy, (b) cocksfoot, (c) fescue, or (d) mixed timothy and cocksfoot. The results in all four groups were similar, and one grass pollen extract was not observed to be superior to another. Frankland and Augustin [6] carried out the first placebo controlled trial of desensitization. Again, patients had grass pollen hay fever, asthma, or both and were treated with either (a) a mixture of timothy and cocksfoot grass extract, (b) an ultrafiltrate of this extract, (c) a purified pollen protein consisting of the material left behind after ultrafiltration, or (d) a placebo consisting of the diluting solution colored with burnt sugar. Two hundred patients were under trial, 50 on each method. Seventy–nine percent of the patients with hay fever had either good or excellent results following pollen treatment, whereas only 33% reported good results after the placebo or the ultra-filtrate. Results with asthma were more striking: 94% of those receiving the active materials had good or excellent results, whereas only 30% of those who received the other two treatments reported good or excellent results.

A similar study was carried out by Johnstone [7] in the treatment of rag-weed rhinitis and asthma. The patients were children and received ragweed pol-len extract in either (a) the highest tolerated dose, (b) doses no higher than 0.5 ml of a 1 to 5000 w/v dilution, (c) doses no higher than 0.1 ml of a 1 to 10 mil-lion w/v dilution or (d) buffered saline. A total of 112 patients were treated, divided randomly among the four groups. Results were evaluated by question-naires answered by the patients' mothers. Treatment in Groups 1 and 2 were significantly better than in Groups 3 and 4, insofar as the symptoms of hay fever were concerned. Symptoms of asthma were improved even more strikingly, and 68% of the individuals in Group 1, 60% of the patients in Group 2 but only 7% of the controls lost their symptoms of asthma. These differences were highly significant. The final conclusion was that the highest tolerated dose provided the best relief of symptoms but at the expense of a higher rate of generalized or systemic reactions to the injections.

Lowell and Franklin [8] organized a careful double-blind study in allergic rhinitis due to ragweed pollen. Patients were divided into two groups at random: Group A was to be treated with allergenic extract, whereas Group B was to be treated nonspecifically with a solution of caramelized glucose containing hista-mine to mimic the local reaction of the true allergen. Group A received ragweed pollen extract along with extract of molds and house dust, where indicated by the patient's sensitivity. Both patients and physicians who performed the evalu-ations were unaware of which treatment patients had received. Injections were extended over a period of nearly 3 yr and patients were observed during this period for symptoms. Assessment of the patient's progress was done at intervals of 1 to 4 wk by physicians in a manner to permit assigning numerical values to the frequency and duration of symptoms and the amount of medication taken. At the outset, the treated group had more severe symptoms than did the un-treated group. However, as time went on, symptoms reported by the treated group became less and less, and during the second and third years, the seasonal peak in symptoms during the ragweed pollination season was significantly more severe in the untreated group than in the treated group. Indeed, the treated group reported almost no rises in symptoms during the period of ragweed pollen exposure. Dosage in this study was variable and depended on the patient's ten-dency to have reactions.

A further double-blind study of the effectiveness and specificity of injec-tion treatments in ragweed hay fever [9] involved 27 patients who were attending the clinic and suffered from ragweed pollen hay fever. These patients were already undergoing treatment, many of them for allergic problems arising from a number of allergens. The patients were divided into two groups at random and one group was continued on a freshly prepared mixture, as before, and acted as the treated group, whereas the other group received a new mixture containing all allergens except ragweed and who now acted as controls. This new treatment was continued from March until October, and symptoms evaluated on the basis of a daily record kept by the patient. During the height of the ragweed season in September, the treated group had significantly less severe symptoms than did the now untreated group. These authors interpreted the findings to indicate that desensitization treatment was highly specific and that in the control group the continued administration of a variety of allergens other than ragweed had not prevented the relapse of their symptoms. At the same time, it was considered evidence that the method had a high relapse rate within a relatively short period of months when injections were discontinued.

These relatively favorable studies seemed to be countered by a 5-yr study of the effectiveness of ragweed hay fever treatment in children [10]. Different numbers of patients were studied each year, ranging from 16 the first year to a high of 68 patients in the fourth year. Patients were assigned to treatment with ragweed pollen extract, or a similarly colored placebo, at random. Dosage was varied according to skin sensitivity and was measured in nitrogen units. Evaluations were by weekly symptom cards filled out by the parents in a form that could be reduced to numbers for statistical analysis. Analysis was mainly concerned with the number of days each patient reported some kind of symptom during the season. No attempt was made to assess the severity or duration of symptoms on a particular day so far as the analysis was concerned. By this count, the number of days on which some symptoms were observed was not different than that for the placebo treated group. It is interesting, however, that of patients who were skin tested before and after treatment, there was a distinct reduction in skin test sensitivity in the treated group but no reduction in the placebo group. These results were interpreted by the authors as indicative of little or no benefit from the injections received. It should be noted, however, that these authors adopted much more restrictive criteria for improvement than had been previously employed.

A. Relation of Dosage to Clinical Efficacy

In 1963 a series of annual studies were initiated at Johns Hopkins to elucidate further some of the clinical and immunologic problems in desensitization treatment [11]. Groups of skin-test positive, ragweed-sensitive hay fever patients who demonstrated histamine release from isolated washed leukocytes in the presence of ragweed extract were subjected to annual study of various treatment regimens with whole ragweed extract or purified allergens obtained from ragweed pollen. Patients were assigned to treatment or placebo groups at random in the earlier studies. The number of patients who completed any particular treatment regimen in any particular year was about 20; that number of patients seemed sufficient to compare with other groups of the same size by appropriate statistical methods. The principal method of evaluation was a daily symptom diary scored twice a day by each patient for specific symptoms of hay fever, i.e., sneezing, stuffy, runny nose, eye symptoms, cough, and antihistamine tablets taken. These results could be reduced to numbers, and the significance of the difference between groups was assessed by nonparametric statistical methods, which make no unnecessary assumptions about equality of variance or normality of distribution [12]. Initially, antigen E of ragweed [13,14] crude extract of ragweed pollen and placebos were compared. Low doses, averaging 32μg of antigen E and 829 protein nitrogen units, in a cumulative annual dose, were employed. At this dosage there was no significant difference between control and treated groups.

In the subsequent year higher doses were given, averaging 250μg of antigen E or 2400 PNU of ragweed extract, and a detectable difference in symptomatology at the height of the season was detected in the two treatment groups. This difference was of borderline significance, having a P value of 0.07 for antigen E and 0.1 for crude extract, respectively (Mann–Whitney U Test). The following year, still larger doses were given, averaging 743μg of antigen E and about 9500 PNU for the two groups; somewhat greater differences emerged, having a P value of 0.05 and 0.016 for the two groups, respectively. Subsequently, [15] many of these same patients were continued on treatment employing booster injections given at six weekly intervals. Still larger doses were administered and clinical results continued to be good, differences between treated and placebo groups having a P value of less than 0.01 in both years.

Because there had been a gradual escalation of dosage in these patients it was not clear whether the results of treatment were strictly dependent on dosage or represented a cumulative effect of several years of treatment. Therefore, it seemed appropriate [16] to select a new hitherto untreated group of patients and administer in a single year of treatment the largest dose previously administered after several years of treatment. There were four groups of patients involved: (a) antigen E; (b) a combination of antigens E and K;* (c) whole crude aqueous extract and (d) placebos containing histamine. A total of 88 patients participated in this study, and clinical results were similar in the three groups of patients treated with antigens of ragweed. For all three methods of treatment, results were significantly better than placebo ($P<0.01$). It appeared from such

_____

*Antigen K is the second most abundant allergen in pollen extracts [17].

study, therefore, that within limits, the results of treatment are dosage dependent and that small doses will achieve less than adequate results. It was also concluded that the principal allergenic protein in the extract, antigen E, accounted for most if not all of the therapeutic activity of the extract. The number of local and systemic reactions that occurred in treated groups served to indicate that the dosage given in this study represents a practical limit to what could be recommended for practice and that methods other than simple repeated dosage, with gradual escalation, would be required for the safe employment of still larger doses in order to determine whether a further increase in dose would result in additional amelioration of symptoms.

B. Efficacy in Children

Another study, using similar methods of evaluation and treatment, was performed by Sadan *et al.* [18] with school-age children as subjects. Thirty-five children were involved, 18 of whom received doses of 17,000 to 31,000 PNU of whole ragweed extract in the preseasonal course and 17 of whom were given placebo injections. Clinical symptomatology was significantly less in the treated group and the degree of clinical improvement seemed somewhat more striking than had been noted in adults; 13 of the 18 treated children had fewer symptoms than any of the controls. This tended to confirm the widespread clinical impression that children respond more readily to desensitization treatment than adults.

C. House Dust

Types of allergy other than those due to seasonal pollen exposure are less completely studied. However, house dust allergy causing asthma has received considerable attention. The effect of extract of house dust in 96 patients studied cooperatively [19] produced comparison results in some 70 patients; 33 treated and 37 controls. The treated patients received 15 injections of commercially produced house dust extract, starting at an initial dose of 0.1 ml of 1:1000 w/v dilution at weekly intervals. The placebo group received 15 injections of a saline solution. Careful attention to blinding, both patients and physicians, was adhered to. Evaluation of results for 6 months through symptom diaries failed to reveal any difference in either symptomatology or occasional studies of expiratory peak flow.

A study of treatment in house dust sensitive patients [20] was performed in which bronchial sensitivity was evaluated. In 7 of the 20 treated patients bronchial tolerance was increased after the injections, whereas tolerance increased in only 4 of the controls. These findings contrast with the 19 of 20 patients who received repeated inhalations of dust extract and in whom bronchial tolerance increased.

A more thorough-going study [21] was carried out in 93 children with asthma showing bronchial reactions to inhalation of house dust extract. The study was completed in 80 patients. Commercial house dust extract labeled *A* had been given to 31 patients, house dust extract labeled *B* to 21 patients, and placebo to 28 patients. Injections were given over a period of 2½ to 3 yr. At the completion of this study, in house dust *A* and house dust *B* treated groups complete bronchial tolerance to house dust provocation had been achieved in 21 and 14 patients, respectively, compared with only 7 in the placebo group. When those with markedly improved bronchial tolerance were included, the figures were 26 of 31, 19 of 21, and 9 of 28, respectively. Thus, both house dust extracts were considered significantly superior to placebo ($P<0.01$). Changes in bronchial sensitivity before and after the injection treatment were compared with clinical improvement as subjectively judged by the patients. While correlation was not perfect, the clinical state tended to match the change in bronchial reactivity. The difference between this study and the previous studies of house dust extract seems to be related to the fact that a much larger dose was given over a much longer period. Some of the variability in the results obtained with house dust extracts may be accounted for by low potency of at least some extracts. May *et al.* [22] found that unusually large amounts (in terms of protein nitrogen) of house dust extracts were necessary to obtain measurable amounts of blocking antibody in the serum of children sensitive to house dust.

Smith [23] reported a double-blind clinical trial of desensitization with extract of *Dermatophagoides pteronyssinus* (the house dust mite) in comparison with placebo in 20 patients. At the end of the period of injections, the patients were asked for a subjective opinion of the treatment and the investigator recorded his own impressions. Significantly more patients in the mite treated group felt better than in the control treated group. Of the patients in the two groups, significantly more in the mite treated group were less breathless during the daytime ($P<0.005$), had fewer attacks of nocturnal breathlessness ($P<0.005$), and used their inhalers less at night ($P<0.01$).

D. Bacterial Vaccines

Killed bacterial vaccines have also long been employed in clinical practice in desensitization regimens. The rationale for this method of treatment arises from the observation that a number of patients with asthma have major attacks arising from or following apparent respiratory infections. On the basis of positive skin test reactions to bacterial extracts, these patients are deemed hypersensitive to bacteria and attempts are made to treat this hypersensitivity by injections of bacterial products. Vaccines are either stock mixtures, containing organisms common in the mouth and throat, such as *Pneumococcus, Streptococcus, Staphylococcus, Neisseria, Klebsiella,* and *Haemophilus* (common gram-negative bacilli are sometimes added) or they are autogenous; i.e., represent organisms actually cultured from swabs or washings of the pharynx. In these patients the infective nature of the exacerbations results from clinical impressions and is not backed up by the complex cultural and serologic techniques employed by investigators of respiratory infections. Hence, the choice of bacterial species for vaccination tends to be haphazard. Furthermore, it may be pointed out that positive skin reactions are a frequent concomitant of infections with bacteria in patients who never have asthma.

Despite these conceptual difficulties with the technique, a number of controlled studies have been carried out on whether one or another variation of the method actually helps patients so treated more than do placebos. In 1955 Frankland *et al.* [24] reported results in 193 patients, 100 treated with an autogenous vaccine prepared from postnasal swabs and 84 controls. Of the vaccine-treated patients, 58% were thought improved, whereas 52.5% of the control patients were improved. The authors point out that patients with mild or episodic asthma tend to improve on supportive and nonspecific treatment and considered the trial inconclusive.

Helander [25] reported a trial of a stock vaccine containing 30% *H. influenzae,* 40% *D. pneumoniae,* 10% *M. catarrhalis,* 10% *K. pneumoniae,* and 10% β-hemolytic streptococci. Among 77 patients in the treated group, 52 (68%) were improved, whereas among 79 placebo-treated patients, 49 (62%) were improved. Again no definite evidence of benefit from bacterial extracts was found.

Johnstone [26] reported results in 118 children with histories of at least three episodes of wheezing and coughing associated with infections or colds in the previous 12 months. The control group (58 patients) was given injections of extracts of inhalant allergens eliciting positive skin reactions. The vaccine treated group (60 patients) received either *Staphylococcus ambotoxoid;* stock vaccine containing *S. aureus, S. pyogenes, S. viridans,* and *H. influenzae;* or an autogenous vaccine. All three vaccine groups were also given injections of the inhalant mixture. In the vaccine treated group, 48 (80%) had fewer episodes of asthma in the following year, whereas 54 (91%) of control group noted a reduction. There was no difference in response to the several vaccine materials employed.

Aas *et al.* [27] , after examining more than 400 children with asthma, could find only 25 who were considered to have isolated bacterial allergies, i.e., symptoms only from infective or bacterial causes. Fifteen patients treated with bacterial vaccine had good results no more often than did 10 control patients.

Although the series was small, there was no evidence that bacterial vaccine was helpful. Reinvestigation of their 25 patients disclosed that 10 had evidence of specific allergy to external allergens at the time of a second look.

Barr *et al.* [28] studied 44 adult patients with asthma aggravated by respiratory infections. He divided these patients into 22 pairs, matched according to age, sex, race, severity and duration of disease, pulmonary function tests, and evidence of hyperplastic sinusitis by x-ray. They were followed through two winters during which they took injections of a stock vaccine consisting of β–hemolytic streptococcus, a–hemolytic streptococcus, *N. catarrhalis, Pneumococcus, S. albus, S. aureus, K. pneumoniae, A. aerogenes, B. proteus, E. coli, P. aeruginosa,* and *H. influenzae.* Evaluations as to symptoms reported, emergency room visits, vital capacity, maximal expiratory flow rate, use of steroids, use of antibiotics, and antiasthma tablets were not significantly different between the two groups. The treated group did use significantly less inhaled bronchodilator medication. Surprisingly, the authors stated that while the study is inconclusive, "the data suggest that the bacterial vaccine was an effective adjunct in the treatment of bronchial asthma."

Fontana *et al.* [29] reported a 2-yr double-blind study to determine the effectiveness of bacterial vaccine in 30 children with infectious asthma. The first year, from October to April, all of the children received buffered saline injections weekly. The second year the children were randomly divided into two groups, one receiving a stock vaccine containing *S. aureus, S. albus, S. viridans, S. haemolyticus, P. aeruginosa,* and *P. mirabilis,* and the other a placebo. A reduction in the incidence of wheezing, infection, and infectious episodes associated with wheezing was observed in a larger percentage of the placebo group than in the vaccine-treated group. The amount of antiasthmatic medication administered during the first and second years was equivalent.

Mueller and Lanz [30] make a distinction between infectious asthma and extrinsic asthma triggered or aggravated by respiratory infection. In the former, symptoms are said to start very early in life, usually before age 5, and to consist entirely of wheezing with respiratory infections, the patient being otherwise symptom-free. Such children usually have negative skin tests to extrinsic allergens and no eosinophilia during infections. In extrinsic asthma with respiratory infections acting as a trigger, positive skin tests to allergens are common, environmental control is helpful, and there are attacks not associated with infection. Eosinophilia continues through infection. According to the authors, infectious asthma accounts for only 25% of childhood asthma associated with infections; the remainder is the extrinsic type. Only prolonged observation will clearly distinguish between the two. Mueller and Lanz's thesis is that only infectious asthma will respond to treatment with bacterial vaccines; hence, earlier studies with the vaccines were bound to be negative. To support their idea, they present a study of 14 patients with infectious asthma, 9 of whom were treated with a stock vaccine of *N. catarrhalis, H. influenzae, K. pneumoniae, S. albus, S. aureus, S. pyogenes, S. viridans,* and *Pneumococcus,* and 5 of whom were treated with placebos. In the 2 yr following the initiation of the study, the number of respiratory infections declined noticeably in the treated group but was unchanged in the untreated group. This is too small a study to be significant statistically, but the authors add another 62 patients treated, without comparison controls, who had less asthma over several years of followup. These data present the usual problem that at least a portion of the observed changes may represent the natural course of the disease.

The studies on bacterial vaccine cited provide little basis for the regular use of such vaccines in either children or adults simply because infections appear to initiate asthmatic attacks. While each of the studies can be criticized for such items as selection of patients, adequacy of the blind technique, dependence on impressions by physicians, and sample size, the almost complete lack of positive results gives little encouragement. Mueller and Lanz's idea that some subgroups of children who will respond more regularly to such treatment can be selected is an interesting one and may deserve further investigation. Their own evidence is less than completely satisfying.

III. Blocking Antibodies

The mechanism by which injections of allergen extracts ameliorate symptoms has been subject to extensive study over many years. Although Noon [1] was mistaken about the nature of disease due to pollen, his rationale for the administration of pollen extract was nevertheless the production of immunologic change in the form of antibodies, which would act as antitoxins. He did not, however, actually demonstrate the presence of serum antibodies as the result of his injections. Indeed, the first report of the development of antibodies as the result of injections was by Cooke and his colleagues [31]. These authors found that the amount of skin sensitizing antibody, as measured by direct Prausnitz–Küstner tests, was practically unchanged by the injections. However, the amount of pollen extract required to neutralize the skin sensitizing antibody in the serum was definitely greater after treatment. This change was attributed to the development, during treatment, of "blocking antibody" that inhibited the reaction between antigen and sensitizing antibody. Furthermore, Cooke and his colleagues [32] showed that injections of pollen extract in normal nonallergic human subjects produced a blocking antibody in the absence of skin sensitizing antibody.

Harley [33,34] observed that in most cases the amount of skin sensitizing antibody in serum was reduced by treatment. Sherman, Stull, and Cooke [35] subsequently did a more extensive study in 55 cases of hay fever and found that the amount of skin sensitizing antibody increased during the first few months of treatment and then subsequently began to decrease. After from 10 to 23 yr of treatment, seven of 29 sera no longer passively sensitized human skin. Eighteen others showed a striking decrease in the amount of skin sensitizing antibody. They confirmed that increases in blocking antibody occurred simultaneously with these changes. Loveless [36] first showed a clear difference between skin sensitizing and blocking antibodies in that blocking antibodies were stable to heat, whereas skin sensitizing antibodies had long been known to be readily denatured by heating. Gordon and his coworkers [37] showed that the heat–stable antibodies could be demonstrated in vitro by hemagglutination of passively sensitized red cells. A variety of attempts, however, to relate the changes in both skin sensitizing and blocking antibody to the results of treatment were not successful [38–40].

A. Histamine Release

Following the observation that specific allergen would induce the release of histamine from specimens of fresh whole blood obtained from an allergic individual, attempts were made to correlate this phenomenon with the results of therapy. Van Arsdel and Middleton [41] noted that the ability of the blood specimen to release histamine was reduced in some patients following therapy but could not correlate this directly with the results of treatment. When a technique for the study of release of histamine from isolated washed human leukocytes in the absence of serum, red cells and platelets was developed by Lichtenstein and Osler [42], it became possible to employ this technique to study and measure accurately the titers of blocking heat stable antibody developed during injection regimen [43].

First application of such technique to desensitization was reported by Lichtenstein, Norman, Winkenwerder, and Osler [44]. In a study in which rather small doses of ragweed pollen extract were given to a series of patients, it was found that there was relatively little change in leukocyte sensitivity as measured by histamine release. Allergic patients who had never received the injections rather regularly had low titers of blocking antibody. However, when injections of pollen extract were initiated, levels of these blocking antibodies began to rise. The titer of blocking antibody peaked within a month or two after the last injection and then began to decline over the next few months. Dosage in this study was too small to observe much clinical effect so no correlation between level of blocking antibody and clinical results could be made. It was noted, however, that the level of symptomatology in patients who did not receive treatment correlated remarkably well with measurements of leukocyte sensitivity by histamine release. It has since become valuable in organizing studies of methods of treatment to use measurements of leukocyte basophil sensitivity to develop matched groups of patients for comparison. In a subsequent study, Lichtenstein, Norman, and Winkenwerder [45] gave larger doses of ragweed antigen E sufficient to achieve a significant difference in symptomatology between patients so treated and patients given placebos. The rises in titers of blocking antibody were greater, but the correlation between blocking antibody titer and the results of treatment, as measured by symptom index obtained from symptom diaries, was not significant.

In children a similar study [18] demonstrated an additional immunologic change, namely, a reduction in basophil sensitivity to pollen extract, that is, larger amounts of extract were required to elicit the release of histamine in isolated leukocyte preparations. In the extreme instance, in some patients, the cells also became less reactive and released a smaller portion of their store of histamine at optimum antigen levels. In the extreme instance leukocytes of a number of patients released essentially no histamine at any concentration of allergen. There was, however, not a good correlation between the results of treatment and this change.

The technique of histamine release could also be used to measure reaginic antibody by passive transfer to preparations of leukocytes from normal nonallergic individuals. Levy and Osler [46] reported a study of the reaginic activity of human sera before and after desensitization treatment, indicating that the level of reaginic antibody might increase moderately shortly after exposure to environmental ragweed. The seasonal rise was somewhat less in the treated group of patients than in a control group. The study in children [18] showed a postseasonal rise in reagin also but with little difference in treated and untreated children.

Using higher doses of either purified allergens or whole ragweed extract than they had used in their earlier studies, Lichtenstein, Norman, and Winkenwerder [16] were able to show that cellular reactivity was reduced in some adult patients who received injections. While many of these patients fared very well during ragweed pollen exposure, cell sensitivity measurements still failed to predict the responses of individual patients on pollen exposure after treatment, even though this test had a high predictive value when no treatment was given. In this study, the development of high titers of blocking antibody correlated significantly with clinical results. There was, however, a sufficiently high rate of exception that tests of blocking antibody by the quantitative technique employed still failed to offer much hope of predicting clinical results in individual patients. Further study in children [47] confirmed that decreased cellular reactivity could be achieved in some but not all individuals under treatment with ragweed pollen extract. At the same time, the postpollen season increase in serum reaginic antibody toward ragweed was suppressed. Total serum IgE levels seemed not to be changed by treatment or by seasonal exposure. Decreased cell sensitivity seemed to be related to lower serum reaginic antibody levels; development, however, of decreased cell *reactivity* (defined as a reduction in the amount of histamine releasable at optimum antigen concentration) seemed to occur by other mechanisms. May *et al.* [48] employed both customary and intensive regimens of treatment with ragweed, *Alternaria,* and house dust extracts and found that changes in cell reactivity were irregular and transient. It is clear that complete desensitization of cells is not regularly achieved by current methods so that the place of such changes in clinical improvement is not clear.

B. Secretory Antibody

A recent study by Platts-Mills and Von Maur [49] in our laboratory shows that ragweed hay fever patients regularly have small amounts of both IgG and secretory IgA antibodies against ragweed antigen in nasal washings. Natural seasonal exposure to ragweed pollen results in a modest rise of these antibodies. After immunotherapy by the parenteral route, the quantity of both antibodies regularly rose in nasal secretions to several times the level induced by natural exposure. No antiragweed IgA was found in the serum and the levels of IgG in serum were not related to those in secretions, so that the antibodies in secretions appear to be synthesized locally. Antibodies in secretions seem to be an ideal first line of defense.

C. IgE Antibodies

The radioallergosorbent technique (RAST) [50] for the accurate measurement of specific IgE antibodies provides a more convenient and accurate technique with which to follow reaginic IgE antibodies to the specific allergen being used in treatment. Lichtenstein and coworkers [51] confirmed that titers of specific IgE antibodies declined gradually in untreated allergic individuals prior to the ragweed season and were boosted by environmental exposure to ragweed pollen. In immunized patients IgE antibodies to ragweed rose at the beginning of treatment but fell as treatment proceeded. By the end of 2 yr the level had decreased in 18 of 19 patients. The increase in blocking (IgG) antibodies during treatment correlated significantly with the decrease in serum IgE antibodies. Sensitivity of basophils to ragweed allergen-induced histamine release correlated significantly with serum IgE antibodies. The decline in IgE antibodies in the treated individual did not appear to predict the amelioration of symptoms that occurred. These authors cautioned against interpreting the fall in IgE antibodies as the result of a rise in IgG antibodies. Changes in IgG antibodies occurred long before any change in IgE was observed.

An important additional finding was reported by Ishizaka and Ishizaka [52] who followed the IgE antiragweed antibody of 5 children through several years of immunization treatment. A slow reduction in IgE antibodies was observed along with a considerable rise in IgG antibodies. When treatment was discontinued, in 3 of the 5 children the subsequent ragweed season caused a considerable rise in serum IgE antibodies against ragweed, which rose to pretreatment levels or above. This tends to explain the treatment relapses often observed clinically [53].

Immunologic changes during immunization treatment can be summarized as follows:

1. There is a rise in serum IgG blocking antibodies shortly after treatment is initiated. In individual patients the rise is roughly proportional to dose. When injections are discontinued, these levels decline over months.

2. Serum IgE antibodies tend to rise initially but then decline slowly as injections are continued. The usual seasonal rise in specific IgE antibodies during exposure is blunted.

3. Basophils tend to show a reduction in sensitivity to the specific allergen, which may be related to changes in serum levels of specific IgE antibodies, i.e., there is less specific IgE antibody on the basophils when serum levels are reduced. Total IgE in serum is usually unchanged.

4. Basophil reactivity may at times be reduced and the amount of histamine released may be less than optimum or nonexistent at optimum concentrations of antigen. This change may not be immunologically specific [54].

IV. Untoward Reactions

Although allergic reactions to injected materials represent the principal hazard in the method of treatment and the principal limitation to rapid increase in dosage, there have been relatively few studies of the immunologic mechanisms involved. The most serious reaction is the immediate "constitutional" or "systemic" reaction that occurs within minutes after the injection and resembles anaphylaxis in every way. Lowell *et al.* [55] set out to induce a systemic reaction in allergic individuals by repeated intravenous injections of increasing amounts of antigen. They found that there was a good correlation between the titer of skin sensitizing antibody and the severity of reaction but a poor correlation with dose required to elicit a reaction. Connell, Sherman, and Myers [56] compared 12 patients who had systemic reactions during the course of therapy with control patients who did not. They found skin-sensitizing antibody titers were higher and blocking antibody titers were lower in the constitutional reaction group. They believed that the greatest risk occurred early in therapy when titers of skin sensitizing antibody might be rising but blocking antibodies had not risen greatly.

The immunologic mechanism of the second kind of reaction, local itchy or painful swellings at the site of injection 4 to 36 hr after injection, has not been studied to the author's knowledge.

A. Long-Acting Materials

As treatment by the injection method rarely produces complete cures of a patient's symptoms, requires a long period of injections, and incurs some risk of allergic reactions, methods of improving the technique have been sought. Stull and his colleagues [57] reported a survey of extracts modified in a variety of ways, including formalinization, irradiation with ultraviolet light, heating, acetylation, and alum precipitation. These extracts were compared in clinical and experimental studies with freshly prepared unmodified extracts. The blocking antibody response in patients with hay fever treated with acetylated, formalinized, or heated extracts was less than in patients treated with alum-precipitated or unmodified extract. None of the modifications eliminated constitutional reactions. Clinical results were best with unmodified extract but seemed to be almost as good with alum-precipitated or formalinized extracts. Heated and acetylated extracts were least satisfactory.

Naterman [58] reported on pollen extracts emulsified in lanolin and olive oil and observed a slow absorption of the material. He was, therefore, able to give larger doses with a reduced number of injections. Clinical results in an uncontrolled trial were good.

Loveless [59,60] used emulsions of pollen extract in mineral oil with similar results. This technique was subsequently extensively tried and evaluated in uncontrolled clinical trials but controlled clinical trials failed to reveal much benefit [61]. The ability of large doses of mineral oil to produce myelomas in mice [62] has been considered an over-riding safety objection with this method.

Fuchs and Strauss [63] prepared an alum-precipitate of pyridine extract of allergen. Clinical results in uncontrolled trials seemed to be successful. In the case of ragweed hay fever, Lichtenstein and his coworkers [64] showed that pyridine extraction denatured the biologically active ragweed allergens and that antibody responses in patients receiving such an extract after alum–precipitation were virtually nil. Starr and Weinstock [65] reported the development of blocking antibodies after treatment with alum–precipitated pyridine extract of timothy grass. They found a rise in blocking antibodies after a series of such injections and noted that such rises showed some correlation with clinical results. This study suggests that the essential antigens of timothy grass are resistant to denaturation by pyridine. There is, however, no systematic study published as to which allergenic proteins can be successfully extracted from crude allergenic materials with pyridine.

Alum–precipitation of water extracts of pollen were reevaluated by Norman *et al.* [66] using ragweed extracts. They found it possible to give a larger dose of extract in a smaller number of injections. Antigen E was found in antigenically active form in the alum–precipitate. When this material was used in comparison with regular aqueous ragweed extract, blocking antibody responses were similar with the two methods and so were clinical results. Subsequently, alum–precipitated extracts for a variety of allergens have been made available for use by physicians.

B. Allergoids

Marsh [67] reopened the question of formalinized extracts employing a mild formalin treatment over many days. Extracts so treated were referred to as *allergoids.* Chromatographic evidence indicated that such treatment resulted in fairly extensive cross-linkage of protein materials contained in the extract. This form of treatment eliminated over 99% of the skin and basophil reactivity of the extract in man [68]. These substances, nevertheless, still showed ability to produce antibody responses of IgG blocking antibodies in both nonallergic man and in animals [69]. Clinical study of allergoids with ragweed pollen (Norman, Marsh, and Lichtenstein, unpublished observations) confirms that larger doses of pollen protein can be given without reaction in the allergoid form than in the unmodified extract form, and that IgG antibody responses and clinical results are at least as good and probably better than those obtained with regular extracts.

Whether chemical modification of allergens can achieve a detoxification sufficient to eliminate the risk of IgE-mediated allergic reactions after parenteral injection while preserving the ability to elicit protective antibody responses remains to be seen.

Recent animal experimentation on IgE antibody formation by Ishizaka *et al.* [70] showed that (as with other types of antibody formation) the T-cell helper function is stimulated by different regions on the antigen E molecule than that which eventually reacts with the IgE antibodies formed by B cells. Furthermore, different populations of T cells appear to serve the helper function for IgE and IgG antibodies to antigen E. Whether such information will eventually lead to more specific interference with IgE antibody production than current methods of injections of antigens remains to be seen. As already noted, methods worked out empirically by allergists many years ago do partially interfere with IgE production and at the same time raise IgG antibodies with a protective function.

V. Standardization

Until the increase in immunologic knowledge discloses ways of specifically controlling immunologic responses in man, immunotherapy as currently employed, is likely to remain a widely used therapeutic method. As already noted, adequate clinical improvement and immunologic change depend on extracts that contain sufficient amounts of the allergens responsible for the disease. The clinician employing extracts for injections has a narrow margin between a dose large enough to induce relief of symptoms and a dose so large as to cause unacceptable allergic reactions to the injected materials. Current methods for standardizing and labeling extracts fail to provide a safe guide to dosage. Baer *et al.* [71] purchased ragweed extract from six different commercial houses and found a 100-fold difference in potency between the most active and the least active extract in terms of skin-test activity and the ability to elicit basophil histamine release. Immunologic determination of antigen E content of the extract by double diffusion in gel was shown to measure accurately the biologic potency of the extracts, whereas measurements of total protein had no relation to biologic activity. Similar observations have been made with several related species of grass and the principal allergen of rye grass referred to as *group I*. Unfortunately, few other purified allergenic proteins are available for use as primary standards in double diffusion methods. As such protein purifications require sophisticated and laborious laboratory techniques, other methods of standardization should be sought. A modification of RAST may be applicable in this regard.

References

1. L. Noon, Prophylactic inoculation against hay fever, *Lancet,* 1:1572–1573 (1911).
2. J. Freeman, Further observations on the treatment of hay fever by hypodermic inoculations of pollen vaccine, *Lancet,* 2:814–817 (1911).
3. R. A. Cooke, Hay fever and asthma. The uses and limitations of desensitization, *N.Y. Med. J.,* 107:577–583 (1918).

4. S. M. Feinberg, R. A. Stier, and W. C. Grater, A suggested quantitative evaluation of the degree of sensitivity of patients with ragweed pollinosis, *J. Allergy,* **23**:387–394 (1952).

5. A. W. Frankland, Seasonal hay fever and asthma treated with pollen extracts, *Int. Arch. Allergy,* **6**:45–52 (1955).

6. A. W. Frankland and R. Augustin, Prophylaxis of summer hay–fever and asthma. A controlled trial comparing crude grass–pollen extracts with the isolated main protein component, *Lancet,* **1**:1055–1057 (1954).

7. D. E. Johnstone, Study of the role of antigen dosage in the treatment of pollenosis and pollen asthma, *J. Dis. Child.,* **94**:1–5 (1957).

8. F. C. Lowell and W. Franklin, A "double blind" study of treatment with aqueous allergenic extracts in cases of allergic rhinitis, *J. Allergy,* **34**:165–182 (1963).

9. F. C. Lowell and W. Franklin, A double–blind study of the effectiveness and specificity of injection therapy in ragweed hay fever, *N. Engl. J. Med.,* **273**:675–679 (1965).

10. V. J. Fontana, L. E. Holt, Jr., and D. Mainland, Effectiveness of hyposensitization therapy in ragweed hay–fever in children, *J.A.M.A.,* **195**: 985–992 (1966).

11. P. S. Norman, W. L. Winkenwerder, and L. M. Lichtenstein, Immunotherapy of hay fever with ragweed antigen E: Comparisons with whole pollen extract and placebos, *J. Allergy,* **42**:93–108 (1968).

12. P. S. Norman, M. B. Rhyne, and D. Mellits, Evaluation of agents for the treatment of seasonal respiratory allergies. In *Clinical Pharmacology.* Vol. 2. Edited by L. Lasagna. Oxford, Pergamon Press, 1966, pp. 639–652.

13. T. P. King and P. S. Norman, Isolation studies of allergens from ragweed pollen, *Biochemistry,* **1**:709–720 (1962).

14. T. P. King, P. S. Norman, and J. T. Connell, Isolation and characterization of allergens from ragweed pollen. II., *Biochemistry,* **3**:458–468 (1964).

15. P. S. Norman, W. L. Winkenwerder, and L. M. Lichtenstein, Maintenance immunotherapy in ragweed hay fever, *J. Allergy,* **47**:273–282 (1971).

16. L. M. Lichtenstein, P. S. Norman, and W. L. Winkenwerder, A single year of immunotherapy for ragweed hay fever, *Ann. Intern. Med.,* **75**:663–671 (1970).

17. T. P. King, P. S. Norman, and L. M. Lichtenstein, Isolation and characterization of allergens from ragweed pollen. IV., *Biochemistry,* **6**:1992–2000 (1967).

18. N. Sadan, M. B. Rhyne, E. D. Mellits, E. Goldstein, D. A. Levy, and L. M. Lichtenstein, Immunotherapy of pollinosis in children. Investigation of the immunologic basis of clinical improvement, *N. Engl. J. Med.,* **280**: 623–627 (1969).

19. P. Forgacs and A. V. Swan, Treatment of house dust allergy, *Br. Med. J.,* **3**:774–777 (1968).

20. M. K. McAllen, Bronchial sensitivity testing in asthma. An assessment of

the effect of hyposensitization in house–dust and pollen–sensitive asthmatic subjects, *Thorax,* 16:30–35 (1961).

21.   K. Aas, Hyposensitization in house dust allergy asthma, *Acta Paediatr. Scand.,* 60:264–268 (1971).

22.   C. D. May, M. Lyman, R. Alberto, and J. Cheng, Immunochemical evaluation of antigenicity of house dust extract, *J. Allergy,* 46:73–89 (1970).

23.   A. P. Smith, Hyposensitization with *Dermatophagoides pteronyssinus* antigen: Trial in asthma induced by house dust, *Br. Med. J.,* 4:204–206 (1971).

24.   A. W. Frankland, W. H. Hughes, and R. H. Gorrill, Autogenous bacterial vaccines in treatment of asthma, *Br. Med. J.,* 2:941–944 (1955).

25.   E. Helander, Bacterial vaccines in the treatment of bronchial asthma, *Acta Allergol.,* 13:47–66 (1959).

26.   D. E. Johnstone, Study of the value of bacterial vaccines in the treatment of bronchial asthma associated with respiratory infections, *Pediatrics,* 24: 427–433 (1959).

27.   K. Aas, P. Berdal, S. D. Henriksen, and O. Gardborg, "Bacterial allergy" in childhood asthma and the effect of vaccine treatment, *Acta Paediatr. Scand.,* 52:338–344 (1963).

28.   S. E. Barr, H. Brown, M. Fuchs, H. Orvis, A. Connor, F. J. Murray, and A. Seltzer, A double–blind study of the effects of bacterial vaccine on infective esthma, *J. Allergy,* 36:47–61 (1965).

29.   V. J. Fontana, A. S. Salanitro, H. I. Wolfe, and F. Moreno, Bacterial vaccine and infectious asthma, *J.A.M.A.,* 193:895–900 (1965).

30.   H. L. Mueller and M. Lanz, Hyposensitization with bacterial vaccine in infectious asthma, *J.A.M.A.,* 208:1379–1383 (1969).

31.   R. A. Cooke, J. H. Barnard, S. Hebald, and A. Stull, Serological evidence of immunity with coexisting sensitization in a type of human allergy (hay fever), *J. Exp. Med.,* 62:733–750 (1935).

32.   R. A. Cooke, M. Loveless, and A. Stull, Studies on immunity in a type of human allergy (hay fever): Serologic response of nonsensitive individuals to pollen injections, *J. Exp. Med.,* 66:689–696 (1937).

33.   D. Harley, Hay–fever. The mechanism of specific desensitisation, *Lancet,* 2:1469–1472 (1933).

34.   D. Harley, Hay fever. (I) The effect of pollen therapy on the skin reactions. (II) A reaction–inhibiting substance in the serum of treated patients, *J. Pathol.,* 44:589–601 (1937).

35.   W. B. Sherman, A. Stull, and R. A. Cooke, Serologic changes in hay fever cases treated over a period of years, *J. Allergy,* 11:225–244 (1940).

36.   M. H. Loveless, Immunological studies of pollinosis. I. The presence of two antibodies related to the same pollen–antigen in the serum of treated hay fever patients, *J. Immunol.,* 38:25–50 (1940).

37.   J. Gordon, B. Rose, and A. H. Sehon, Detection of "non–precipitating" antibodies in sera of individuals allergic to ragweed by an in vitro method, *J. Exp. Med.,* 108:37–51 (1958).

38. J. T. Connell and W. B. Sherman, Skin sensitizing antibody titer. III. Relationship of the skin–sensitizing antibody titer to the intracutaneous skin test, to the tolerance of injections of antigens, and to the effects of prolonged treatment with antigen, *J. Allergy*, **35**:169–176 (1964).

39. M. H. Loveless, Immunological studies of pollinosis, IV. The relationship between thermostable antibody in the circulation and clinical immunity, *J. Immunol.*, **47**:165–180 (1943).

40. C. E. Arbesman, S. Z. Kantor, D. Rapp, and N. R. Rose, Immunologic studies of ragweed–sensitive patients. III. Clinical aspects: The relationship of reagin and hemagglutinating antibody titers to results of hyposensitization therapy, *J. Allergy*, **31**:342–350 (1960).

41. P. P. Van Arsdel, Jr. and E. Middleton, Jr., The effect of hyposensitization on the *in vitro* histamine release by specific antigen, *J. Allergy*, **32**:348–356 (1961).

42. L. M. Lichtenstein and A. G. Osler, Studies on the mechanisms of hypersensitivity phenomena. IX. Histamine release from human leukocytes by ragweed pollen antigen, *J. Exp. Med.*, **120**:507–530 (1964).

43. L. M. Lichtenstein and A. G. Osler, Studies on the mechanisms of hypersensitivity phenomena. XII. An in vitro study of the reaction between ragweed pollen antigen, allergic human serum, and ragweed sensitive human leukocytes, *J. Immunol.*, **96**:169–179 (1966).

44. L. M. Lichtenstein, P. S. Norman, W. L. Winkenwerder, and A. G. Osler, In vitro studies of human ragweed allergy: Changes in cellular and humoral activity associated with specific desensitization, *J. Clin. Invest.*, **45**:1126–1136 (1966).

45. L. M. Lichtenstein, P. S. Norman, and W. L. Winkenwerder, Clinical and in vitro studies on the role of immunotherapy in ragweed hay fever, *Am. J. Med.*, **44**:514–524 (1968).

46. D. A. Levy and A. G. Osler, Studies on the mechanisms of hypersensitivity phenomena. XVI. *In vitro* assays of reaginic activity in human sera: Effect of therapeutic immunization on seasonal titer changes, *J. Immunol.*, **99**:1068–1077 (1967).

47. D. A. Levy, L. M. Lichtenstein, E. O. Goldstein, and K. Ishizaka, Immunologic and cellular changes accompanying the therapy of pollen allergy, *J. Clin. Invest.*, **50**:360–369 (1971).

48. C. D. May, M. Lyman, R. Alberto, and N. Aduna, Immunochemical effects of injection therapy with allergens by customary and intensive dosage regimens in children, *Pediatrics*, **49**:536–546 (1972).

49. T. A. E. Platts–Mills, R. K. von Maur, K. Ishizaka, P. S. Norman, and L. M. Lichtenstein, IgA and IgG anti–ragweed antibodies in nasal secretions: Quantitative measurements of antibodies and correlation with histamine release, *J. Clin. Invest.*, (submitted for publication).

50. L. Wide, H. Bennich, and S. G. O. Johansson, Diagnosis of allergy by an in vitro test for allergen antibodies, *Lancet*, **2**:1105–1107 (1967).

51. L. M. Lichtenstein, K. Ishizaka, P. S. Norman, A. K. Sobotka, and B. M. Hill, IgE antibody measurements in ragweed hay fever. Relationship to

clinical severity and the results of immunotherapy, *J. Clin. Invest.*, **52**: 472–482 (1973).

52.   K. Ishizaka and T. Ishizaka, Role of IgE and IgG antibodies in reaginic hypersensitivity in the respiratory tract. In *Asthma: Physiology, Immunopharmacology, and Treatment.* Edited by K. F. Austen and L. M. Lichtenstein. New York, Academic Press, 1973, pp. 55–68.

53.   P. S. Norman, Specific therapy in allergy. Pro (with reservations), *Med. Clin. North Am.*, **58**:111–125 (1974).

54.   L. M. Lichtenstein and D. A. Levy, Is 'Desensitization' for ragweed hay fever immunologically specific?, *Int. Arch. Allergy Appl. Immunol.*, **42**: 615–626 (1972).

55.   F. C. Lowell, W. Franklin, J. W. Schiller, and E. M. Follensby, Acute allergic reactions induced in subjects with hay fever and asthma by intravenous administration of allergens with observations on blood clot lysis, *J. Allergy*, **27**:369–376 (1956).

56.   J. T. Connell, W. B. Sherman, and P. A. Myers, Antibody studies in constitutional reactions resulting from injections of ragweed pollen extract, *J. Allergy*, **33**:365–377 (1962).

57.   A. Stull, R. A. Cooke, W. B. Sherman, S. Hebald, and S. F. Hampton, Experimental and clinical study of fresh and modified pollen extracts, *J. Allergy*, **11**:439–465 (1940).

58.   H. L. Naterman, The treatment of hay fever by injections of pollen extract emulsified in lanolin and olive oil, *N. Engl. J. Med.*, **218**:797–802 (1938).

59.   M. H. Loveless, Application of immunologic principles to the management of hay fever, including preliminary reports on the use of Freund's adjuvant, *Am. J. Med. Sci.*, **214**:559–567 (1947).

60.   M. H. Loveless, Repository immunization in pollen allergy, *J. Immunol.*, **79**:68–79 (1957).

61.   P. S. Norman, W. L. Winkenwerder, and B. C. D'Lugoff, Controlled evaluations of repository therapy in ragweed hay fever, *J. Allergy*, **39**:82–92 (1967).

62.   M. Potter and C. R. Boyce, Induction of plasma–cell neoplasms in strain BALB/C mice with mineral oil and mineral oil adjuvants, *Nature*, **193**: 1087-1087 (1962).

63.   A. M. Fuchs and M. B. Strauss, The clinical evaluation and the preparation and standardization of suspensions of a new water–insoluable whole ragweed pollen complex, *J. Allergy*, **30**:66–82 (1959).

64.   L. M. Lichtenstein, P. S. Norman, and W. L. Winkenwerder, Antibody response following immunotherapy in ragweed hay fever: Allpyral vs. whole ragweed extract, *J. Allergy*, **41**:49–57 (1968).

65.   M. S. Starr and M. Weinstock, Studies in pollen allergy. III. The relationship between blocking antibody levels and symptomatic relief following hyposensitisation with Allpyral in hay fever subjects, *Int. Arch. Allergy*, **38**:514–521 (1970).

66. P. S. Norman, W. L. Winkenwerder, and L. M. Lichtenstein, Trials of alum-precipitated pollen extracts in the treatment of hay fever, *J. Allergy Clin. Immunol.*, **50**:31-44 (1972).

67. D. G. Marsh, Preparation and properties of 'Allergoids' derived from native pollen allergens by mild formalin treatment, *Int. Arch. Allergy Appl. Immunol.*, **41**:199-215 (1971).

68. D. G. Marsh, L. M. Lichtenstein, and D. H. Campbell, Studies on 'Allergoids' prepared from naturally occurring allergens. I. Assay of allergenicity and antigenicity of formalinized rye Group I component, *Immunology*, **18**:705-722 (1970).

69. D. G. Marsh, L. M. Lichtenstein, and P. S. Norman, Induction of IgE-mediated immediate hypersensitivity to Group I rye grass pollen allergen and allergoids in non-allergic man, *Immunology*, **22**:1013-1028 (1972).

70. K. Ishizaka, T. Kishimoto, G. Delespesse, and T. P. King, Immunogenic properties of modified antigen E. I. Presence of specific determinants for T cells in denatured antigen and polypeptide chains, *J. Immunol.*, **113**: 70-77 (1974).

71. H. Baer, H. Godfrey, C. J. Maloney, P. S. Norman, and L. M. Lichtenstein, The potency and antigen E content of commercially prepared ragweed extracts, *J. Allergy*, **45**:347-354 (1970).

23

Transplantation of the Lung

JOHN R. BENFIELD

University of California at Los Angeles
School of Medicine and Harbor General Hospital
Torrance, California

I. Introduction

Organ transplantation was the dream of imaginative scientists for generations before Medawar established the immunologic basis of allograft rejection in 1943 [1]. Despite the skepticism amassed from work with animals, Murray, Merrill and Harrison [2] had the courage to accomplish the first successful human kidney allograft between identical twins in 1954. Now, less than 20 yr later, the Organ Transplantation Registry of the American College of Surgeons and the National Institutes of Health reports on 12,389 human kidney transplants accomplished up to 1972, and a major factor limiting the number of kidney transplants is the availability of grafts [3]. When renal transplant recipients are fortunate enough to obtain transplants, the chance for primary graft survival for 3 yr or longer is about 60%, and the chance for recipient survival is approximately 10% greater [3,4]. Long-term unqualified success from 8 to 17.5 yr has been achieved [5,6]. While it is certainly true that hemodialysis has played a vital

Supported in part by Research Grant HL 13077, National Heart and Lung Institute of the National Institutes of Health, and by grants from the American Heart Association and the Los Angeles County Heart Association.

role in the development of kidney transplantation, and that the success rate is as yet suboptimal, there is general agreement that renal transplantation has become a therapeutic life-saving modality. Thus, successful organ transplantation has become a reality during our generation.

Lung transplantation has not achieved the same growth as kidney grafting. Since the number of patients with far advanced, irreversible, progressive respiratory insufficiency is so large, the potential applicability for lung allografting exceeds that for kidney transplantation. Therefore, it is important critically to examine the reasons for the lag of lung transplantation behind kidney transplantation and to identify the progress made. It seems even more important to pinpoint barriers that must be overcome to advance lung transplantation from its current investigational status to that of greater clinical applicability.

A. Historical Landmarks

It would be superfluous to fully reiterate data presented in previous reviews [7-12] but certain historic highlights merit particular note. Juvenelle [13] has been credited most often with the initial success in the technical accomplishment of lung autografting or reimplantation. Although reported at different times, several groups almost simultaneously were successful in demonstrating that one reimplanted lung alone can provide sufficient respiratory function to sustain life in dogs [14-17]. That fact, more so than trying to assign credit accurately to any one group of investigators, is of historic importance. Meshalkin [18] in the Soviet Union was the first to take lung autografting into the clinical arena in an effort to treat otherwise intractable asthma. While the results of his trials do not support the rationale with which they were undertaken, Meshalkin proved that pulmonary reimplantation can be accomplished successfully in humans. Meanwhile, Lower and Shumway, [19] showed that total cardiopulmonary grafting in dogs is compatible with graft function and life of the recipient. In 1963 Hardy [20] took the giant step of attempting to use lung allografting for the treatment of a man with end-stage respiratory insufficiency. Others followed suit with regard to trying unilateral allografts in man, but Cooley [21] was the first to use total cardiopulmonary replacement in an infant. Evidence suggesting that bilateral lung transplantation might be more successful than unilateral grafting began to accumulate, and as a result of this and factors particular to his patient, Haglin [22] was the first to utilize bilateral staged lung transplantation in a human. His efforts did not succeed, but Alican and Hardy [23] were able to demonstrate the potential feasibility of the approach in the laboratory by showing that bilateral simultaneous lung transplantation in dogs is compatible with survival. The distinction of having come closest to successful human lung transplantation belongs to Derom and his coworkers [24] at the University of

Ghent in Belgium. Their patient lived with his pulmonary allograft over 10 months and during this period it became clear that the pulmonary allograft was his only functioning lung tissue. Significant palliation was achieved and the feasibility of lung transplantation in man was demonstrated. However, the counterbalance of adverse experiences with other clinical trials unintentionally generated an unfortunate sense of skepticism regarding the promise of the future [25].

B. The Current Major Obstacle

Why is this chapter included in a monograph that focuses on the pulmonary response to immunologic challenges? Clearly this is recognition of the fact that the immunologic response of homograft rejection is the major residual barrier to successful lung transplantation. To be sure, there are other obstacles that will be discussed, but experimental evidence and clinical experience strongly suggest that they can be surmounted currently, or within the near future. The purpose of this summary is to analyze the past and to suggest approaches to the future.

II. The Reimplantation Response

The reimplantation or autotransplantation response can be defined as changes resulting from excision and orthotopic replacement of lungs. This response has been studied in a variety of species, but the preponderance of work has been done with dogs. Efforts to minimize species differences between experimental animals and man have relied principally upon primates [26-28]. Unilateral, left lung autografts wherein the severed pulmonary arteries, mainstem bronchi, and pulmonary veins (atrial cuff) each were reconstituted in one suture line have been most extensively studied. Other preparations utilized for evaluating reimplantation response include labor and bilobar autografts, bilateral lung autotransplants, and reimplanted heart-lung units [19,23,26,29-33]. In most instances, there has been no effort to reestablish bronchial artery flow, but Haglin's group developed a technique for doing so [22]. It seems clear from the variety of preparations just sketched that to derive a distillate from them to describe the reimplantation response is complex. Nevertheless, certain common denominators emerged.

A. Technique

The technical details of accomplishing lung reimplantation are important, and those who are not surgeons, nevertheless, need to be cognizant of this fact. For example, increased pulmonary vascular resistance to the point that precluded autografted lungs from sustaining life was thought to be a part of the reimplantation response [34]. Then it became clear that this problem was negligible in primates where the operation was technically less demanding than in dogs from which almost all previous data had come [35]. Next it was recognized that the venous or atrial cuff anastomosis was subject to stenosis because of technical imperfections [36]. When operative and study techniques employed for lung reimplants were refined to the level that permitted exclusion of preparations with imperfect anastomoses [37], it became apparent that pulmonary vascular resistance and blood flow after reimplantation were entirely compatible with normal or near-normal function [29,38-41]. Unilateral and bilateral autografts were shown to be able to sustain life [16,23,26]. Similarly, arterial and bronchial anastomoses were transiently thought to be serious impediments to success, but it is now clear that neither of these suture lines is necessarily a problem.

The bronchial anastomosis is worthy of special comment because there is a residual difference of opinion as to whether or not the bronchial vessels need to be sutured. This difference is based upon laboratory data and bronchial anastomotic complications that occur in human allograft recipients [22,25]. By serial photofiberoptic bronchoscopic observation the evolution of bronchial anastomoses and the distal bronchial mucosa in 47 dogs, including 10 reimplant recipients were followed [42]. All dogs except one autograft recipient had a degree of bronchial stenosis caused by postoperative edema at some time during the postoperative period. However, half of the reimplants never had significant stenosis, and the narrowing that occurred in the remaining half was almost, without exception, entirely transient. It was maximal on the third postoperative day, usually well along towards reversal at the end of the first postoperative week, and generally entirely gone within 3 wk after autografting. There was no evidence of inadequate blood supply either early or late after grafting, and the incidence of bronchial anastomotic leak was 6%. These leaks were appreciated only by bronchoscopy and not by chest x-ray films. They did not cause apparent signs or the death of the animals. Thus, it is likely that there is no need for bronchial artery transplants and it appears that the bronchial anastomosis is not necessarily an impediment to successful lung grafting.

B. Surmounted Barriers

It could be argued that the reimplantation response is inconsequential and no longer an impediment to successful lung transplantation. The factors upon which this viewpoint could be based are as follows:

1. Skilled surgeons throughout the world have learned to accomplish the arterial, bronchial and venous (atrial cuff) anastomosis with precision and regularity without technical imperfections.

2. The best available evidence indicates that the vascular bed of reimplanted lungs can return essentially to normal or near normal, except perhaps at very high blood flows [39,40,43].

3. The ventilatory mechanics of reimplanted lungs return essentially to normal [38,39,41].

4. There appears to be no long-term ventilatory vascular imbalances as sequellae to lung autografting [38,39].

5. Bronchial circulation and mucociliary clearance are only temporarily impaired. Both these important functions return rapidly to normal [44,46].

6. Quantitative surfactant studies show essentially no difference between reimplanted lungs and normal controls [47,48].

7. Dogs can survive bilateral simultaneous pulmonary autografting, or unilateral reimplantation followed by ablation or excision of the contralateral lung [15,16,23,49].

One cannot dismiss the importance of the reimplantation response on these grounds, since there is necessarily a vital transition period between the completion of pulmonary autografting and the end points just enumerated. Indeed, the period of most critical need for human transplant recipients coincides with that of the transient and significant abnormalities that follow lung grafting prior to return to essential normality [25,29,50]. We shall therefore examine the reimplantation responses as a function of time.

C. Barriers to be Surmounted

Lung Preservation

These efforts clearly aim to delay or to abrogate that component of the reimplantation response which is the consequence of ischemic damage. Therefore, analysis of temporal influences upon the response can begin by considering those experiments relevant to reimplantation. Although some investigators have achieved a degree of success with lung preservation experiments [51,52], there is as yet no generally acceptable method for preserving lung grafts. During reimplantation, methods for preserving grafts in optimum condition have varied from simply minimizing normothermic ischemic times to rather elaborate hypothermic perfusion with rhythmic ventilation. Although most investigators have felt it advisable to clear blood from the grafts by flushing the vascular beds at the onset of the ischemic interval, it appears that this is not indicated [53,54]. For example, in 23 preservation experiments, simple flushing of the pulmonary vascular bed with low molecular-weight dextran or millipore filtered plasma at pressures of 15 cm H_2O resulted in significant increases in pulmonary water. When these grafts were then maintained at $4°C$ and rhythmically ventilated either with or without perfusion, ventillation, oxygen uptake, and compliance of the grafts were regularly impaired. The grafts preserved without perfusion were apparently damaged less than those that had been perfused, and one can conclude that vascular flushing and perfusion of lung grafts by the tested techniques is deleterious. Furthermore, one can infer that at least a part of the so-called reimplantation response may indeed be initiated during the first several minutes wherein the vascular bed of the extracorporeal graft is flushed. We therefore avoid flushing or perfusing grafts, feeling that these well-intentioned efforts may actually hasten the reimplantation response.

The second temporal element is the duration of ischemia during the operation. It appears that more than 4 hr of ischemia are not tolerated while 1 hr or less is well-accepted [55,56]. By measuring the rate of oxidative metabolism of [^{14}C]-labeled glucose and acetate substrates and glucose utilization, we have been able to obtain quantitative correlation with previously empiric observations indicating that the maximum period of tolerable normothermic ischemia is from 2 to 4 hr, and that hypothermia adds perhaps 2 hr more to the period wherein excised lungs are potentially useful as grafts [57,58]. For example, during observations upon hypothermic ($4°C$) lung slices at intervals during the first 24 hr after excision, glucose consumption began descending sharply and significantly as compared to baselines within 30 min after excision. Although the oxidation rates of [^{14}C]-labeled glucose and acetate substrates remained stable and not significantly different from baseline values during the first 2 to 4 hr after excision, by 6 hr after the onset of ischemia, they had descended to levels significantly less than baseline. From these observations and those of Von Wichert [59], one can safely conclude that, like the method of extracorporeal handling, the duration of the ischemic interval is at least a major contributor to the severity of the reimplantation response.

D. The Evolution of the Reimplantation Response

This has been studied through serial application of a variety of techniques. These include differential bronchospirometry, angiography, inhalation and perfusion lung scanning, measurement of pulmonary water, and anatomic studies at both the light and electron microscopy levels [29,39,50,60-64]. A number of important contributions have tested the reimplant function by contralateral pulmonary artery occlusion, either acutely or gradually [43,49,65]. Recently, through the use of radionuclide labeled microspheres, studies of the reimplantation response have been extended to include evaluation of the distribution of blood flow among the lobes of reimplanted lungs [66].

Despite the fact that lung function appears to return to normal or near normal levels within 3 to 6 wk after technically perfect autografting by measurements that have been made [29], there are important transient abnormalities. For example, even after the atrial cuff suture technique, which virtually assures the absence of outflow obstruction, there is a transient increase in vascular resistance and a decrease in blood flow to reimplanted lungs at resting cardiac outputs [66]. Ventilation–perfusion imbalances and decreased compliance, as well as centrally located coalescing alveolar infiltrates, have been observed in the early period after autografting, and almost invariably there has been a period of bronchial suture line edema that has already been described [42,50]. While long-term studies (2.5 to 4 yr after reimplantation) indicate that there is remarkable return towards normality, including the ability to maintain normal responsiveness to decreases in alveolar oxygen tensions, these data do not obviate concern regarding the early postoperative period [39].

In general, it appears that lung reimplants function at maximal, near normal levels immediately after operation. Within the first 3 days there are significant manifestations of the reimplantation response, and these manifestations are consistent in timing, severity, and recovery rate with postoperative edema in the bronchial suture line. Recovery of function is generally well underway by the end of the first postoperative week, and it is usually complete and at near–normal levels at some time between the third and sixth postoperative week.

In addition to functional considerations, another important aspect of the reimplantation response that concerns the potential success of clinical lung transplantation is the influence reimplantation might have upon the ability of recipients to resist postoperative pneumonia. Based upon studies with experimentally induced lobar pneumonias in dogs, my colleagues and I concluded that the ability of grafted lungs to confine pneumonitis is impaired as compared to controls [67]. Nevertheless, the therapeutic response to specific antibiotic treatments was prompt eradication of sensitive organisms. Thus, while the reimplantation response includes abnormal susceptibility to pulmonary infection, this potential pitfall apparently can be overcome.

The degree to which the reimplantation response is the result of denervation, mechanical postoperative changes, pulmonary reaction to trauma, severance of lymphatics, and other complex factors has not been fully sorted out. From the goal–directed viewpoint, it seems safe to conclude that the first postoperative week will probably be critical, and it is during this period that transient auxiliary respiratory support and precise antibiotic therapy might well be required, even in the absence of transplantation rejection phenomena. Despite this, it is clear

that the reimplantation response does not preclude successful therapeutic human
lung transplantation.

III. The Allograft Response

Are allografts of lungs different from those of other organs? To answer this question, one must attempt to separate lung allograft responses, which are a consequence of tissue rejection, from other manifestations of the reimplantation response. One must accept that it may not be entirely possible to dissect lung
rejection changes from abnormalities that accompany autografting, and that
there may be uncertainties in interpolations from results in animals to predict
what can be accomplished in humans. These uncertainties shall be approached
by commenting initially upon what is known about the lung allograft response
in animals, and thereafter by analyzing information derived from lung transplantation experience in humans.

A. Heterotopic Allografts

The technique of heterotopic lung transplantation has been useful for studies
seeking to answer two important questions regarding the allograft response. The
first was suggested by unexplained abnormalities in the lungs of canine lung allograft recipients [68]. Is lung allograft rejection necessarily noxious to the recipient's own lungs? When heterotopic pulmonary homotransplants were placed into
the systemic circulation in the groin and the recipients followed serially by differential bronchospirometry of their own lungs as rejection of the extrathoracic
lung homografts was proceeding, no abnormalities in the pulmonary function of
the recipients were found [69]. These recipients were then sacrificed 9 to 30
days after heterotopic lobar homotransplantation. The expected macroscopic
and microscopic signs of graft rejection were found in lung lobes transplanted to
the groins, but the recipient's intact, unoperated, intrathoracic lungs were normal.
The second question addressed through the use of heterotopic transplants is:
how promptly does the allograft response begin and what is the nature of its earliest manifestations? Heart–lung units from puppies were transplanted into the
necks of adult dog recipients and the grafted lungs biopsied at intervals from 30
min to 4½ hr after transplantation [70]. Although there was variation in the
time of onset of the allograft response, light and electron microscopy revealed a
regular pattern of early rejection in lung transplants analogous to that previously
described for renal transplants. In the lungs there was margination of leukocytes,
sticking of lymphocytes to endothelial cells, progressive disintegration of neutrophils, swelling and exfoliation of endothelial cells from basement membranes of

pulmonary capillaries, and platelet aggregation. The result was obstruction of pulmonary capillaries by ballooned-out epithelial cells, cellular debris, and fibrin. Thus, heterotopic lung allograft experiments indicated that the allograft response begins promptly and it does not necessarily involve the recipient's own lungs.

B. Morphology

The importance of understanding morphologic signs of rejection in lung allografts was appreciated over 10 yr ago when perivascular mononuclear infiltrates, intra-alveolar edema, and terminal massive pulmonary necrosis and hemorrhage were described as hallmarks of the allograft response [71,72]. Examples are shown in Figures 1 and 2. These observations have been refined and extended, and in 1972 they were the subject of an international symposium [64]. It became clear that the morphology of the allograft response is not only a function of rejection and the passage of time, it also includes manifestations that are part of the pulmonary response to injury and inflammation. For example, my colleagues and I found that the lungs of allograft recipients studied by light micros-

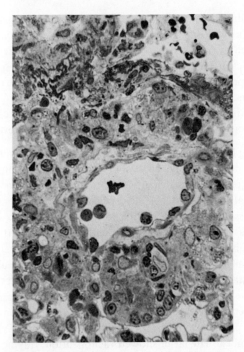

FIGURE 1 Light micrograph showing perivascular collection of mononuclear cells characteristic of rejection. 400X.

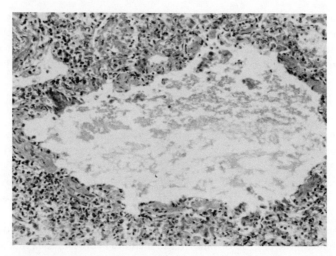

FIGURE 2 Diffuse leukocytic infiltration extending through lung parenchyma and disrupting vessel walls. 175X.

copy, either terminally or postmortem, showed similar changes in the grafts and in the recipient's own contralateral lungs [68]. In both, extensive inflammation was accompanied by hemorrhage, necrosis, and atelectasis. Perivascular infiltration of mononuclear cells, the hallmark of rejection in other organs, was difficult to assess in the presence of organizing pneumonia. It became apparent that serial morphologic observations at both the light and electron microscopy levels were required to clarify evolution of the allograft response and to determine whether or not morphology could serve as a diagnostic guide to the severity of rejection.

Serial lung biopsies after lung allografting between immunologically matched beagle dogs that survived 40.3 (19 to 97) days permitted observations during allograft responses sufficiently slow to allow some conclusions [73]. It became clear that the morphologic diagnosis of rejection rests upon the classic finding of perivascular round cell infiltration. The alveolar exudation, which has been described as an integral and perhaps pathognomonic part of rejection, was seen but it was also seen occasionally in the lungs contralateral to the allografts [68]. These changes were like those seen in other forms of pulmonary injury and in the end stages of pneumonia. By ultrastructural studies, the earliest changes were swelling of the Type I alveolar cells and cytoplasmic vacuolization in the capillary endothelial cells [74]. Examples are shown in Figures 3 and 4. Later there was progressive infiltration of macrophages and Type II alveolar cells increased in number. The latter showed vacuolization, fraying and membrane disruption of their lamellar inclusions. Examples are shown in Figures 5 and 6. A decrease in the relative number of Type II cell inclusions and extensive

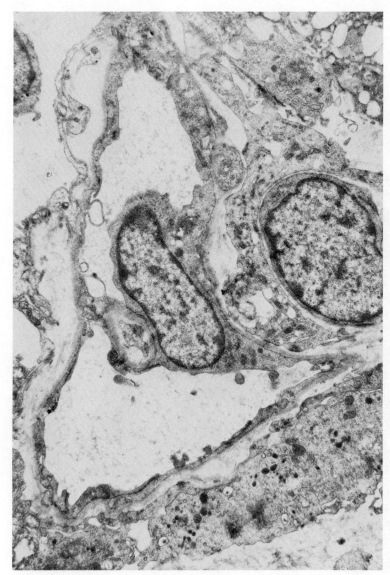

FIGURE 3 Electron microscopic section of pulmonary vessel, 4 days post–transplantation, showing swollen endothelial cell (En) and intraluminal adhesions. 8500X.

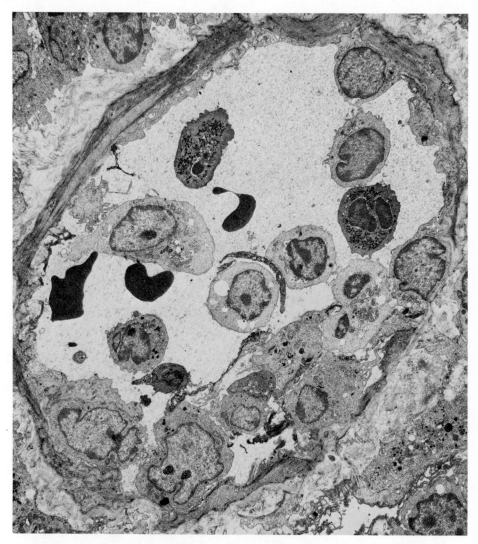

FIGURE 4 Engorged blood vessel containing red blood cells (rbc), polymorpho-nuclear leukocytes (PMN), and lymphocytes (Ly), 8 days post–transplantation. Endothelial cells in various stages of disruption and intravascular sloughing are shown. Note perivascular collagen accumulation (Co). 3200X.

endothelial damage were observed in preterminal biopsies. In considering the relative value of light microscopy and ultrastructural observations, it became clear that the former provided practical information regarding the degree of rejection changes and the latter were more useful in understanding morphologic mechanisms [75].

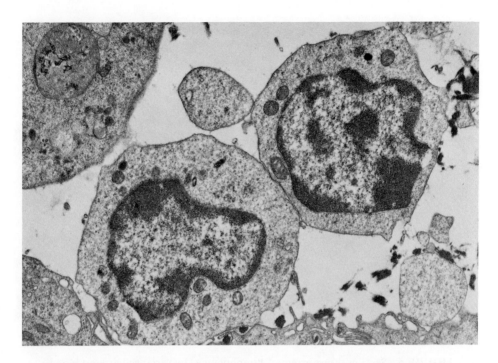

FIGURE 5 Electron micrograph of 2 lymphocytes in lung interstitium, 30 days post–transplantation. Nuclei (nu) show infoldings and chromatin margination characteristic of normal circulating lymphocytes. Cytoplasm contains few organelles. 12,000X.

Refinement of the morphologic description of the allograft response is being sought. Based upon sequential biopsies from lung allografts in T-cell deprived dogs, the consequences of cellular rejection as compared to rejection mediated by humoral factors may have been separated [76,77]. Cellular rejection was felt to be represented by perivascular mononuclear cuffing and by cellular debris in destroyed grafts. Humoral rejection was manifested by the destruction of vascular epithelium and when the grafts were destroyed, there was hemorrhagic alveolar necrosis in which the alveoli were stuffed with erythrocytes in the absence of mononuclear cell infiltration. Despite these refinements, recent attention to fine structural changes as seen with scanning electron microscopes [78], and evidence suggesting that antibody–producing cells in lung transplants can be identified [79], it seems clear that the allograft response needs to be viewed from perspectives additional to those of morphology.

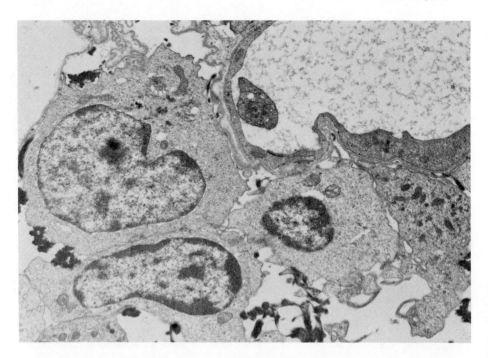

FIGURE 6   Section shows group of lymphocytes (Ly) arranged around blood vessel (BV). Cell at upper left has large nucleus and abundant cytoplasm, resembling a monocyte. 8700X.

C. The Bronchi

Bronchial Changes

Changes of the allograft response are worthy of comment because the bronchial anastomoses has been troublesome [80,81]. Not infrequently, it has been the cause of death in human recipients [82,83]. The endobronchial changes of the reimplant response have been summarized earlier, and both the transient nature of these changes, as well as the general adequacy of the bronchial blood supply, even without bronchial artery transplants, was stressed [42]. The allograft response of the bronchi in dogs was different. During allograft rejection in recipients without immunosuppression progressive bronchostenosis occurred regularly at the suture line. In some allograft recipients treated with immunosuppression, bronchostenosis was reversible but reversibility was never observed in nonimmunosuppressed recipients. Either grossly or on biopsies, the bronchial mucosa itself did not regularly reflect the allograft response. Anastomotic disruption was not a significant problem but it was clear that progressive bronchial stenosis is a feature of lung transplant rejection.

D. Physiology

The Physiology of Allografts

These have been studied by a variety of techniques, ranging from differential bronchospirometry to studies of blood flow and vascular resistance in transplants during acute or gradual occlusion of the contralateral pulmonary arteries. Ventilation–perfusion (V/Q) relationships were measured by lung scanning techniques as well as by more classic means, and V/Q indexes derived from inhalation-perfusion scans were used as indicators of the severity of the allograft response [61,85,87]. There is general agreement that impaired ventilation and perfusion are regularly demonstrable in failing allografts and that the severity of the deficits is related to the severity of the allograft response. While changes both in blood flow and ventilation reflect the allograft response, the rates of decrease often seem to be disparate. Inhalation and perfusion lung scanning have been found to be among the most practical means to calculate a V/Q index that correlates quite reliably with that calculated from data obtained by differential spirometry. Further transplant deterioration manifested by V/Q derangements was characterized by decreasing V/Q indexes [61,73]. One can conclude that physiologic parameters can quantitate the functional deficit due to allograft responses, but there is no evidence that they can either differentiate rejection from infection or define the immunologic consequences of lung transplantation.

E. Monitoring

The need to diagnose and monitor rejection is not unique to lung transplants, but there are specific aspects of it that pertain only to pulmonary allografts. For example, abnormalities that are either part of the reimplantation response or the result of pneumonia need to be separated from true allograft responses. Optimum immunosuppressive and antibiotic therapy depend upon this separation. The two general approaches, which have been used in animals in search of accurate diagnosis of allograft responses, have been trials with immunoassays and experiments wherein coexisting graft rejection and pneumonia were studied.

Concerning the question of clearly separating pneumonitic changes from allograft responses, experiments in which lobar pneumonias were induced in transplants provide some insight [67]. These showed that, as compared to controls, both the allograft and the reimplant responses decrease the lung's ability to confine experimental pneumonias to the inoculated lobes. They further showed that endobronchial pus was a feature of pneumonia, which was absent from rejecting allografts free of pneumonia. Cultures from endobronchial specimens were less precise than cultures of tissue obtained by lung biopsies, with regard to identifying offending bacteria. It was apparent that with the use of cultures obtained from bronchoscopies and from lung biopsies, pneumonia could be diagnosed precisely even in the presence of graft responses. While histologic features of the allograft response and far advanced pneumonias overlapped, it was clear that biopsies were sometimes the only method for identifying causative infectious organisms. Most important perhaps, it was proven that specific antibiotic therapy administered promptly could eradicate pneumonitis due to previously inoculated organisms, even during progressive graft rejection. Therefore, while lung biopsies cannot be regularly or frequently obtained from human recipients, they will occasionally be advisable more as a guide to antibiotic therapy than as indicators of the degree of rejection.

Information regarding the immunologic characterization of the lung allograft response is still primitive. In part, this is because the science of histocompatibility matching and the detection of early rejection changes by monitoring immune responses may have reached a plateau, and in part, because lung grafts are difficult experimental preparations. While the reimplant response can be minimized in laboratories in which lung transplantation is seriously studied, the combination of reimplantation and allograft responses is still formidable. Few laboratories with the expertise to overcome the reimplant response possess similar expertise in immunology. Conversely, leading immunologic laboratories tend to have little specific interest and no experience in lung transplantation.

Survival of lung allograft recipients is an important baseline in considering the efficacy of methods seeking to detect and modify rejection. Mongrel recipients of allografts from mismatched donors survived about 10 (7 to 16) days without immunosuppressives [88]. Beagles prospectively typed for lymphocytic antigens, using II lymphotoxic sera and erythrocytic antigens A, C and D, survived 98 (31–229) days. The two longest survivors in the series were sacrificed. Although there is one remarkably successful series wherein 13 of 22 randomly chosen immunosuppressed mongrel recipients survived 210 (33 to 941) days [86], experience in most laboratories more closely approximates ours in which the survival of randomly chosen mongrels was 14.7 (2 to 72) days [89]. Our beagle recipients typed for 15 lymphocytic antigens, survived 22 (11 to 68) days without immunosuppression, and 40.3 (19 to 97) days when immunosuppressives were used [73]. However, the interpretation of survival statistics from our laboratory must be viewed in light of the fact that none of the experiments from which they derive sought to test survival; all of them involved serial and multiple invasive tests that unquestionably shortened the lives of the grafts and the recipients. Currently, we have decreased the number of invasive tests, and the mean survival of our matched recipients exceeds 65 days. One can conclude that immunosuppression of lung allograft recipients significantly prolongs both graft and host survival and that further prolongation can be achieved when prospective donors and recipients are matched. Lest the reader despair at the statistics just given, it should be noted that they are far better than those achieved with canine renal allograft recipients when kidney transplantation entered the clinical arena.

Although it has been suggested that the allograft response can be detected and monitored by radiologic and currently standard clinical means [90,91], our laboratory experience and a review of lung transplant efforts in humans convinced us that the most accurate monitoring of rejection most probably lies in the immunologic realm [25]. We therefore studied some of the immunologic responses of beagle left lung allograft recipients whose grafts came from histocompatible donors, with and without immunosuppression [73]. Immunosuppression was accomplished with azathioprine 5 mg/kg-day and prednisolone 1 mg/kg-day. Donor skin fibroblasts propogated in tissue culture were labeled with [^{51}Cr] as target cells for an in vitro cytotoxicity assay using recipient lymphocytes as effector cells. Recipient lymphocytotoxicity toward donor cells could be detected as soon as 10 days after transplantation, thereafter it was present only variably. The effect of serum on this cytotoxicity was assessed by suspending the recipient lymphocytes both in pretransplant and autochthonous plasma. A small increment in cytotoxicity ($7 \pm 4.2\%$) was noted in autochthonous plasma, suggesting the presence of cytotoxic antibodies. There was no evidence for the development of blocking antibody activity. Although lymphocytes that killed donor skin cells appeared after lung transplantation, the correlation with rejection was not sufficiently constant to warrant firm conclusions. A significant but transitory decrease in serum total hemolytic complement was found 10 days after transplantation. Gamma globulin binding to transplanted lung detectable by immunofluorescense (IF) occurred in only 10% of biopsies taken 10 days or later after transplantation. Despite the fact that our data suggested that IF can be detected more regularly within 3 days of transplantation when the recipients are not immunosuppressed than when they are immunosuppressed, we concluded that dogs rarely develop antilung antibodies detectable by IF. The experience of others [79,92] suggests that immunoglobulins, particularly γM, can be identified quite regularly in lung allografts, but this method does not promise to be a practical parameter with which to monitor the allograft response. We also tested the effect of lung allografting on reactive blastogenesis by dog leukocytes and found that the incorporation of [^{3}H] thymidine into nucleated blood cells of controls and graft recipients was highly variable and without correlation with rejection [93]. To date our experience with mixed lymphocyte culture (MLC) techniques and rosette inhibition has also not provided the accurate monitoring required for allograft response, but we nevertheless remain convinced that serologic testing will ultimately prove at least as important as anatomic and physiologic parameters for defining the severity of allograft responses and differentiating them from reimplant responses and supervening infections.

F. Immunosuppression

Immunosuppression of lung allograft recipients to prolong graft function and survival, has been accomplished with azathioprine and corticosteroids in most laboratories, although results relying primarily or exclusively upon methotrexate have rarely been exceeded [94,95]. Antilymphocyte serum (ALS) has been used as adjunctive therapy, and other immunosuppressives have also been employed. More recently there have been experiments wherein lung allografts were given to T-cell deprived mongrel recipients [76,77]. The effects of thymectomy were augmented by giving antithymocyte serum (ATS). Although still based upon a relatively small series of experiments, it was concluded that T-cell deprivation is compatible with long-term survival (greater than 20 wk) of mongrel lung allograft recipients. T-cell deprivation made the recipients unresponsive to cellular aspects of lung rejection, but it was also associated with a high incidence of viral infections after lung transplantation. In view of the long-term survival achieved with simple pharmacologic immunosuppression in mongrel recipients in one laboratory [86], these exciting results must still stand the test of time. Further comparison with other methods of modifying the allograft response and the ability of T-cell deprived recipients to withstand bacterial pneumonias probably should be tested. Despite these reservations, experiments alluded to are very important in that they represent a needed new research direction in efforts to abrogate lung allograft responses.

G. State of the Art

In concluding this section, I will briefly answer the opening question concerning the comparison between lung allografts and transplants of other organs. Other than the lung's inherent fragility and susceptibility to infection, there is no reason to consider lung transplants more prone to failure than allografts of other organs. From a series of 43 simultaneous lung and kidney transplants in matched beagle recipients, we have evidence to support this viewpoint [96], and from data relevant to the allograft response summarized earlier, there is no evidence to the contrary. We therefore concluded that lung transplants can enjoy the same degree of success as other organ grafts, although the hazards of the reimplantation response and pneumonias require special attention.

IV. Human Lung Transplantation

A. The World Experience

The Organ Transplant Registry of the American College of Surgeons and the National Institutes of Health currently has 32 human lung transplants on record [97]. There is preliminary, as yet unconfirmed, information about three additional efforts. Collective reviews were published when there had been 23 and 27 human recipients, respectively, and a separate review, which focused on postmortem microscopic findings after 25 human lung transplantations, was compiled [12,25,98]. In addition, there have been individual reports by a number of investigators and each of these has made significant contributions. The purpose here is neither to update these reviews in detail nor summarize their contents. Instead, experience of the past will be analyzed with a view to the lessons it seems to teach and in prelude to projections into the future.

If one makes the unmodified observation that of 32 known human lung transplants, only one recipient survived longer than 6 months, and that most of the remaining recipients died within 30 days of transplantation, the picture seems hopelessly discouraging. On the other hand, the patient with the best result to date derived true palliation during a 10–month period wherein the transplant sustained his life [24]. One might also contrast the facts that only one of the first 23 recipients survived longer than 30 days after transplantation, while 2 of the next 9 recipients lived longer than 30 days. Of these 9 patients, one was lost during the operation and 2 others had either a bilateral lung transplant or a heart–lung unit graft, and one could cogently argue that these 3 patients should be considered separately from the total group of 9 in that they may represent special considerations of operative technique and judgment that do not necessarily apply to unilateral lung transplantation. This line of reasoning leaves 6 unilateral lung transplant recipients within the last 3 yr, in whom there were no apparent technical problems during operation, for consideration and contrast with the first 23 patients. The salient observation is that 2 of the 6 were well along the road to success, with minimal morphologic evidence of graft rejection, when they succumbed to a delayed bronchial anastomotic breakdown [82,83,91]. If laboratory experience with animals can be extrapolated to humans, this complication is largely preventable. These data suggest that clinical trials within the past 3 yr came much closer to success than those during the preceeding 7 yr, and that they approached being quite encouraging.

Considering the group of 32 recipients, the major problems encountered during the postoperative period were progressive respiratory insufficiency despite the transplants, disruptions of bronchial anastomoses, graft rejection, and pneumonias. These occurred in various combinations, and each warrants some comments. Postoperative respiratory insufficiency was primarily introduced and exacerbated by the recipients' own lungs contralateral to the transplants in at least seven patients [25]. Examples of this were patients with chronic obstructive disease in whom the transplants were more compliant than their own remaining lungs, as a result of which their own lungs over-expanded with compression of the grafts. Equally serious were discrepancies between the vascular resistances of the grafts and the contralateral lungs. For instance, one patient with primary pulmonary hypertension had a single lobar transplant which could not tolerate the share of cardiac output to which it was subjected as soon as blood flow to the transplant was initiated.

These problems of ventilatory-vascular imbalance which became apparent in the 1970 review have received considerable attention since then, and to obviate or deal with them, 2 of the 9 subsequent human transplants received either a bilateral lung transplant [22] or a heart-lung unit (C. Barnard, Capetown). General agreement that patients with restrictive lung disease are optimum candidates for unilateral lung transplantation emerged, but it is also evident that patients with chronic obstructive lung disease need not necessarily be excluded from eligibility for lung transplantation [99].

B. Analysis of Longest Survivors

Considerable perspective can be gained by analyzing the experience of those whose recipients received transplants that functioned for more than 30 days. Patients operated upon by Derom, Veith, and Cullum survived for from 2 to more than 10 months [24,82,83,91,100,101]. Derom and Cullum's patients had restrictive lung disease, and Veith's patient had obstructive lung disease with a restrictive component. Each of these recipients had end-stage respiratory insufficiency, and each had received maximal benefit from available treatment short of transplantation. The donors of each graft had suffered cerebral deaths, and the transplants were harvested after 14 to 50 hr of artificial ventilation. In each instance the duration of graft ischemia was short, ranging from 35 to 100 min. It is noteworthy that Cullum's recipient had been considered a candidate for transplantation for 9 months, and that during this period only four lungs of donors with compatible blood groups became available. The first three potential grafts were refused on the basis of tissue typing, preexisting infection, or general poor condition of the donors. When the fourth donor was accepted, there was some reluctance because HLA typing had revealed three major mismatches. Veith's recipient had two major and two minor mismatches of the 10 HLA compatibilities tested, and there were four of the 12 major mismatches between Derom's donor and recipient. All three recipients had right lung transplants and two required about 2 hr of atriofemoral cardiopulmonary bypass. It is clear that operative techniques did not present particularly difficult problems and that the readiness of the transplant groups permitted them to respond effectively and rapidly when suitable donors became available. If one can assume a well-coordinated lung transplant team, the limiting factor regarding the conduct of the operation appears to be the availability of donors; the key point regarding recipients is proper selection.

Recipients who lived beyond the first postoperative month varied in age from 23 to 53 yr. More important, they were apparently free of cancer or significant diseases involving organ systems other than the lungs. Both Derom and Cullum chose recipients with restrictive lung disease, e.g., silicosis and fibrosing alveolitis, respectively, for reasons well-expressed by Bates [102]. Previously, in 1968 K. A. Wasserman of our group had predicted that successful unilateral lung transplants would most likely be achieved first in recipients with restrictive disease because he recognized that perfect ventilatory-vascular balance between unilateral transplant and the recipient's own contralateral lung might be difficult to achieve, and that imbalances either in vascular resistance or in airway mechanics, which would divert blood or air away from the transplant, could be disastrous. Conversely, he postulated that if the recipient's own lungs were less compliant than those of the graft, and the transplant vascular resistance was less than that of the other lung, then the transplant would be favored during the postoperative period and little if anything would be lost by diverting blood and air away from the recipient's own diseased and insufficient lung. Both Derom's patient and Cullum's followed the latter pattern. In both instances, postoperative studies proved there was preferential perfusion and ventilation to the transplants, and their lung allografts alone, in fact, supported the life of the recipients to the point where Derom's patient returned home transiently and Cullum's recipient was approaching discharge to a new life when he unexpectedly succumbed. Notwithstanding, Veith's important experience in which he showed that a single lung allograft can be of therapeutic value in emphysematous patients, the clinical experience reported by Derom and Cullum is such that potential recipients with restrictive disease seem far more favorable than those with primarily chronic obstructive disease.

An axiom, which emerges from the postoperative period of the three recipients who survived the longest, is that postoperative management is at least as important to long-term success as the conduct of the transplant and the selection of recipients. In recipients whose selection eliminates or minimizes the physiologic problems of ventilatory-vascular imbalance between the two lungs, the salient diagnostic and therapeutic question during the postoperative period revolves around infection and rejection. Derom's patient died after 10 months, during which he suffered one episode of rejection 5 days after transplantation and another episode 5 months postoperatively. An episode of gram–negative sepsis occurred 3 wk after transplantation. The first rejection episode responded to treatment within 24 hr after prednisolone was increased from 50 mg daily to 300 mg per day. The second episode was also controlled by increasing cortico-steroid therapy and by giving antilymphocytic globulin. The final episode, which led to death, was interpreted as bronchopneumonia due to gram–negative bacte-ria superimposed upon chronic rejection. Cullum's patient also had a complex postoperative course, which was reported in admirable detail [83,100,101]. During the postoperative period of 53 days, exercise tolerance as compared to preoperative status improved markedly but there were many periods of illness. Antilymphocyte globulin (ALG) and large doses of intravenous prednisolone were used episodically to combat rejection. There were significant side effects to the ALG, and despite the first clinical use of rosette inhibition tests after lung transplantation, it is apparent that accurate diagnosis of rejection and its differ-entiation from infection were limited. The patient died when a peribronchial abscess resulted in a fistula between the bronchus and the pulmonary artery. The histologic features of rejection in the graft were mild and there was minimal evidence of infection. The findings raised the important unresolved question of whether or not the allograft was in the process of developing the recipient's orig-inal disease. Veith's patient also suffered multiple (at least seven) apparent epi-sodes of rejection, and these were treated with 1–g doses of methyl prednisolone, given at 12–hr intervals for 2 to 4 days [91]. At the time of reporting, the patient was 3.6 months postoperative (approximately 105 days). If each of the seven epi-sodes of presumed rejection required 3 days of treatment with massive doses of prednisolone, then at least 21 days or 20% of the postoperative days included therapy with 2 g methyl prednisolone per day. Clearly, the intervening days were required so that dosage could be tapered, and it appears evident the medication required could have contributed significantly to impaired healing of the bronchial anastomosis, which ultimately led to the patient's death.

C. Clinical Monitoring

The signs and symptoms of lung allograft rejection have been commented upon by Derom whose experience along these lines exceeds that of anyone else [24, 90]. On day 5 after transplantation, the recipient complained of dyspnea and general malaise. He was febrile (39.2°C) and new reticular infiltrates appeared in the chest x–ray film. The antibiotics were changed and the dose of prednisol-one increased to 300 mg. Within 24 hr, the patient improved. Based upon this and subsequent similar episodes, Derom concluded that the symptoms of rejec-tion are principally general malaise, dyspnea accompanied by a fall in Pao₂ and a productive cough. His experience was the first to show that rejection crises after lung transplantation in humans are reversible, and his group also showed that supervening infections of the graft can be controlled with the judicious use of antibiotics. The clinical observations of Veith and Cullum agree with Derom's. Cullum's group used the rosette inhibition test and differential circulating lymphocyte counts in search of additional means whereby rejection could be differentiated from infection [100]. They commented that the distinguishing clinical and radiologic features between rejection and infection were "unhelpful and even confusing," and their experience suggested the feasibility of predicting lung allograft rejection on the basis of assays of the immunologic response of recipients and their grafts. The message seems clear. Rejection could not be differentiated from infection precisely, and therapy for rejection was somewhat of an art rather than an exact science, which it optimally should be.

Veith and Hagstrom summarized histologic findings from 23 patients after reviewing microscopic findings in the lungs [98]. They considered 18 patients as having had sufficiently long clinical courses so that the morphology of their grafts was helpful. Shilkin and Reid [83] reported pathologic findings in the patient operated upon by Cullum, and Derom described the morphology of chronic rejection as seen in his patient [24]. An important common denominator between these reports is the relative paucity of evidence for far-advanced or end-stage rejection in any of the grafts. Thus, in the three patients who survived 2 to 10 months and in those who succumbed earlier in the postoperative period, the rejection problem seems to have been quite well controlled at the time of death. Even though Derom's 10-month survivor had chronic rejection, it is noteworthy that the rejection changes in his graft were predominantly peribronchial rather than perivascular and that bronchopneumonia superimposed upon chronic rejection was thought to be the cause of death.

D. Lessons From Personal Experience

During the past 5 yr our group has been consulted regarding five patients whom we accepted for transplantation. Brief consideration of why these patients never received transplants and their preterminal periods adds perspective to the question of lung transplantation. One patient with apparently preterminal restrictive lung disease initially accepted transplantation but subsequently decided against it. Although she never returned to a life she considered satisfactory or comfortable, she nevertheless unexpectedly survived for 1.6 yr thereafter. This experience points out the inherent uncertainties in selecting potential recipients. The next four potential recipients died before appropriate donors became available. This underscores the fact that organ availability is a serious limiting factor. One potential recipient suffered a cerebral air embolus during transseptal cardiac catheterization of the left atrium. Although this was recognized and the patient recovered from it, the increased risk pulmonary cripples incur during left heart catheterization came to fore. The most recent potential recipient, a patient of Dr. Robert Bartlett (University of California, Irvine), had acute respiratory insufficiency from amniotic fluid emboli. Her disease reached the point where she required prolonged extracorporeal oxygenator support, without which she clearly would have succumbed. Although no donor became available in time, this patient is an excellent example of the potential supplementary use of lung transplantation and extended extracorporeal oxygenation.

These experiences, our own and those of others, tell us that lung transplantation not only requires accurate selection of recipients and precise guidelines to postoperative management, but also organs for grafting and the wider availability of safe, effective auxiliary methods of mechanical oxygenation. They also strongly suggest that clinical success to the level of cadaver kidney transplants may be considerably closer than superficial review would indicate.

V. The Future

A. General Approach

During the developmental stages of any ultimately successful therapeutic method, the earliest clinical trials are clearly investigational. It could be argued that the extensive work in lung transplantation laboratories throughout the world has reached a plateau, and that further experiments with animals are not necessary so long as there are no substantive advances in the general immunology and immunotherapy of allograft rejection. It could further be argued that lung grafts are too complicated to warrant immunologic experiments with them, and that it is wasteful to study them when experiments with simpler grafts can be conducted. If these arguments are accepted it would delay clinical success in lung transplantation by many years because it would scuttle much of the expertise that currently exists in a few selected lung transplant centers while breakthroughs from basic science immunologists are awaited. Instead, the particular tasks of lung transplantation laboratories need to be identified and attacked in a more concerted manner and with less duplication of effort than in the past. The concerted research approach should have the following foci:

1. Diagnosis and treatment of lung allograft rejection.

2. Development of lung preservation and storage techniques.

3. Coordination between biologic prolonged respiratory support (transplantation) and artificial methods (oxygenators).

4. Development of a carefully coordinated prospectively planned series of clinical trials.

The Diagnosis and Treatment of Lung Allograft Rejection

This should be approached by applying immunoassay methods developed in transplant systems simpler than lung grafts to assess lung transplants. It is now possible quite regularly to obtain canine survivors with functioning grafts in excess of 2 months duration. It is also possible to produce experimental pneumonia in allograft recipients and to treat it effectively. These two facts achieved quite recently should be combined to develop means for accurately differentiating allograft rejection from infection. The investigational approach should use serologic, physiologic, and anatomic methods, keeping in mind that direct diagnostic access to the airways has not been fully exploited. For example, it seems conceivable that sophisticated analysis of exfoliated cells from the tracheobronchial tree of lung allografts could be indicators of the severity of the allograft response. Whatever the means, accurate guidelines for the diagnosis, prevention, and therapy of transplant rejection need to be developed.

Lung Preservation and Storage Techniques

The availability of organs will be a limiting factor in lung transplantation, just as it already is a major limiting factor in therapeutic human renal transplantation. The empiric approach taken to lung preservation experiments in the past should be relegated to a secondary role. The inherent fragility of lungs demand special attention beyond that necessary for preserving kidney grafts. The metabolic requirements of extracorporeal lungs must be studied further, and practical assays of lung graft viability need to be developed. Only then can we realistically expect to develop lung preservation and storage techniques.

Extracorporeal oxygenators for prolonged respiratory support are appropriately receiving considerable attention. Just as dialysis has not replaced renal transplantation, so oxygenators are not likely to obviate the need for lung grafting. The research capabilities and technical skills required for work with prolonged extracorporeal oxygenation are different from those currently necessary for lung transplantation research. As our own experience showed, it is inevitable that lung transplanters will turn to oxygenator teams for help and that the converse will also be true. Indeed, such interaction would seem to be a requisite for the success of either approach, and the laboratory is the milieu in which to develop the dual attack.

Clinical Trials

As the renal transplant experience has amply shown, there is no substitute for clinical trials and the state of the art of the laboratory cannot fully predict the feasibility of successful human transplants. And yet, how can one justify further clinical trials when only one human lung transplant recipient to date has achieved success? In the laboratory, lung transplants are currently more successful than renal transplants were when clinical trials with kidney grafting started. In the clinical setting, justification rests upon frank admission that the clinical trials so far done have only occasionally been prospectively planned by multidisciplinary teams with laboratory backgrounds in lung transplantation adhering to rigid recipient and donor selection criteria. Based upon the analysis of available data concerning recipients who survived longer than 30 days, we suggest the following approach for clinical trials in *selected* centers for the near-term future:

The recipients should be as follows:

1. Patients under age 50, with primary totally or near totally disabling respiratory disease, without significant unrelated complicating illness.

2. Patients whose physiologic studies indicate that the course of their disease has been relentlessly downhill and unresponsive to therapy, and that their life expectancy is less than 2 months under the direction of an internist skilled in the management of their disease. *We consider patients with restrictive lung disease prime candidates, and for the time being exclude patients with chronic obstructive disease.*

3. Patients who pass a psychiatric evaluation that indicates they are suited for an experimental operation, the success of which remains to be proven. Patients and their families must be able to cope with frequently trying postoperative management problems.

B. Current Attitude

The complexity of human lung transplantation is such as to defy complete prospective discussion here. However, two imperatives need to be stressed. First, the graft must be viable and not apparently incompatible for the recipient. Second, the clinical experiment must be conducted with the same requirements for evaluation as those of a well-designed laboratory experiment. For that purpose the recipient selection and transplant committees should be separate and

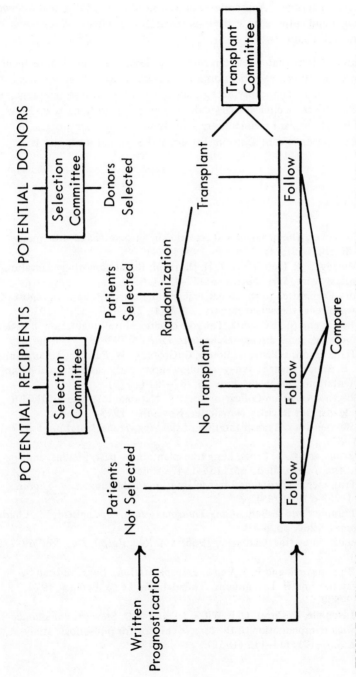

FIGURE 7 Clinical lung transplant trials should seek to evaluate the efficacy of the method by following a research plan similar to that depicted here. Selection of recipients and donors should be made by physicians other than the transplant surgeons.

independent of each other. Appropriate controls need to be studied and followed with equal vigor and enthusiasm as the lung transplant recipients. A suggested plan is outlined in Figure 7.

Our group differentiates between actively seeking lung transplant recipients and being prepared to proceed under optimum circumstances. Well organized teams with appropriate laboratory background and continuing research programs can justifiably undertake clinical trials under the proper conditions now. However, before lung transplant recipients are actively sought, further progress in accurately monitoring rejection, storing organs, and oxygenator support is necessary.

References

1. P. B. Medawar, The behavior and fate of skin autografts and skin homo-grafts in rabbits, *J. Anat.*, **78**:176–199 (1944).
2. J. E. Murray, J. P. Merrill, and J. H. Harrison, Renal homotransplantation in identical twins, *Surg. Forum*, **6**:432–439 (1955).
3. Advisory Committee to the Renal Transplant Registry, The 11th report of the human renal transplant registry, *J.A.M.A.*, **226**:1197–1204 (1973).
4. F. D. Belzer and S. L. Kountz, The role of clinical transplantation in patients with end–stage renal disease, *Transplant. Proc.*, **5**:793–797 (1973).
5. C. G. Halgrimson, I. Penn, A. Booth, C. Groth, C. W. Putnam, J. Corman, and T. E. Starzl, Eight to ten–year follow–up in early cases of renal homo-transplantation, *Transplant. Proc.*, **5**:787–791 (1973).
6. J. J. Bergan. American College of Surgery, National Institutes of Health Organ Transplant Registry Newsletter, November 1973.
7. D. A. Blumenstock, Transplantation of the lung, *Transplantation*, **5**:917–928 (1967).
8. E. D. Robin and C. E. Cross, Lung transplantation—past, present, and future, *Ann. Intern. Med.*, **65**:1138–1147 (1966).
9. M. J. Trummer, Experimental transplantation of the lung, *Ann. Thorac. Surg.*, **1**:203–219 (1965).
10. M. J. Trummer and P. Berg. *Lung Transplantation.* Springfield, Ill., Charles C. Thomas, 1968, pp. 6–10.
11. F. J. Veith, Lung transplantation 1968, *Am. Rev. Respir. Dis.*, **98**:769–775 (1968).
12. D. A. Blumenstock and F. J. Veith, Transplantation. *Lung.* Edited by J. S. Najarian and R. L. Simmons. Philadelphia, Lea & Febiger, 1972, pp. 569–587.
13. A. A. Juvenelle, C. Citret, C. E. Wiles, Jr., and J. D. Stewart, Pneumonec-tomy with reimplantation of the lung in the dog for physiologic study, *J. Thorac. Surg.*, **21**:111–115 (1951).

14. G. E. Duvoisin, W. S. Fowler, and F. H. Ellis, Jr., Reimplantation of the dog lung with survival after contralateral pneumonectomy, *Surg. Forum,* 15:173-175 (1964).

15. L. P. Faber, A. L. Pedreira, P. H. Pevsner, and E. J. Beattie, The immediate and long-term physiologic function of bilateral reimplanted lungs, *J. Thorac. Cardiovasc. Surg.,* 50:761-768 (1965).

16. N. Lempert and D. A. Blumenstock, Survival of dogs after bilateral reimplantation of the lungs, *Surg. Forum,* 15:179-181 (1964).

17. S. L. Nigro, R. H. Evans, J. R. Benfield, O. Gago, W. A. Fry, and W. E. Adams, Physiologic alterations of cardiopulmonary function in dogs living one and one-half years on only a reimplanted right lung, *J. Thorac. Cardiovasc. Surg.,* 46:598-605 (1963).

18. E. N. Meshalkin, V. S. Sergievskii, G. L. Feofliov, G. A. Savinski, and A. V. Baeva, First attempts at surgical treatment of bronchial asthma by the method of pulmonary autotransplantation, *Eksp. Khir. Anesteziol.,* 9:26-33 (1964).

19. R. R. Lower, R. C. Stofer, E. J. Hurley, and N. E. Shumway, Complete homograft replacement of the heart and lungs, *Surgery,* 50:842-845 (1961).

20. J. D. Hardy, W. R. Webb, M. L. Dalton, Jr., and G. R. Walker, Lung homotransplantation in man, *J.A.M.A.,* 186:1065-1074 (1963).

21. D. A. Cooley, R. D. Bloodwell, G. L. Hallman, J. J. Nora, G. M. Harrison, and R. D. Leachman, Organ transplantation for advanced cardiopulmonary disease, *Ann. Thorac. Surg.,* 8:30-42 (1969).

22. J. Haglin, In a report of the lung transplantation workshop 1970, *Ann. Thorac. Surg.,* 12:347-358 (1971).

23. F. Alican, M. Cayirili, E. Isin, and J. D. Hardy, One-stage replantation of both lungs in the dog, *J.A.M.A.,* 215:1303-1306 (1971).

24. F. Derom, F. Barbier, S. Ringoir, J. Versieck, G. Rolly, G. Berzsenyi, P. Vermeire, and L. Vrints, Ten-month survival after lung homotransplantation in man, *J. Thorac. Cardiovasc. Surg.,* 61:835-846 (1971).

25. C. R. H. Wildevuur and J. R. Benfield, A review of 23 human lung transplantations by 20 surgeons, *Ann. Thorac. Surg.,* 9:489-513 (1970).

26. A. R. Castenada, O. Arnar, P. S. Habelman, J. H. Moller, and R. Zamura, Cardiopulmonary autotransplantation in primates, *J. Cardiovasc. Surg.* (Turino), 13:523-531 (1972).

27. J. J. Haglin and O. Arnar, Pulmonary function in the baboon with lung reimplantation and subsequent contralateral pneumonectomy: Four-year follow-up. In *The Baboon in Medical Research.* Vol. 2. Austin, University of Texas Press, 1968.

28. W. L. Joseph and D. L. Morton, Immediate function with survival after left lung autotransplantation and contralateral pulmonary artery ligation in the baboon, *J. Thorac. Cardiovasc. Surg.,* 60:859-865 (1970).

29. J. R. Benfield, T. Isawa, J. C. Nemetz, D. E. Johnson, and G. V. Taplin, Immediate, early, and prolonged lung function after autotransplantation, *Arch. Surg.,* 101:52-55 (1970).

30. C. E. Huggins, Reimplantation of lobes of the lung: An experimental technique, *Lancet,* **2**:1059–1062 (1959).

31. J. T. T. Yeh, H. Manning, L. T. Ellison, and R. G. Ellison, Anatomic and physiologic consideration in pulmonary lobar reimplantation, *Surg. Forum,* **17**:211–213 (1966).

32. M. I. Perelman and J. J. Rabinovitch, Methods and technique of experimental autotransplantation of a lung lobe, *J. Thorac. Cardiovasc. Surg.,* **59**:275–282 (1970).

33. P. Vuillard, P. Gadot, P. Radice, P. LaMothe, L. Fischer, J. Belleville, F. Lesbroc, T. Wiesandenger, A. Brune, J. Falconnet, and J. Descotes, Simultaneous bilateral pulmonary homograft in the dog, *Presse Med.,* **77**: 1725–1726 (1969).

34. S. L. Nigro, R. H. Evans, O. Gago, and W. E. Adams, Altered physiology of the pulmonary vascular bed: A factor in decreased function of the reimplanted lung, *Dis. Chest,* **46**:317–320 (1964).

35. J. Haglin and O. Arnor, Physiologic studies of the baboon living on only the reimplanted lung, *Surg. Forum,* **15**:175–176 (1964).

36. J. R. Benfield and B. S. Coon, The role of the left atrial anastomosis in pulmonary reimplantation, *J. Thorac. Cardiovasc. Surg.,* **53**:626–684 (1967).

37. T. T. Flaherty, A. B. Crummy, and J. R. Benfield, The angiographic demonstration of left atrial anastomosis in pulmonary reimplantation and transplantation, *J. Thorac. Cardiovasc. Surg.,* **55**:797–799 (1968).

38. J. S. Brody, A. B. Fisher, C. D. Park, R. W. Hyde, and J. A. Waldhausen, Factors influencing function of the autotransplanted lung, *J. Appl. Physiol.,* **29**:587–592 (1970).

39. G. M. Tisi, M. J. Trummer, A. J. Cuomo, W. L. Ashburn, and K. M. Moser, Long–term autotransplanted canine lungs: Baseline ventilatory and hemodynamic function, *J. Appl. Physiol.,* **32**:113–120 (1972).

40. O. A. Wagner, G. S. M. Cowan, and H. L. Edmunds, Lobar pulmonary arterial blood flow in reimplanted canine lungs, *J. Thorac. Cardiovasc. Surg.,* **65**:171–179 (1973).

41. C. R. H. Wildevuur, H. Heemstra, G. J. Tammeling, C. Hilvering, H. G. D. Bouma, F. ten Hoor, L. A. Scherpenisse, J. W. Kleine, N. G. M. Orie, and J. N. Homan van der Heide, Long–term observations of the changes in pulmonary arterial pressure after reimplantation of the canine lung, *J. Thorac. Cardiovasc. Surg.,* **56**:799–808 (1968).

42. K. Shimada, G. Gondos, and J. R. Benfield, Photofiberoptic bronchoscopic findings during lung transplant rejection, *Arch. Surg.,* **106**:774–778 (1973).

43. P. A. Ebert and B. H. Hudson, Pulmonary hemodynamics following lung autotransplantation, *J. Thorac. Cardiovasc. Surg.,* **62**:188–192 (1971).

44. R. M. Stone, R. J. Ginsberg, R. F. Colapinto, and F. G. Pearson, Bronchial artery regeneration after radical hilar stripping, *Surg. Forum,* **17**:109–110 (1966).

45. L. H. Edmunds, Jr., R. J. Stallone, P. D. Graf, S. S. Sagel, and R. H. Greenspan, Mucus transport in transplanted lungs in dogs, *Surgery,* **66**: 15–22 (1969).

46. H. Morinari, K. Shimada, G. V. Taplin, D. E. Johnson, and J. R. Benfield, Bronchial mucous transport after lung autotransplantation in dogs, *J. Thorac. Cardiovasc. Surg.,* **67**:484–490 (1974).

47. J. A. Drews, D. F. Tierney, and J. R. Benfield, Effect of lung transplantation on surfactant, *Surg. Forum,* **24**:334–336 (1973).

48. J. A. Drews, D. F. Tierney, and J. R. Benfield, Effect of immunosuppression upon surfactant, *Surgery,* **76**:80–87 (1973).

49. F. J. Veith, K. Richards, S. Siegelman, W. Rosh, and J. W. C. Hagstrom, Effects of lung transplantation and simultaneous ligation of the opposite pulmonary artery after 2–14 months, *Eur. Surg. Res.,* **2**:153 (1970).

50. S. S. Sigelman, S. B. Sinha, and F. J. Veith, Pulmonary Reimplantation response, *Ann. Surg.,* **177**:30–36 (1973).

51. A. A. Garzon, C. Cheng, J. Pangan, and K. E. Karlson, Hyporthermic hyperbaric lung preservation for 24 hours with reimplantation, *J. Thorac. Cardiovasc. Surg.,* **55**:546–554 (1968).

52. F. Largiader, W. G. Manax, G. W. Lyons, and R. C. Lillehei, In vitro preservation of canine heart and lung, *Arch. Surg.,* **91**:801–804 (1965).

53. J. T. Castagna, E. Shors, and J. R. Benfield, The role of perfusion in lung preservation, *J. Thorac. Cardiovasc. Surg.,* **63**:521–526 (1972).

54. G. H. Stevens, J. D. de Moura Rangel, Y. Yakerski, M. N. Sanchez, and E. W. Fonkalsrud, Evaluation in dogs of various techniques of perfusion to preserve the lung. In *Organ Perfusion and Preservation.* Edited by J. E. Norman. New York, Appleton–Century–Crofts, Inc., 1968, p. 229.

55. J. Homatas, L. Bryant, and B. Eiseman, Time limits of cadaver lung viability, *J. Thorac. Cardiovasc. Surg.,* **56**:132–140 (1968).

56. F. J. Veith, S. B. P. Sinha, J. S. Graves, S. J. Boley, and J. C. Dougherty, Ischemic tolerance of the lung, *J. Thorac. Cardiovasc. Surg.,* **61**:804–810 (1971).

57. W. L. Joseph and D. L. Morton, Influence of ischemia and hypothermia on the ability of the transplanted primate lung to provide immediate and total respiratory support, *J. Thorac. Cardiovasc. Surg.,* **62**:752–762 (1971).

58. K. Shimada, W. D. Davidson, and J. R. Benfield, Metabolic changes in ischemic lungs for evaluation of graft viability, *J. Thorac. Cardiovasc. Surg.,* **66**:137–144 (1973).

59. P. Von Wichert, Studies on the metabolism of ischemic rabbit lungs: Conclusions for lung transplantation, *J. Thorac. Cardiovasc. Surg.,* **63**: 284–291 (1972).

60. M. J. Trummer and A. H. Christiansen, Radiologic and functional changes following autotransplantation of the lung, *J. Thorac. Cardiovasc. Surg.,* **49**:1006–1014 (1965).

61. T. Isawa, J. R. Benfield, J. Castagna, D. E. Johnson, and G. V. Taplin, Functional assessment of canine lung transplants by radioisotope lung scanning procedures, *Am. Rev. Respir. Dis.,* **103**:76–84 (1971).

62. P. Ketonen, S. Mattila, L. Siirila, and K. E. Kreus, Distribution of pulmonary blood flow before and after autotransplantation measured with xenon–133, *Scand. J. Thorac. Cardiovasc. Surg.,* **4**:102–106 (1970).

63. G. S. M. Cowan, Jr., L. H. Edmunds, Jr., and A. J. Erdmann, III. Analysis of weight gain in reimplanted dog lungs. *Surg. Forum*, 24:269–271 (1973).

64. C. R. H. Wildevuur. *Morphology in Lung Transplantation*. New York, S. Karger, 1972.

65. C. L. Huang, A. P. Norico, and R. R. Baker, Changes in pulmonary blood flow produced by autotransplantation of the left lung and placement of an Ameroid constrictor on the right pulmonary artery, *J. Thorac. Cardiovasc. Surg.*, 62:131–137 (1971).

66. O. A. Wagner, S. M. Cowan, and L. H. Edmunds, Lobar pulmonary arterial flow in reimplanted canine lungs, *J. Thorac. Cardiovasc. Surg.*, 65:171–179 (1973).

67. P. Schick, J. R. Benfield, B. Gondos, B. Hayakawa, E. Shors, K. Shimada, and M. E. Peter, Experimental lobar pneumonia in canine lung grafts, *Surgery*, 75:348–366 (1974).

68. B. Gondos, P. White, and J. R. Benfield, Histologic changes associated with rejection of canine lung transplants, *J. Thorac. Cardiovasc. Surg.*, 62:183–187 (1971).

69. W. D. Schwindt and J. R. Benfield, Autogenous and homologous heterotopic pulmonary lobar transplants, *J. Surg. Res.*, 8:267–273 (1968).

70. B. A. Warren and A. H. B. De Bond, The ultrastructure of early rejection phenomena in lung homografts in dogs, *Br. J. Exp. Pathol.*, 50:593–599 (1969).

71. B. A. Barnes, M. H. Flax, and G. Barr, Experimental pulmonary homografts in the dog. I. Morphologic studies, *Transplantation*, 1:351–364 (1963).

72. B. A. Barnes and M. H. Flax, Experimental pulmonary homografts in the dog. II. Modification of the homograft response by B.W. 57–322, *Transplantation*, 2:343–356 (1964).

73. J. R. Benfield, G. N. Beall, G. Gondos, M. E. Peter, K. Shimada, and P. Schick, Serial observations on immunologically matched lung allografts, *J. Thorac. Cardiovasc. Surg.*, 64:907–921 (1972).

74. B. Gondos, P. White, and J. R. Benfield, Ultrastructural alterations in canine lung allografts, *Am. J. Pathol.*, 64:373–386 (1971).

75. B. Gondos, K. Shimada, M. E. Peter, and J. R. Benfield, Light and electron microscopic findings in canine lung transplants. In *Morphology in Lung Transplantation*. Edited by C. R. H. Wildevuur. The Netherlands, S. Karger, 1972, P. 73.

76. C. R. H. Wildevuur, A. A. Van Der Broek, and C. R. Jerusalem, Prolonged lung allograft survival in "T–cell" deprived (TD) dogs, *Eur. Surg. Res.*, 5:Suppl.:50–51 (1973).

77. C. R. H. Wildevuur. Personal communication. (1973).

78. Y. Kondo, D. Turner, V. G. Lockard, C. Hallford, and J. D. Hardy, Scanning electron microscopy of canine lung transplants, *J. Thorac. Cardiovasc. Surg.*, 65:940–950 (1973).

79. S. Fujimura, V. Rosen, G. E. Adomian, W. W. Parmley, C. Suzuki, and J. M. Matloff, Cellular characteristics of the rejection response to canine lung allotransplants, *J. Thorac. Cardiovasc. Surg.,* **65**:438–448 (1973).

80. F. J. Veith and K. Richards, Improved technique for canine lung transplantation, *Ann. Surg.,* **171**:553–558 (1970).

81. M. J. Andrews and F. G. Perason, Relation of bronchial arterial circulation, and other factors, to the transient defect in oxygen uptake following autotransplantation of the canine lung, *Can. J. Surg.,* **16**:97–109 (1973).

82. F. J. Veith. Personal communication. (1973).

83. K. B. Shilkin and L. Reid, Pathologic findings after right lung transplantation in a patient with fibrosing alveolitis, *J. Clin. Pathol.,* **25**:674–679 (1972).

84. F. J. Veith, K. Richards, and P. Lalezari, Protracted survival after homotransplantation of the lung and simultaneous contralateral pulmonary artery ligation, *J. Thorac. Cardiovasc. Surg.,* **58**:829–836 (1969).

85. C. L. Pio Roda, J. D. Strandberg, J. W. Baker, and R. R. Baker, Serial changes in pulmonary blood flow during acute rejection of a lung allograft, *J. Thorac. Cardiovasc. Surg.,* **65**:88–93 (1973).

86. A. A. Garzon, S. K. Dutta, C. Okadigwe, N. Paley, S. Goldstein, S. Minkowitz, and K. E. Karlson, Functions of canine lung allografts, *J. Thorac. Cardiovasc. Surg.,* **65**:76–87 (1973).

87. J. D. Strandberg, C. L. Pio Roda, and R. R. Baker, Lung allografts in calves, *Arch. Surg.,* **106**:196–200 (1973).

88. D. Blumenstock, E. Wells, C. Sanford, and M. De Gillio, Allotransplantation of the lung in beagle and mongrel dogs prospectively typed for lymphocytic antigens, *Transplantation,* **11**:192–194 (1971).

89. J. R. Benfield, T. Isawa, J. T. Castagna, P. H. White, and B. Gondos, Canine lung allografts during rejection, *Proc. Soc. Int. Chirurgie,* **31**:277 (1972).

90. F. Derom, L'immunodepression en transplantation pulmonaire, *Minerva Chir.,* **26**:735–738 (1971).

91. F. J. Veith, S. K. Koerner, L. A. Attai, P. Barfeld, S. J. Boley, A. Bloomberg, M. Everhard, J. Anderson, B. Pollara, R. Steckler, H. Nagashima, S. Siegelman, P. Lalezari, and M. L. Gliedman, Single lung transplantation in emphysema, *Lancet,* **1**:1138–1139 (1972).

92. S. Fujimura, T. Nakada, Y. Kawakami, T. Sukeno, M. Yoneti, G. Okinawa, W. Kagami, and C. Suzuki, Detection of immunoglobulins by fluorescent antibody method in canine lung allotransplantation, *Tohoku J. Exp. Med.,* **101**:183–198 (1970).

93. G. N. Beall, J. R. Benfield, and K. Shimada, The effect of lung allografting on reactive blastogenesis by dog leukocytes, *Transplantation,* **16**:263–265 (1973).

94. D. A. Blumenstock, J. A. Collins, E. D. Thomas, and J. W. Ferrebee, Homotransplantation of the lung in dogs treated with methotrexate, *Surg. Forum,* **12**:121–122 (1961).

95.   D. A. Blumenstock, O. V. Grosjean, H. P. Otter, and M. A. Mulder,
      Experimental allotransplantation of the lung, *J. Thorac. Cardiovasc. Surg.*,
      54:807–814 (1967).
96.   J. R. Benfield and M. E. Peter, Simultaneous lung and kidney grafts in
      canine recipients. Unpublished data.
97.   Advisory Committee to the Organ Transplant Registry: The Eleventh
      report of the human organ transplant registry, *J.A.M.A.*, **226**:1197–
      1204 (1973).
98.   F. J. Veith and J. W. C. Hagstrom, Alveolar manifestations of rejection:
      An important cause of poor results with human lung transplantation,
      Ann. Surg., **175**:336–348 (1972).
99.   F. J. Veith, S. K. Koerner, S. S. Siegelman, M. Torres, P. A. Bardfeld,
      L. A. Attai, S. J. Boley, T. Takaro, and M. L. Gliedman, Single lung
      transplantation in experimental and human emphysema, *Ann. Surg.*, **178**:
      463–476 (1973).
100. P. A. Cullum, M. Bewick, K. Shilkin, D. E. H. Tee, P. Ayliffe, D. C. S.
      Hutchison, J. W. Laws, S. A. Mason, L. Reid, P. Hugh–Jones, and A. M.
      MacArthur, Distinction between infection and rejection in lung trans-
      plantation, *Br. Med. J.*, **2**:71–74 (1972).
101. P. Hugh–Jones, A. M. MacArthur, P. A. Cullum, S. A. Mason, W. A.
      Crosbie, D. C. S. Hutchison, M. C. Winterton, A. P. Smith, B. Mason, and
      L. A. Smith, Lung transplantation in a patient with fibrosing alveolitis,
      Br. Med. J., **3**:391–398 (1971).
102. D. V. Bates, The other Lung, *N. Eng. J. Med.*, **282**:277–279 (1970).

24

Transfer Factor in Diseases of the Lung

ANTONIO CATANZARO

University of California at San Diego School of Medicine
San Diego, California

LYNN SPITLER

University of California School of Medicine
San Francisco, California

I. Cell-Mediated Immunity in Lung Disease

A. Introduction

Transfer factor is a very potent molecule that may have far-reaching effects on the understanding of certain diseases of the lung. Perhaps more importantly, transfer factor brings to clinical medicine a new modality of therapy—immunotherapy. Before speculating on the possible effects of transfer factor, a brief overview of some aspects of cell-mediated immunity and diseases of the lung may add perspective.

As will become clear to the reader, the data available often provides no more than hints or suggestions of defects in thymus-derived lymphocyte (T-cell) function in pulmonary granulomatous diseases. Clinical use of transfer factor in

This study was supported by National Institutes of Health Grant, Pulmonary SCOR, HL–14169 and AI–CA–10686, and United States Public Health Service Career Development Award 1–K4–A143012.

these diseases has been limited. In this setting it is difficult to factually discuss the role of transfer factor in diseases of the lung. Instead, Dr. Spitler and I will speculate rather freely in an effort to spur further studies that might elucidate the role of cell-mediated immunity and transfer factor in these diseases. The group of lung diseases characterized by a granulomatous reaction will be discussed. Tuberculosis, coccidioidomycosis, histoplasmosis, North American blastomycosis and South American blastomycosis will be considered individually below. At the outset, however, it is pertinent to emphasize some of the many similarities exhibited between microorganisms that produce these diseases. The organisms discussed herein are slow to multiply and lack a potent mechanism for invading the physical barriers provided. They cannot penetrate the skin or mucous membrane; they are swept away by the ciliary blanket from the upper airway. Only when they reach the alveoli can infection occur. The unique interface between man and his environment provided by the alveolar membrane becomes the stage upon which the cell-cell interactions begin. The alveolus is the only place in the body where the host is not protected from the environment by a thick layer of cells or an elaborate mechanism for the physical removal of contaminating microorganisms. Particles that reach the alveoli are removed by phagocytosis by macrophages and polymorphonuclear neutrophils. These cells join the lymph in its journey to the lymph nodes. There the long chain of cellular events begin.

The host response to infection reveals more similarities: (a) a clinically detectable illness occurs only in a fraction of those infected; (b) dissemination of infection is common, often with little clinical symptomatology; (c) a latent, symptom-free period may be followed by reactivation of disease; or (d) a chronic active form of the disease may develop; and (e) cell-mediated immunity has a role in each infection.

B. Infection Due to Intracellular Organisms

Tuberculosis

The primary defenses against this organism, like others discussed in this section, are the physical barrier of the skin and mucous membrane and the mucociliary blanket of the airways. Mycobacteria that reach alveoli, regardless of the lack of prior exposure to the organism, are ingested by macrophages [2]. The virulence of strains of mycobacteria is directly related to their rate of growth within macrophages [3,4]. The role of the immune response or acquired immunity in resistance to disease has been difficult to define. A vigorous antibody response does not offer the host protection from infection, nor does it influence the course of disease [5]. The contribution of delayed hypersensitivity is less clear. Many of the destructive features of the disease are associated with granuloma formation and lymphocyte interaction with infected macrophages [6,7]. Delayed hypersensitivity to tuberculin has proven to be a useful tool clinically in the diagnosis of tuberculosis [8]. While lack of delayed hypersensitivity to tuberculin, as detected by skin test, is often associated with more extensive disease; this is not always the case [9]. The relationship between protective immunity and delayed hypersensitivity remained obscure for years. As our understanding of cell-mediated immunity increased, so has our ability to bring together an understanding that delayed hypersensitivity and acquired cellular resistance are different manifestations of the same immunologic process. As reviewed in detail by Mackaness and Blanden [10], the specifically sensitized T cell initiates the elaboration of many chemical mediators and the participation of nonsensitized monocytes. When the challenge is a soluble protein injected into the skin, delayed hypersensitivity is measured as an inflammatory reaction in the skin. When the challenge is a Mycobacterium within a macrophage, the same mediators and nonsensitized monocytes participate in an effort to kill the mycobacteria, contain the infection, or both.

Occasionally, delayed hypersensitivity and resistance are dissociated. In some animal models, a negative skin test to tuberculin has been observed even when peripheral lymphocytes respond to tuberculin sensitivity [10]. Conversely, the relationship between protective immunity of vaccine-induced delayed hypersensitivity and host resistance has been far from absolute [10].

There is some evidence to support the contention that active tuberculosis develops in individuals who have some impairment in the ability to mount a cell-mediated immune response [11]. Howard *et al.* [12] described distinctive clinical and histopathologic differences in patients with tuberculosis who did not develop cell-mediated immunity to tuberculin. Looking at patients who did not react to 10 mg of old tuberculin, they showed great numbers of mycobacteria in their sputum, extensive recent spread of disease was apparent on x-ray, and peripheral white counts were high and nearly devoid of lymphocytes. Six patients who died of progressive tuberculosis were reported. The histopathology was of great interest, particularly in the area of recent spread where no granuloma or tissue necrosis was found. The findings were described as "an acute exudative pulmonary response similar to what one might expect in acute pneumococcal pneumonia" [12]. Whitcomb and Rocklin [13] reported a patient with progressive tuberculosis who received vigorous antituberculous treatment but whose disease progressed. The patient had a profound defect in cell-mediated immunity on in vitro testing. When that defect was reversed with transfer factor, the patient eventually was able to control the infection. A report by Thomas *et al.* [11] suggests that defective T-cell function may play a role in most patients with tuberculosis. They found that the response to PHA was significantly lower in tuberculous patients, irrespective of the state of activity. Differences were not great, but were significant ($P<0.01$) [11].

Atypical Tuberculosis

This type involves the same basic protective mechanisms. Disease due to *Mycobacterium intracellulare* (Battey Disease) is of particular interest. In huge areas of the southeastern United States infection with *M. intracellulare* is highly endemic [14]. While many cases of *Battey disease* develop, they represent a very small fraction of those infected [15]. Individuals who develop disease are selected largely on host factors, such as ethnic background (more common in whites), socioeconomic status, and age [15]. Such patients often fail to demonstrate a vigorous delayed hypersensitivity response to an antigen derived from the cell wall of *M. intracellulare* (PPD B) [16].

Coccidioidomycosis

As with other intracellular microbial pathogens discussed in this section, the physical barriers provided by the integument mucous membrane or mucociliary blanket offer what appears to be complete protection from *Coccidioides immitis*. Infection occurs only when the airborne spores reach the alveoli [17] where they mature into spherules. As cell-mediated immunity develops, specific immunologically mediated killing probably begins, and granuloma formation contains the infection. Coccidioidin is a filtrate of lysed mycelia of *C. immitis*, which has been used as antigen to study the development of cell-mediated immunity to *C. immitis*. The southwestern United States contains large areas of high endemicity. In fact, 90% of the residents in areas of highest endemicity become infected by *C. immitis* [18]. Clinical disease, by contrast, is uncommon [19]. Pulmonary symptoms are noted in 30% to 40% of recent exposures only if the clinical condition is closely monitored [18,20]. Dissemination beyond the lungs probably occurs in less than 0.5% [21]. The role of cell-mediated immunity is suggested by the observation that 50% of patients with disseminated disease fail to develop delayed hypersensitivity to intradermal coccidioidin [17,22]. More importantly, a worse prognosis is associated with a negative skin test [17]. More recently we have shown that patients with chronic infection due to *C. immitis* have abnormal T-cell function in response to both mitogen and specific antigen [23]. The in vitro culture of peripheral blood lymphocytes shows that the response to PHA is blunted quantitatively and is abnormal in its time course.

The response to coccidioidin was negative by lymphocyte transformation in 10 of 18 patients (even when skin test with coccidiodin was positive) as well as in 5 of 6 with a negative skin test. T cells, as identified by rosette formation with sheep red blood cells, were not reduced in number in most patients; nor was the number of B cells, identified by immunofluorescence, abnormal. The plasma of patients was not suppressive to normal immune T cells. However, the reduced reactivity of T cells to mitogen and antigen is not fixed. Normal T-cell function was restored in some patients after prolonged standard medical therapy and in others after the administration of transfer factor. Occasionally, T-cell reactivity was recovered with no treatment at all [24].

Histoplasmosis

The pathogenesis of this infection began to unravel with the introduction of histoplasmin as a skin testing agent [25]. This extract of the fungus provided the antigen for studies of the host immune response to infection. Cell-mediated immunity, as measured by histoplasmin skin tests, develops promptly in 90% of cases of acute primary histoplasmosis. Of residents in endemic areas, 95% have a positive skin test with histoplasmin [26]. Pathologic and radiologic studies demonstrated that infection nearly always results in dissemination; and that dissemination is often asymptomatic [27]. Protection from disease after reexposure is nearly absolute. Recovery from primary histoplasmosis is associated with cell-mediated immunity to histoplasmin. Clinically significant disseminated histoplasmosis tends to occur in individuals with impaired cell-mediated immunity, i.e., lymphoreticular malignancy, corticosteroid treatment, advanced age, or infancy [28,29]. Humoral antibody responses to histoplasmin can be detected by complement fixation. Complement fixing antibody is usually present, but neither the presence nor the titer of the antibody is associated with immunoprotection [30]. Chronic pulmonary histoplasmosis develops in a very small fraction of the exposed population. These patients have local pulmonary infection for many months. A defect in cell-mediated immunity can be demonstrated in some patients with this form of histoplasmosis [31]. Another study demonstrated a defect in a fraction of patients with chronic pulmonary histoplasmosis [32]. Reduced T-cell reactivity can be documented by a reduction in the frequency of histoplasmin skin test positivity. A serum factor that can depress the response of normal sensitized lymphocytes to histoplasmin has been found in patients with disseminated and chronic pulmonary histoplasmosis [31]. Lymphocyte cultures demonstrate a cellular defect in addition to the serum factor. Reduced reactivity of T cells to PHA and candida antigen, as well as to histoplasmin, has been found to be independent of the serum factor [31,33]. The cause of reduced T-cell reactivity in these patients is not known; however, it obviously affects cell-mediated immunity in general. Most importantly, the defect is reversible; for when patients achieve cure, either following therapy with amphotericin or spontaneously, T-cell reactivity also returns to normal [34].

Blastomycosis (Paracoccidioidomycosis)

Efforts to delineate the full spectrum of human infections due to *Paracoccidioides brasiliensis* have been frustrated by the lack of a reliable antigenic marker. Many antigen preparations have been used and the results vary. All studies tend to indicate, however, that there are endemic areas of paracoccidioidal infection [35]. In certain populations, particularly among persons engaged in agriculture and cattle raising, reactor rates as high as 43% have been observed [36]. These studies, in conjunction with pathologic and radiologic studies, support the concept of a primary lesion in the lung and hematogenous dissemination to viscera and skin; dissemination is often asymptomatic. Clinical disease can be subdivided as follows: (a) acute pulmonary, (b) chronic pulmonary, (c) acute disseminated, (d) chronic disseminated, and (e) associated forms [37]. Humoral antibody to antigenic fractions of *P. brasiliensis* can be demonstrated by immunoelectrophoresis or complement fixation. Such antibody was found in 25 of 26 confirmed cases of paracoccidioidomycosis [38]. No correlation with severity of disease or prognosis could be established. Skin tests with several antigens of *P. brasiliensis* are frequently negative [35]. Mendes and Raphael [39] demonstrated that 73% of patients with paracoccidioidomycosis could not be sensitized to dinitrochlorobenzene, raising the question of a possible defect in cell–mediated immunity in patients suffering from the disease. Skin tests to tuberculosis, trichophyton, and candida were negative in 54% to 64%. Furthermore, Mendes *et al.* [40] demonstrated that [^{3}H] thymidine response to PHA was reduced in 6 of 10 cases. A plasma factor could not be demonstrated to effect the in vitro cultures. Skin allograft survival was tested in 7 patients. Five were rejected in 7 to 8 days, 1 survived 17 days, and another, 60 days. Impairment of cell–mediated immunity also has been demonstrated in patients with paracoccidioidomycosis. Patients effected with the lymphatic form have a more severe defect in cell–mediated immunity.

Cryptococcosis

The pathologic interaction between man and *Cryptococcus neoformans* has not been defined in detail but appears to be similar to that of other intracellular pathogens discussed earlier [41]. The organism gains entry into the body through the lungs. While the frequency of dissemination is unclear, hematogenous spread to skin, bones, abdominal viscera, and the central nervous system does occur [42]. The site of the initial pulmonary infection may be contained by granuloma formation, or acute or chronic pneumonia may develop. Healing usually occurs without calcification or residual destruction of underlying parenchyma. Frequently, the pulmonary focus is healed at the time extrapulmonary cryptococcal disease is diagnosed clinically. Studies to define the full scope of human infection with the organism have been hampered because the antigen extracts of *C. neoformans* have been complex and lack specificity.

Using lymphocyte stimulation in response to heat-killed *C. neoformans*. Diamond and Bennett [43] observed marked stimulation of lymphocytes from persons who had been exposed to *C. neoformans* but did not develop disease. Patients with disease had a lesser response to the antigen (*P*<0.005). Depression was specific and not seen in the response of patients to SKSD in a similar system. This study may suggest that an impaired response to T cells may be associated with the occurrence of *C. neoformans* dissemination [43].

C. Diseases of Unknown Etiology

Sarcoidosis

Despite intensive investigation, sarcoidosis remains a disease of unknown etiology. Even though granuloma formation is a major feature of this disease, the presence of defective delayed hypersensitivity has been recognized in these patients as early as 1905 when it was noted that the frequency of positive delayed hypersensitivity to tuberculin was greatly reduced in patients with sarcoidosis compared with the general population [44]. It was further observed that many patients with sarcoidosis could not develop delayed hypersensitivity to tuberculin even after repeated innoculation with BCG [45]. Reduced skin test reactivity in sarcoidosis subsequently has been demonstrated to be a general phenomenon affecting the response to candida, mumps virus, and trichophyton [46-48]. A skin homograft rejection was delayed to 4 wk in a patient with active sarcoidosis in contrast to 11 to 14 days in normal subjects [49]. Attempts to induce contact sensitivity with dinitrochlorobenzene and paradinitrodiphenylaniline have been unsuccessful in 71% of patients with sarcoidosis compared with 14% of the control subjects [50]. On the basis of these data, it can be concluded that patients with sarcoidosis have a defect in cell-mediated immunity. Where that defect is and its relationship to the pathogenesis of this disease remain to be elucidated.

Studies of lymphocytes in short-term cultures have been undertaken by several groups. It has been found that lymphocytes from patients with active sarcoidosis undergo blastic transformation more readily than do control cells, without stimulation. Specifically, in unstimulated cultures Lawgner *et al.* [51] found 6.8% blasts on day 3, 11.5% blasts on day 5, and 20% blasts on day 7 in patients with sarcoidosis. Healthy donor's lymphocytes underwent blastic transformation in only 2.4% to 2.8% on each of these days. Interestingly, many studies using the incorporation of radiolabeled thymidine have found no increased incorporation in unstimulated cultures [52]. Lawgner et al. [51] found a decrease in the incorporation of uridine into mRNA in lymphocytes from patients with sarcoidosis (0.6% versus 19.6% in normal subjects), but incorporation of thymidine into DNA was normal. Whether or not this blastic transformation in unstimulated cultures is on an immunologic basis is a moot question. Production of migration inhibitory factor under these circumstances may or may not be on an immunologic basis. Response to PHA in culture is depressed in lymphocytes from patients with sarcoidosis. This diminished response is evident whether blast transformation [53], leucine incorporation into protein, thymidine incorporation into DNA [52], or uridine incorporation into RNA is measured.

The specific response to PPD has been used to investigate lymphocyte function in vitro and in vivo. Patients with sarcoidosis, who have a positive skin test to tuberculin, can provide lymphocytes that react normally in vitro; that is, upon stimulation by PPD they undergo increased incorporation of thymidine [54]. They also can produce blastogenic factor upon stimulation by PPD. Patients with sarcoidosis, who have a negative skin test to tuberculin, are more confusing. Blast transformation has been reported to occur in this group with PPD (26.3% as compared with 17.5% in controls) but thymidine incorporation has not been increased above control levels in several studies [55].

Even more complex is the paradoxic skin test response. Patients with active sarcoidosis and a negative skin test may react to the antigen when cortisone is mixed with the antigen. Fifty percent of nonreactors to both tuberculin and candida demonstrate this paradoxic skin test response [56]. This finding is difficult to explain in view of the many actions that cortisone has. One mechanism might be some kind of unmasking or derepression of expression of sensitized lymphocytes. Efforts to demonstrate a repressor cell in the circulation of patients with active sarcoidosis have not been successful in a series of cell–transfer experiments.

Urbach et al. [57] injected into the skin of a recipient with a positive tuberculin skin test, leukocytes from 50 ml of blood from a patient with active sarcoidosis and a negative tuberculin test; a tuberculin skin test applied 18 hr later was 24 X 22 mm compared with a simultaneous control of 10 X 10 mm. These investigators also confirmed the observation that leukocytes from normal subjects sensitized to PPD could transfer local tuberculin sensitivity to patients with active sarcoidosis. Systemic transfer did not occur, however [57].

Transfer factor alone also can transfer local, but not systemic tuberculin sensitivity to patients with sarcoidosis [58]. Kohout [59] examined the affect of increasing the number of cells transferred. He took blood from normal subjects with tuberculin sensitivity, isolated the leukocytes, washed, and injected the cells into patients with active sarcoidosis and a negative tuberculin skin test. When the leukocytes from 25 ml of blood were transferred, 6 of 6 recipients demonstrated local but no systemic transfer. When the leukocytes from 50 ml of blood were transferred, 1 of 14 also demonstrated systemic sensitization that persisted for 4 wk. When the leukocytes from 400 ml of blood were transferred, 12 of 12 developed systemic sensitization that persisted for 4 wk; in 8 of 12, it persisted for 3 months [59]. One may conclude that transfer of delayed hypersensitivity to patients with sarcoidosis is difficult but can be accomplished. Normal sensitized lymphocytes have difficulty expressing their immunologic potential in the milieu provided by patients with sarcoidosis. That difficulty can be overcome by testing in close proximity to the transfer or by massive increases in the number of cells used to accomplish transfer.

The "defect" may be in the form of circulating molecules that affect lymphocyte function or cells that interact with the specifically sensitized lymphocyte. More likely, the effector cells needed to respond to the mediators released by specifically sensitized T-cells may be ineffective.

Studies of skin reactive factor by Gross [56] are revealing. He prepared this lymphokine by stimulating normal cells with concanavalin A for 24 hr. This prepared supernatant, when injected into normal skin, produced induration in 93% of normal subjects. None of the 8 patients with sarcoidosis had induration at the site of injection with the lymphokines. Six of the 8 did respond to lymphokines mixed with 1.25 mg cortisone acetate [56]. These findings suggest that the action of cortisone is not on the immunologically specific interaction between antigen and sensitized T cell, but rather on the nonspecific amplification system.

Many have questioned the specificity and mode of action of the Kveim antigen in patients with sarcoidosis. The interaction of Kveim antigen and lymphocytes is poorly understood. This material is handled differently than other delayed hypersensitivity immunogens. No induration is seen at 48 hr; instead, granuloma formation occurs weeks later. Delayed hypersensitivity to tuberculin never results in granuloma formation either in normal or patients with sarcoidosis. If the Kveim reaction represents delayed hypersensitivity, why is there no reaction at 48 hr? Many efforts to detect lymphocyte stimulation by Kveim antigen have been futile. Incorporation of leucine, thymidine, and uridine have been studied with no stimulation observed [60-62]. Silzbock [62] thought blastic transformation was stimulated by Kveim in patients with sarcoidosis. In fact, the data show that Kveim antigen was inhibiting to both normal and sarcoid cells. The effect was less marked on sarcoid cells. Both cultures with Kveim added showed less blast transformation than did cultures without additive [62]. On the other hand, release of migration-inhibition factor is stimulated by Kveim in patients with sarcoidosis and a positive Kveim test [63]. Lebacq [63a] did demonstrate that leukocytes from patients with active sarcoidosis and a positive Kveim test could transfer a positive Kveim test to three normal subjects.

II. Transfer Factor

A. Introduction

Our current understanding of delayed sensitivity was begun in 1942 when Landsteiner and Chase [64] reported experiments showing that this type of immunity could be transferred in animals with living white cells. Lawrence [65,66] subsequently demonstrated that whole cells could be used to transfer delayed sensitivity to tuberculin and to streptococci in man.

Lawrence [67] was then able to show that delayed sensitivity to streptococcal M substance and tuberculin could be transferred with extracts prepared from leukocytes by distilled water lysis or by freezing and thawing. This important observation was relatively ignored for the next 15 yr, mainly because of two major problems pertaining to transfer factor:

1. Transfer of delayed sensitivity could not readily be achieved in experimental animals with the use of leukocyte extracts, leading many to question the validity, or the significance, or both of the observed transfers in man.

2. The state of scientific knowledge with regard to cellular immunology and molecular biology was too primitive at the time of the original description of transfer factor to permit understanding regarding the possible mechanism of action of transfer factor.

Thus, transfer factor was not used prophylactically or therapeutically in patients until 1969, when my colleagues and I used it to induce cellular immunity in a patient with the Wiskott–Aldrich syndrome [68]. Transfer factor has now been used in a variety of conditions, including the Wiskott–Aldrich syndrome [69,70], severe combined immunodeficiency disease [71,75], mucocutaneous candidiasis [72,76-80], coccidioidomycosis [24,81,82], tuberculosis [13], and malignancy [83,88]. Our group has also published a preliminary report indicating the results of transfer factor therapy in a variety of other conditions, including varruca vulgaris, keratoacanthoma, aphthous stomatitis, ataxia telangiectasia, partial Di George syndrome, dysgammaglobulinemia, linear morphia, Behcet's disease, Nezelof syndrome [89].

The results of transfer factor therapy indicate that it is clearly possible to transfer skin test reactivity and in vitro parameters to patients lacking these responses. At times there is dissociation between the various modalities transferred; for example, in a number of immunodeficiency diseases it has been observed that skin test reactivity and the production of migration-inhibition factor to specific antigen may be transferred, whereas lymphocyte stimulation in response to the same antigen remains negative. The question of clinical benefit is much more difficult to evaluate. The response often appears dramatic to physicians dealing with the patients. Proof of the therapeutic efficacy of transfer factor will await controlled double-blend studies, which are currently being designed.

B. Chemical Characterization of Transfer Factor

The characterization of transfer factor has been hindered tremendously by the lack of a reproducible animal or in vitro test system for transfer factor activity; thus all information currently available with regard to the characterization of transfer factor has been derived from tedious and difficult studies of the transfer of reactivity in human subjects.

Lawrence [67] demonstrated very early that transfer factor resists enzymatic treatment with pancreatic deoxyribonuclease (DNAse) or with pancreatic ribonuclease A (RNAse). Subsequent studies have clearly confirmed that transfer factor is not inactivated by DNAse and, indeed, DNAse is used in the routine preparation of transfer factor in many laboratories. The fact that transfer factor resists pancreatic ribonuclease has been confirmed in our own laboratory and, in addition, my colleagues and I found that the transfer factor resists degradation with both Tl and pancreatic RNAse at low molarity, which breaks down the majority of single stranded RNA used in the control [90]. Lawrence [91] reported that transfer factor is in fact inactivated by pronase. Our studies indicate that a peptide is indeed involved in the activity of transfer factor.

Lawrence and Zweiman [92] found that transfer factor is inactivated by heating it at 56°C for 30 min. This statement comes from a study of local transfer of reactivity in patients with sarcoidosis. Our own studies using systemic transfers in normal human subjects indicate that transfer factor is heat-stable and resists heating at 56°C for 1 hr and even 80°C for 1 hr [90].

The low molecular weight of transfer factor was initially inferred by the observation that it is dialyzable [93]. This observation has been confirmed by a number of laboratories, and, in fact, dialysis is one of the routine procedures currently used in most laboratories for the preparation of transfer factor.

Column fractionation studies performed by a number of investigators indicate that transfer factor is retained on a Sephadex G25 column, suggesting that its molecular weight is under 10,000 [93,95]. Baram *et al.* [94] found two fractions capable of transferring sensitivity. One was a high molecular-weight fraction that contained IgG and other globulins, lipoprotein, and ribose; the other fraction was of lower molecular weight and was a polynucleotide containing adenine, guanine, and cytosine, but no uracil. They did not find amino acids in this fraction, which contradicts our findings, suggesting that a peptide is involved in transfer factor activity. Neidhart *et al.* [95] found that the transfer factor eluted at four-fifths the void volume from a Sephadex G25 column, thus suggesting that the transfer factor is not solely a polypeptide, since it would be unusual for most polypeptides to adhere to a Sephadex column. It may indicate that the fraction contains other agents, such as a polynucleotide, or that it is rich in aromatic amino acids.

The authors' studies indicate that transfer factor contains deoxyribose, polynucleotides, and polypeptides, but not cyclic AMP; however, it still remains to be seen which of these components is the active agent.

C. Animal Models and In Vitro Tests

The discouraging results of attempts to transfer delayed sensitivity in experimental animals have been reviewed by Bloom and Chase [96]. Recently, however, a number of investigators reported success in transferring reactivity with leukocyte extracts in experimental animals.

Baram and Condaulis [97] were the first to successfully transfer cell-mediated immunity in an animal. Macaca mulatta were immunized with keyhole limpet hemocyanin. They were able to demonstrate in vitro as well as in vivo transfer of initiated thymidine response to keyhole limpet hemocyanin using nondialyzable keyhole limpet hemocyanin–transfer factor.

Burger and associates reported success in transferring sensitivity to dinitrochlorobenzene between animals [98,99]. Maddison *et al.* [100] reported transfer of sensitivity with leukocyte extracts to monkeys. Librud *et al.* [101] reported transfer of sensitivity to rat coccidiosis. These reports have yet to be confirmed in other laboratories, and it is not known, at this time, whether these models will be sufficiently sensitive and reproducible to permit progress in the characterization of transfer factor.

An in vitro model has been described in which dialyzable transfer factor is added to nonsensitive lymphocytes in vitro [102]. Conversion of reactivity is a measure of the ability of these lymphocytes to then respond to specific antigen by increased DNA synthesis, as measured by radioactive thymidine incorporation. This model was worked out only after years of disappointing study, and it has been suggested that part of the reason for past failures to transfer reactivity in vitro were based on the method by which transfer factor was prepared. Specifically, it was found that the water used in the dialysis of transfer factor contains an inhibitor that prevents the lymphocyte response following the addition of transfer factor and antigen to the cultures. Accordingly, transfer factor was dialyzed against culture medium, and it was this preparation that permitted the observation of in vitro transfer of reactivity. It will be of great interest to see whether or not this model will prove useful in the characterization of transfer factor.

D. Specificity of Transfer

Strong evidence suggesting that transfer factor does confer specific reactivity on the recipient came from studies of the transfer of homograft sensitivity. Thus, the administration of transfer factor from a donor sensitized to one individual confers accelerated rejection of a skin graft obtained from that individual, but not from another individual to whom the donor was not sensitized [103]. Our own studies suggested that the reactivity transferred is specific, since recipients never showed conversion of reactivity to antigens to which the donor was not sensitized, with one minor exception [69]. On the other hand, Lawrence [104] did observe transfer of reactivity to coccidioidin in some recipients of transfer factor prepared from donors who appeared to be negative to coccidioidin. We also observed conversion of reactivity following the administration of transfer factor from donors who showed no reactivity to coccidioidin either in vivo or in vitro.

It is clear that nonspecific effects may occur following the administration of transfer factor. This is not unexpected, since it is known that the crude transfer factor preparation contains polynucleotides and it is well-recognized that polynucleotides can have a nonspecific effect of increasing cellular immunity in vivo and in vitro. The observation of nonspecific effects of transfer factor, therefore, does not negate the possibility that there also may be specific effects of transfer factor.

Three types of evidence have demonstrated the nonspecific effects of transfer factor:

>   1.   It has been reported that reactivity to PHA may increase following the administration of transfer factor [24,105].

2. Administration of transfer factor from donors not known to be sensitive to dinitrochlorobenzene may cause conversion of skin test reactivity from negative to positive in recipients with immunodeficiency diseases who were previously exposed to dinitrochlorobenzene [106].

3. There may be an increase in reactivity in mixed leukocyte culture following the administration of transfer factor [107].

Although the above studies do suggest that transfer factor may have specific as well as nonspecific effects, the answer to this question has not been definitively resolved. We are aware of studies in two separate laboratories that appear to clearly document that transfer factor may confer specific reactivity. Unfortunately, at the time this manuscript was prepared, neither of these studies had been published, either in abstract or in munuscript form and accordingly, cannot be included herein. However, it can be anticipated that more information regarding the subject will soon be forthcoming.

E. Therapeutic Uses

The therapeutic use of transfer factor is predicated on the following important principles:

1. Transfer factor is exceedingly potent. The amount necessary to transfer skin test reactivity is the amount derived from 0.1 ml of packed leukocytes. This is the amount contained in approximately 10 ml of blood (for therapeutic purposes, the dose of transfer factor utilized is far greater than the amount necessary for conversion of skin test reactivity).

2. Systemic reactivity occurs in the recipient. Accordingly, if transfer factor is administered subcutaneously over the deltoid, skin test reactivity may be measured in the opposite forearm, and will be positive if the transfer is successful.

3. Not only is skin test reactivity transferred, but in vitro tests of cellular immunity also shows conversion. In normal subjects, conversion of lymphocyte stimulation and production of migration–inhibition factor to specific antigens occur in patients with defects in cellular immunity. These results are variable, and there may be conversion of reactivity as measured by one test, such as migration–inhibition factor; whereas, reactivity as measured by another test, such as lymphocyte stimulation, may remain negative.

4. Antibody formation is not transferred.

As indicated above, there may be both specific and nonspecific effects following the administration of transfer factor. It is not known whether the clinical benefit observed following the administration of transfer factor to patients with defects in cellular immunity results from specific transfer of reactivity or from the nonspecific effects of transfer factor. In preliminary studies it seemed reasonable to use transfer factor derived from donors showing strong reactivity to specific antigens to determine whether or not clinical benefit would be observed. Thus, in the treatment of patients with coccidioidomycosis, donors were selected who showed strong reactivity to coccidioidin by both in vivo and in vitro testing. As indicated below, in the preliminary study, transfer factor from coccidioidin-positive individuals did appear to have a beneficial clinical effect in some of the patients treated. A controlled double-blind study has now been designed, which will include an evaluation of the therapeutic effects of transfer factor from coccidioidin-negative donors and a control group treated with placebo. Until more information is available on this subject, it would seem preferable to choose as donors individuals who react strongly to the specific antigen to which the patient is not responding. However, in instances in which a donor with appropriate immunity is not available, as for patients with disseminated viral infections, it may be reasonable to administer transfer factor from donors not known to have specific reactivity to the antigen involved because it is possible that the nonspecific effects of transfer factor may prove beneficial.

Selection of Patients

The following groups of patients may reasonably be considered candidates for transfer factor therapy.

1. Those with congenital defects of cellular immunity

2. Those with disseminated intracellular infections

3. Those with diseases of unknown etiology which may have an infectious basis

4. Those with malignancy

With regard to patients with congenital defects in cellular immunity, it was thought that those with combined immunodeficiency disease who lack T cells (thymic-derived lymphocytes) would not respond to transfer factor therapy. Such therapy was administered to patients with combined immunodeficiency disease thought to lack T cells, and we found that the administration of transfer factor in these patients can cause conversion of skin test reactivity and production of migration inhibitory factor. Accordingly, it seems that our knowledge of the cause of this disease and/or the mechanism of action of transfer factor are inadequate. Accordingly, beneficial results may result even in patients thought to lack T cells. Thus, it is possible that responses may be observed in other patients with congenital deficiencies of T cells, such as those with Nezelof's and Di George syndrome as well.

In patients with disseminated intracellular infections, the question is frequently raised as to whether it is reasonable to treat patients with transfer factor if their skin test is positive. As reviewed above, many diseases are known to be associated with a defect, but even when defects are described, the patients often do not fall into well-defined groups. The reason may be that the defect, if present, is operative at an as yet undefined site. Possibilities include an aberrant mechanism for handling a particular class antigen or expression of cell mediated immunity. A stem cell may be missing or ineffective and the tests discussed herein may imperfectly reflect the cellular defect. Certainly, testing of cellular immunity provides some information regarding these patients, and it is most helpful to evaluate skin test reactivity, lymphocyte stimulation, production of migration inhibitory factor, and inhibition of leukocyte migration in patients with disseminated infections.

In the final analysis, a return to the bedside is indicated. The clinical course will usually provide clues regarding the capacity of the patient to rid himself of the particular infection. If his antimicrobial management has been excellent but he is unable to make a recovery, one must question the function of systems that bear those functions. In the case of intracellular infections, a careful examination of cell-mediated immunity is indicated. If such an examination is unproductive, the reason may be the inadequacy of the test systems. Faced with the dual problem of inadequate test systems and a lack of knowledge regarding the site of action of transfer factor, the possible beneficial effect of transfer factor cannot be excluded. Then a decision regarding the use of transfer factor must be made on the basis of risk to the patient versus likelihood of benefit. At the same time, maximizing the yield of useful information that may be transferred to other patients, or other diseases, or both, must be considered carefully. To this end, clinical and immunologic effects, both in vivo and in vitro, must be monitored carefully. In normal subjects, these tests of cellular immunity usually correlate with one another; however, in patients with infectious diseases, they frequently do not correlate with one another and which correlate is important in clearing the infection is not known. However, it appears likely that the patient who has a continuing disseminated intracellular infection probably has a defect in cellular immune response, even though his skin tests, lymphocyte stimulation, and migration-inhibition factor may be positive to that antigen. Thus, while the usual policy is to reserve transfer factor for the treatment of patients who have clearly demonstrated a defect in cellular immunity, as manifested by negative responses on all tests, it may be reasonable to administer this therapy on a trial basis to patients who do show some degree of reactivity on the tests, if they are showing a poor biologic response to the infection as indicated by ongoing infection.

There are a number of diseases in which the cause is unknown, but which may have an infectious basis. One example of this category of disease is rheumatoid arthritis; another is aphthous stomatitis. Although the general level of cellular immunity is normal in these patients, one may postulate that they have an ongoing infection with an unrecognized agent to which most normal subjects have been exposed and developed immunity. Accordingly, it may be reasonable, in some of these patients to administer, as a therapeutic trial, transfer factor from normal subjects in an attempt to reconstitute cellular immune responses to the unrecognized organism.

Timing and Dosage Administration of Transfer Factor

The reactivity transferred to normal subjects frequently is long-lived and had been observed to remain positive as long as 2 yr; however, in patients with immunodeficiency diseases, reactivity remains positive for varying lengths of time, and sometimes may be quite transient. Accordingly, it seems reasonable to follow cellular immune responses serially and to administer the transfer factor when these responses decline following administration. This interval may vary with different disease states; for example, in patients with the Wiskott–Aldrich syndrome, it appears that the administration of transfer factor once every 6 months may be sufficient. However, in patients with disseminated coccidioidomycosis, reactivity may diminish as promptly as within 1 or 2 wk.

Information regarding the dose of transfer factor necessary is anecdotal at best. We have arbitrarily used the amount derived from 5×10^8 lymphocytes as one dose of transfer factor, and many other laboratories have used a similar amount. At times we have not noted conversion of reactivity in our patients following the administration of this dose of transfer factor, but we have observed conversion when larger doses were administered. It is our impression that the doses of transfer factor currently being used are at the lower limits of efficacy for patients with infectious diseases, and that increasing the dose and the frequency of administration may well improve the clinical results in these patients.

III. The Role or Potential Role of Transfer Factor
in Treatment of Lung Diseases

We have discussed several diseases of the lung in which impaired cell–mediated immunity appears to be part of the problem. Transfer factor is known to be a potent agent capable of transferring cell–mediated immunity to humans previously lacking that type of response. Therefore, many have been anxious to bring this molecular form of therapy to the bedside. Many obstacles have been, and are still, in the way. As indicated in Section I, our understanding of the defect in cell–mediated immunity in these diseases is quite incomplete. The actions and limitations of transfer factor have been difficult to delineate because of obvious limitations imposed by working with humans.

The use of transfer factor in human infections underscores questions about its dose, duration of transfer, specificity, and so on. Evaluation of the effect of transfer factor on human infections is further complicated by the use of antibiotics. When is it ethical or wise to withhold antibiotics? When is the patient's prior course used as the baseline for comparison? What is the cumulative effect over time, with or without antibiotics? How can controls be selected when patients with severe infection and defective cell–mediated immunity are few and the defect is often at what appears to be different levels? Is transfer factor more fairly used as an adjunct to antibiotic therapy? What end point should be used to judge the effect of transfer factor? The course of this disease is variable and usually nonfatal.

A. Tuberculosis

Whitcomb and Rocklin [13] treated the first case of tuberculosis with transfer factor. Their patient was extremely unusual. She had progressive primary tuberculosis; that is, with what appeared to be her first encounter with *M. tuberculosis,* she developed progressive disease. Extensive infiltrative lesions in both lungs revealed acid fast bacilli (AFB) and noncaseating granuloma on biopsy. Tuberculin skin test (5 tuberculin U) produced 15 mm induration at 48 hr. Despite treatment, at the onset of her illness, with isoniazid, para–aminosalicylic acid (PAS), and streptomycin, her lesions progressed. Her course was complicated from the onset by pancytopenia and splenomegaly. Prednisone, 60 mg per day, was also administered.

In vitro tests showed that her peripheral lymphocytes, as well as splenic lymphocytes, responded to PHA but not to PPD or streptokinase–streptodornase. After 2 months, the three–drug program produced no improvement and after 2 months her antituberculosis drug program was changed to INH, rifampin, and ethambutal. Prednisone, 60 mg per day, was continued. The disease progressed and 4 months later her sputum became positive for the first time. Sensitivity studies demonstrated *M. tuberculosis*, sensitive to all drugs in her regimen. Dialyzable transfer factor from donors with strong tuberculin sensitivity was prepared from 250 ml blood. Four such doses were given at roughly 1-wk intervals, followed by two more doses several months later. Shortly after the first course of transfer factor therapy was completed, the patient developed a subcutaneous abscess over the sternum. This was presumed to be a dissemination of tuberculosis, and pyrazinamide (PZA) and streptomycin were added to the antituberculosis regimen. Streptomycin was promptly discontinued. Within 4 to 6 wk after the first course of transfer factor therapy, the patient began to improve clinically. Her cell-mediated immunity, including skin test, [^{3}H] thymidine incorporation, and production of migration-inhibition factor in response to tuberculin became and remained positive. Her clinical condition continued to improve, she developed negative sputum for *M. tuberculosis*, and roentgenographs stabilized as her chest lesions healed [13].

This patient was unusual in that she demonstrated severe progressive tuberculosis unresponsive to antituberculous drugs and failed to show a cell-mediated immune response to tuberculin. Her case can be very instructive with regard to the role of cell-mediated immunity in controlling infection and the reconstitution of that immunity with transfer factor.

One must wonder whether minor degrees of impaired cell-mediated immunity may play a role in cases of tuberculosis that involve less progressive disease. In fact, when we consider that disease develops in only 80 per 100,000 infected individuals per year [8], one must question protective mechanisms lacking in the 80 who develop the disease. As discussed in the section on immunity and tuberculosis, some patients with active tuberculosis have a negative skin test to tuberculin and many react to a lesser extent than do normal subjects to PHA. Certainly, these patients might be considered candidates for therapy with transfer factor. If other assays of cell-mediated immunity are applied, such as cytotoxicity, more subtle defects may be found. The mode of action of transfer factor is, of course, unknown. It follows that the abnormality in cell-mediated immunity that best identifies patients likely to respond to transfer factor is also unknown. The relevance of an abnormal laboratory study should be determined by the patient's clinical course. It has always been traditional in medicine to try a new form of treatment on the most desperately ill patients, and later offer the advantage of the new therapy to patients who are less sick.

The current treatment of atypical tuberculosis is particularly unsatisfactory. Treatment programs are long and complicated, using many drugs and frequently including surgery. The experimental use of a new form of therapy seems justified under these circumstances.

B. Coccidioidomycosis

In this disease, the use of transfer factor is quite attractive. Standard therapy
with amphotericin is long, difficult to administer, and associated with significant
toxicity. An unfavorable clinical course is more likely when the skin test with
coccidioidin is negative [17]. As discussed in Section I, many patients with
coccidioidomycosis whose response to the invading fungus is less than adequate
have a reduced T-cell reactivity to PHA and coccidioidin [23]. This may be the
case even when the skin test to coccidioidin is positive.

Graybill [81] treated three patients with progressive coccidioidomycosis
with transfer factor from donors with strong cell-mediated immunity to coccidioidin. Each had had extensive therapy with amphotericin and persistent active
disease. Two had negative skin tests, [^{3}H] thymidine incorporation, and production of migration-inhibition factor in response to coccidioidin. Following the
administration of several doses of transfer factor, all in vitro parameters of cell-
mediated immunity became reactive to coccidioidin. Two patients had dramatic
clinical improvement; one went into remission. The other patients had a strongly
positive skin test and a negative migration-inhibition factor and [^{3}H] thymidine
incorporation on exposure to coccidioidin. Infection became worse and spread
despite vigorous therapy with amphotericin. After two doses of transfer factor,
the in vitro tests became positive. Clinical improvement was not noted at the
time of the report [81].

We have administered transfer factor to 7 patients with coccidioidomycosis.
The primary criterion for patient selection was a "poor biologic response" to *C.
immitis.* It is difficult to give a concise definition of what is meant by a "poor
biologic response to cocci." But a little clinical information will make it clear.
Over a period of 2 to 20 yr, 4 of 7 patients had persistent or recurrent infection.
In 2 of 7, the rate of progression of disease was alarming. A patient with miliary
disease had fungimia, an ominous clinical finding. All patients had amphotericin
prior to the administration of transfer factor. Over prolonged periods, 4 to 7 had
had huge doses. Each had extensive disease. Table 1 provides some clinical
detail.

Transfer factor was administered by subcutaneous injection. The frequency of administration and the total number of injections varied according
to the immunologic response. T-cell reactivity to coccidioidin in vivo and in
vitro as well as response to PHA are listed before and after transfer factor in
Table 2. Skin test with coccidioidin was positive in 3 of 7 before and in 7 of 7
after transfer factor. Release of migration-inhibition factor in response to coccidioidin was detected in 2 of 7 before and in 5 of 7 after transfer factor. Thymidine incorporation following stimulation with coccidioidin produced a stimulation index (SI) greater than 2 in 1 of 7 before transfer factor; after transfer

TABLE 1 **Characterization of Patients with Coccidioidomycosis**

Patient	Age	Sex	Organ involvement
A. C.	51	M	Acute miliary
R. H.	33	M	Pulmonary Sinus tract Lymph nodes
H. O.	7	F	Extensive pulmonary Bone Sinus tract
H. F.	38	F	Pulmonary Extensive sinus tract Lymph nodes
H. M.	59	M	Progressive pulmonary
J. K.	14	M	Pulmonary Pleura Pericardium
W. S.	53	M	Pulmonary Bone

factor all had SI greater than 2. The one patient who had an SI greater than 2 before transfer factor had a significantly greater SI after therapy than before. Thymidine incorporation following stimulation with PHA produced an SI greater than 30 in only 1 out of 6 before transfer factor; after transfer factor, SI was greater than 30 in 5 of 7. Immunologic improvement was often transient, but could be maintained with repeated doses of transfer factor. Each patient had a favorable clinical response to transfer factor as measured by fever, exercise tolerance, healing of infected wounds, clearing of pulmonary infiltration and decrease in complement-fixation titers to coccidioidin. In 4 of 7, improvement was transient or incomplete. We have observed a fairly close correlation between immunologic and clinical events. In vitro monitoring and repeated doses are often needed. Many questions remained regarding the need for specific transfer factor, patient selection, and a host of other things [108]. Analysis of serial response to coccidioidin in [³H] thymidine incorporation and production of migration-inhibition factor has revealed several important points. Conversion is most apt to occur following the initial administration of transfer factor. In certain patients, large doses may be needed to attain that conversion. [³H] thymidine and, to a lesser extent, production of migration-inhibition factor in response to coccidioidin, which becomes positive after transfer factor, tends to revert back to negative within 4 days to 4 months. When in vitro tests have reverted to negative, much more intense administration of transfer factor is required to regain a

TABLE 2 Immunologic Response to Transfer Factor

Patient	Skin test response Coccidioidin Before TF[a]	Skin test response Coccidioidin After TF	Migration-inhibition factor Coccidioidin Before TF	Migration-inhibition factor Coccidioidin After TF	Lymphocyte stimulation index Coccidioidin Before TF	Lymphocyte stimulation index Coccidioidin After TF	Lymphocyte stimulation index PHA[b] Before TF	Lymphocyte stimulation index PHA[b] After TF
A. C.	−	+	−	−	1	8	8	1
R. H.	+	+	−	+	1	4	1–2	15–150
H. O.	+	+	+	+	1	8	12–16	100–271
H. F.	+	+	+	+	1	5	5–10	40–110
H. M.	−	+	−	+	1	4	1–2	1–5
J. K.	−	+	−	+	6	22	130	170
W. S.	−	+	−	−	1.6	8	-	260

[a]TF = transfer factor.
[b]PHA = phytohemagglutination.

positive response, if it can be reachieved at all. The best clinical response is seen in patients who have maintained positive in vitro tests most of the time. A large initial dose of transfer factor followed by repeat doses at variable periods is recommended [104].

Turning to the larger question, all patients with clinical coccidioidomycosis may be termed to have a "poor biologic response to *C. immitis*" since no more than 5% of the infected population develops clinically diagnosable disease. Many of these patients do, indeed, have reduced T-cell reactivity.

We have demonstrated that this reduced T-cell reactivity may be temporary. It may return to normal long after cure has been established by conventional therapy; or it may return to normal promptly after the administration of coccidioidin plus transfer factor [24]. Whether or not transfer factor from a coccidioidin-negative donor would also be effective is not known. The course of disease in coccidioidomycosis is quite variable. Especially in milder cases, the effect of therapy is difficult to observe. A larger double-blind controlled study is urgently needed.

C. Histoplasmosis, Blastomycosis and Cryptococcosis

These all demonstrate sufficient evidence of a defect in cell-mediated immunity to warrant considering therapy with transfer factor. This consideration is further spurred by the fact that current therapy is confined to the use of systemic or intrathecal amphotericin. Because of the toxic effects of the drug, it is reserved only for gravely ill patients, because these patients often have a defect in the function of nonspecific effector cells, such as monocytes and macrophages.

The data cited in the previous section would indicate that receptor lymphocytes are available and transfer factor may be able to "turn them on" to the infecting fungus and effect improved clinical response.

D. Sarcoidosis

As yet we are not aware of any experience with the use of transfer factor to treat sarcoidosis. Previous studies in this disease have been directed toward answering the question of whether or not reactivity to standard antigens could be transferred to these patients. They were not attempts at therapy. It is well-recognized that a defect in cellular immunity exists in many patients with sarcoidosis. A number of lines of evidence suggest an infectious etiology for this disease, although a specific agent has yet to be isolated. The majority of patients recover, perhaps by developing immunity to the unrecognized agent. Those patients could be used as donors of white cells for the preparation of transfer factor for therapy of the small group of patients who develop progressive disease.

E. Conclusion

Thus, experience with the use of transfer factor in the therapy of granulomatous diseases of the lungs is limited, but the results of therapy with transfer factor appears encouraging. A small number of patients with disseminated progressive disease is unresponsive to standard forms of therapy. Since most infections with these organisms are self-limited, frequently inapparent, it seems reasonable to reserve the use of transfer factor for patients who demonstrate a poor biologic response to infection, as evidenced by the development of disseminated disease. It may be unwise at this stage to withhold therapy with an agent or standard drugs known to be effective in those diseases, but the addition of transfer factor to the regimen may prove to shorten the period of disability and the length of amphotericin therapy. Controlled studies will be necessary to establish the answer to these questions.

References

1. G. M. Green, In defense of the lung, *Am. Rev. Respir. Dis.*, **102**:691–703 (1970).
2. A. R. Rich. *The Pathogenesis of Tuberculosis*. Springfield, Ill., Thomas, 1951, pp. 287–297.
3. E. Suter, The multiplication of tubercle bacilli within normal phagocytes in tissue culture, *J. Exp. Med.*, **96**:137–150 (1952).
4. M. Berthrong and M. A. Hamilton, Normal guinea pig monocytes with tubercle bacilli of different virulence, *Am. Rev. Tuberc.*, **77**:436–449 (1958).
5. S. Raffel, The mechanism involved in acquired immunity to tuberculosis. In *Experimental Tuberculosis*. 1955, pp. 261–279.
6. A. R. Rich. *The Pathogenesis of Tuberculosis*. Springfield, Ill., Thomas, 1951, pp. 740–746.
7. M. B. Lurie. *Resistance to Tuberculosis*. Cambridge, Mass., Harvard Press, 1964, p. 27.
8. P. Q. Edwards, Story of the tuberculin skin test from an epidemiological viewpoint, *Am. Rev. Respir. Dis.*, **81**:1–47 (1960).
9. D. C. Kent and R. Schwartz, Active pulmonary tuberculosis with negative tuberculin skin reactions, *Am. Rev. Respir. Dis.*, **95**:411–418 (1967).
10. G. B. Mackaness and R. V. Blanden, Cellular immunity, *Prog. Allergy*, **11**: 89–140 (1967).

11. W. Thomas, S. Naiman, and D. Clement, Lymphocyte transformation by phytohemagglutinin: II. In the tuberculous patient, *Can. Med. Assoc. J.,* **97**:836–840 (1967).

12. L. W. Howard, M. D. Klopfenstein, W. J. Steininger, and C. E. Woodruff, The loss of tuberculin sensitivity in certain patients with active pulmonary tuberculosis, *Chest,* **57**:530–534 (1970).

13. M. E. Whitcomb and R. E. Rocklin, Transfer factor therapy in a patient with progressive primary tuberculosis, *Ann. Intern. Med.,* **79**:161–166 (1973).

14. L. B. Edwards, L. Haywood, L. F. Affronti, and C. E. Palmer, Sensitivity profiles of mycobacterial infection, *Bull. Int. Union Tuberc.,* **32**:384–394 (1962).

15. R. F. Corpe, Clinical aspects, medical and surgical, in the management of Battey–type pulmonary diseases, *Dis. Chest,* **45**:380–382 (1964).

16. M. Zack, L. Fulkerson, G. Hartshorve, E. Kennedy, and E. Stein, Clinical evaluation of stabilized and non–stabilized PPD–B in patients with group III atypical mycobacteria, *Chest,* **63**:348–352 (1973).

17. M. J. Fiese. *Coccidioidomycosis.* Springfield, Ill., Charles Thomas, 1958.

18. C. E. Smith, R. R. Beard, E. G. Whiting, and H. G. Rosenberger, Varieties of coccidioidol infection in relations to the epidemiology and control of the diseases, *Am. J. Public Health,* **36**:1394–1402 (1946).

19. C. E. Smith, D. Pappagianis, H. B. Levine, and M. Saito, Human coccidioidomycosis, *Bacteriol. Rev.,* **25**:310–317 (1962).

20. W. A. Winn, Coccidioidomycosis, *J. Chronic Dis.,* **5**:430–444 (1957).

21. J. L. Converse and R. E. Reed, Experimental epidemiology of coccidioidomycosis, *Bacteriol. Rev.,* **30**:678–687 (1966).

22. K. T. Maddy, A study of one hundred cases of disseminated coccidioidomycosis in the dog, *Proceedings Symposium Coccidioidomycosis.* In *U.S. Public Health Service Publication 578,* 1957, pp. 107–118.

23. A. Catanzaro, L. E. Spitler, and K. M. Moser, Cellular immune response in coccidioidomycosis, *Cell. Immunol.,* **15**:360–371 (1975).

24. A. Catanzaro, L. E. Spitler, and K. M. Moser, Recovery of T–cell reactivity, *Fed. Proc.,* **33**:790 (1974) (abstr.).

25. C. W. Emmons, B. J. Olson, and W. W. Eldridge, Studies of the role of fungi in pulmonary disease, *Pub. Health Rep.,* **60**:1383–1394 (1945).

26. P. Q. Edwards and C. E. Palmer, Nationwide histoplasmin sensitivity and histoplasma infection, *Pub. Health Rep.,* **78**:241–259 (1963).

27. M. Straub and T. Schwartz, The healed primary complex in histoplasmosis, *Am. J. Clin. Pathol.,* **25**:727–741 (1955).

28. N. A. Nelson, H. L. Goodman, and H. L. Oster, The association of histoplasmosis and lymphoma, *Am. J. Med. Sci.,* **223**:56–65 (1957).

29. P. Holland and N. Holland, Histoplasmosis in early infancy, *Am. J. Dis. Child.,* **112**:412–421 (1966).

30. S. B. Salvin, Resistance of animals and man to histoplasmosis. In *Histoplasmosis.* Edited by H. C. Sweaney. Springfield, Ill., Charles Thomas, 1960, pp. 99–112.

31.   W. M. Newberry, Jr., J. W. Chandler, Jr., T. Chin, and C. H. Kirkpatrick,
      Immunology of the mycoses. I. depressed lymphocyte transformation in
      chronic histoplasmosis, *J. Immunol.*, **100**:436–443 (1968).
32.   R. H. Alford and R. A. Goodwin, Patterns of immune response in chronic
      pulmonary histoplasmosis, *J. Infect. Dis.*, **125**:269–275 (1972).
33.   C. H. Kirkpatrick, J. W. Chandler, T. K. Smith, and W. M. Newberry, Cel-
      lular immunologic studies in histoplasmosis. Thomas, Springfield, Ill.,
      Proceedings Second National Conference on Histoplasmosis, 1971, p. 371.
34.   R. H. Alford and R. A. Goodwin, Variation in lymphocyte reactivity to
      histoplasmin during the course of chronic pulmonary histoplasmosis, *Am.
      Rev. Respir. Dis.*, **108**:85–92 (1973).
35.   I. A. Conti-Diaz, Skin tests with paracoccidioidin and their importance,
      Pan American Health Organization Scientific Publication 254, 1972,
      pp. 197–202.
36.   A. M. Restrepo, S. Robeledo, M. Ospina, and A. Corea, Distribution of para-
      coccidioidin sensitivity in Columbia, *Am. J. Trop. Med.*, **17**:25–37 (1968).
37.   H. W. Mumay, M. L. Littman, and R. B. Roberts, Disseminated paracoccid-
      ioidomycosis (South American Blastomycosis) in the United States, *Am.
      J. Med.*, **56**:209–220 (1974).
38.   L. A. Yarzobal, J. M. Torres, M. Josef, F. Vigna, A. Da Luiz, and S.
      Andrieu, Antigenic mosaic of paracoccidiodes brasiliensis, Pan American
      Health Organization Scientific Publication 254, 1971, pp. 239–244.
39.   E. Mendes and A. Raphael, Impaired delayed hypersensitivity in patients
      with South American Blastomycosis, *J. Allergy*, **47**:17–22 (1971).
40.   N. F. Mendes, C. C. Musatti, R. C. Leao, E. Mendes, and C. K. Naspitz,
      Lymphocyte culture and skin allograft survival in patients with South
      American blastomycosis, *J. Allergy Clin. Immunol.*, **48**:40–45 (1971).
41.   W. M. Newberry, J. E. Walter, J. W. Chandler, and F. E. Tosh, Epidemio-
      logic study of cryptococcus neoformans, *Ann. Intern. Med.*, **67**:724–732
      (1967).
42.   J. P. Utz, Cryptococcosis. In *Immunologic Diseases.* Vol. I. Boston,
      Mass., Little, Brown & Co., 1971.
43.   R. D. Diamond and J. E. Bennett, Disseminated cryptococcosis in man:
      Decreased lymphocyte transformation in response to cryptococcus neo-
      formans, *J. Infect. Dis.*, **127**:694–697 (1973).
44.   C. Boeck, Fortgesetzte Untersuchungen uber das multiple begigne sarkoid,
      Arch. Dermatol. Syphilol. (Wein), **73**:71–86 (1905).
45.   P. D'Arcy Hart and D. N. Mitchell, Lymphocyte sensitization, *Br. Med. J.*,
      3:246 (1971) (abstr.).
46.   C. J. Friou, A study of the cutaneous reactions to oidiomycin, tricophytin,
      and mumps skin test antigens in patients with sarcoidosis, *Yale J. Biol.
      Med.*, **24**:533–539 (1952).
47.   M. Sones and H. L. Israel, Altered immunologic reactions in sarcoidosis,
      Ann. Intern. Med., **40**:260–268 (1954).
48.   E. L. Quinn, D. C. Bunch, and E. M. Yagle, The mumps skin test and com-
      plement fixation test as a diagnostic aid in sarcoidosis, *J. Invest. Dermatol.*,
      24:595–598 (1955).

49. R. F. Elton and J. H. Andrew, Homograft survival in sarcoidosis, *Arch. Dermatol.,* **94**:403–405 (1966).

50. O. P. Sharma, D. G. James, and R. A. Fox, A correlation of in vivo delayed–type hypersensitivity with in vitro lymphocyte transformation in sarcoidosis, *Chest,* **60**:35–37 (1971).

51. A. Lawgner, D. Moskalewska, and M. Proniewska, Studies of the mechanism of lymphocyte transformation inhibition in sarcoidosis, *Br. J. Dermatol.,* **81**:829–834 (1969).

52. M. Topilsky, L. E. Siltzback, M. Williams, and P. R. Glade, Lymphocyte response in sarcoidosis, *Lancet,* **117**:120 (1972).

53. K. Prague, In vitro cultured lymphocytes in sarcoidosis. Fourth International Conference on Sarcoidosis, 1967, p. 276.

54. E. A. Caspary and E. J. Field, Lymphocyte sensitization in sarcoidosis, *Br. Med. J.,* **2**:143–145 (1971).

55. J. P. Girard, M. F. Poupon, and P. Press, Culture of peripheral blood lymphocytes from Sarcoidosis response to mitogenic factor, *Int. Arch. Allergy,* **41**:604–619 (1971).

56. N. J. Gross, The paradoxical skin response in sarcoidosis, *Am. Rev. Respir. Dis.,* **107**:798–801 (1973).

57. F. Urbach, M. Sones, and H. L. Israel, Passive transfer of tuberculin sensitivity to patients with sarcoidosis, *N. Engl. J. Med.,* **247**:294–297 (1952).

58. H. S. Lawrence and B. Zweiman, Transfer factor deficiency response—a mechanism of anergy in Boeck's Sarcoidosis, *Trans. Am. Physiol.,* **81**:240–248 (1968).

59. J. Kohout, Passive transfer of delayed type sensitivity in sarcoidose. Rapp IV. Conference International, 1967, pp. 287–290.

60. T. Izumi, B. S. Nelson, and E. Ripe, In vitro lymphocyte reactivity to different Kviem preparation in patients with sarcoidosis, *Scand. J. Respir. Dis.,* **54**:123–127 (1973).

61. E. A. Caspary and E. J. Field, Lymphocyte sensitization, *Br. Med. J.,* **3**:369–370 (1971).

62. L. E. Siltzbock, P. R. Glade, Y. Hirshout, L. Vilira, I. S. Gelikogla, and K. Hirschhorn, In vitro stimulation of peripheral lymphocytes in sarcoidosis. Fifth International Conference on Sarcoidosis. Edited by L. Levinsky and F. Macholda. Prague, University Karlova, 1969, pp. 217–220.

63. J. Williams, E. Pioli, D. J. Jones, and M. Digheru, The K MIF (Kviem–induced macrophage migration inhibition factor) test in sarcoidosis, *J. Clin. Pathol.,* **25**:951–954 (1972).

63a. E. Lebacq and H. Verhaegen, Passive transfer of the Kveim reaction to normal subjects by means of leukocytes of sarcoidosis patients, *Int. Arch. Allergy,* **24**:209–214 (1964).

64. K. Landsteiner and M. W. Chase, Experiments on transfer of cutaneous sensitivity to simple compounds, *Proc. Soc. Exp. Biol. Med.,* **49**:688–690 (1942).

65. H. S. Lawrence, The cellular transfer of cutaneous hypersensitivity to tuberculin in man, *Proc. Soc. Exp. Biol. Med.,* **71**:516–522 (1949).

66. H. S. Lawrence, The cellular transfer in humans of delayed cutaneous reactivity to hemolytic streptococci, *J. Immunol.*, **68**:159–178 (1952).

67. H. S. Lawrence, The transfer in humans of delayed skin sensitivity to streptococcal M. substance and to tuberculin with disrupted leukocytes, *J. Clin. Invest.*, **34**:129–230 (1955).

68. A. S. Levin, L. E. Spitler, D. P. Stites, and H. H. Fudenberg, Wiskott–Aldrich syndrome, a genetically determined cellular immunologic deficiency: Clinical and laboratory responses to therapy with transfer factor, *Proc. Natl. Acad. Sci.*, **67**:821–828 (1970).

69. L. E. Spitler, A. S. Levin, D. P. Stites, H. H. Fudenberg, B. Pirofsdy, C. S. August, E. R. Stiehm, W. H. Hitzig, and R. A. Gatti, The Wiskott–Aldrich syndrome results of transfer factor therapy, *J. Clin. Invest.*, **51**:3216–3224 (1972).

70. M. Ballow, B. Dupont, and R. A. Good, Autoimmune hemolytic anemia in Wiskott–Aldrich syndrome during treatment with transfer factor, *J. Pediatr.*, **83**:772–780 (1973).

71. W. H. Hitzig, H. P. Fontanellaz, U. Muntener, S. Paul, L. E. Spitler, and H. H. Fudenberg, Transfer factor: Immunologische grundlagen und therapeutische erfahrungen, *Schweiz. Med. Wochenschr.*, **102**:1237–1243 (1972).

72. L. E. Spitler, A. S. Levin, and H. H. Fudenberg, Human lymphocyte transfer factor, *Methods Cancer Res.*, **8**:59–106 (1973).

73. L. E. Spitler, A. S. Levin, and H. H. Fudenberg, Transfer factor II. Results of therapy. Second International Conference on Immunodeficiency Disease. Edited by R. Good. St. Petersburg, Fla., National Foundation, 1974. In press.

74. J. R. Montgomery, M. A. South, and R. Wilson, Study of a gnotobiotic child with severe combined immunodeficiency, *Clin. Res.*, **21**:118 (1973) (abstr.).

75. R. M. Goldlum, R. A. Lord, E. Dupree, A. C. Weinberg, and R. S. Goldman, Transfer factor induced delayed hypersensitivity in x–linked combined immunodeficiency, *Cell. Immunol.*, **9**:297–305 (1973).

76. C. H. Kirkpatrick, R. R. Rich, and T. K. Smith, Effect of transfer factor on lymphocyte function in anergic patients, *J. Clin. Invest.*, **51**:2948–2958 (1972).

77. H. F. Pabst and R. Swanson, Successful treatment of candidiasis with transfer factor, *Br. Med. J.*, **2**:442–443 (1972).

78. M. L. Schulkind, W. H. Adler, W. A. Altemeier, and E. M. Ayoub, Transfer factor in the treatment of chronic mucocutaneous candidiasis, *Pediatr. Res.*, **5**:379–464 (1971).

79. R. A. Rocklin, R. A. Chilgren, R. Hong, and J. R. David, Transfer of cellular hypersensitivity in chronic mucocutaneous candidiasis monitored in vivo and in vitro, *Cell. Immunol.*, **1**:290–299 (1970).

80. R. D. Feigin, P. G. Shackelford, S. Eisen, L. E. Spitler, L. K. Pickering, and D. C. Anderson, Treatment of mucocutaneous candidiasis with transfer factor, *Pediatrics*, **53**:63–70 (1974).

81. J. R. Graybill, J. Silva, Jr., R. H. Alford, and D. E. Thor, Immunologic and clinical improvement of progressive coccidioidomycosis following administration of transfer factor, *Cell. Immunol.,* 8:120–135 (1973).

82. A. Catanzaro, L. E. Spitler, and K. M. Moser, Defective cellular immunity in patients with coccidioidomycosis, *Am. Rev. Respir. Dis.,* 107:1084 (1973) (abstr.).

83. A. F. LoBuglio, J. A. Neidhart, R. W. Hilberg, E. N. Metz, and S. P. Balcerzak, The effect of transfer factor therapy on tumor immunity in alveolar soft part sarcoma, *Cell. Immunol.,* 7:159–165 (1973).

84. A. S. Levin, L. E. Spitler, J. Wybran, V. S. Byers, and H. H. Fudenberg, Treatment of Osteogenic sarcoma (OS) with tumor specific dialyzable transfer factor (TF), *Clin. Res.,* 21:648 (1973) (abstr.).

85. L. E. Spitler, J. Wybran, H. H. Fudenberg, A. S. Levin, M. Lewis, and L. Horn, Transfer factor therapy of malignant melanoma, *Clin. Res.,* 21:654 (1973) (abstr.).

86. L. J. Brandes, D. A. G. Galton, and E. Wiltshaw, New approach to immunotherapy of melanoma, *Lancet,* 2:293–295 (1971).

87. R. B. Thompson, Lymphocyte transfer factor, *Eur. J. Clin. Biol. Res.,* 16: 201–204 (1971).

88. H. Oettgen, L. Old, J. Farrow, F. Valentine, S. Lawrence, and L. Thomas, Effects of transfer factor in cancer patients, *J. Clin. Invest.,* 1:71a (1971) (abstr.).

89. L. E. Spitler, A. S. Levin, and H. H. Fudenberg, Transfer factor II. Results of therapy. Second International Conference on Immunodeficient Disease. St. Petersburg, Fla., National Foundation, 1974. In press.

90. L. E. Spitler, D. Webb, C. VonMuller, and H. H. Fudenberg, Studies on the characterization of transfer factor, *J. Clin. Invest.,* 52:80a (1973) (abstr.).

91. H. S. Lawrence, The transfer of hypersensitivity of the delayed–type in man. *Cellular and Humoral Aspects of the Hypersensitive State.* New York, N. Y., Hoeber, 1959, pp. 279–318.

92. H. S. Lawrence and B. Zweiman, Transfer factor deficiency response: A mechanism of anergy in Boeck's sarcoid, *Trans. Assoc. Am. Physicians,* 81:240–248 (1968).

93. H. S. Lawrence, S. Al–Askar, J. David, E. C. Franklin, and B. Zweiman, Transfer of immunological information, *Trans. Assoc. Am. Physicians,* 76: 84–91 (1963).

94. P. Baram, L. Yuan, and M. M. Mosko, Studies on the transfer of human delayed–type hypersensitivity. (1) Partial purification and characterization of two active components, *J. Immunol.,* 97:407–420 (1966).

95. J. A. Neidhart, R. S. Schwartz, P. E. Hurtubise, S. G. Murphy, E. N. Metz, S. P. Balcerzak, and A. F. LoBuglio, Transfer factor: Isolation of a biologically active component, *Cell. Immunol.,* 9:319–323 (1973).

96. B. R. Bloom and M. W. Chase, Transfer of delayed–type hypersensitivity: A critical review and experimental study in the guinea pig, *Prog. Allergy,* 10:151–255 (1967).

97. P. Baram and W. Condoulis, The in vitro transfer of delayed hypersensitivity to rhesus monkeys and human lymphocytes with transfer factor obtained from Rhesus monkey peripheral white blood cells, *J. Immunol.*, **104**:769–779 (1970).

98. D. R. Burger and W. S. Jeter, Cell–free passive transfer of delayed hypersensitivity to chemicals in guinea pigs, *Infect. Immun.*, **4**:575–580 (1971).

99. D. R. Burger, W. S. Cozine, and D. J. Hinrichs, The passive transfer of chemical hypersensitivities in rabbits, *Proc. Soc. Exp. Biol. Med.*, **136**: 1385–1388 (1971).

100. S. E. Maddison, M. D. Hicklin, B. P. Conway, and I. G. Kagan, Transfer factor: Delayed hypersensitivity to Schistosoma mansoni and tuberculin in macaca mulatta, *Science*, **178**:757–759 (1972).

101. E. M. Librud, H. F. Pabst, and W. D. Armstrong, Transfer factor in rat coccidiosis, *Cell. Immunol.*, **5**:487–489 (1972).

102. M. S. Ascher, W. J. Schneider, F. T. Valentine, and H. S. Lawrence, In vitro properties of leucocytes dialysis containing transfer factor, *Proc. Natl. Acad. Sci.*, **71**:1178–1182 (1974).

103. H. S. Lawrence, F. T. Rapaport, J. M. Converse, and W. S. Tillett, Transfer of delayed hypersensitivity to skin homografts with leukocyte extracts in man, *J. Clin. Invest.*, **39**:185–198 (1960).

104. F. T. Rapaport, H. S. Lawrence, J. W. Millar, D. Pappagianis, and C. E. Smith, The immunologic properties of coccidioidin as a skin test reagent in man, *J. Immunol.*, **84**:368–373 (1960).

105. A. Catanzaro, L. E. Spitler, and K. M. Moser, Immunotherapy of coccidioidomycosis, *J. Clin. Invest.*, **54**:690–701 (1974).

106. C. Griscilli, J. P. Revillard, H. Betuel, C. Herzog, and J. L. Touraine, Transfer factor therapy in immunodeficiencies, *Biochem. Med.*, **18**:220–227 (1973).

107. M. Ballow, et al., Immunodeficiencies in man. Second International Conference Immunodeficiency Disease. St. Petersburg, Fla., National Foundation, 1974, in press.

108. A. Catanzaro, L. E. Spitler, H. Einstein, and K. M. Moser, Transfer factor therapy of coccidioidomycosis, *Am. Rev. Respir. Dis.*, **109**:724 (1974) (abstr.).

AUTHOR INDEX

Numbers in brackets are reference numbers and indicate that an author's work is referred to although his name is not cited in the text. Italic numbers give the page on which the complete reference is listed.

A

Aas, K., 468[21], 469[27], *480*
Aberman, A., 281[73], *286*
Abramson, N., 162[15], 171[15], *173*
203[60], *209,* 338[18], *351*
Ackroyd, J. F., 261[11], 265[11], *282*
Ada, G. L., 74[1], 75[1], 77[24], *97, 98*
Adams, W. E., 486[17], 488[34], *513, 514*
Addington, W. W., 291[20], *325*
Adinolfi, M., 19[57], *26,* 155[28], *158*
Adkinson, J., 423, *441*
Adler, W. H., 528[78], *546*
Adomian, G. E., 497[79], 501[79], *517*
Aduna, N., 474[48], *481*
Affronti, L., G., 522[14], *543*

Agus, S. G., 255[50], *259*
Aiuti, F., 9[25], *24,* 155[27], *158*
Akazaki, K., 44[43], 45, *55*
Alarcón, D. G., 278[65], *285*
Alarcon-Segovia, D., 247[15,17], 249[15], *257,* 278[64,65], *285*
Al-Askar, S., 529[93], 530[93], *547*
Alberto, R., 468[22], 474[48], *480, 481*
Alexander, E. R., 102[10], 110[10], *126*
Alford, R. H., 13[48], *26,* 388[69], *403,* 523[32,34], 528[81], 538[81], *544, 546*
Alican, F., 486–489[23], *513*
Allen, H. D., 200[48], *208,* 349[36], *352*
Allen, J. C., 339[19], *351*
Alling, D. W., 19[55], *26*
Allison, A. C., 118, 120[61,67], *129, 130,* 182[13], 184[13], 185[13], *187*

Alper, C. A., 162[15], 171[15], *173,*
    194[19], 195[19], 203[60],
    204[62], *207, 209,* 338[18],
    340[30], 341[31], 343[30],
    351, 352
Altermeier, W. A., 380[31], *400,*
    528[78], *546*
Altman, L. C., 163[54], 170[102],
    175, 178
Altose, M. D., 9[22], 10[22], *24*
Altounyan, R. E. C., 454[61], *458*
Amache, N., 268[22], *283*
Ammann, A. J., 196[24,25,30,34],
    197[24,30], 198[30], 201[24],
    207, 350[39], *352*
Amos, D. B., 215[45], *224*
Amos, F. B., 438[38], *443*
Amsbaugh, D. F., 415[39], *418*
Anacker, R. L., 61[15], 65[15], *70*
Anand, S. C., 219[77], *226*
Andermann, F., 200[53], *209*
Andersen, B. R., 162[19], 171[19],
    173
Andersen, H. A., 269[34], 271[34],
    273[37], *284*
Andersen, V., 302[80], *328,* 349[37],
    352
Anderson, D. C., 528[80], *546*
Anderson, G. R., 392[88,90], *404*
Anderson, J., 501[91], 504[91],
    506[91], *517*
Anderson, J. A., 217[69], *226*
Anderson, R. E., 294[31], *325*
Anderson, S. A., 385[55], *402*
Andrew, J. H., 525[49], *545*
Andrews, E. J., 44[37], *55*
Andrews, M. J., 498[81], *517*
Andrieu, S., 524[38], *544*
Ansell, G., 261[7], 281[85], *282, 286*
Arai, S., 117[56], *129*
Arbesman, C. E., 281[83], *286,*
    298[48], 299[57], *326, 327,*
    472[40], *481*
Archer, G. T., 295[35], 296[35],
    298[50], 299[56], *325, 326*

Archer, R. K., 299[6], 307[61,112,
    113,114], 313[61], 318[61, *327*
    330
Armstrong, D., 184[25], *188*
Armstrong, W. D., 76[19], *98,*
    530[101], *548*
Arnar, O., 487[26,27], 488[26,35],
    513, 514
Arnason, B. G., 311[135], 314[135],
    331
Aronson, J. D., 411[17], *417*
Arora, S., 220[98], *228*
Arquembourg, P., 46[51], *55*
Arrobio, J. O., 131[1,2,3], 139[8,9,
    10], *140, 141,* 376[6], 379[25],
    380[25], 382[25], 396[101,105],
    398, 399, 405
Artenstein, M. S., 155[32], *159*
Ascher, M. S., 530[102], *548*
Ashburn, W. L., 488–491[39], *514*
Ashenbruker, H., 301[77], 302[77],
    328
Askonas, B. A., 29[2], *52*
Astrap, T., 166[66], *176*
Athens, J. W., 171[105], *178,* 255
    [39], *258,* 301[77], 302[77], *328*
Atkinson, J. P., 8[14,15], 19[15], *24,*
    255[46], *259*
Attai, L. A., 501[91], 504[91,99],
    506[91], *517, 518*
August, C. S., 199[44], *208,* 528[69],
    531[69], *546*
Augustin, R., 463, *479*
Austen, K. F., 162[26,27], 163[37,
    47], 165[26,27,57,59,60], 168[72,
    73], 169[81,82,83,84], *173, 174,*
    175, 176, 177, 214[36], *224,* 303
    [83], 307[83], 309[83], 308[118],
    310[128,130], 311[7,134], 314[128,
    130,134], *328, 330, 331,* 447[19,
    20,21,22], 446[19,20], 448[29,31,
    32,33,34], 450[20], 451[20,21,39,
    40], 452[44,49], *455, 456, 459*
Austen, W. G., 447[21], 451[21], *455*
Austrian, R., 413[30], *417*

Austwick, P. K. C., 44[40], *55*
Averbeck, A. K., 196[27], *207*
Ayer, L. N., 184[32], *188*
Ayliffe, P., 504[100], 506[100], 507[100], *518*
Ayoub, E. M., 62[18], 63[18], 68 [18], *70,* 528[78], *546*

B

Babbitt, L. H., 103[16], 106[16], *127*
Bacal, H. L., 200[53], *209*
Bachmann, R., 196[33], *207*
Baehner, R. L., 203[59], *209,* 298[51], *326*
Baer, H., 478, *483*
Baeva, A. V., 486[18], *513*
Baggenstoss, A. H., 254[35], *258*
Baker, J., 409[9], 415[9], *416*
Baker, J. R., 282[96], *287*
Baker, J. W., 499[85], *517*
Baker, P. J., 415[39], *418*
Baker, R. F., 184[35], *188*
Baker, R. R., 489[65], 499[85,87], *516,517*
Balcerzak, S. P., 528[83], 530[95], *547*
Balestra, S. T., 196[28], 197[28], 201[28], *207*
Balfour-Lynn, L., 454[69], *459*
Ballieis, R. E., 413[34], *418*
Ballow, M., 528[70], 532[107], *546, 548*
Balow, J. E., 255[42], *259*
Banaszak, E. F., 230[12,13], 232–234 [12,13], 237[12,13], *241*
Bane, H. N., 220[103], *228,* 453[53], *458*
Bang, B. G., 31[14], 52[14], *53*
Bang, F. B., 31[14], 52[14], *53*
Bankier, J. D. H., 454[63], *458*
Baram, P., 530, *547*
Barandun, S., 342[33], *352*
Barbaro, A. M., 356[8], *372*

Barbier, F., 486[24], 503[24], 504 [24], 506[24], 507[24], *513*
Barboriak, J. J., 217[70], *226,* 230 [2,5,12], 232[2,5,12], 233[2,5, 12], 234[2,5,12], 237[2,5,12], 238[2,20,22], *240, 241*
Barfeld, P. A., 501[91], 504[91,99], 506[91], *517, 518*
Barnard, J. H., 471[31], *480*
Barnes, B. A., 493[71,72], *516*
Barnes, B. D., 340[25], *352*
Barnett, E. V., 196[32], *207*
Barnett, M., 217[67], *226*
Barnhart, M. I., 295[37], *325*
Barr, G., 493[71], *516*
Barr, S. E., 470[28], *480*
Barrett, C. D., Jr., 392[90], *404*
Barton, R. M., 292[21], *325*
Barza, M., 355[3], 356[9], 357[9, 14], *371, 372*
Baskerville, A., 182[8], 183[16], 184[8,16], 185[16], *187*
Basten, A., 301[78], 308[78,120,121, 123], 311[120], 314[78,120,121, 123], *328, 330*
Bauer, H., 338[16], *351*
Baum, J., 162[7], 170[7], *172*
Baum, S. G., 385[58], *402*
Baumann, M. C., 454[76], *459*
Baumann, M. L., 453[55], *458*
Bauserman, S. C., 238[21], *241*
Bays, R. P., 277[61], *285*
Bazarel, M., 439, *443*
Beakey, J. R., 369[46], *374*
Beall, G. N., 494[73], 499[73], 500 [73], 501[73,93], *516, 517*
Beard, R. R., 522[18], *543*
Beare, A. S., 390[78,79,80], 391[79, 83], 392[80], 394[98], *404, 405*
Beattie, E. J., 486[15], 489[15], *513*
Beaudry, C., 282[87], *286*
Beaver, P. C., 290[9], 292[25,26], *324, 325*
Becker, E. L., 170[99,100,101], *177, 178,* 448[29], *456*

Beckman, B. L., 102[6], *126*
Beebe, G. W., 384[51], *402*
Beem, M., 378[22], *399*
Beers, R. F., Jr., 281[82], *286*
Beeson, P. B., 301[78], 302[81], 308
[78,120,121,122,124,125], 311
[120], 314[78,120,121,122,124,
125], *328, 330, 331*
Begley, J., 412[21], *417*
Bell, J. A., 378[21], *399*
Bell, R. J. M., 290[13], *324*
Bellanti, J. A., 139[10], *141*, 155[32],
159, 338[16], *351*, 380[26], 382
[26], 383[48], *400, 401*
Belleville, J., 487[33], *514*
Belmaker, E. Z., 195[22], *207*
Belzer, F. D., 485[4], *512*
Benacerraf, B., 44[31], *54*, 77[23],
98, 215[48], *225*
Benditt, E. P., 47[68], *56*
Benfield, J. R., 486–492[17,25,29,36,
37,42,46,47,48,53,58,61,67,68,69],
494[68,73,74], 496[75], 498–504
[25,42,67,73,74,89,93,96], *513–
518*
Bennett, J. E., 201[55], *209*, 525[43],
544
Bennich, H. H., 214[32], *224*, 446[9–
13,15], *454, 455*, 474[50], *481*
Benveniste, J., 450[35], *456*
Berat, N. M., 349[37], *352*
Berdal, P., 469[27], *480*
Berenberg, J. A., 162[21], 165[21],
173
Berg, T., 214[32,34], *224*
Bergan, J. J., 485[6], *512*
Berge, E., 394[99], *405*
Bergeron, M. G., 357[14], *372*
Bergman, R. K., 305[104], *329*, 409,
416
Berk, J. E., 290[8], *324*
Berke, R. A., 214[29], 218[29], *223*
Bernhard, W. G., 413[33], 415[33],
418
Bernstein, R. A., 453[58], *458*
Berry, R. W., 170[95], *178*

Berthrong, M., 520[4], *542*
Berzsenyi, G., 486[24], 503[24], 504
[24], 506[24], 507[24], *513*
Betuel, H., 532[106], *548*
Bewick, M., 504[100], 506[100],
507[100], *518*
Biagi, G. L., 356[8], *372*
Bias, W. B., 215[44], *224*, 438[37],
443
Biberfeld, G., 10[35], *25*, 105[20],
106[21,22,23,27], 117[57], 124
[20], 125[71, *127, 129, 130,* 151
[18], *158*, 381[33], *400*
Biberfeld, P., 125[71], *130*
Bien, Z., 293[28], *325*
Bienenstock, J., 9[26], 10[34], 19
[62], *24, 25, 26,* 30[4,5,6], 31
[5,6], 38[6,18,19], 40–50[5,6,18,
19,20,23,29,30,32,45,54,57,58,65,
67,69,81,89], *52–57,* 60[2,3], 67
[28], *69, 71,* 82[41], 92[41], *99,*
111[47,48], 112[48], 114[48],
116[48], *129,* 151[17], 156[36],
158, 159, 381[34], *400*
Bierman, C. W., 454[71], *459*
Biggar, W. D., 46[55], *56,* 192, *205*
Bilbo, R. E., 212[11], 221[11], *222*
Biliotti, G., 217[68], *226*
Bilodeau, M., 368[30], 369[30],
371[30], *373*
Birnbaum, G. L., 182[4], *187*
Bishop, C. R., 171[105], *178*
Black, J. H., 423[15], *441*
Black, J. W., 220[100], *228,* 452[43],
457
Blaese, M., 170[102], *178*
Blair, A. M. J. N., 446[7], *454*
Blake, J. T., 10[29], *24,* 146[13],
157
Blanc, W. A., 50[90], *58*
Blanden, R. V., 521[10], *542*
Blandford, G., 138[6], *141*
Blank, N., 282[90], *287*
Blatt, I. M., 248[25], *258*
Blatt, N., 368[36], 369[36], 371[36],
373

Blecher, T. E., 195[21], *207*
Blizzard, R. M., 170[93], *177*
Bloch, K. J., 216[58], *225*
Block, E. R., 367[29], *373*
Block, K. J., 448[28], *456*
Blomgren, S. E., 278[69], 279[69], *286*
Bloodwell, R. D., 486[21], *513*
Bloom, B. R., 10[38], *25,* 61[9,11, 12], 62[12], *69, 70,* 152[26], *158,* 530, *547*
Bloom, H. H., 378[20], *399*
Bloomberg, A., 501[91], 504[91], 506[91], *517*
Blumenstock, D. A., 486[7,12,16], 488[16], 489[16], 500[88], 502 [94,95], 503[12], *512, 513, 517, 518*
Blumenthal, M. N., 215[45], 217[66], *224, 226,* 281[81], *286*
Boat, T. F., 198[41], *208*
Bockman, D. E., 38, *53,* 193[5], *206*
Boeck, C., 525[44], *544*
Bogartz, I. J., 281[76], *286*
Boggs, D. R., 171[105], *178,* 255[39], *258*
Bohrud, M. G., 218[72], *226,* 251[33], *258*
Bokisch, V. A., 165[56], *175*
Bolano, C., 194[17], *206*
Boley, S. J., 489[56], 501[91], 504 [91,99], 506[91], *515, 517, 518*
Booth, A., 485[5], *512*
Booth, B. H., 309[127], 314[127], *331*
Borel, H., 194[19], 195[19], *207*
Borel, J. F., 163[29,30,36], 166[29, 30], *174*
Borman, G. S., 385[60], *402*
Bottcher, E., 251[31], *258*
Bouchard, R., 47[71], *56*
Bouma, H. G. D., 488[41], 489[41], *514*
Bourne, H. R., 450[38], 451[41,42], 452[42], *456, 457*
Bowerman, C. I., 230[8], 232–234[8],

[Bowerman, C. I.]
237[8], *241*
Boxerbaum, B., 205[67], *209*
Boyce, C. R., 476[62], *482*
Boyd, G., 454[63], *458*
Boyden, S., 161[1], 171[1], *172*
Boyer, M. H., 301[78], 308[78,121, 122], 314[78,121,122], *328, 330*
Brain, J. D., 8[17], *24,* 45[48], *55*
Branch, L. B., 220[100], *228*
Brandes, L. J., *547*
Brandt, C. D., 131[1,2,3], 137[5], 139[8,9,10], *140, 141,* 376[6], 379[25], 380[25], 382[25,36,37], 386[36,37], 396[101,105], *398, 399, 400, 405*
Brashear, R. E., 269[35], 271[35], *284*
Braun, D. G., 50[90], *58*
Brayton, R. G., 171[104], *178*
Brazin, H., 86[48], *100*
Bredt, W., 102[3], 123[3], *126*
Brettner, A., 261[6], *282*
Bringhurst, L. S., 230[9], 232–234[9], 237[9], *241*
Brinkman, G. L., 47[59], *56*
Brobst, M., 376[12], *399*
Brody, A. W., 17[53], *26*
Brody, J. S., 488[38], 489[38], *514*
Brooks, G. F., 408[1], *416*
Brooks, N., 47[59], *56*
Broome, J., 307[113], *330*
Bro-Rasmussen, F., 302[80], *328*
Brostoff, J., 217[62], *225*
Brough, J. A., 197[37], *208*
Brown, A. L., 184[23], *188,* 247[15], 249[15], *257*
Brown, E., 46[57], *56*
Brown, E. A., 262[12], *283*
Brown, E. J., 19[62], *26*
Brown, H., 470[28], *480*
Brown, R. K., 340[25], *352*
Brown, W. T., 199[43], *208*
Brundelet, P. J., 31, 42[11], 44[11], *53*
Brune, A., 487[33], *514*

Brunner, H., 106[24], 107[24], 108
    [41], 124[70], *127, 128, 130,* 382
    [43], 387[64], 397[64,108], *401,*
    402, 405
Brunner, K. T., 61[10], *69*
Brusch, J., 357[14], *372*
Bruton, O. C., 336[3], *350*
Bryant, D. H., 217, *225*
Bryant, L., 489[55], *515*
Bryant, V., 47[59], *56*
Buchanan, T. M., 408[1], *416*
Buckland, R., 384[50], *301*
Buckley, C. E., III, 438, *443*
Buckley, J. J., 292[27], *325*
Buckley, R. H., 193[10], 195[22],
    197, 198[40], *206, 207, 208,* 214,
    223, 336[6,7], 337[6,10,15], 338
    [6,15], 344[7], 345[7], 349[15],
    350[15], *350, 351*
Buechner, H. A., 230[10], 232–234
    [10], 237[10], *241*
Buescher, E. L., 380[31], 385[56],
    389[74], 390[75], *400, 402, 403*
Bull, C. G., 413[32], *418*
Bunch, D. C., 525[48], *544*
Burger, D. R., 530[98,99], *548*
Burke, B. A., 193[6], *206*
Burnet, F. M., 47, *56*
Burnet, M. E., 359[25], 360[25],
    361[25], *373*
Burns, M. W., 217[61], *225*
Burns, W. A., 274[44], *284*
Burrell, R. G., 281[86], *286*
Busbee, D. L., 3[5], 7[5], 18[5], *23*
Bushnell, L. S., 368[40], 369[40],
    371[40], *373*
Busse, W. W., 214[30], 218[30], *223,*
    425[20], *442*
Butcher, B., 213[26], *223*
Butler, W. T., 13[48], *26,* 76[14],
    85[14], 95[14], *98,* 225[45], *259*
Butz, O., 230[10], 232–234[10],
    237[10], *241*
Byers, L. A., 8[18], *24*
Byers, V. S., *547*
Bynoe, M. L., 390[78], *404*

Byrd, R. B., 278[68], *285*
Byrne, J. P., Jr., 281[80], *286*
Byrne, R. N., 230[9], 232–234[9],
    237[9], *241*

C

Cabezas, G. A., 219[86], *227*
Cacey, J., 230[11], 232–234[11],
    237[11], *241*
Cade, J. F., 212[12], *222*
Cain, W. A., 196[24,25], 197[24],
    201[24], *207*
Caldwell, J. R., 238[19], *241*
Callerame, M. L., 50[91], *58,* 218,
    226
Camargo, E., 131[2], 139[8], *140,*
    141, 379[25], 380[25], 382[25],
    396[101], *399, 405*
Cambridge, B. S., 340[27], *352*
Campbell, D. H., 75[3], 76[3], *97,*
    477[68], *483*
Canchola, J. G., 137[5], *141,* 382
    [37], 386[37], *400*
Cantor, C. R., 170[96], *178*
Cantrell, E. T., 3[5], 7[5], 18[5], *23*
Capitano, M. A., 199[46], 200[46],
    208
Carbone, P. P., 106[25], *127,* 143[3],
    157
Cardell, B. S., 212[9], 218[9], *222*
Carlens, O., 31, *53*
Carnright, D. V., 453[59], *458*
Carr, R. H., 425[20], *442*
Carrington, C. R. B., 248[23], 249[30],
    258, 290[2], 297[2,20], 293[2],
    324, 325
Carryer, H. M., 214[33], *224*
Carter, G. R., 44[34], *54*
Cartwright, G. E., 171[105], *178,* 255
    [39], *258,* 277[53], *285,* 301[77],
    302[77], 321[152], *328, 332*
Casey, M. J., 385[57], *402*
Caspary, E. A., 140[12], *141,* 526[54],
    527[61], *545*
Cassell, H., 184[26], *188*

Castagna, J. T., 489[53,61], 500[89], *515, 517*
Castenada, A. R., 487[26], 488[26], *513*
Castro-Murillo, E., 213[211], *223*
Catanzaro, A., 522[23], 523[24], 528 [24], 531[24,105], 538[23], 539 [24], *543, 548*
Cate, R. R., 107[33], *128,* 380[30], 389[30], 390[76], *400, 403*
Cathey, W. J., 277[53], *285,* 321 [152], *332*
Cavanaugh, J. J. A., 213[19], *223*
Cayirilli, M., 486–489[23], *513*
Cebra, J. J., 48, *57*
Cerilli, G. J., 200[52], *209*
Cerottini, J. C., 61[10], *69*
Chakera, T. M. H., 277[52], *285*
Chakrin, L., 86[47], *100*
Chalhub, E. G., 393[92,96], 394[92, 96], 395[92], *404, 405*
Chamberlain, D. W., 38, 44[16], *53, 68[30], 71,* 80, *99*
Chandler, J. W., Jr., 523[31,33], 524 [41], *544*
Chang, Y., 377[15], *399*
Channell, S., 454[60], *458*
Chanock, R. M., 102[1,4,5], 106[24], 107[24,29,32,33], 108[35,41], 124[70], *126, 127, 128, 130,* 131 [1,2,3], 136[4], 137[5], 139[8,9, 10], *140, 141,* 375–380[1,5,6,7, 10,11,15,19,20,21,23,25,26,27,28, 29,30], 382[25,26,27,28,36,37,38, 42,43], 383[27,48], 385[7,54,57], 386[27,36,37,38], 387[64,65], 388[67,69], 389[29,30], 390[76], 393[92,93,94,96], 394[94,96], 395[92], 396[101, 102, 103, 104, 105], 397[106,107,108], 398[28, 64], *398–405*
Chanock, V., 396[104], *405*
Chase, M. W., 528[64], 530, *545, 547*
Chaves-Carballo, E., 411[19], *417*
Chawla, P. L., 268[23], *283*
Chen, J. L., 196, *207,* 454[65], *458*

Cheng, C., 489[51], *515*
Cheng, F. H., 238[21], *241*
Cheng, J., 468[22], *480*
Cherayil, G. D., 230[4], 232–235[4], 237[4], 238[4], *240*
Chester, E. H., 221[107], *228*
Chiampi, P. N., 305[102], *329*
Chikkappa, G., 301[74], *327*
Chilgren, R. A., 528[79], *546*
Chin, J., 386[61], *402*
Chin, T., 523[31], *544*
Chinitz, H., 428, *442*
Chinn, S., 384[50], *401*
Chou, C. T., 40[21], 41[21], *54*
Christian, C. L., 193[12], *206,* 304[28], *352*
Christiansen, A. H., 489[60], *515*
Chu, L. W., 380[30], 389[30], *400*
Chung, E., 321[150], *332*
Churg, J., 248[21,22], 249, 254[29], *257, 258*
Chusid, M. J., 294[32], *325*
Cinader, B., 40[21], 41[21], *54*
Citret, C., 486[13], *512*
Citro, L. A., 290[4], 293[4], *324*
Clancy, R. L., 38[19], 40[20], 41 [23], 42[19,29,30], 43[30], 45 [45], 46[58], 47[58], 48[20,72], 49[20], *53–56*
Clark, E., 246[9], *257*
Clark, R. A., 162[2,6,10,16], 163 [55], 165[16], 170[6,10], 171 [55], *172, 173, 175*
Clarke, J. A., Jr., 425[18], *442*
Clarke, P. S., 454[72], *459*
Clarysse, A. M., 277[53], *285,* 321[152], *332*
Clement, D., 521[11], 522[11], *543*
Clements, J. A., 21[63], *26*
Cleveland, W. W., 199[43], *208*
Cline, M. J., 7[12], 8[12,13,19], *23, 24, 100,* 168[80], *177,* 295[39], 298[46], 299[52], *326*
Clough, J. D., 49[79], *57*
Clyde, W. A., Jr., 10[34], *25,* 50[89], *57,* 82[41], 92[41], *99,* 102[2],

[Clyde, W. A., Jr.]
105[17], 106[17], 107[31], 108
[37,40], 109[40,42,43,44,45], 110
[40], 111[48], 112[48,51], 114
[48], 116[48], 117[51,53], 118
[60], 121[53], 124[60], *126–129*
151[17], *158*, 181[2], 184[28],
186, 188, 382[41], *401*
Coates, H. V., 378[23], *399*
Coca, A. F., 212, *223*, 420, 421[2],
425[18], *441, 442*
Cochrane, C. G., 162[24], 163[24,46],
165[46], 171[24], *173, 175*, 218,
226, 244, 248[20], *256, 257*, 310
[131], 314[131], 320[148], *331,
332*, 420[1], 434[1], *441*, 450[35],
456
Codling, B. W., 277[52], *285*
Coffey, R. G., 220[101,103], *228*,
453[52,53,59], *458*
Coggeshall, L. T., 182[5], *187*
Cohen, A. B., 7[12], 8[12], 9[21],
17, 18[54], *23, 24, 26, 100*, 168
[80], *177*
Cohen, E. P., 219[95], *227*
Cohen, H. I., 232[15], 233[15], 234
[15], 237[15], *241*
Cohen, M., 219[94], 221[106], *227,
228*
Cohen, S., 48[76], *57*, 168[74], 169
[89], *176, 177*, 303[85], 311[85],
312[85,136], 313[85], *328, 331*
Cohen, S. G., 298[49], 305[102,103],
306[49,105,107], 307[115], 318
[141], 321[153], *326, 329, 332*
Cohn, E. S., 340[25], *352*
Cohn, Z. A., 5[8], 21[65], *23, 27*,
76[17], *98*
Colapinto, R. F., 489[44], *514*
Cole, A. M., 184[30,38], *188, 189*
Cole, G. A., 65[22], *70*
Colebatch, H. J. H., 219[76], *226*
Coleman, M. T., 221[108], *228*
Colinet, G., 394[99], *405*
Collan, Y., 47, *56*
Collen, H. R., 162[8], *172*

Colley, D. G., 303[86], 313[86,137],
328,331
Collier, A. M., 102[2], 103[13], 109
[42,43,44,46], *126, 128*, 382[40],
401
Collins, J. A., 502[94], *517*
Colten, H. R., 204[62], *209*
Combs, J. W., 47[68], *56*
Conant, R. M., 378[19], *399*
Condemi, J. J., 50[91], *58*, 218[72,
73], *226*, 278[69], 279[69], *286*
Condoulis, W., 530, *547*
Connell, J. T., 466[14], 472[38], 476,
479,482
Connioly, N. M., 454[69], *459*
Connor, A., 470[28], *480*
Connor, J. D., 408[2], *416*
Constantopoulous, A., 197[38], *208*
Conti-Diaz, J. A., 524[35], *544*
Converse, J. M., 531[103], *548*
Converse, J. L., 522[21], *543*
Conway, B. P., 530[100], *548*
Cooch, J. W., 385[56], *403*
Cooke, R. A., 212, *223*, 274[39], *284*,
420, 421[2], 422[12], *441*, 463,
471[31,32,35], 476[51], *478,
480, 482*
Cookson, D. V., 219, *227*
Cooley, D. A., 486, *513*
Coombs, R. R. A., 244, *256*, 316
[139], 318[139], 322[139], *331*
Coon, B. S., 488[36], *514*
Cooney, M. K., 379[24], *399*
Cooper, G. N., 50[84], *57*
Cooper, M. D., 38, 50[85,86,88], *53,
57*, 193[5], *206*, 336[9], 350[40],
351, 353
Corea, A., 524[36], *544*
Corley, R. B., 438[38], *443*
Corman, J., 485[5], *512*
Cornwall, H. J., 184[29], *188*
Corpe, R. F., 522[15], *543*
Coryllos, P. N., 182[4], *187*
Costea, N., 102[9], 105[9], *126*
Cotton, E. K., 360[27], *373*
Cotton, G. S., 184[27], *188*

Cottrell, T. S., 274[15], *285*
Couch, R. B., 103[14], 106[24], 107 [24,33], *126, 127, 128,* 170[90] *177,* 382[43], 387[63], 390[75], *401, 402, 403*
Court, S. D. M., 139[7], *141*
Cowan, G. S. M., Jr., 488[40], 489[40, 63], 491[66], *514, 516*
Cox, J. S. G., 454[74,75], *459*
Cozine, W. S., 530[99], *548*
Craig, S. W., 48, *57*
Crain, J. D., 340[30], 343[30], *352*
Credle, W. F., Jr., 3[3]. *23*
Criep, L. H., 261[10], *282*
Crofton, J. W., 290[1], 293[1], 294 [1], *324,* 357[15], *372*
Cronkite, E. P., 300[63], 301[76], *327, 328*
Crosbie, W. A., 504[101], 506[101], *518*
Cross, C. E., 486[8], *512*
Cross, T., 230[11], 232–234[11], 237[11], *241*
Crowder, J. G., 145[10], *157*
Crowley, J. H., 162[4], *172*
Crummy, A. B., 488[37], *514*
Cullum, P. A., 504[100, 101], 506 [100,101], 507[100], *518*
Cumming, C., 385[54], *402*
Cunningham, A. J., 89[49], *100*
Cuomo, A. J., 488–491[39], *514*
Curelaru, Z., 255[11], *258*
Curran, W. L., 182[8], 183[16], 184 [8,16], 185[16], *187*
Curran, W. S., 7[9], *23*
Curry, J. J., 212[10], *222*
Czarnecki, S. E., 247[18], *257*

D

Dacie, J. V., 105[19], *127*
Dajani, A. S., 108[40], 109[40], 110 [40], *128,* 184[28], *188*
Dale, D. C., 8[20], *24,* 182[12], 185 [12], 186[43], *187, 189,* 255[43, 52], *259,* 294[32], 301[75], *325,*

[Dale, D. C.] *327,* 366[28], *373*
Dalmasso, A. P., 19[58,61], *26,* 155 [29], *158*
Dalton, A. C., 298[48], *326*
Dalton, M. L., Jr., 486[20], *513*
Da Luiz, A., 524[38], *544*
Damodaran, V. N., 185[39], *189*
Danaraj, T. J., 292[25], *325*
Daneau, D., 368[31], 369[31], 371 [31], *373*
Daniele, R. P., 9[22], 10[22], *24*
Darbyshire, J. H., 181[3], *187*
D'Arcy Hart, P., 525[45], *544*
Darlington, D., 47[61], *56*
Dauer, C. D., 377[13], *399*
Davenport, F. M., 383[44,45], 392 [88,89,90,91], *401, 404*
David, J., 529[93], 530[93], *547*
David, J. R., 61[13], *70,* 163[33], 169[75], *174, 176,* 268[21], 271 [21], *283,* 528[79], *546*
David, R. B., 269[34], 271[34], *284*
Davidson, M., 298[47], *326*
Davidson, W. D., 489[58], *515*
Davie, J. M., 10[29], *24,* 146[13], *157*
Davies, A. J. S., 308[123], 314[123], *330*
Davies, P. D. B., 261[4], *282*
Davies, S. E., 454[70], *459*
Davis, S. D., 50[87], *57,* 124[68], *130,* 195, *207*
Dawkins, A. T., 383[46], *401*
Day, N. K., 171[106], *178*
Day, R. P., 42[30], 43[30], 47[65,67, 69], *54, 56*
de A. Cardoso, R. R., 220[103], *228*
Deak, B. D., 432[29], *442*
De Bernardo, R., 446[16], 450[36], *455, 456*
De Bond, A. H., 492[70], *516*
de Bracco, M., 171[106], *178*
de Cardosa, R. R., 453[53], *458*
Decker, J. L., 162[16], 165[16], *173,* 255[50], *259*
Dees, S. C., 214, *223*

De Gillio, M., 500[88], *517*
Degre, M., 182[7], 184[36], 185[36], *187, 188*
De Groot, W. J., 212[4], *222*
De Kock, M. A., 219[76], *226*
de Koning, J., 349[38], *353*
Delespesse, G., 477[70], *483*
Delves, D. M., 358[20], 359[20], 360 [20], 361[20], *372*
D'Lugoff, B. C., 476[61], *482*
De Masi, C. J., 269[30], *283*
De Meo, A. N., 162[19], 171[19], *173,* 221[106], *228*
de Moura Rangel, J. D., 489[54], *515*
Denhy, F. W., 181[2], 184[28], *186, 188*
Denny, F. W., 105[17], 106[17], 107 [31], 108[40], 109[40,42,43], 110[40], 118, 120[62], *127, 128, 129,* 182[13], 184[13], 185[13], *187*
Derbyshire, J. B., 44[41], *55*
De Remee, R. A., 269[33], 271[33], 273[37], *284*
Derom, F., 486[24], 501[90], 503 [24], 504[24], 506[24,90], 507 [24], *513, 517*
Derouaux, G., 340[25], *352*
de St. Growth, S. Fazekas, 382[39], *401*
Descotes, J., 487[33], *514*
De Swarte, R. D., 261[2], 264[2], 266[2], *282*
Devlin, H. B., 10[28], *24,* 145[7,9], 146[7], 152[7], *157*
De Weck, A. L., 261[9], 264[9], 266[9], *282*
Diaconita, G., 291[15], *324*
Diamond, P., 269[26], *283*
Diamond, R. D., 525[43], *544*
Dick, E. C., 221[106], *228,* 378[19], *399*
Dicke, K. A., 349[38], *353*
Dickie, H. A., 230[7], 232–235[7], 237[7], 238[7], *241*
Dibella, F., 453[48], *457*

Diener, E., 76[19], *98*
Di George, S. M., 199[42], *208*
Digheru, M., 528[63], *545*
Dines, D. E., 269[33], 271[33], *284*
Dingle, J. H., 103[15], 107[31], *127, 128*
Dinsdale, F., 44[36], 45, *54*
Dixon, F. J., 244, 246[12], 248[20], *256, 257*
Dixon, J. A., 44[40], *55,* 281[80], *286*
Doershuk, C. F., 198[41], *208*
Dohner, V. A., 282[92], *287*
Dolovich, J., 47[67], *56*
Donalley, H. H., 425[18], *442*
Donnelley, M., 382[39], *401*
Donohugh, D. L., 292[23], *325*
Dooren, L. J., 349[38], *352*
Dorner, M. M., 194[20], *207*
Dorsey, F. C., 438[38], *443*
Dougherty, J. C., 489[56], *515*
Dougherty, S. F., 47[66], *56*
Douglas, R. G., Jr., 394[97], *405*
Douglas, S. D., 194[13], 200[13], *206*
Dow, C., 182[8], 183[16], 184[8], 185[16], *187*
Dowling, H. F., 368[36], 369[36], 371[36], *373*
Drachman, R. H., 204, *209*
Drash, A. L., 453[58], *458*
Dreesen, L. J., 120[66], *130*
Drever, J. C., 454[60], *458*
Drews, J. A., 489[47,48], *515*
Driesbach, M. E., 303[88], *328*
Duberstein, J. L., 281[72], *286*
Dubiski, S., 40[21], 41[21], *54*
Dudding, B. A., 390[75], *403*
Dudgeon, J. A., 194[16], 196[16], *206*
Dukor, P., 244[5], *257*
Dumonde, D. C., 217[65], *226*
Duncan, W. A. M., 452[43], *457*
Dupont, B., 349[37], *352,* 528[70], *546*
Dupree, E., 204[65], *209,* 528[75], *546*

Durant, C. J., 452[43], *457*
Dutta, S. K., 500[86], 502[86], *517*
Dutton, R. W., 77, *98*
Duvoisin, G. E., 486[14], *513*
Dvorak, H. F., 266[13], *283*
Dworski, M., 412[21], *417*
Dwyer, J. E., 155[33],

E

Eaton, M. D., 108[38], 109[38], *128*
Ebert, P. A., 489[43], 490[43], *514*
Eddie, D. S., 19[59], *26,* 155[30], *158*
Eddleston, A. L., 46[52], *55*
Eddy, B. E., 385[60], *402*
Edfors-Lubs, M. L., 213, *223*
Edgren, G., 422[9], *434*
Edmondson, W. P., 380[29], 389[29], *400*
Edmunds, L. H., Jr., 488[40], 489[40, 63], 491[66], *514, 516*
Edwards, E. A., 392[91], *404*
Edwards, L. B., 522[14], *543*
Edwards, P. Q., 521[8], 523[26], 537[8], *542, 543*
Eggleston, P. A., 454[71], *459*
Ehrenreich, B., 76[17], *98*
Eickhoff, T. C., 360[27], *373*
Eidelman, S., 50[87], *57*
Eidinger, D., 120[63], *130,* 300[68], *327*
Eijsvoogel, V. P., 348[38], *353*
Einstein, H., 539[108], *548*
Eiseman, B., 489[55], *515*
Eisen, A. H., 200[53], *209,* 300[62], 318[62], *327*
Eisen, S., 528[80], *546*
Eisner, E. V., 267[19], *283*
Eknoyan, G., 162[20], 171[20], *173*
Eldering, G., 409, 415[9], *416*
Eldridge, F., 232[15], 233[15], 234 [15], 237[15], *241*
Eldridge, W. W., 523[25], *543*
Elin, R. J., 8[20], *24,* 186[43], *189,* 366[28], *373*

Eller, J. J., 221[105], *228,* 386[62], *402*
Elliott, R. C., 3[3], *23*
Ellis, E. F., 221[105], *228,* 341[32], *352*
Ellis, F. H., Jr., 486[14], *513*
Ellison, L. T., 487[31], *514*
Ellison, R. G., 487[31], *514*
Ellman, L., 163[40], *174,* 310[130], 314[130], *331*
Elsom, K. A., 291[17], *324*
Elton, R. F., 525[49], *545*
Emanuel, D. A., 230[8], 232–234[8, 16], 237[8,16], *241*
Emery, J. L., 44[36], 45, *54*
Emmons, C. W., 523[25], *543*
Enquist, R. W., 281[75], *286*
Enta, T., 219[94], *227*
Eppinger, H., 425[21], *442*
Epstein, S. W., 454[64], *458*
Erdmann, A. J., III, 489[63], 491[66], *516*
Estensen, R. D., 170[98], *178*
Esterly, J. R., 274[45], *284*
Evans, A. S., 376[12], *399*
Evans, L., 339[24], 340[24], *352*
Evans, R. H., 217[63], *226,* 486[17], 488[34], *513, 514*
Everhard, M., 501[91], 504[91], 506[91], *517*
Ezeoke, A., 319[143], *332*

F

Faber, L. P., 486[15], 489[15], *513*
Faber, V., 349[37], *352*
Fackton, M. A., 453[58], *458*
Fahey, J., 248[22], *258*
Fairchild, G. A., 182[11], *187*
Falconnet, J., 487[33], *514*
Falk, G. A., 148[14], *157*
Falliers, C. J., 220[103], *228,* 453 [53], *458*
Fallis, B. D., 151[16], *158*
Fariss, B., *55,* 183[18], *187*
Fariss, F., 81[32], *99*

Farr, R. S., 212, 216[59], *222, 225*
Farrow, J., 528[88], *547*
Fauci, A. S., 248[24,26], 249[24], 254[24], 255[24,43,51,52], *258, 259,* 321[149], *332*
Faulk, W. P., 42[24], *54,* 336[9], *351*
Faux, J. A., 217[65], *226*
Feigenberg, D. S., 290[12], *324*
Feigin, R. D., 528[80], *546*
Feinberg, S. L., 423[16], *441*
Feinberg, S. M., 463, *479*
Feingold, D. S., 368[40], 369[40], 371[40], *373*
Feldman, J. D., 246[12], *257*
Felton, L. D., 415[37], *418*
Fenner, F. J., 75[7], *97*
Feofliov, G. L., 486[18], *513*
Fernald, G. W., 10[34], *25,* 50[89], *57,* 82[41], 92[41], *99,* 105[17], 106[17,26], 111[48], 112[48], 114[48], 116[48,52], 117[52,53, 55], 118[59,60,62], 120[62], 121 [52,53], 124[60], *127, 129,* 151 [17], *158,* 382[41], 388[70], *401, 403*
Ferrebee, J. W., 502[94], *517*
Fichtelius, K. E., 47[62], *56*
Fiegenberg, D. L., 282[98], *287*
Field, E. J., 140[12], *141,* 526[54], 527[61], *545*
Fiese, M. J., 522[17], 538[17], *543*
Filip, D. J., 277[57], *285*
Filler, R. M., 199[44], *208*
Finegold, M. J., 183[17], *187*
Fink, J. N., 217[70], *226,* 230[2,3,4, 12,13,14], 232–235[2,3,4,12,13, 14,17,18], 237[2,3,4,12,14], 238 [2,4,20,22], *240, 241*
Finke, S. R., 219[91], 220[91], *227*
Finland, M., 368[35], 369[35], *373,* 413, 415[36,38], *417, 418*
Finlay-Jones, L. R., 274[49], *284*
Finley, T. N., 7[9,11], 8[13,18,19], 9[21], 20[11], 21[11], *23, 24*
Fireman, P., 453[58], *458*
Fischer, K., 339[22], *352*

Fischer, L., 487[33], *514*
Fisher, A. B., 488[38], 489[38], *514*
Fisher, M. W., 145[9,10], *157,* 357 [10], 358[10], 359[10], 360[10], 361[10], 362[10], *372*
Fishman, A. P., 9[24], *24,* 75[8], *97*
Fishman, R. A., 356[5], 357[5], 358[5], *371*
Flaherty, T. T., 488[37], *514*
Flaks, A., 44, *55*
Flanagan, T. D., 169[89], *177*
Flax, M. H., 493[71,72], *516*
Fleischman, R. W., 282[96], *287*
Fliedner, T. M., 301[76], *328*
Fogel, B. J., 199[43], *208*
Follensby, E. M., 475[55], *482*
Fonkalsrud, E. W., 489[54], *515*
Fonke, S. R., 453[57], *458*
Fontana, V. J., 465[10], 470, *479, 480*
Fontanellaz, H. P., 528[71], *546*
Ford, M., 120[65], *130,* 182[14], *187*
Ford, R. J., Jr., 81[37], 86[37], 89 [37,50], 90, 92, *99, 100*
Forgacs, P., 467[19], *479*
Foroozan, P., 200[51], *208*
Fotino, M., 215[43], *224,* 434[36], 437[36], *443*
Fotino, R. H., 434[36], 437[36], *443*
Foucard, T., 214[34], *224*
Fowler, T., 343[35], *352*
Fowler, W. S., 486[14], *513*
Fox, H. H., 376[11], *399*
Fox, J. P., 182[6], *187,* 379[24], *399*
Fox, R. A., 525[50], *545*
Foy, H. M., 102[10], 107[30], 110[10], 124[68], *126, 127, 130,* 376[9], 379[9], *399*
Fradelizi, D. P., 40[21], 41[21], *54*
Frai, M., 166[63], 167[63], *176*
Francis, T., Jr., 376[2], 377[2], 392 [88], *398, 404*
Frand, U. I., 281[73], *286*
Frank, M. M., 8[14,15], 19[15,55,56], *24, 26,* 163[40,41–44,48,55],

[Frank, M. M.]
171[55], *174, 175,* 255[46], *259*
Frankel, A., 170[102], *178*
Frankland, A. W., 463[5,6], 469[24], *479, 480*
Franklin, E. C., 529[93], 530[93], *547*
Franklin, W., 454[66], *458,* 464, 475 [55], *479, 482*
Freeman, J., 462, *478*
Freestone, D. S., 384[50], *401*
Frenkel, J. K., 184[34], *188*
Friday, G. A., 453[58], *458*
Fridy, W. W., 221[108], *228*
Friedewald, W. T., 108[25], *128,* 387 [65], 388[69], *403*
Friedman, A., 384[49], *401*
Friedman, L., 182[15], *187*
Friedman, M., 282[94], *287*
Friedman, M. H., 184[25], *188*
Friedman, P. J., 249[30], *258*
Frimodt-Möller, C., 292[21], *325*
Friou, C. J., 525[46], *544*
Frommel, D., 40[22], 49[80], *54, 57*
Fruchtman, M. H., 213[20], *223*
Fry, W. A., 486[17], *513*
Fuchs, A. M., 470[28], 476, *480, 482*
Fudenberg, B. R., 339[21], *351*
Fudenberg, H. H., 42[24], *54,* 194[13, 15], 196[32], 200[13,49], *206, 207, 208,* 246[10], *257,* 336[8,9], 337[11,12,14], 339[20,21], 340 [12,20], 341[20], 342[12], 344 [14], 349[12], *351,* 528[68,69,71, 72,89], 529[90], 531[69], *546, 547*
Fujimura, S., 497[79], 501[79,92], *517*
Fuld, S. L., 107[29], *127,* 387[65], *403*
Fulginiti, V. A., 192[2], *205,* 221 [105], *228,* 386[62], *402*
Fulk, R. V., 383[46,47], *401*
Fulkerson, L., 522[16], *543*
Furlong, S. L., 184[27], *188*
Furstenberg, A. C., 248[25], *258*

G

Gabrielsen, A. E., 255[49], *259*
Gacot, P., 487[33], *514*
Gaensler, E. A., 291[20], *325,* 369 [46], *374*
Gaffney, J., 61[11], *69*
Gago, O., 486[17], 488[34], *513, 514*
Gaither, T. A., 19[55], *26,* 163[40], *174*
Galant, S. P., 219[78], *226*
Gale, J. L., 102[8], 124[8], *126*
Galindo, B., 10[30], *24,* 151[19], *158*
Gallin, J. I., 162[2,3,17], 163[2,34, 55], 165[58], 166[70], 167[71], 168[34,79], 170[92,94,103], 171[94], *172-178*
Galton, D. A. G., *547*
Gamba, M. F., 356[8], *372*
Gambrill, M. R., 255[48], *259*
Ganellin, C. R., 452[43], *457*
Garancis, J. C., 230[4], 232-235[4], 237[4], 238[4], *240*
Gard, F. R. N., 340[25], *352*
Gardborg, O., 469[27], *480*
Gardner, P. S., 139[7], *141*
Gartmann, J., *374*
Garvey, J. S., 75[3], 76[3], *97*
Garzon, A. A., 489[51], 500[86], 502[86], *515, 517*
Gaskell, J. F., 183[21], *188*
Gaskin, F., 170[96], *178*
Gatti, R. A., 192[1], 193[8], 200[48], *205, 206, 208,* 349[36], *352,* 528 [69], 531[69], *546*
Gatto, L., 306[105], *329*
Gauld, R. L., 385[55], *402*
Gauldie, J., 49[82], *57*
Gault, E. W., 292[24], *325*
Gear, J. S. S., 204[62], *209*
Gebbie, T., 454[68], *459*
Geer, J. C., 299[59], *327*
Geiger, H., 171[106], *178*
Gelfand, E. W., 194[19], 195[19], *207,* 214[36], *224*

Gelikogla, I. S., 527[62], *545*
Gell, P. G. H., 244, *256*, 316[139], 318[139], 322[139], *331*
Gengozian, N., 145[11], *157*
Gerber, M. A., 50[93], *58*, 218[74], *226*
Gerbrandy, J. L. F., 48[75], *57*
Gershon-Cohen, J., 230[9], 232–234 [9], 237[9], *241*
Geuning, C., 368[31], 369[31], 371[31], *373*
Gewurz, H., 162[13,22,23], 163[50, 51], 171[13], *172, 173, 175*, 193[12], *206*
Gharpure, M. A., 396[102], *405*
Ghossein, N. A., 321[151], *332*
Gibbons, R. J., 155[35], *159*
Gibbs, J. H., 170[93], *177*
Giddens, W. E., 44[33,34,39], *54, 55*
Gigli, I., 163[37], 168[73], *174, 176*, 311[134], *331*
Gilden, R. V., 389[72], *403*
Gill, V., 377[15], *399*
Gillespie, E., 452[46,47], *457*
Gillespie, J. M., 340[25], *352*
Ginsberg, R. J., 489[44], *514*
Giraldo, B., 281[81], *286*
Girard, J. P., 526[55], *545*
Giroux, M., 368[30], 369[30], 371 [30], *373*
Gitlin, D., 194[14], *206*
Glade, P. R., 61[12], 62[12], *70*, 526 [52], 527[62], *545*
Glascock, H. W., Jr., 269[25], *283*
Glasgow, L. A., 63[19], *70*, 182[7], *187*
Glasser, R. M., 300[64], 301[64], *327*
Gleich, G. J., 196, *207*, 214[33,39,40], *224*, 296[44], *326*, 337[13], 349 [13], *351*
Glenn, W., 170[90], *177*
Glennon, J. A., 219[89], *227*, 453 [56], *458*
Glexen, W. P., 181[2], *186*
Glezen, P., 388[70], *403*
Glick, B., 120[66], *130*

Gliedman, M. L., 501[91], 504[91,99], 506[91], *517, 518*
Glueck, M. A., 269[32], *284*
Glynn, A. A., 19[57], *26, 155[28], *158*
Gnabasik, F. J., 145[9], *157*
Godfrey, H., 478[71], *483*
Godfrey, S., 454[69], *459*
Godleski, J. J., 8[17], *24*, 45[48], *55*
Godman, G. D., 248[21,22], *257, 258*
Goetzl, E. J., 162[26], 165[26], 168 [72,73], 169[81], *173, 176, 177*, 310[130], *331*, 450[34], *456*
Goff, A. M., 291[20], *325*
Golbert, T. M., 320[147], *332*
Gold, E., 290[10], *324*
Gold, W. M., 219[78,80], *226*
Goldberg, I. S., 369[43], *374*
Goldberg, L. S., 194[13], 196[32], 200[13], 201[56], *206, 207, 209*
Goldberg, N. D., 170[98], *178*
Golde, D. W., 8[13,18,19], *23, 24*
Goldis, G., 291[15], *324*
Goldblum, R. M., 528[75], *546*
Goldman, A. L., 281[75], *286*
Goldman, A. S., 204[65,66], *209*
Goldman, G. C., 277[56], *285*
Goldman, R. S., 528[75], *546*
Goldstein, E. O., 467[18], 473[18,47], *479, 481*
Goldstein, I. M., 166[63,67], 167[63, 71], *176*
Goldstein, S., 500[86], 502[86], *517*
Gondos, B., 491[67], 492[68], 494 [68,74], 496[75], 499[67], 500 [89], *516, 517*
Gondos, G., 488[42], 491[42], 494 [73], 498[42], 499[73], 500[73], 501[73], *514, 516*
Good, J. T., 184[34], *188*
Good, R. A., 40[22], 46[52,55], 49 [80], *54, 55, 56, 57*, 162[13], 171 [13,106], *172, 178*, 192[1,3], 193 [6,7,12], 196[24,25], 197[24], 200[7,48], 201[24], 203[58], *205-209*, 255[49], *259*, 336[8,9], 349

[Good, R. A.]
    [36,37], *351, 352,* 528[70], *546*
Goodburn, G. M., 108[39], 109[39],
    128
Goodfriend, L., 215[44], *224,* 438
    [37], *443,* 446[6], *454*
Goodlin, R. C., 339[23], *352*
Goodman, D. M. P., 453[48], *457*
Goodman, H. C., 336[8], *351*
Goodman, H. L., 523[28], *543*
Goodman, J. R., 42[24], *54*
Goodrich, B. E., 290[6], *324*
Goodwin, R. A., 523[32,34], *544*
Gordon, J., 472[37], *480*
Gordon, M. E., 290[4], 293[4], *324*
Gorrill, R. H., 469[24], *480*
Götze, O., 163[38], *174*
Graf, P. D., 219[86], *227, 514*
Graham, J. R., 277[59,60], *285*
Graham, M. L., 411[20], 412[20],
    417
Grant, I. W. B., 454[60], *458*
Grater, W. C., 463, *479*
Graves, J. S., 489[56], *515*
Graw, R. G., 8[20], *24,* 182[12], 185
    [12], 186[43], *187, 189,* 366[28],
    373
Grayston, J. T., 102[10], 107[30],
    110[10], *126, 127,* 376[9], 379
    [9], *399*
Graybill, J. R., 528[81], 538[81],
    546
Green, G. M., 8[16], *24,* 45[49], *55,*
    76[12], 79[12,27], 84[27], *98,*
    99, 144[4], *157,* 183[20], *188,*
    542
Greenberg, H. B., 106[24], 107[24],
    127, 380[28], 382[28,43], 387
    [64], 397[64], 398[28], *400, 401,*
    402
Greenberg, M. L., 300[63], 301[74],
    327
Greene, B. M., 313[137], *331*
Greene, L. T., 369[41], *374*
Greenfield, S., 368[40], 369[40],
    371[40], *373*

Greenspan, R. H., *514*
Gregory, R. G., 197[36], *208*
Greisman, S. E., 151[25], 152[25],
    158
Grey, H. M., 193[4], *206*
Grieco, M. H., 151[22], *158,* 219[96],
    228
Griffin, L. M., 269[29], *283,* 291[19],
    325
Grimley, P. M., 215[46], *224*
Griscelli, C., 532[106], *548*
Grosjean, O. V., 502[95], *518*
Gross, N. J., 526[56], 527, *545*
Gross, R., 300[67], *327*
Groth, C., 485[5], *512*
Grubbs, G. E., 385[60], *402*
Grubek, H., 186[41], *189*
Grumet, F. C., 432[32], *442*
Gowans, J. L., 80[30], *99*
Guerra, M. C., 356[8], *372*
Gundelfinger, B. F., 380[29], 389
    [29], *400*
Gupta, S., 220[98], *228*
Gustafson, G. T., 295[41], *326*
Gutekunst, R. R., 107[29], *127.* 376
    [11], 387[65], *399, 403*
Guthnow, C. G., Jr., 453[48], *457*
Gwaltney, J. M., Jr., 378[19], *399*
Györkey, F., 274[43], 275[43], *284*

H

Haab, O. P., 301[77], 302[77], *328*
Haase, A. T., 387[63], *402*
Habelman, P. S., 487[26], 488[26],
    513
Hadden, J. W., 46[52], *55*
Hafez, F. F., 359[25], 360[25], 361
    [25], *373*
Haggard, M. E., 197[36], *208,* 274[50],
    284
Haglin, J. J., 486, 487[22,27], 488[22,
    35], 504[22], *513, 514*
Hagstrom, J. W. C., 489[49], 490[49],
    503[98], 507[98], *515, 518*
Hagy, G. W., 214[42], *224*

Hahn, G. W., 281[74], *286*
Hailey, E. J., 269[25], *283*
Halgrimson, C. G., 485[5], *512*
Hall, C. E., 379[24], *399*
Hall, D. L., 47[71], *56*
Hall, T. S., 390[79,80], 391[79], 392 [80], *404*
Hall, W. H., 394[97], *405*
Hallford, C., 497[78], *516*
Hallgren, J., 217[66], *226*
Hallman, G. L., 486[21], *153*
Halmagyi, D. F. J., 75[5], *97*
Halpern, B. N., 268[20,22], *283*
Halprin, G. M., 359[26], 360[26], *373*
Ham, A. W., 52, *58*
Hamburger, R. N., 439, *443*
Hamilton, M. A., 520[4], *542*
Hamilton-Smith, S., 384[50], *401*
Hammond, R. C., 184[31], *188*
Hamparian, V. V., 378[19], *399*
Hampton, S. F., 476[51], *482*
Hamre, D., 378[19], *399*
Han, T., 268[23], *283*
Hanessian, S., 145[8], *157*
Hanifin, J., 298[46], *326*
Hanks, J. H., 5[7], *23*
Hanna, J., 182[8], 183[16], 184[8, 16], 185[16], *187*
Hansen, L. A., 196[31], *207*
Hardin, J. H., 295[40], *326*
Harding, J. D. J., 183[22], *188*
Hardy, J. D., 486-489[23], 497[78], *513, 516*
Hardy, W. R., 294[31], *325*
Hargreave, F. E., 217[65], *226*
Harkleroad, L. E., 282[95], *287*
Harle, T. S., 277[57], *285*
Harley, D., 471, *480*
Harper, L. O., 281[86], *286*
Harris, E. A., 454[68], *459*
Harris, H. B., 162[9], 169[85], 171 [9], *172, 177*
Harris, J. O., 7[10], 18[10], *23*, 46 [51], *55*
Harris, R. D., 282[89], *287*

Harrison, E. G., Jr., 273[37], *284*
Harrison, G. M., 486[21], *513*
Harrison, J. H., 485[2], *512*
Hartshorve, G., 522[16], *543*
Haskell, T. H., 145[8], *157*
Hasleton, P. S., 274[40], *284*
Hauptman, S. P., 17[52], 19, 21[52], *26*
Hauser, R. E., 42[28], 45[28], 46[28], *54,* 81[36], 86[36], 87[36], 89 [36], 90, 96[36], *99*
Hausman, M. S., 163[54], *175*
Hayakawa, A., 107[28], *127*
Hayakawa, B., 491[67], 499[67], *516*
Hayek, Von, H., 81, *99*
Hayes, K., 194[16], 196[16], *206*
Haywood, L., 522[14], *543*
Heard, B. E., 274[39], *284*
Heath, R. B., 138[6], *141*
Hebald, S., 471[31], 476[51], *480, 482*
Heckenlively, J. R., 281[74], *286*
Heckman, M. G., 143[2], *157*
Hedley-Whyte, J., 368[40], 369[40], 371[40], *373*
Heemstra, H., 488[41], 489[41], *514*
Heffelfinger, J. C., 392[90], *404*
Heffron, R., 412[26], 415[26], *417*
Heidelberger, M., 413[33], 415[33], *418*
Heilman, D. H., 255[48], *259*
Heinemann, H. O., 75[8], *97*
Heiner, D. C., 197, *208,* 339[24], 340 [24], *352*
Heiner, G. G., 383[46], *401*
Heitzman, E. R., 261[6], *282*
Helander, E., 469, *480*
Heller, P., 102[9], 105[9], *126*
Helms, C., 380[28], 382[28], 398 [28], *400*
Henderson, E. S., 166[66], *176*
Henderson, L. L., 214[33], *224*
Hennessy, H. V., 392[88,90,91], *404*
Henney, C. S., 10[31,32], *25,* 42[25], 48[25], *54,* 60[7,8], 61[7,11,14], 62[7,14,18], 63[18], 65[22], 68

[Henney, C. S.]
  [7,14,18], *69, 70,* 81[33], *99,* 118
  [59], *129,* 341[32], *352,* 381[35],
  400
Henriksen, K., 349[37], *352*
Henriksen, S. D., 469[27], *480*
Henry, C., 77[26], 87[26], *98*
Hensle, T., 281[70], *286*
Hensley, G. T., 230[4,14], 232[4,14],
  233[4,14], 234[4,14], 235[4],
  237[4,14], 238[4,22], *240, 241,*
  282[93], *287*
Henson, P. M., 420[1], 434[1], *441,*
  450[35], *456*
Heremans, J. F., 10[40], 12[40], 13
  [46], *25,* 86[48], *100,* 196[31],
  207
Herick, van, W., 108[38], 109[38],
  128
Herion, J. C., 300[64], 301[64], *327*
Hers, J. F. Ph, 103[12], *126*
Hersh, E. M., 106[25], *127*
Herzenberg, L. A., 339[23], *352*
Herzog, C., 532[106], *548*
Hess, L., 425[21], *442*
Hewitt, W. F., 269[25], *283*
Hicklin, M. D., 530[100], *548*
Hierholzer, J. C., 221[108], *228*
Hijmans, W., 349[38], *352*
Hilberg, R. W., 528[83], *547*
Hill, B. M., 214[37], *224,* 470[51],
  481
Hill, D. J., 212[3], *222*
Hill, H. R., 170[98], *178*
Hill, J. H., 166[69], *176*
Hilleman, M. R., 384[49], 385[55],
  401, 402
Hilvering, C., 488[41], 489[41], *514*
Hindle, W., 277[62], *285*
Hinrichs, D. J., 530[99], *548*
Hinuma, Y., 117[56], *129*
Hirsch, J. G., 163[31], 166[31], *174,*
  295[35], 296[35], 298[50], *325,*
  326
Hirschhorn, K., 527[62], *545*
Hirshout, Y., 527[62], *545*

Hirst, G. K., 390[81], 391[82], *404*
Hitzig, W. H., 199[45], *208,* 336[8,9,],
  351, 528[69,71], 531[69], *546*
Hjorth, T., 290[3], *324*
Hobbs, J. R., 319[143], *332*
Hodes, D. S., 131[2], 139[9], *140, 141,*
  379[25], 380[25], 382[25], 393
  [94], 396[105], 397[106], *399,*
  405
Hodges, R. G., 413[33], 415[33],
  418
Hodges, R. T., 44[40], *55*
Hoehne, J. H., 214[30], 218[30], *223*
Hoffman, L. S., 221[105], *228*
Hoffstein, S., 167[71], *176*
Hogan, J., 170[98], *178*
Hogben, C. A., 355[2], 356[2], 357
  [2], 358[2], *371*
Hogg, J. C., 47[71], *56*
Hoigné, R., 266[16], *283*
Holland, N., 523[29], *543*
Holland, P., 523[29], *543*
Hollander, D., 254[36], *258*
Holle, B., 48[74], *57, 68, 71,* 81[35],
  95[35], 96[35], *99*
Hollers, J. C., 204[65], *209*
Holmes, B., 46[55], *56*
Holmes, R. A., 230[2], 232[2], 233
  [2], 234[2], 237[2], 238[2], *240*
Holt, L. E., Jr., 465[10], *479*
Holub, M., 42[28], 45[28], 46[28],
  54, 81[36], 86[36], 87[36], 89
  [36], 90, 96[36], *99*
Holzinger, E. A., 184[33], *188*
Homan van der Heide, J. N., 488[41],
  489[41], *514*
Homatas, J., 489[55], *515*
Hong, R., 40[22], 49[80], *54, 57,*
  196[24,25,30,34], 197[24,30],
  198[30], 200[48], 201[24], *207,*
  208, 349[36], *352,* 528[79], *546*
Honsinger, R. W., Jr., 296[43], 302
  [43], *326*
Hook, W. A., 47[66], *56*
Hoor, ten, F., 488[41], 489[41], *514*
Horn, L., *547*

Horn, R. G., 248[26], *258*
Hornbeck, C., 409[9], 415[9], *416*
Hornbrook, M. M., 446[1], *454*
Horner, G. J., 75[5], *97*
Hornick, R. B., 151[25], 152[25], *158,* 383[46,47], *401*
Horowitz, A. L., 282[94], *287*
Horswood, R. L., 106[24], 107[24], 108[41], *127, 128,* 382[43], 387 [64], 397[64,107,108], *401, 402, 405*
Hougard, K., 302[80], *328*
Housley, E., 212[2], *222*
Housworth, J., *399*
Howard, L. W., 521[12], *543*
Howard, W. A., 217[69], *226*
Howell, J. B. L., 454[61], *458*
Hsu, H. S., 185[40], *189*
Hsu, S. H., 215[44], *224,* 438[37], *443*
Huang, C. L., 489[65], *516*
Huber, G. L., 7[9], *23*
Huber, M. G., 383[47], *401,* 453[55], 454[76], *458, 459*
Hubner, K. F., 145[11], *157*
Hubscher, T., 300[62], 318[62], *327*
Hudson, B. H., 489[43], 490[43], *514*
Hudson, G., 300[69,71], 301[69], *327*
Huebner, R. J., 376[7], 380[30], 385 [7, 54, 57], 389[30,71,72], *398, 400, 402, 403*
Huggins, C. E., 487[30], *514*
Hughes, W. H., 469[24], *480*
Hugh-Jones, P., 504[100, 101], 506 [100, 101], 507[100], *518*
Hume, E. B., 383[47], *401*
Humphrey, J. H., 29[1,2], *52,* 446[12, 13], *455*
Humphrey, W., 432[30,31], *442*
Hunsicker, L. G., 163[47], *175*
Hunt, W. B., 84, *100*
Hunter, R. L., 45[46], *55*
Huntley, C. C., 198, *208*
Hurley, E. J., 486, 487[19], *513*

Hurtubise, P. E., 530[95], *547*
Hutchison, D. C. S., 500[100], 506 [100,101], 507[100], *518*
Huygelen, C., 394[99], 395[100], *405*
Hyde, R. W., 394[97], *405,* 488[38], 489[38], *514*
Hyde, S., 162[20], 171[20], *173*

I

Imagawa, D., 184[32], *188*
Ingelfinger, F. J., 291[17], *324*
Ingling, A. L., 184[31], *188*
Ingold, A., *374*
Ingraham, J. S., 75, *97*
Ingram, R. H., 221[108], *228*
Inoue, S., 219[90], *227*
Isawa, T., 487-491[29,61], 500[89], *513, 515, 517*
Ishikawa, T., 298[48], 299[57], *326, 327*
Ishizaka, K., 14[50], *26,* 50[91,92,95], *58,* 196[24,25], 197[24], 201[24], *207,* 214[37,40], 215[47,49,50], 218[73], *224, 225, 226,* 446[1,2,4, 11,15,16,18,19], 447[19, 23-27], *454, 455, 456,* 470[51], 473[47], 474[49], 475, 477[70], *481, 482, 483*
Ishizaka, T., 215[47], *224,* 446[1,2,4, 11,15,16,19], 447[19,23-27], *454, 455, 456,* 475, *482*
Isin, E., 486-489[23], *513*
Isliker, H., 342[33], *353*
Israel, H. L., 254[37], *258,* 269[26], *283,* 525[47], 526[57], *544, 545*
Israel, K. S., 269[35], 271[35], *284*
Isuchi, T., 107[28], *127*
Itkin, I. H., 219[77], *226*
Izumi, T., 527[60], *545*

J

Jackson, A. E., 151[16], *158*
Jackson, G. G., 368[36], 369[36],

[Jackson, G. G.]
371[36], *373,* 389[73], *403*
Jacobs, F. M., 219[85], *227*
Jacobs, J. C., 203[61], *209,* 338[17], *351*
Jacobsen, R., 378[20], *399*
Jacobson, E. B., 49[78], *57*
Jager, B. V., 343[34], *352*
James, D. G., 525[50], *545*
James, W. D., 102[5], 106[24], 107 [24], 108[41], *126, 127, 128,* 376 [11], 382[43], 387[64], 388[67], 397[64], *399, 401, 402, 403*
Jandl, J. H., 162[15], 171[15], *173,* 203[60], *209,* 338[18], *351*
Janeway, C. A., 194[14], 199[44], *206, 208,* 340[30], 341[31], 343 [30], *352*
Janower, M. L., 269[32], *284*
Jansen, V., 303[89], *328*
Jarrett, W. F. H., 47[63], *56*
Jeffries, B. C., 131[3], *141,* 376[6], *398*
Jeffries, B. D., 131[1], *140*
Jenkins, P. A., 230[6], 232-234[6], 237[6], *240*
Jenkins, V. K., 304[95,96], 314[95], 315[95,96], 309[96], *329*
Jensen, K. E., 137[5], *141,* 387[65], *403*
Jericho, K. W. F., 44[35,40,41], *54, 55*
Jerne, N. K., 77[26], 87[26], *98*
Jerusalem, C. R., 497[76], 502[76], *516*
Jeter, W. S., 530[98], *548*
Jeunet, F., 342[33], *352*
Job, C. K., 292[24], *325*
Johanson, W. G., 368[37,38], *373*
Johansson, S. G. O., 50[91], *58,* 214 [31,32,34], 218[73], *224, 226,* 446[9,10,11,12,13,15], *454, 455,* 474[50], *481*
John, T. J., 103[16], 106[16], *127*
Johnson, D. E., 487-491[29,46,61], *513, 515*

Johnson, J. E., III, 7[10], 10[37], 18 [10], *23, 25,* 48[73], *56,* 62[18], 63[18], 68[18], *70,* 81[34], 95 [34], *99,* 213[20], *223*
Johnson, J. S., 13[47], *26,* 145[12], *157,* 255[51], *259*
Johnson, K. M., 107[32], *128,* 378[20. 21], *399*
Johnson, V., 411[20], 412[20], *417*
Johnston, H. S., 47, *56*
Johnston, J., 299[56], *326*
Johnston, N., 9[26], *24,* 30]4,6], 31 [6], 38[6], 44[6], 45[6], *52, 53,* 60[2], 67[28], *69, 71,* 111[47], *129,* 156[36], *159*
Johnston, R. B., Jr., 162[15], 171[15], *173,* 203[60], 204, *209,* 298[51], *326,* 338[18], *351*
Johnstone, D. E., 464, 469, *479, 480*
Jones, D. J., 528[63], *545*
Jones, G. R., 282[97], *287*
Jones, J. E. T., 44[41], *55*
Jones, S. E., 282[90], *287*
Jordan, W. S., Jr., 103[15], *127,* 378 [19], *399*
Jose, D. G., 193[8], *206*
Josef, M., 524[38], *544*
Josefsson, B., 295[41], *326*
Joseph, W. L., 487[28], 489[57], *513, 515*
Jost, M. C., 196[28], 197[28], 201 [28], *207*
Joyner, J. W., 386[62], *402*
Juhl, F., 349[37], *352*
Jurgenson, P. F., 62[18], 63[18], 68 [18], *70*
Juvenelle, A. A., 486, *512*

K

Kabat, E. A., 194[20], *207,* 413[28,29], *417*
Kabe, J., 62[17], *70*
Kagami, W., 501[92], *517*
Kagan, I. G., 530[100], *548*
Kagumba, M., 205[67], *209*

Kahn, D. D., 184[33], *188*
Kahnt, F. W., 340[25], *352*
Kajani, M. K., 277[54], *285*
Kalica, A. R., 124[70], *130*
Kaliner, M. A., 446[40], 447[20],
    450[20], 451[20,39,40], 452[44],
    453[49], *455, 457*
Kalsow, C., 355[1], 357[1], 358[1],
    371
Kaltreider, H. B., 10[27], *24,* 42[27],
    46[27], 48[27], *54,* 67[27], 67
    [29], *71,* 75[6], 81[38,39], 82
    [39], 83[39], 84[39,42], 86[38,
    39], 87[38], 89[39], 90[6,38],
    92[6], 94[6], 95[38], *97, 99, 100*
Kamp, G. H., 369[42], *374*
Kane, M. A., 163[43,44], *174*
Kantor, M., 306[105], *329*
Kantor, S. Z., 472[40], *481*
Kapikian, A. Z., 378[19,21], 380[27],
    382[27,36,38], 383[27], 386[27,
    36,38], *399, 400*
Kaplan, A. P., 162[17,26,27], 165[26,
    27,58,59,60], 171[17], *173, 175,*
    319[144], *332*
Kaplan, B. I., 246[9], *257*
Kaplan, H., 217[63], *226*
Kaplan, J. M., 247[18], *257,* 359[23],
    372
Kaplan, M. E., 19[58,61], *26,* 155[29],
    158
Karakitas, K., 213[25], *223*
Karliner, J. S., 281[71], *286*
Karlson, A. G., 184[23], *188*
Karlson, K. E., 489[51], 500[86],
    502[86], *515, 517*
Karnovsky, M. L., 488[31], *456*
Karpati, G., 200[53], *209*
Karpouzas, J., 197[38], *208*
Kasel, J. A., 383[46,47], 387[63],
    393[96], 394[96], *401, 402, 405*
Kass, E. H., 45[49], *55*
Kass, W. H., 183[20], *188*
Kato, J., 107[28], *127*
Katz, D. H., 44[31], 49[83], *54, 57,*
    77[23], *98,* 215[48], *225*

Katz, S., 281[73], *286*
Kauffman, G., 415[37], *418*
Kaufman, D. M., 281[72], *286*
Kaufman, P., 415[40], *418*
Kavets, J., 384[52], *402*
Kawai, T., 46[51], *55*
Kawakami, Y., 501[92], *517*
Kay, A. B., 162[27], 165[27], 169
    [82,83,84], *173, 177,* 303[83,84],
    307[83,116], 309[83,116], 310
    [84,133,128], 314[128,133], *328,
    330, 331,* 448[33], *456*
Kay, H. E. M., 199[43,44], *208*
Kay, J. M., 274[40], *284*
Kayman, E. H., 213[22], *223*
Kayman, H., 425[23], 439[23], *442*
Kazemi, H., 212[7], *222*
Keightley, R., 350[40], *353*
Keimowitz, R. I., 10[39], 12[39],
    15[39], *25*
Keller, C., 219[92], *227*
Keller, H. L., 162[14], *173*
Keller, H. U., 163[29], 166[29], *174,*
    310[132], 314[132], *331*
Keller, R., 155[33], *159*
Kelman, G. R., 212[5], *222*
Kemper, J. W., 254[35], *258*
Kendal, A. P., 392[89], *404*
Kendig, E. L., 412[22], *417*
Kennard, H. E., 302[79], *328*
Kennedy, E., 522[16], *543*
Kenny, G. E., 102[6,8,10], 107[30],
    110[10], 124[8,68], *126, 127, 130*
    376[9], 378[9], 379[9], *399*
Kent, D. C., 219[83], *227,* 521[9],
    542
Kerbel, R. S., 120[63], *130*
Kerby, G. R., 3[1], *23*
Kern, J., 389[72], *403*
Kessler, G. F., 219[80], *227*
Ketonen, P., 489[62], *515*
Kevy, S. V., 194[14], *206*
Kilbourne, E. D., 384[53], 391[85],
    402, 404
Kilburn, K. H., 79[28], *99*
Killingback, P. G., 446[7], *454*

Kim, H. W., 131[1,2,3], 137[5], 139 [8,9,10], *140, 141,* 376[6], 379 [25], 380[25], 382[25,36,37], 385[54], 386[36,37], 393[95], 397[101,105], 397[106], *398, 399, 400, 402, 405*

Kimball, H. R., 162[2,6,10,16], 165 [16], 170[6,10], *172, 173*

Kincade, P. W., 50[85,86], *57*

Kinder, P. H., 454[62], *458*

King, T. P., 466[13,14,17], 477[70], *479, 483*

Kirk, D. L., 411[17], *417*

Kirkpatrick, G. H., 162[10], 163[34], 168[34,79], 170[10], 171[34], *172, 174, 177,* 194[17], 200[50], 201[55], *206, 208, 209,* 219[92], *227,* 319[142], *332,* 523[31,33], 528[76], *544, 546*

Kirkpatrick, J. A., 199[46], 200[46], *208,*

Kirschner, R. H., 274[45], *284*

Kirschstein, R. L., 120[65], *130,* 182 [14], 186[42], *187, 189*

Kirshman, H., 282[98], *287,* 290[12], *324*

Kiser, R., 212[4], *222*

Kishimoto, T., 215[50], *225,* 477[70], *483*

Kistler, P., 342[33], *352*

Kitayama, T., 107[28], *127*

Kjeldgaard, J. M., 281[74], *286*

Klastersky, J., 368[31], 369[31], 371[31], *373*

Klein, E., 31, 33[8], 38[8], *53,* 60[1], *69*

Klein, J., 432[29], *442*

Kleine, J. W., 488[41], 489[41], *514*

Klimerman, J. A., 170[103], *178*

Klopfenstein, M. D., 521[12], *543*

Knapp, P. H., 219[93], *227*

Knight, E. J., 80[30], *99*

Knight, V., 107[32], *128,* 170[90], *177,* 387[63], 390[76], *402, 403*

Knopf, H. L. S., 380[27], 382[27,42], 383[27], 386[27], *400, 401*

Kobayshi, N., 62[17], *70*

Koblenzer, P. J., 162[11], 171[11], *172*

Koch, C., 349[37], *352*

Kochwa, S., 50[93], *58,* 218[74], *226*

Koch-weser, J., 302[82], *328*

Koerner, S. K., 501[91], 504[91,99], 506[91], *517, 518*

Koffler, D., 246[11], *257*

Kofman, S., 368[36], 369[36], 371 [36], *373*

Kofoed, M. A., 308[119], *330*

Kohler, P. F., 193[11], *206*

Kohout, J., 526, 527[59], *545*

Kok-Jensen, A., 277[63], *285*

Kondo, Y., 497[78], *516*

Kory, R. C., 368[39], 369[39], *373*

Koop, W. L., 200[51], *208*

Kosek, J. C., 232[15], 233[15], 234 [15], 237[15], *241*

Koss, I. G., 274[47], *284*

Kostage, S. T., 298[49], 306[49,107], *326, 329*

Koster, F. T., 65[24], *70*

Kountz, S. L., 485[4], *512*

Kovacs, B. A., 446[6], *454*

Kravetz, A. M., 107[32], *128*

Kremer, W., 293[28], *325*

Kreus, K. E., 489[62], *515*

Krieger, I., 197[37], *208*

Kronenberg, R., 269[28], *283*

Krovetz, C. J., 193[6], *206*

Kuhn, C., 81[37], 86[37], 89[37,50], 90, 92, *99, 100*

Kundur, V., 213[21], *223*

Kunin, C. M., 357[13], *372*

Kunkel, H. G., 194[20], 196[31], *207,* 246[10,11], *257,* 336[8,9], 339[19], *351*

Kustner, H., 421[7], *441*

Ky, N. T., 268[22], *283*

Kyselka, L., 67[29], *71*

L

Lachmann, P. J., 230[6], 232-234[6],

[Lachmann, P. J.]
237[6], *240,* 310[133], 314[133],
331
Ladman, A. J., 7[9,11], 20[11], 21
[11], *23, 24*
Lagunoff, D., 47[68], *56*
Lalezari, P., 501[91], 504[91], 506
[91], *517*
La Mothe, P., 487[33], *514*
Landa, J., 3[2], *23*
Landau, L. I., 212[3], *222*
Landreth, K., 120[66], *130*
Landsteiner, K., 528[64], *545*
Lane, S. R., 217[69], *226*
Langmuir, A. D., 377[14], *399*
Langner, A., 525, 526, *545*
Lanz, M., 470, *480*
La Plante, L., 282[87], *286*
Lapp, N. L., 281[86], *286*
Largiader, F., 489[52], *515*
La Raia, P. J., 451[39], *457*
Lawrence, H. S., 46[50], *55,* 168[77,
78], *177,* 526[58], 528[88], 529,
530[93,102], 531[103,104], 541
[104], *545, 547, 548*
Lawrence, M., 212[7], *222*
Laws, J. O., 44, *55*
Laws, J. W., 504[100], 506[100],
507[100], *518*
Lawson, D., 356[6,7], 357[6], 359
[7], 360[6], 361[7], *372*
Lawton, A. R., 50[85,88], *57,* 193[5],
206, 350[40], *353*
Lawton, B. R., 230[8], 232-234[8,16]
237[8,16], *241*
Laxdal, S. D., 203[58], *209*
Lazarus, L., 217[61], *225*
Leachman, R. D., 486[21], *513*
Leake, E. S., *55,* 81[32], *99,* 183[18],
187, 274[41], *284*
Leao, R. C., 524[40], *544*
Le Compte, P. R., 277[59], *285*
Leder, R., 238[19], *241*
Lee, E. H., 447[23], *456*
Lee, S. L., 278[67], *285*
Lee, Y. K., 389[72], *403*

Leeuwer, W. S. V., 293[28], *325*
Lefeoe, N. M., 454[67], *459*
Lehrer, R. I., 298[46], *326*
Lehrer, R. J., 295[39], *326*
Leichner, J. P., 255[48], *259*
Leikin, S., 140[11], *141,* 217[69],
226
Leikin, S. L., 162[8], *172*
Lempert, N., 486[16], 488[16], 489
[16], *513*
Lener, W. F., 340[25], *352*
Lennette, E. H., 378[19], 386[61],
389[72], *399, 402, 403*
Lepper, M. H., 368[36], 369[36],
371[36], *373*
Lepow, I. H., 169[87], *177*
Leonard, E., 248[22], *258*
Lerner, A. M., 143[1], 151[1,23],
157, 158
Lesbroc, F., 487[33], *514*
Leskowitz, S., 213[19,22,23,24], *223,*
425[23], 439[24], *442*
Leslie, G., 213[26], *223*
Leu, R. W., 46[52], *55*
Leuchars, E., 308[123], 314[123],
330
Levin, A. S., 200[49], *208,* 337[11],
351, 528[68,69,72,89], 531[69],
546, 547
Levin, D. C., 249[27], *258*
Levin, W. C., 197[36], *208*
Levine, B. B., 215[43], *224,* 266[17],
283, 425, 426[25], 428[26,27],
431[26], 433[33,34], 434[35,36],
437[36], 439[24], *442, 443*
Levine, G., 212[2], *222*
Levine, H. B., 522[19], *543*
Levinthal, B. G., 106[25], *127*
Levy, D. A., 196, *207,* 446[5], *454,*
467[18], 473[18,46,47], 475[54],
479, 481, 482
Lewis, M., *547*
Lichtenstein, L. M., 214[37], *224,*
446[14,16], 450[36,37,38], 451
[41,42], 452[42,46,47], *455, 456,*
457, 465[11], 466[15,16,17],

[Lichtenstein, L. M.]
467[18], 470[51], 472[42-44],
473[[16,18,45,47], 474[49], 475
[54], 476[64], 477[66,68,69]
478[71], *479, 481, 482, 483*
Lieberman, P., 86, *100*
Lieberman, R., 432[30,31], *442*
Liebow, A. A., 248[23], 249[30],
251[32], 254[32], *258,* 290[2],
291[2], 293[2], *324*
Lietze, A., 60[4], *69*
Lillehei, R. C., 489[52], *515*
Lillie, M. G., 184[31], *188*
Limas, C., 338[16], *351*
Linaris, L. I., 182[15], *187,* 453[58],
458
Lind, K., 124[69], *130*
Lindeneg, O., 177[63], *285*
Lindsay, M., 19[57], *26,* 155[28],
158
Lindsay, J. R., 184[26], *188*
Ling, I., 76[15], *98*
Linger, J. D., 143[2], *157*
Lipman, R. P., 109[45], *128*
Litt, M., 299[53,55], 304[53,98,99,
100], 307[100], 306[106,108,109,
110], 311[98], 313[138], 318[98],
326, 329, 330, 331
Little, T. W. A., 183[22], *188*
Littler, W. A., 274[40,48], *284*
Littman, M. L., 524[37], *544*
Liu, C. H., 105[18], *127,* 340[25],
352
Liveright, J. L., 290[1], 293[1],
294[1], *324*
Lo Buglio, A. F., 528[83], 530[95],
547
Lockey, S. D., Jr., 219[89], *227,*
453[56], *458*
Lockward, V. G., 497[78], *51*
Loegering, D. A., 296[44], *326*
Loewinsohn, E., 411[20], 412[20],
417
Löffler, W., 290[5], *324*
Logsdon, P. J., 220[101], *228,* 453
[52,59], *458*

Logue, G. L., 277[57], *285*
Lokich, J. J., 282[91], *287*
Long, D. J., 390[76], *403*
Lopez, M., 454[66], *458*
Loosli, C. G., 184[35], *188*
Lord, R. A., 204[65], *209,* 528[75],
546
Louie, J. S., 201[56], *209*
Lourenco, R. C., 76[11], 79[11], *98,*
369[43], *374*
Louria, D. B., 171[104], *178,* 281[70],
286
Love, J. W. P., 380[29], 389[29], *400*
Loveless, M. H., 471[32], 472[39],
476, 480, 481, 482
Lowell, F. C., 212[7], 213[19,23],
222, 223, 415[36], *418,* 454[66],
458, 464, 475[55], *479, 482*
Lower, R. R., 486, 487[19], *513*
Luce, R. R., 124[68], *130*
Luckey, H. H., 385[54], *402*
Ludwig, W., 380[29,30], 389[29,30],
400
Lundstedt, C., 65[21], *70*
Lurie, M. B., 521[7], *542*
Lutz, W., 357[10], 358[10], 359[10],
360[10], 361[10], 362[10], *372*
Luzzati, A. L., 49[78], *57*
Lybass, T. G., 221[105], *228*
Lyerly, A. D., 198[40], *208*
Lyman, M., 468[22], 474[48], *480,
481*
Lynch, H., 17[53], *26*
Lyons, G. W., 489[52], *515*
Lyons, H. A., 212[6], *222*

M

Maassab, H. F., 376[2], 377[2], 390
[80], 392[80,88,89,90,91], *398,
404*
Mac Arthur, A. M., 504[100,101],
506[100,101], 507[100], *518*
Maciver, A. M., 230[11], 232-234[11],
237[11], *241*
Mackaness, G. B., 10[33], *25,* 46[53],

[Mackaness, G. B.]
  55, 65[23,24,25,26], 66[25,66],
  70, 84, 100, 151[20], 156[20],
  158, 411[13], 416, 521[10], 542
Mac Kay, M., 340[27], 352
Mac Klem, P. T., 212[2], 222
Macklin, C. C., 44[44], 55
Mac Leod, C. M., 412[27], 413[33],
  415[33], 417, 418
Mac Leod, P., 212[2], 222
Mac Nab, G. M., 204[62], 209
Maddison, S. E., 530, 548
Maddocks, J. L., 358[19], 361[19],
  372
Maddy, K. T., 522[22], 543
Madoff, I. M., 291[20], 325
Magoffin, R. L., 386[61], 402
Mahon, W. E., 230[6], 232-234[6],
  237[6], 240, 281[85], 286
Maini, R. N., 217[65], 226
Mainland, D., 465[10], 479
Maisel, J. C., 103[16], 106[16], 127
Malawista, S. E., 166[68], 176
Maldonado, J. E., 296[44], 326
Malley, A., 217[67], 226
Malone, D. N. S., 282[97], 287
Maloney, C. J., 478[71], 483
Mammen, R. E., 392[91], 404
Manax, W. G., 489[52, 515
Maner, A. M., 301[77], 302[77], 328
Mann, J. J., 383[46], 401
Mann, P. E. G., 9[21], 24
Mann, P. R., 299[60], 313[60], 327
Manning, H., 487[31], 514
Manning, R. T., 254[36], 258
Mansy, A. M., 376[9], 379[9], 399
Marchalonis, J. J., 75[2], 97
Marcoux, J. P., 214[33], 224
Margolis, S., 450[37], 456
Markowski, B., 199[44], 208
Marks, A., 291[20], 325
Marks, M. I., 360[27], 373
Marmary, Y., 255[41], 258
Marmion, B. P., 108[39], 109[39],
  128
Marschke, G., 369[45], 374

Marsh, D. G., 215[44], 224, 438,443,
  477[67,68,69], 483
Martin, R., 162[20], 170[90], 171[20],
  173, 177
Martin, R. R., 3[4,5], 7[4,5], 10[4],
  12[4], 15[4], 18[4,5], 23, 168[76],
  177
Martinez-Tello, F. J., 50[90], 58
Mason, B., 504[101, 506[101], 518
Mason, S. A., 504[100,101], 506[100,
  101], 507[100], 518
Masson, P. L., 10[40], 12[40], 25
Mathe, A. A., 219[93], 227
Mathé, G., 412[24], 417
Mathews, K. P., 213[35], 223
Matloff, J. M., 497[79], 501[79], 517
Matsaniotis, N., 197[38], 208
Matsumoto, K., 117[56], 129
Matthews, L. W., 198[41], 205[67],
  208, 209
Matthews, M. J., 274[44], 284
Mattila, S., 489[62], 515
Maxwell, J. H., 248[25], 258
May, C. D., 468, 474, 480, 481
May, J. E., 19[56], 26, 163[40,41,43,
  44,48], 174, 175
May, J. R., 356[4], 358[4,19,20,21],
  359[4,20,22], 360[4,20,21,22],
  361[19,20], 362[22], 371, 372,
  374
Mayer, K., 274[47], 284
Mayer, M. M., 413[28,29], 417
Mays, B. B., 182[9], 183[9], 187
McAllen, M. K., 465[20], 479
McCarroll, J., 182[11], 187
McCarter, J. H., 218, 226
McCarthy, D. S., 293[30], 320[30,
  146], 325, 332
McCombs, R. P., 243[1], 244[8], 246
  [8], 247[8,16], 252[16], 254[16],
  256, 257
McCormick, J. N., 42[24], 54
McCourtie, D. R., 454[67], 459
McCowan, J. M., 380[31], 400
McCracken, G. H., Jr., 359[23], 372
McDevitt, H. O., 428, 432[29,32], 442

McFadden, E. R., 212[4,6], *222*
McFarland, W., 274[44], *284*
McFarlin, D. E., 200[54], 201[54], *209*
McGarry, M. P., 304[95,96], 309[96], 314[95], 315[95,96], *329*
McGregor, D. D., 65[24], *70*
McIntosh, K., 221[105], *228*
McKee, C. M., 413[32], *418*
McLaughlin, J. A., 303[92], *328*
McMahan, H. E., 243[1], *256*
McMahan, R., 102[10], 107[30], 110 [10], *126, 127,* 376[9], 379[9], *399*
McMahon, S. M., 359[26], 360[26], *373*
McNiell, R. S., 219, *228*
McQuillin, J., 139[7], *141*
McRae, J., 75[5], *97*
Medawar, P. B., 485[1], *512*
Meiklejohn, G., 108[38], 109[38], *128,* 386[62], *402*
Meisner, P., 454[62], *458*
Melamed, M. R., 274[47], *284*
Mellits, D., 466[12], 467[18], 473 [18], *479*
Melmon, K. L., 261[1], *282,* 450[38], 451[41], *456, 457*
Melnick, J. L., 378[19], 389[72], *399, 403*
Meltzer, S. J., 420[5], *441*
Melvin, I. G., 412[21], *417*
Mencado, B., 171[106], *178*
Mendell, N. R., 215[45], *224*
Mendes, E., 524, *544*
Mendes, N. F., 524, *544*
Menzel, A. E. O., 446[2], *454*
Merckx, J. J., 184[23], *188*
Mergenhagen, S. E., 162[22,23], 163 [39,49,50,51,54], *173, 174, 175,* 193[12], *206*
Merigan, T. C., 232[15], 233[15], 234[15], 237[15], *241*
Merler, E., 194[14], *206,* 340[30], 341 [31], 343[30], *352*
Merrill, J. P., 485[2], *512*

Meshalkin, E. N., 486, *513*
Metz, E. N., 528[83], 530[95], *547*
Metzgar, R. S., 117[55], *129*
Metzger, H., 215[46], *224*
Meuwissen, H. J., 200[48], *208,* 349 [36], *352*
Mickenberg, I. D., 295[33], 298[33], *325*
Middleton, E., Jr., 219[91], 220[91,101, 103], *227, 228,* 453[52,53,57,59], *458, 472, 481*
Mihm, M. C., Jr., 266[13], *283*
Millar, J. W., 531[104], 541[104], *548*
Miller, H. R. P., 47[63], *56*
Miller, J. F. A. P., 77, *98*
Miller, M. E., 162[9,11,18], 171[9,11], *172, 173,* 203[61], *209,* 336[4], 338[17], *350, 351*
Miller, T., 112[50], *129*
Miller, W. C., 281[76], *286*
Miller, W. F., 368[34], 369[34], *373*
Miller, W. S., 31, *53*
Miller, W. T., 290[4], 293[4], *324*
Mills, J. E., 219[79], *227,* 382[42], 393[93], 396[104], *401, 404, 405*
Milne, C. M., 19[57], *26,* 155[28], *158*
Mims, L. H., 49[79], *57*
Min, K. W., 274[43], 275[43], *284*
Minamitani, M., 386[62], *402*
Minden, P., 216[59], *225*
Minkowitz, S., 500[86], 502[86], *517*
Minning, W., 290[7], *324*
Minor, T. E., 221[106], *228*
Minuse, E., 392[88,90,91], *404*
Mishell, R. I., 77, *98*
Mitchell, D. N., 525[45], *544*
Mitchell, G. F., 77, *98,* 432[32], *442*
Mitchell, J. R., 392[90,91], *404*
Mitchell, R. H., 382[38], 386[38], *400*
Mitchison, N. A., 77[25], *98*
Mittelman, D., 340[25], *352*
Miura, K., 62[17], *70*

Miyamoto, J., 62[17], *70*
Mizutani, H., 107[28], *127*
Moe, H., 31, *53*
Moffatt, B., 300[65], *327*
Mogabgab, W. J., 108[36], *128,* 378
 [19], 387[66], *399, 403*
Moller, J. H., 487[26], *513*
Moloney, W. C., 292[91], *287*
Monhanty, S. A., 184[31], *188*
Montgomery, J. R., 166[65], 168[65],
 176, 546
Moore, M., 282[90], *287*
Moore, N., 454[65], *458*
Moore, V. L., 217[70], *226,* 238[20],
 241
Moran, F., 454[63], *458*
Moreno, F., 470[29], *480*
Morgan, J. E., 302[81], *328*
Morgan, T. E., 21[64,66], *27*
Morinari, H., 489[46], *515*
Morse, S. I., 409[4,5,6], 410[11],
 416
Morton, D. L., 487[28], 489[57],
 513, 515
Morton, V., 184[25], *188*
Moschella, S. L., 277[56], *285*
Moser, K. M., 488-491[39], *514,* 522
 [23], 523[24], 528[24,82], 531
 [24,105], 538[23], 539[108],
 541[24], *543, 547, 548*
Moskalewska, D., 525[51], 526[51],
 545
Mosko, M. M., 530[94], *547*
Mostow, S. R., 391[86], *404*
Mouawad, E., 368[31], 369[31],
 371[31], *373*
Mouton, R. F., 340[25], *352*
Mouton, R. P., 413[34], *418*
Mowatt, A. J., 162[7], 170[7], *172*
Mueller, H. L., 470, *480*
Mufson, M. A., 377[15], *399*
Muggia, F. M., 321[151], *332*
Muir, D. C. F., 269[27], *283*
Mukhopadhyay, M. G., 321[150], *332*
Mulder, M. A., 502[95], *518*
Muller, S. A., 214[38], *224*

Müller-Eberhard, H. J., 162[24], 163
 [24,36,38,46], 165[46,56], 171
 [24], *173, 174, 175,* 193[11], *206,*
 244[4], 246[10], *256, 257,* 310
 [131], 314[131], *331*
Muls, N. A. J., 413[34], *418*
Mumay, H. W., 524[37], *544*
Munoz, J., 305[104, *329,* 409, *416*
Muntener, U., 528[71], *546*
Murphy, B. R., 131[2], *140,* 379[25],
 380[25], 382[25], 393[92,94,96],
 394[92,96,97], 395[92], *399, 404,*
 405
Murphy, R. C., 448[31], *456*
Murphy, S. G., 530[95], *547*
Murray, F. J., 470[28], *480*
Murray, J. E., 485[2], *512*
Murray, M. J., 47[63], *56,* 269[28],
 283
Murray, R., 378[18], 384[18], *399*
Musatti, C. C., 524[40], *544*
Myers, P. A., 476, *482*
Myrvik, Q. N., 10[30], *24, 55,* 84,
 100, 151[19], *158,* 183[18], *187,*
 202[57], *209*
Myrvik, W., 81[32], *99*

N

Nadel, J. A., 219[76,81,82,84,85,86],
 226, 227
Naff, G. B., 166[61], *176*
Nagaishi, C., 75[9], 78[9], 80, 81[9],
 82[9], *97,* 156[37], *159*
Nagashima, H., 501[91], 504[91],
 506[91], *517*
Nagayama, E., 107[28], *127*
Naiman, S., 521[11], *543*
Naimark, A., 21[67], *27*
Nakada, T., 501[92], *517*
Nakamura, K., 107[28], *127,* 391[84],
 404
Nakamura, T., 117[56], *129*
Nash, D. R., 42[26], 48[26,74], *54,*
 57, 68, *71,* 81[35], 95[35], 96[35,
 51], *99, 100*

Naspitz, C. K., 524[40], *544*
Naterman, H. L., 476, *482*
Nathan, D. G., 203[59], *209*
Nattarrlarrier, L., 297[45], *326*
Neidhart, J. A., 528[83], 530[95], *547*
Nelson, B. S., 527[60], *545*
Nelson, H. S., 220[99,100], *228*
Nelson, M., 299[56], *326*
Nelson, N. A., 523[28], *543*
Nemetz, J. C., 487-491[29], *513*
Neva, F. A., 319[144], *332*
Newball, H. H., 3[6], 8[6,14,15], 10[6], 12[6], 15[6], 18[6], 19[15], *23, 24,* 148[15], 155[15], *158,* 357[16], *372*
Newberry, W. M., Jr., 523[31,33], 524[41], *544*
Newcomb, R. W., 14[50], *26,* 50[95], *58,* 214[40], *224*
Newman, L. J., 169[87], *177*
Newman, S. L., 204[64], *209*
Nicklaus, T. M., 269[31], *284*
Niewoehner, D. E., 221[107], *228*
Nigro, S. L., 486[17], 488[34], *513, 514*
Nitz, R. E., 385[56], *402*
Noda, M., 62[17], *70*
Noguchi, P., 186[42], *189*
Noon, L., 462, 471, *478*
Nopajaroonsri, C., 38[16], 44[16], *53,* 68[30], *71,* 80[29], *99*
Nora, J. J., 486[21], *513*
Nordin, A. A., 77[26], 87[26], *98*
Noreen, H., 215[45], *224*
Norico, A. P., 489[65], *516*
Norman, A. P., 213[27], *223*
Norman, M. E., 162[11,18], 171[11], *172, 173*
Norman, P. S., 214[37], *224,* 454[65], *458,* 465[11], 466[12,13,14,15,16, 17], 470[51], 472[44], 473[16, 45], 474[49], 475[53], 476[61, 64], 477[66,69], 478[71], *479, 481, 482, 483*
North, D., 112[50], *129*

North, R. J., 63[20], *70*
Nossal, G. J. V., 74[1], 75[1], 77[24], *97, 98*
Novack, S. N., 254[38], 255[38], *258*
Novey, H. S., 214[29], 218[29], *223*
Nowell, P. C., 255[47], *259*
Nugent, C. G., 107[30], *127*
Nusinoff, S. R., 393[92,94,96], 394[92,96], 395[92], *404, 405*

O

Ochs, H., 124[68], *130*
O'Donnell, T. V., 454[68], *459*
Offen, C. D., 166[65], 168[65], 169[65], *176*
Ogilvie, C., 274[48], *284*
Ohman, J. L., 212[7], 216[58], *222, 225,* 448[28], *456*
Okinaka, A. J., 148[14], *157*
Okon, M., 186[41], *189*
Okudaira, H., 215[49], *225*
Okumura, K., 215[51,52,54,55,56], 216[57], *225*
Okuno, Y., 391[84], *404*
Oliner, H., 274[38], *284*
Oliver, J., 214[35], *224*
Olsen, C. R., 219[76], *226*
Olsen, G. N., 62[18], 63[18], 68[18], *70*
O'Neill, E. F., 358[18], 368[18], 369[18], 371[18], *372*
Oppenheim, E., 291[16], *324*
Oppenheim, J. J., 47[66], *56,* 140[11], *141,* 217[69], *226*
Orange, R. P., 446[19,20], 447[19,20, 21], 448[31,32], 450[20], 451[20, 21,39,40], *455, 456, 457*
Orgel, H. A., 213[27], *223*
Osler, A. G., 446[5,14], *454, 455,* 472[42,43,44], 473, *481*
Orvis, H., 470[28], *480*
Osada, Y., 304[93], 305[93], 313[93], *329*
Osgood, E. E., 300[66], *327*
Oski, F. A., 162[9], 171[9], *172*

Osler, A. G., 163[42], 166[63], 167 [63], *174, 176*
Oster, H. L., 523[28], *543*
Ostertag, M., 425[17], *441*
Oswald, N. C., 290[1], 293[1], 294 [1], *324*
Otter, H. P., 502[95], *518*
Ottinger, B., 415[37], *418*
Ouellette, J. J., 221[104,106], *228*

P

Pabst, H. F., 528[77], 530[101], *546, 548*
Pacheco, G., 292[25], 319[144], *325, 332*
Padgett, G. A., 170[103], *178*
Pain, M. C. F., 212[12], *222*
Paine, J. R., 369[44], *374*
Page, A. R., 162[13], 171[13], *172*
Palade, G. E., 295[42], *326*
Paley, N., 500[86], 502[86], *517*
Palmer, C. E., 522[14], 523[26], *543*
Palmer, J. G., 300[64], 301[64], *327*
Palmer, K. N. V., 212[5], *222*
Pangan, J., 489[51], *515*
Pappagianis, D., 522[19], 531[104], 541[104], *543, 548*
Pappenheimer, A. M., 168[77], *177*
Parish, W. E., 216, 217, *225*, 299[58], 304[101], 307[58,101,117], 310 [129], 313[58], 314[129], *327, 329, 330, 331*, 446[8], *454*
Park, B. H., 192, *205*, 349[37], *352*
Park, C. D., 488[38], 489[38], *514*
Parker, C. D., 212[11], 221[11], *222*
Parker, C. W., 261[8], *282*, 453[51,54, 55], 454[54,76], *457, 458, 459*
Parmely, M. J., 281[78], *286*
Parmley, W. W., 497[79], 501[79], *517*
Paronetto, F., 50[93], *58*, 218[74], *226*, 246[13], *257*
Parrott, R. H., 131[1,2,3], 137[5], 139[8,9,10], *140, 141*, 376[5,6], 378[21], 379[25], 380[25], 382

[Parrott, R. H.]
[25,36,37], 385[54], 386[36,37], 393[95], 396[105], 397[106], *398-400, 402, 405*
Parsons, E. M., 452[43], *457*
Parvu, M., 297[45], *326*
Passalera, A., 217[68], *226*
Patchefsky, A. S., 254[37], *258*
Patterson, G. D., 369[42], *374*
Patterson, H., 86[47], *100*
Patterson, J. F., 243[1], *256*
Patterson, R., 233[17], *241*, 309 [127], 314[127], 320[127], *331, 332*
Pearson, C. M., 254[38], 255[38], *258*
Pearson, F. G., 489[44], *514*
Pearson, R. S. B., 212[9], 218[9], *222*, 454[62], *458*
Peckinpaugh, R. O., 392[91], *404*
Pedreira, A. L., 486[15], 489[15], *513*
Peetermaris, J., 394[99], *405*
Pence, H., 217[63], *226*
Pendharker, M. B., 368[39], 369[39], *373*
Penn, I., 485[5], *512*
Pennington, J. E., 8[20], *24*, 143[3], *157*, 182[12], 185[12], 186[43], *187, 189*, 357[11], 359[11,24], 363[11,24], 366[11,28], 367[11, 29], *372, 373*
Pepys, J., 217[65], *226*, 230-235[1, 6], 237[1,6], 238[1], *240*, 281 [14], *286*, 291[18], 293[29,30], 320[29,30,146], *324, 325, 332*, 454[73], *459*
Perason, F. G., 498[81], *517*
Pereira, H. G., 387[63], *402*
Pereira, R. M., 199[46], 200[46], *208*
Perelman, M. I., 487[32], *514*
Perera, A. B., 319[143], *332*
Perey, D. Y. E., 9[26], *24*, 30[5,6], 31[5,6], 38[6,19], 40[20,22], 42 [19,30], 43[30], 44[5,6,32],

[Perey, D. Y. E.]
45[6], 48[20,32], 49[20,80,81,82, 83], 50[81], *53, 54, 57,* 60[2], 67[28], *69, 71,* 111[47], *129,* 156 [36], *159*
Perez-Guerra, F., 282[95], *287*
Perkins, J. C., 380[27], 382[27], 383 [27], 386[27], *400*
Perkins, H. A., 337[12], 340[12], 342[12], 349[12], 350[39], *351, 353*
Perlman, F., 217[67], *226*
Pernis, B., 61[16], *70*
Persner, P. H., 486[15], 489[15], *513*
Peter, M. E., 491[67], 494[73], 496 [75], 499[67,73], 500[73], 501 [73], 502[96], *516, 518*
Peters, G. A., 214[33], *224*
Petersen, V., 86[47], *100*
Petty, T. L., 219[95], *227*
Pfuetze, B., 220[100], *228*
Phelan, P. D., 212[3], *222*
Phelps, P., 163[28], *173*
Phillips, C. A., 378[19], *399*
Phillips, J. K., 163[39,50,51], *174, 175*
Phillips-Quagliata, J. M., 428[27], *442*
Picken, J. J., 221[107], *228*
Pickering, L. K., 528[80], *546*
Pickering, R. J., 162[13], 171[13], *172,* 193[12], *206*
Pieper, W., 308[119], *330*
Pierce, A. K., 151[16], *158,* 182[9], 183[9], *187,* 368[37,38], *373*
Pierce, D. E., 238[19], *241*
Pierce, N. F., 155[34], *159*
Pierson, R. N., 219[96], *228*
Pierson, W. E., 454[71], *459*
Pietra, G. G., 9[24], *24*
Pihl, E., 295[41], *326*
Pikering, C. A. C., 454[73], *459*
Pines, A., 368[33], 369[33], *373*
Piper, P. J., 452[45], *457*
Pioli, E., 528[63], *545*
Pio Roda, C. L., 499[85,87], *517*
Pirofsky, B., 193[4], *206,* 528[69],

[Pirofsky, B.]
531[69], *546*
Pi-Sunyer, F. X., 219[96], *228*
Pittman, M., 409[8], 410[8], *416*
Pitts, T. W., 8[20], *24,* 182[12], 185 [12], *187,* 366[28], *373*
Plackett, P., 102[7], 105[7], *126*
Platts-Mills, T. A. E., 474[49], *481*
Plotz, P. H., 255[50], *259*
Plucinski, K., 368[33], 369[33], *373*
Pollack, J. D., 388[68], *403*
Pollara, B., 501[91], 504[91], 506 [91], *517*
Pollard, M., 44[42], 45[42], *55*
Polmar, S. H., 196[28,29], 197[28], 198[41], 201[28], *207, 208*
Ponzio, N. M., 304[97], 314[97], 315[97], *329*
Portier, P., 420, *441*
Posner, E., 277[62], *285*
Potter, M., 476[62], *482*
Poupon, M. F., 526[55], *545*
Powell, D. A., 118[60], 124[60], *129*
Prague, K., 526[53], *545*
Prausnitz, C., 421[7], *441*
Prendergast, R. A., 13[49], *26,* 60[6], 65[22], *69, 70*
Prentice, R., 360[27], *373*
Prescott, B., 102[4,5], *126,* 387[65], *403,* 415[37], *418*
Press, P., 526[55], *545*
Prevatt, A. L., 230[10], 232–234[10], 237[10], *241*
Pride, N. B., 454[62], *458*
Priest, R. E., 219[95], *227*
Prignot, J., 10[40], 12[40], *25*
Proniewska, M., 525[51], 526[51], *545*
Pruzansky, J. J., 233[17], *241*
Purcell, R. H., 380[26,29], 382[26], 389[29], *400*
Putnam, C. W., 485[5], *512*
Pyles, G., 131[1], 137[5], 139[8], *140, 141,* 382[37], 386[37], 396 [101], *400, 405*

Q

Quie, P. G., 170[98], *178,* 203[58], 209
Quigley, T. B., 302[79], *328*
Quinn, E. L., 525[48], *544*

R

Raab. S. O., 301[77], 302[77], *328*
Raafat, H., 368[33], 369[33], *373*
Rabellino, E., 193[4], *206*
Rabinovich, S., 412[25], *417*
Rabinovitch, J. J., 487[32], *514*
Rabson, A. R., 204[62], *209*
Rackemann, F. M., 423[14], 435[14], *441*
Rademaker, M., 212[8], *222*
Radice, P., 487[33], *514*
Radl, J., 349[38], *353*
Raff, M., 300[68], *327*
Raffel, S., 521[5], *542*
Rajewsky, K., 77[25], *98*
Ramirez, M. A., 421[6], *441*
Ramirez, R. J., 358[18], 368[18,52], 369[18,32], 371[18], *372, 373*
Randhawa, H. S., 185[39], *189*
Rankin, J., 230[7], 232[7], 233[7], 234[7], 235[7], 237[7], *241*
Rapaport, F. T., 531[103,104], 541 [104], *548*
Raphael, A., 524, *544*
Rapp, D., 472[40], *481*
Rapp, F., 389[72], *403*
Rapp, H. J., 389[72], *403*
Rasmussen, H., 453[48], *457*
Ratnoff, O. D., 166[61], *176*
Razin, S., 124[70], *130*
Rebuck, J. W., 162[4], *172*
Reed, C. E., 212[11], 214[30], 218 [30], 219, 221[11, 104, 106], *222, 223, 227, 228,* 233[17], *241,* 425 [20], *442,* 453[56], *458*
Reed, N. D., 415[39], *418*
Reed, R. E., 522[21], *543*
Reeder, W. H., 290[6], *324*

Rees, R. J. W., 411[15], 412[15], *417*
Reese, D. L., 305[103], *329*
Regan, W., 145[8], *157*
Regula, H., 357[17], 360[17], 366 [17], *372*
Reid, J. L., 131[1], *140*
Reid, L., 498[83], 503[83], 504[83, 100], 506[83,100], 507, *517, 518*
Reinarz, J. A., 197[36], *208*
Remington, J. S., 60[4], *69*
Remmer, H., 266[14], *283*
Remold, H. G., 163[33], *174*
Renold, A. E., 302[79], *328*
Restrepo, A. M., 524[36], *544*
Revillard, J. P., 532[106], *548*
Reynolds, H. Y., 3[6], 8[6,14,15,20], 10[6,28], 12[6,43], 13[47], 15[6], 18[6], 19[15], *23, 24, 25, 26,* 46 [56], *56,* 143[3], 145[5,6,7,12], 146[5,7], 148[5,15], 149[6], 152 [7], 155[5,15,34], *157-159,* 182 [12], 185[12], 186[43], *187, 189,* 335[1,2], *350,* 357[11,16], 359[11, 24], 363[11,24], 366[11,28], 367 [11,29], *372, 373*
Rhodes, J. M., 76[15], *98*
Rhyne, M. B., 466[12], 467[18], 473 [18], *479*
Ribi, E., 61[15], 65[15], *70*
Ricci, M., 217[68], *226*
Rich, A. R., 520[2], 521[6], *542*
Rich, R. R., 201[55], *209,* 528[76], *546*
Richards, K., 489[49], 490[49], 498 [80], *515, 517*
Richardson, J. B., 47[71], *56*
Richerson, H. B., 238[21], *241,* 340 [29], 341[29], *352*
Richet, C., 420, *441*
Richman, D., 394[97], *405*
Richman, S., 282[89], *287*
Ricks, J., 86[47], *100*
Riddle, J. M., 295[37], *325*
Riester, S. K., 409[4], *416*
Rifkind, D., 107[32], *128*

Riggs, D. A., 300[66], *327*
Riggs, J. L., 389[72], *403*
Riley, J. F., 317[140], *331*
Rindge, B., 376[6], *398*
Ringoir, S., 486[24], 503[24], 504 [24], 506[24], 507[24], *513*
Ripe, E., 527[60], *545*
Ritzman, S. E., 197[36], *208*
Rivera, E. C., 339[23], *352*
Rivero, I., 278[67], *285*
Rizzo, A. P., 298[49], 306[49,107], *326, 329*
Roan, J., 182[11], *187*
Robb, P., 200[53], *209*
Robbins, J. B., 19[59], *26,* 155[30], *158,* 193[7,9], 194[9], 198[40], 199[9], 200[7], *206, 208*
Robeledo, S., 524[36], *544*
Roberts, D. H., 181[3], *187*
Roberts, M., 233[17], *241*
Roberts, R. B., 524[37], *544*
Roberts, T. M., 290[1], 293[1], 294 [1], *324*
Robertson, D. G., 454[64], *458*
Robertson, J. S., 301[76], *328*
Robertson, O. H., 182[5,6], *187*
Robin, E. D., 486[8], *512*
Rockey, J. H., 196[31], *207*
Rocklin, R. A., 528[79], *546*
Rocklin, R. E., 217[63], *226,* 268[21], 271[21], *283,* 521, 528[13], 536 [13], 547[13], *543*
Rodin, A. E., 274[50], *284*
Rogers, A. W., 47[61], *56*
Rogers, D. E., 376[4], 377[4], *398*
Roitt, I. M., 217[62], *225,* 336[8], *351*
Rolly, G., 486[24], 503[24], 504 [24], 506[24], 507[24], *513*
Rolph, W. B., 438[38], *443*
Romagnani, S., 217[68], *226*
Romansky, M. J., 377[15], *399*
Rook, A. J., 261[11], 265[11], *282*
Root, R. K., 162[10], 170[10], *172,* 295[33], 298[33], *325*
Rose, B., 212[8], 218[8], *222,*

[Rose, B.]
300[68], *327,* 466[6], *454,* 472 [37], *480*
Rose, D. K., 454[67], *459*
Rose, G. A., 247, 248, 249[14], *257*
Rose, H. D., 143[2], *157,* 368[39], 369[39], *373*
Rose, J., 281[70], *286*
Rose, N. R., 472[40], *481*
Rosen, F. S., 162[15], 171[15], *173,* 194[14,19], 195[19], 199[14], 203[60], 204[62], *206, 207, 208, 209,* 336[8,9], 338[18], 340[30], 341[31], 343[30], *351, 352*
Rosen, V., 497[79], 501[79], *517*
Rosenbaum, M. J., 392[91], *404*
Rosenberger, H. G., 522[18], *543*
Rosenow, E. C., III, 261[3], 269[33], 271[31], 275[3], *282, 284*
Rosenstreich, D. L., 10[29], *24,* 146 [13], *157*
Rosenthal, A. S., 10[29], *24,* 146[13], *157,* 170[92], *177,* 248[26], 255 [42], *258, 259*
Rosenthal, S. R., 411[20], 412[20], *417*
Rosh, W., 489[49], 490[49], *515*
Ross, H., 182[10], *187*
Rossen, R. D., 13[48], *26,* 76[14], 85[14], 95[14], *98,* 255[45], *259*
Roth, J., 196[34], *207*
Rothenberg, S. P., 274[51], *285*
Rouse, B. T., 120[64], *130*
Rowlands, D. R., Jr., 9[22], 10[22], *24*
Rowe, D. S., 14[51], *26,* 50[94], *58,* 214[41], *224,* 336[8], *351*
Rowe, W. P., 376[7], 385[7,58], *398, 402*
Roy, J. C., 368[30], 369[30], 371 [30], *373*
Royal, A. S., 50[88], *57*
Rubin, B. A., 385[57], *402*
Rubin, P., 248[25], *258*
Rubio, F., Jr., 274[38], *284*
Rudders, R. A., 282[93], *287*

Ruddy, S., 163[37,47], *174, 175,* 311
   [134], 314[134], *331*
Rudzik, O., 38[18,19], 40[20], 42
   [19,30], 43[30], 46[58], 47[18,
   58,65], 48[20], 49[20], *53, 54, 56*
Ruegsegger, J. M., 415[38], *418*
Ruff, L. C., 238[20], *241*
Ruff, L. L., 217[70], *226*
Ruikka, I., 269[36], 271[36], *284*
Russell, P. K., 76[19], *98,* 390[75],
   403
Ruth, W. E., 3[1], *23,* 200[50], *208*
Ryan, G. B., 244[7], *257*
Ryan, J. W., 9[23], *24*
Rylander, R., 181[1], 182[1], 183[1],
   186
Ryning, F., 17[53], *26*
Rytömaa, T., 295[38], 300[70],
   301[70], *326, 327*

S

Saarimaa, H., 269[36], 271[36], *284*
Sabesin, S. M., 299[54], *326*
Sackner, M. A., 3[2], *23*
Sagel, S. S., *514*
Saggers, B. A., 356[6,7], 357[16],
   359[7], 360[6], 361[7], *372*
Saenz, C., 162[20], 171[20], *173*
St. Pierre, R. L., 200[52], *209*
Saito, M., 522[19], *543*
Salanitro, A. S., 470[29], *480*
Salem, H., 219[84], *227*
Salisbury, B. G., 9[22], 10[22], *24*
Salmon, P. F., 151[22], *158*
Salmon, S. E., 10[27], *24, 42*[27], 46
   [2], 48[27], *54,* 67[27,29], *70, 71,*
   81[38,39], 82[39], 83[39], 84[39,
   42], 86[38,39], 87[38], 89[39],
   90[38], 95[38], *99, 100,* 340[30],
   343[30], 350[39], *352, 353*
Salvaggio, J. E., 213, *223,* 425, 439
   [23], *442*
Salvaggio, S., 46[51], *55*
Salvin, S. B., 523[30], *543*
Sampson, J. J., 247[18], *257*

Samter, M., 261[8], 266[15], 281[82],
   282, 283, 286, 308[119], 309[126],
   314[126],318[126], *330, 331*
Samuelson, T., 356[9], 357[9], *372*
Sanchez, G. A., 411[19], *417*
Sanchez, M. N., 489[54], *515*
Sandberg, A. L., 163[42], *174*
Sandhy, D. K., 185[39], *189*
Sandhy, R. S., 185[39], *189*
Sanford, C., 500[88], *517*
Sanford, J. P., 151[16], *158,* 182[9],
   183[9], *187,* 368[37,38], *373*
Sanyal, R. K., 220[98], *228*
Sapp, T. M., 305[102,103], 306[107],
   307[115], *329, 330*
Sarauw, A., 369[45], *374*
Sarkany, I., 268[24], *283*
Savinski, G. A., 486[18], *513*
Schade, H., 213, *223*
Schanzer, B., 278[68], *285*
Scherpenisse, L. A., 488[41], 489[41],
   514
Scheukin, M., 338[16], *351*
Schick, P., 491[67], 494[73], 499[67,
   73], 500[73], 501[73], *516*
Schieble, J. H., 378[19], 386[61],
   399, 402
Schild, G. C., 384[50], *401*
Schiller, J. W., 475[55], *482*
Schimke, R. N., 194[17], *206*
Schiffer, L. M., 300[63], *327*
Schlueter, D. P., 217[70], *226,* 230[2,
   14,20], 232-234[2,14,18,20], 237
   [2,14], 238[2,20], *240, 241*
Schmid, F. R., 254[34], *258*
Schmid, K., 340[25], *352*
Schmidt, A. P., 337[13], 349[13],
   351
Schmidt-Nowara, W., 212[7], *222*
Schneider, W. J., 530[102], *548*
Schoeler, K., 31, 42[12], 45[12], *53*
Schonauer, T., 162[11], 171[11],
   172
Schreffler, D. C., 432[29], *442*
Schulkind, M. L., 19[59], *26,* 155
   [30], *158,* 528[78], *546*

Schull, W. J., 248[25], *258*
Schultz, M. G., 193[9], 194[9], 199 [9], *206*
Schumacher, M. J., 343[35], *352*
Schüppel, R., 266[14], *283*
Schur, P. H., 194[19], 195[19], *207*
Schwaber, J. R., 291[20], *325*
Schwartz, D. P., 197, *207*
Schwartz, I. R., 277[54], *285*
Schwartz, M., 213, *223,* 421[8], 423-425[8], 434[8], *441*
Schwartz, M. S., 171[104], *178*
Schwartz, R., 274[38], *284*
Schwartz, R. S., 521[9], 530[95], *542, 547*
Schwartz, T., 523[27], *543*
Schwarz, M. I., 277[58], *285*
Schwindt, W. D., 492[69], *516*
Scott, D. J., 281[85], *286*
Seaman, A. J., 300[66], *327*
Sears, J. W., 197, *208*
Seebach, von, H. B., 31, 42[12], 45 [12], *53*
Seebohm, P. M., 340[29], 341[29], *352*
Seeman, P. M., 295[42], *326*
Segal, M. S., 369[46], *374*
Sehon, A. H., 472[37], *480*
Sell, K. S., 50[88], *57*
Seligmann, M., 336[8,9], *351*
Sellick, H., 219[79,82], *227*
Seltzer, A., 470[28], *480*
Seltzer, H. S., 248[25], *258*
Sen, D. K., 220, *228*
Senterfit, L. B., 107[29], *127,* 376 [11], 387[65], 388[68], *399, 403*
Seravalli, E., 10[36], *25,* 151[21], *158*
Serfling, R. E., 377[13], *399*
Sergievskii, V. S., 486[18], *513*
Settipane, G. A., 214[42], *224*
Severson, C. D., 281[78], *286*
Shackelford, P. G., 528[80], *546*
Shahidi, N. T., 275[19], *283*
Shanmugaratnam, K., 292[25], *325*
Sharma, H. M., 269[35], 271[35], *284*

Sharma, O. P., 525[50], *545*
Sharp, P. M., 3[4], 7[4], 10[4], 12 [4], 15[4], 18[4], *23*
Sharon, M., 44[42], 45[42], *55*
Sharon, N., 44[42], 45[42], *55*
Sheard, P., 446[7], *454*
Shearer, L. A., 386[61], *402*
Sheffer, A. L., 214[36], *224*
Shelanski, M. M., 170[95,96,97], *178*
Sheldon, W. H., 308[122], 314[122], *330*
Sherman, W. B., 213[15], *223,* 471, 472[38], 476[56,57], *480, 481, 482*
Sherwood, R. W., 385[56], *402*
Shilkin, K. B., 498[83], 503[83], 504 [83,100], 506[83,100], 507[100], *517, 518*
Shimada, K., 488[42], 489[46,58], 491 [42,67], 494[73], 496[75], 498 [42], 499[67,73], 500[73], 501 [73,93], *514, 515, 516, 517*
Shin, H. S., 162[23], 163[50,51], 169[84], *173, 175, 177*
Shope, R. E., 184[37], *189*
Shors, E., 489[53], 491[67], 499 [67], *515, 516*
Shortman, K. D., 76[19], *98*
Showell, H. J., 170, *177*
Shulman, N. R., 266[18], *283*
Shultz, J. A., 184[34], *188*
Shumway, N. E., 486, 487[19], *513*
Shur, P. H., 246[11], *257*
Sieber, O. F., 386[62], *402*
Siegel, M., 278[67], *285*
Siegelman, S. S., 489[49,50], 501 [91], 504[91,99], 506[91], *515, 517, 518*
Siirila, L., 489[62], *515*
Siltzback, L. E., 526[52], 527[62], *545*
Silva, J., Jr., 528[81],
Silverman, M., 454[69], *459*
Silverstein, D., 296[43], 302[43], *326*
Simon, A. H., 384[51], *402*

Simon, G. T., 38[16], 44[16], *53,*
68[30], *71,* 80[29], *99,* 293[29],
320[29], *325*
Simons, M. J., 343[35], *352*
Simson, F. W., 31, *53*
Simonsson, B. G., 219[85], *227*
Simpson, R. W., 390[81], *404*
Singal, D., 40[20], 47[69], 48[20,
72], 49[20], *53, 56*
Singer, S. H., 120[65], *130,* 182[14],
186[42], *187, 189*
Singh, S. B., 117[54], *129*
Sinha, S. B. P., 489-491[50,56], *515*
Siskind, G. W., 148[14], *157*
Slavin, R., 233[17], *241*
Slepushkin, A. N., 390[80], 392[80],
404
Slocumb, C. H., 254[35], *258*
Small, P. A., 60[5], *69*
Smalley, R. V., 274[42], *284*
Smiddy, J. F., 3[1,3], *23*
Smith, A. P., 468, *480,* 504[101],
506[101], *518*
Smith, C. B., 106[25], 108[35], *127,
128,* 380[26], 382[26], 383[48],
387[65], 388[69], *400, 401, 403*
Smith, C. E., 522[18,19], 531[104],
541[104], *543, 548*
Smith, C. W., 204[65,66], *209*
Smith, D. T., 412[23], *417*
Smith, D. W., 411[18], 412[18], *417*
Smith, I. M., 412[25], *417*
Smith, J. W., 282[94], *287,* 453[51,
52], 454[54], *457, 458*
Smith, L. A., 504[101], 506[101],
518
Smith, T. J., 380[31], *400,* 420, *441*
Smith, T. K., 523[33], 528[76], *544,
546*
Smith, U., 9[23], *24*
Smith, W. G., 274[41], *284*
Smithwick, E., 217[64], *226*
Smorodincev, A. A., 392[87], *404*
Snell, G. D., 432[29], *442*
Snider, G. S., 368[39], 369[39], *373*
Snyder, A. B., 269[31], *284*

Snyder, E., 359[23], *372*
Snyderman, R., 162[8,22], 163[39,
42,49,50,51,54], 170[102], *172,
173, 174, 175, 178,* 193[12], *206*
Sobeslavsky, O., 102[4,5], *126*
Sobotka, A. B., 214[37], *224,* 470
[51], *481*
Sokal, J. E., 268[23], *283*
Solberg, L. A., 184[36], 185[36],
188
Solomon, A., 13[49], *26,* 60[6], *69*
Solomon, S., 151[24], *158*
Somerson, N. L., 388[67,68], *403*
Sones, M., 525[47], 526[57], *544,
545*
Sonosaki, H., 48[76], *57*
Soothill, J. F., 194[16], 195[21], 196
[16], *206, 207,* 213[27], *223*
Soothill, J. R., 336[8,9], *351*
Soriano, R. B., 204[66], *209*
Sorkin, E., 162[14,25], 163[29,36],
166[29], 169[86], *173, 174, 177,*
310[132], 314[132], *331*
Sosman, A. J., 230[2,5], 232[2,5],
233[2,5,18], 237[2,5], 238[2],
240
Soto, C. S., 215[47], *224,* 447[27],
456
South, M. A., 204[66], *209, 546*
Southern, P. M., 151[16], *158,* 182[9],
183[9], *187*
Spaich, D., 425[17], *441*
Spain, W. C., 422[12], *441*
Spaulding, H., 226[100], *228*
Spears, G. F. S., 454[68], *459*
Spector, S. L., 212, *222*
Spector, W. G., 183[19], 185[19],
188, 244[7], *257*
Speirs, E. E., 303[89], 304[94], *328,
329*
Speirs, R. S., 303[87,88,89,90,91,92],
304[93,94,95,96,97], 305[93],
306[90], 309[96], 313[87,93],
314[95,97], 315[95,96,97], *328,
329*
Spencer, C. S., 48[73], *56,* 81[34],

[Spencer, C. S.]
91[34], *99,* 238[19], *241*
Spencer, H., 30, *52,* 247, 248, 249
[14], *257*
Spencer, J. C., 10[37], *25*
Spicer, S. S., 295[40], *326*
Spieler, P. J., 166[67], *176*
Spier, R., 369[44], *374*
Spink, W. W., 281[81], *286*
Spitler, L. E., 200[49], *208,* 522[23],
523[24], 528[24,68,69,71,72,80,
82,89], 529[90], 531[24,69,105],
538[23], 539[108], 541[24], *543,*
546, 547, 548
Spitz, E., 214[36], *224*
Spitzer, R. E., 163[45], *174*
Spradbrow, P. B., 184[38], *189*
Spring, W. C., 415[36], *418*
Spring-Stewart, S., 393[94], *405*
Spry, C. J. F., 300[72], 301[72,73],
302[73], 308[72,73,122], 314
[122], *327, 330*
Stallone, R. J., *514*
Stallones, R. A., 385[55], *402*
Stamm, S. J., 454[71], *459*
Standord, R. E., 282[92], *287*
Stanley, E. D., 389[73], *403*
Stanton, J. A., 269[27], *283*
Stanworth, D. R., 446[12,13], *455*
Starr, M. S., 477, *482*
Starzecki, B., 75[5], *97*
Starzl, T. E., 485[5], *512*
Stashak, P. W., 415[39], *418*
Stecher, V. J., 162[25], *173*
Stechschulte, D. J., 303[83], 307[83],
328, 448[33], 452[44], *456, 457*
Stechschulte, P. E., 169[83], *177*
Steckler, R., 501[91], 504[91], 506
[91], *517*
Steele, R. W., 338[16], *351*
Steerman, R. L., 162[8], *172*
Steger, L., 184[25], *188*
Stein, E., 522[16], *543*
Steinberg, A. D., 255[50], *259,* 281
[71], 282[88], *286, 287*
Steinberg, P., 107[29], *127,* 387[65],

[Steinberg, P.]
397[107,108], *403, 405*
Steininger, W. J., 521[12], *543*
Stember, R. H., 215[43], *224,* 425,
434[36], 437[36], 439[24], *442,*
443
Stenhouse, A. C., 377[16], *399*
Stern, R. C., 198[41], *208*
Sterner, G., 106[23], 125[71], *127,*
130
Stevens, G. H., 489[54], *515*
Stewart, J. D., 486[13], *512*
Stewart, S. M., 357[10], 358[10],
359[10,25], 360[10,25], 361[10,
25], 362[10], *372, 373*
Stickler, G. B., 269[34], 271[34],
284
Stiehm, E. R., 192[2], 194[15], 200
[51], *205, 206, 208,* 337[14], 339
[20], 340[20], 341[20], 344[14],
351, 528[69], 531[69], *546*
Stier, R. A., 463, *479*
Stifler, W. C., Jr., 422, *441*
Stimpfling, J. H., 432[29], *442*
Stites, D. P., 528[68,69], 531[69],
546
Stitzel, A. E., 163[45], *174*
Stofer, R. C., 486, 487[19], *513*
Stokes, C. R., 213[27], *223*
Stokes, P. E., 171[104], *178*
Stone, R. M., 489[44], *514*
Stone, S. P., 200[47], *208,* 214[38],
224
Stott, E. J., 378[19], *399*
Strachan, A. S., 31, *53*
Strandberg, J. D., 499[85,87], *517*
Straub, M., 523[27], *543*
Strauss, E., 413, *417*
Strauss, L., 246[13], 249, *257, 258*
Strauss, M. B., 476, *482*
Strauss, W. G., 269[29], *283,* 291[19],
324
Strober, W., 49[79], *57,* 200[54],
201[54], *209,* 340[26], *352*
Stroud, R., 171[106], *178*
Struth, A. G., 204[64], *209*

Stryckmans, P. A., 300[63], *327*
Stuart-Harris, C. H., 376[3], 377[3], *398*
Stull, A., 471[31,32,35], 476[51], *480, 482*
Suby, H. I., 277[59], *285*
Sukeno, T., 501[92], *517*
Sulitzeanu, B. D., 29[1], *52*
Sullivan, A. L., 215, *224*
Summers, R., 220[100], *228*
Sunderman, F. W., 290[14], *324*
Sunderman, F. W., Jr., 290[14], *324*
Surgenor, D. M., 340[25], *352*
Surprenant, E. L., 214[29], 218[29], *223*
Suter, E., 520[3], *542*
Suzuki, C., 497[79], 501[79,92], *517*
Svegaard, A., 349[37], *352*
Swan, A. V., 467[19], *479*
Swanson, R., 528[77], *546*
Swarson, R., 360[27], *373*
Swedlund, H. A., 196[27], *207*
Swedlund, H. H., 214[33], *224*
Sweetnam, M. T., 277[62], *285*
Swenson, E. W., 7[9,10], 18[10], *23,* 62[18], 63[18], 68[18], *70*
Switzer, W. P., 184[24], *188*
Symmers, W. St. C., 278[66], 282[99], *285, 287*
Szentivanyi, A., 219, *227,* 425[19], 439[19], *442,* 453[50], *457*
Szidon, J. P., 9[24], *24*
Szymanska, D., 186[41], *189*

T

Tada, T., 50[92], *58,* 215[51-55], 216[56,57], *225*
Takaro, T., 504[99], *518*
Talbot, C. H., 309[127], 314[127], *331*
Tam, E. M., 60[6], *69*
Tamlyn, T. T., 151[22], *158*
Tammeling, G. J., 488[41], 489[41], *514*
Tamplin, B., 219[84], *227*

Tamura, E., 107[28], *127*
Tan, E. M., 13[49], *26*
Taniguchi, M., 215[51,53], 216[56], *225*
Taplin, G. V., 487-491[29,46,61], *513, 515*
Taranta, A., 10[36], *25,* 151[21], *158*
Taswell, H. F., 337[13], 349[13], *351*
Tauber, A. I., 452[44], *457*
Taylor, B., 213, *223*
Taylor, G., 118, 120[62], *129*
Taylor, H. C., 411[17], *417*
Taylor, R. B., 77[25], *98*
Taylor-Robinson, D., 118, 120[61,62], *129,* 182[13], 184[13], 185[13], *187*
Tee, D. E. H., 504[100], 506[100], 507[100], *518*
Tennant, F. S., Jr., 281[77], *286*
Tennenbaum, J. I., 200[52], *209*
Teres, D., 368[40], 369[40], 371[40], *373*
Terrel, E. E., 182[15], *187*
Terry, W. D., 194[18], 195[18], 196 [28,29], 197[28], 201[28], *206, 207*
Tevethia, S. S., 117[54], *129*
Thiede, W. H., 230[12,13], 232-234 [12,13], 237[12,13], *241*
Thomas, E. D., 502[94], *517*
Thomas, G. D., 368[38], *373*
Thomas, L., 298[47], *326,* 528[88], *547*
Thomas, W., 521[11], 522[11], *543*
Thompson, G. R., 282[96], *287*
Thompson, H., 184[29], *188*
Thompson, J. S., 230[10], 232-234 [10], 237[10], *241,* 281[78], *286*
Thompson, R. A., 310[133], 314[133], *331*
Thompson, R. B., *547*
Thompson, R. E., 10[28], 12[43], *24, 26,* 46[56], *56,* 145[5,6,7], 146[5, 7], 148,[5], 149[6], 152[7],

[Thompson, R. E.]
155[7], *157,* 335[1,2], *350*
Thor, D. E., 528[81], 538[81], *546*
Thorn, G. W., 302[79], *328*
Thorne, M. G., 411[20], 412[20], *417*
Thurman, G. B., 338[16], *351*
Tierney, D. F., 184[32], *188,* 489[47, 48], *515*
Tierney, E. L., 393[94], *405*
Tillett, W. S., 531[103], *548*
Tillotson, J. R., 143[1], 151[1,23], *157, 158,* 368[35], 369[35], *373*
Tisi, G. M., 489-491[39], *514*
Tivey, H., 300[66], *327*
Togo, Y., 383[46,47], *401*
Tokiwa, Y., 219[84], *227*
Tomasi, T. B., Jr., 13[44,45,49], 17 [52], 19, 21[52], *25, 26,* 46[54], *56,* 60[3,6], *69,* 82[40], *99,* 112 [49], *129,* 246[10], *257,* 381[34], *400*
Tomioka, H., 446[16,18], *455*
Toogood, J. H., 454[67], *459*
Top, F. H., Jr., 380[31], 390[75], *400, 403*
Topilow, A. A., 274[51], *285*
Topilsky, M., 526[52], *545*
Torisu, M., 168[74], *176,* 312[136], *331*
Tormey, D. C., 277[58], *285*
Torres, E. J., 60[5], *69*
Torres, M., 504[99], *518*
Torres, J. M., 524[38], *544*
Tosh, F. E., 524[11], *544*
Touraine, J. L., 532[106], *548*
Townley, R. G., 17[53], *26*
Travis, L. B., 274[50], *284*
Trenkner, E., 186[41], *189*
Trentin, J. J., 304[95,96], 309[96], 314[95], 315[95,96], *319*
Trier, J. S., 200[51], *208*
Truitt, G. L., 10[33], *25,* 65[25], 66 [25], *70,* 151[20], 156[20], *158*
Trummer, M. J., 486[9,10], 489-491 [39,60], *512, 514, 515*

Tuchman, H., 290[11], *324*
Tucker, A. D., 76[13], 79[13], *98*
Tucker, D. N., 380[27], 382[27], 383 [27], 386[27], *400*
Tully, J. G., 184[25], *188*
Turk, A., 474, *481*
Turner, D., 497[78], *516*
Turner, F. N., 75[6], 90[6], 92[6], 94[6], *97*
Turner, H. C., 389[72], *403*
Turner, K., 50[84], *57*
Turner, M. W., 213[27], *223*
Turner, M. X., 303[90,92], 306[90], *328*
Tyrrell, D. A. J., 378[19], 384[50], 390[78,80], 391[84,86], 392[80], *399, 402, 404*

U

Unanue, E. R., 76[18], *98*
Undery, D., 76[13], 79[13], *98*
Unger, G., 230[3], 232[3], 233[3], 234[3], 237[3], *240*
Unger, J. D., 230[3], 232[3], 233[3], 234[3], 237[3], *240*
Urbach, F., 526[57], *545*
Uroma, E., 340[25], *352*
Utz, J. P., 524[42], *544*
Uvnas, B., 448[30], *456*

V

Vaerman, J. P., 13[46], *25,* 337[14], 344[14], *351*
Vaissalo, T., 269[36], 271[36], *284*
Valentine, F. T., 46[50], *55,* 528[88], 530[102], *547, 548*
Valentine, M. D., 448[32], *456*
Vallet, L., 340[27], *352*
Van Arsdel, P. P., Jr., 296[43], 302 [43], *326,* 454[71], *459,* 472, *481*
Van Bekkum, D. W., 349[38], *353*
Van Dellen, R. G., 214[33], *224*
Van Der Broek, A. A., 497[76], 502 [76], *516*

Van der Veen, J., 376[8], 379[8],
  399
Vander Veer, A., 422, *441*
Vandiviere, H. M., 412[21], *417*
Van Dura, E. A., 48[75], *57*
Van Furth, R., 9[25], *24*, 155[27],
  158
Van Kirk, J. E., 382[42], *401*
Van Loghem, E., 349[38], *353*
Van Melve, T., 454[65], *458*
Vannier, W. E., 13[48], *26*
Verdaman, T. H., 120[66], *130*
Varekamp, H., 293[28], *325*
Vargosko, A. J., 376[6], 385[54],
  398, 402
Van Rood, J. J., 347[38], *353*
Vascoboinic, E., 394[99], *405*
Vasquez, J. J., 218, *226*
Vaughan, J., 50[91], *58*
Vaughan, W. T., 423[15], *441*
Vaughn, J. H., 218[72,73], *226*, 278
  [69], 279[69], *286*
Vaz, N. M., 426[25], 428[26,27],
  431[26], 433[33], *442*
Vazquez, J. J., 246[12], 248[20],
  257
Veith, F. J., 486[11,12], 489-491[49,
  50,56,80,82], 501[91], 503[12,
  82,98], 504[82,91,99], 506[91],
  507[98], *512, 515, 517, 518*
Velo, G. P., 183[19], 185[19], *188*
Vercauteren, R., 295[36], *325*
Vermeire, P., 486[24], 503[24], 504
  [24], 506[24], 507[24], *513*
Vernon-Roberts, B., 76[16], *98*
Versieck, J., 486[24], 503[24], 504
  [24], 506[24], 507[24], *513*
Verwey, W. F., 355[1], 357[1,12],
  358[1], *371, 372*
Vigna, F., 524[38], *544*
Vilira, L., 527[62], *545*
Viola, M. V., 321[150], *332*
Virchow, C., 14[51], *26*, 50[94], *58*,
  214[41], *224*
Viswanathan, R., 319[145], *332*
Vivona, S., 384[51], *402*

Vogel, H., 290[7], *324*
Von Maur, R. K., 474[49], *481*
Von Muller, C., 529[90], *547*
Von Wichert, P., 489, *515*
Vossen, J. M., 349[38], *353*
Vosti, K. L., 60[4], *69*
Voyce, M. A., 195[21], *207*
Vrints, L., 486[24], 503[24], 504
  [24], 506[24], 507[24], *513*
Vuillard, P., 487[33], *514*
Vyas, G. N., 337[11,12], 340[12],
  342[12], 349[12], *351*

W

Waaij, van der, D., 349[38], *353*
Wagner, O. A., 488[40], 489[40],
  491[66], *514, 516*
Wahren, B., 214[34], *224*
Waindorff, J. A., 425[22], *442*
Wakim, K. G., 247[17], *257*, 278[64],
  285
Waksman, B. H., 244, *257*, 311[135],
  314[135], *331*
Waldhausen, J. A., 488[38], 489[38],
  514
Waldman, R., 213[20], *223*
Waldman, R. H., 10[31,32,37], 14[51],
  25, 26, 42[25], 48[25,73], 50[94],
  54, 56, 58, 60[5,7], 61[7,14], 62
  [7,14,18], 68[7,18], *69, 70*, 81
  [33,34], 95[34], *99*, 118[59], *129*,
  214[41], *224*, 238[19], *241*, 381
  [35], 383[46], *400, 401*
Waldmann, T. A., 196[28,29], 197[28],
  200[54], 201[28,54], *207, 209*,
  340[26], *352*
Walker, G. R., 486[20], *513*
Walker, J. L., 452[45], *457*
Walker, W. H. C., 195[21], *207*
Wall, R. L., 274[42], *284*
Wallace, J. H., 5[7], *23*
Walls, B. E., 388[67], *403*
Walls, R. S., 308[123,124,125], 314
  [123,124,125], *330, 331*
Walsh, R. E., 282[95], *287*

Walter, J. E., 524[41], *544*
Walzer, P. D., 193[9], 194[9], 199[9], *206*
Wanner, A., 3[2], *23*
Wara, D. W., 350[39], *353*
Ward, H. N., 281[79], *286*
Ward, H. P., 282[92], *287*
Ward, L. E., 247[17], *257*
Ward, P. A., 162[21,24], 163[24,32, 33,52,53], 165[21], 166[32,62, 64,65,69], 168[32,65,74], 169[53, 65,87,88,89,], 170[32,99,100,101], 171[24,53,107], *173-178*, 244[4]. 255[40], *256, 258*, 303[85], 306 [111], 310[111,131], 312[85,136], 313[85], 314[131], *328, 330, 331*
Wardell, J., Jr., 86[47], *100*
Warfield, M. S., 385[55], *402*
Warner, H. R., 171[105], *178*
Warner, N. L., 120[64], *130*
Warr, G. A., 3[4,5], 7[4,5], 10[4], 12[4], 15[4], 18[4,5], *23,* 168 [76], *177*
Warrell, D. A., 454[64], *458*
Warren, B. A., 492[70], *516*
Wasserman, S. E., 450[34], *456*
Wasserman, S. I., 168[73], 169[81], *176,* 310[130], 314[130], *331*
Watson, D., 145[8], *157*
Watson, K. A., 412[21], *417*
Weaver, D. K., 203[59], *209*
Webb, D., 529[90], *547*
Webb, J. K. G., 292[24], *325*
Webb, W. R., 486[20], *513*
Webster, R. G., 377[17], 378[17], *399*
Wedgwood, R. J., 336[9], *332*
Wehrle, P. F., 408[3], *416*
Weigle, W. O., 248[20], *257*
Weinberg, A. C., 528[75], *546*
Weiner, E., 5[8], *23*
Weingarten, R. J., 292[22], *325*
Weinstein, L., 355[3], 356[9], 357 [9,14], 358[3], *371, 372*
Weinstock, M., 477, *482*
Weiss, A. P., 162[17], 171[17], *173*

Weiss, H., 282[98], 290[12], *324*
Weissman, G., 166[63,67], 167[63, 71], *176,* 244[5], 255[44], *257, 259*
Wells, E., 500[88], *517*
Welsh, R. A., 299[59], 313[59], *327*
Wenck, U., 303[87], 313[87], *328*
Wenzel, F. J., 230[8], 232-234[8,16], 237[8,16], *241*
Wenzel, R. P., 380[27], 382[27], 383 [27], 386[27], *400*
Werb, Z., 21[65], *27*
West, B. C., 294[32], *325*
Western, K. A., 193[9], 194[9], 199 [9], *206*
Wetherbee, R. E., 381[32], *400*
Weyman-Rzucidlo, D., 186[41], *189*
Whang-Peng, J., 140[11], *141*
Whatley, S., 120[66], *130*
Whitcomb, M. E., 261[5], 277[58], *282, 285,* 521, 528[13], 536[13], 537[13], *543*
White, A., 145[10], *157*
White, P. H., 492[68], 494[68,74], 500[89], *516, 517*
White, R. J., 107[29], *127,* 376[11], *399*
Whitehair, C. K., 44[33,34], *34*
Whiting, E. G., 522[18], *543*
Whitman, V., 198[41], *208*
Whur, P., 47, *56*
Wicher, K., 281[83], *286,* 299[57], *327*
Wickramasinghe, S. N., 300[65], *327*
Widdecombe, J. G., 219[79,81,82,83], *227*
Wiebel, R. E., 384[49], *401*
Wide, L., 446[10], *455,* 474[50], *481*
Wiener, E., 255[41], *258*
Wiesandenger, T., 487[33], *514*
Wieser, O., 357[17], 360[17], 366 [17], *372*
Wigley, F. M., 213[20], *223*
Wiik, A., 349[37], *352*
Wildevuur, C. R. H., 487-489[25,41, 64], 493[64], 497[76,77], 501[25],

[Wildevuur, C. R. H.]
502[76,77], 503[25], 504[25],
513, 514, 516
Wiles, C. E., Jr., 486[13], *512*
Wilkins, J., 408[3], *416*
Willett, F. M., 291[16], *324*
Williams, H. R., Jr., 355[1], 357[1,12],
358[1], *371, 372*
Williams, J., 528[63], *545*
Williams, M., 526[52], *545*
Williams, R. C., 155[35], *159*
Wilson, A. F., 214[29], 218[29], *223*
Wilson, I. D., 19[60], *26*, 155[31],
159
Wilson, M. S., 217[67], *226*
Wilson, R., *546*
Wiltshaw, E., *547*
Windhorst, D., 171[106], *178*
Winkelstein, J. A., 204, *209*
Winkenwerder, W. L., 465[11], 466
[15,16], 472[44], 473[16,45],
476[61,64], 477[66], *479, 481,
482, 483*
Winn, W. A., 522[20], *543*
Winterton, M. C., 504[101], *518*
Wintrobe, M. M., 171[105], *178*, 255
[39], *258*, 301[77], 302[77], 321
[152], *328, 332*
Witebsky, E., 369[44], *374*
Wochtel, H. L., 247[18], *257*
Wolfe, H. I., 470[29], *480*
Wolff, S. M., 170[103], *178*, 248[24,
26], 249[24], 254[24], 255[24,50,
51,52], *258, 259*, 294[32], 295[33],
298[33], 301[75], 321[151], *325,
327, 332*
Wolfson, J. J., 203[58], *209*
Won, W. D., 182[10], *187*
Wong, V. G., 255[50], *259*
Wood, C. B. S., 214[35], *224*
Wood, D., 220[100], *228*
Wood, S. C., 131[3], *141*, 377[15],
399
Wood, S. H., 60[5], *69*
Wood, W. B., 415, *418*
Woodend, W. G., 396[103], *405*

Woodhour, A. F., 384[49], *401*
Woodin, W. G., 261[6], *282*
Woodliff, H. J., 274[49], *284*
Woodruff, C. E., 521[12], *543*
Woodson, M., 19[58,61], *26*, 155[29],
158
Wordburg, M. A., 438[38], *443*
Worthington, J. W., 247[17], *257*,
278[64], *285*
Wray, B. B., 195[22], *207*
Wright, D. G., 166[68,70], *176*, 290
[10], *324*
Wright, N. G., 184[29], *188*
Wright, P. F., 139[9], *141*, 396[102,
103,104,105], *405*
Wu, L. Y. F., 350[40], *353*
Wundt, W., 357[17], 360[17], 366
[17], *372*
Wünschmann, B., 166[66], *176*
Wyatt, J. H., 76[13], 79[13], *98*
Wybran, J., *547*

Y

Yagle, E. M., 525[48], *544*
Yakerski, Y., 489[54], *515*
Yakulis, V. J., 102[9], 105[9], *126*
Yamomoto, K., 61[15], 65[15], *70*
Yarzobal, L. A., 524[38], *544*
Yeh, J. T. T., 487[31], *514*
Yoffey, J. M., 42[24], *54*
Yoneti, M., 501[92], *517*
Yoshida, T., 48[76], *57*, 168[74],
176, 312[136], *331*
Youmans, A. S., 411[14], *416*
Youmans, G. P., 411[14], *416*
Young, J. E., 357[10], 358[10], 359
[10], 360[10], 361[10], 362[10],
372
Young, R. D., 385[60], *402*
Young, S. H., 217[64], *226*
Yount, W. J., 194[20], *207*
Yu, D. Y. C., 219[78,80], *226*
Yuan, L., 530[94], *547*
Yunginger, J. W., 214[39], *224*
Yunis, E. J., 215[45], 217[66], *224*,

[Yunis, E. J.]
226, 350[40], *353*
Yurchak, A. M., 281[83], *286*

Z

Zack, M., 522[16], *543*
Zaky, D. A. 394[97], *405*
Zamura, R., 487[26], *513*
Zbar, B., 389[72], *403*
Zeek, P. M., 247[19], *257*
Zeiss, C. R., 233[17], *241*
Zhdanov, V. M., 390[77], 394[77], *403*

Zigmon, S. H., 163[31], 166[31], *174*
Zimmerman, A. L., 60[4], *69*
Zimmerman, J., 217[64], *226*
Zipursky, A., 19[62], *26,* 46[57], *56*
Zucker-Franklin, D., 295[34], 298 [47], *325, 326*
Zurier, R. B., 166[67], *176*
Zvaifler, N. J., 166[64], *176*
Zweiman, B., 526[58], 529, 530[93], *545, 547*
Zwi, S., 219[76], *226*

SUBJECT INDEX

A

Activated macrophages, 153
Adenovirus, 380
Adenyl cyclase, 450
Adjuvants for vaccines, 384
Alpha 1-antitrypsin, 11, 17
Allergic granulomatosis, 249
Allergic rhinitis, 419
Allergy
  to drugs (hypersensitivity, 262
  genetics, 213, 412
  genetics in mouse model, 426
Alveolar macrophages
  afferent limb of immunity, 84
  human respiratory, size, 5
  in immunodeficiency, 202
  intracellular survival of organisms,
    184
  phagocytosis of *pseudomonas,* 144
  receptors, 7
Antibiotics
  aerosol usage, 368
  concentration in sputum and bron-
    chial secretions (Table),
    364

Antibodies
  functions of immunoglobulin
    classes, 192
  homocytotropic, 215, 216, 305,
    446
  local respiratory to respiratory
    syncytial virus, 139
  to mycoplasma in humans, 107,
    124
  to mycoplasma in respiratory tract,
    105, 106
  opsonic activity of IgG and IgA,
    149
  to *pseudomonas* in rabbits, 146
  serum antibodies to viruses, 379
  in serum to respiratory syncytial
    virus, 136
Antilymphocyte serum, 118
Asthma, 211, 419, 445
  autonomic mechanisms, 219
  cause of hypersensitivity lung dis-
    ease, 229
  infections, 221
  pathology and physiology, 212,
    218
  pulmonary eosinophilia, 292

[Asthma]
    release of mediators, 445
Aspergillus, 232
    pulmonary hypersensitivity, 293
Atopy, 212, 213
    definition of, 420
Autoimmunity in IgA deficiency, 197

B

Basophils, 215
    IgE binding, 446
B-cells (dog lung), 83
β-adnergic blockade in asthma, 453
Blocking antibody
    IgG following immunotherapy, 474
    in vitro, 472
    in vivo, 472
Blood-bronchus barrier, 356
Bone marrow transplantation, 337,
    349
Bronchiolitis, due to respiratory syncy-
    tial virus, 136
Bronchoalveolar junction, to demarcate
    upper and lower respiratory
    tract, 78
Bronchial lavage
    procedure, 4
        in animals, 81
        in humans, 4
Bronchospasm related to drugs, 281
Busulfan-lung, 275

C

Cell-mediated immunity
    in allergic diseases, 217
    in blastomycosis, 524
    in cryptococcosis, 524
    in histoplasmosis, 523
    to mycoplasma infections, 106
    in rabbit respiratory tract to
        Pseudomonas, 151
    in respiratory tract (review), 61
    in sarcoidosis, 525
    in tuberculosis, 520

[Cell-mediated immunity]
    viral and mycoplasma infection,
        381
Chemotaxis, 161, 170
    of eosinophils, 302
Chronic granulomatous disease, 202
Clearance of particles from respiratory
    tract, 78
Cold-hemagglutinins, 105
Complement
    chemotactic factors, 163, 203
        in immunodeficiency, 203
    phagocytosis, 203
        receptors on alveolar macro-
        phages, 8
    quantitation in bronchial fluids, 19
        in human respiratory tract, 10
Cyclic AMP, 450
Cyclic GMP, 451
Cyclic nucleotides, 170
    in asthma, 220
Cyclophosphamide, 254
    as cause pulmonary disease, 275
Cystic fibrosis, 17
    serum inhibitor, 205
Cytology
    for diagnosis of busulfan or cyclo-
        phosphamide lung, 276

D

Diplococcus pneumoniae, 184
Disodium chromoglycate, 454
Drug-induced pulmonary disease,
    Table of, 270
Drug induced systemic lupus erythe-
    matosus, 277

E

Eosinophils
    cellular mechanisms, 314
    chemotaxis of, 302
    chemotactic factors for (ECF-A,

[Eosinophils]
    ECF-C, ECF-p, ESP, 303
    inhibition of allergic inflammation, 299
    kinetics of, 300
    phagocytosis, 297
    in pulmonary diseases, 290
    releasing factor, 302
Eosinophil chemotactic factor of
    anaphylaxis, 448
Experimental models
    for IgE (reagin), 426
    for mycoplasma disease, 108
    for pheumonia, 181
    Pseudomonas infections in rabbits, 143
    to study eosinophilia, 308

F

Fetal liver transplant, 350
Fibrinolytic system
    in chemotaxis, 165

G

Gamma globulin, intravenous preparations, 342
Gamma globulin therapy, 340
Genetic recombinant virus, 391
Granulocyte transfusion in experimental pneumonia, 185
Granulomatous response in lung, 248

H

Histamine, 446, 448, 472
Histamine sensitizing factor, 409
Hypersensitivity to drugs, as drug allergy, 262
Hypersensitivity pneumonitis, 230
    due to aspergillus, 293
    etiologic agents, 230
    immunologic features, 237
    pulmonary function, 233

I

Immune deficiency, 191
    and cell mediated immune functions, 198
    hypogammaglobulinemia, 336
    lack of immunoglobulin and antibodies, 193
    passive antibody therapy, 336
    therapy by cellular reconstitution, 337
Immune response to pneumococcal polysaccharides, 415
Immune response gene
    in man, 433
    in mice, 428, 432
Immunization with BCG, 411
Immunoglobulin A
    histamine release, 474
    IgA producing cells in BALT, 43, 48
    in immunodeficiency, 195, 336
    local immunity in viral disease, 381
    T-cells and IgA synthesis, 49
Immunoglobulin E
    in allergic diseases, 214, 215, 419
    in BALT, 50
    in human respiratory secretions, 15
    in immunodeficiency, 195
    mediator release in asthma, 446, 474
Immunoglobulin G
    in BALT, 43, 49
    biologic properties of subclasses, 194
    mediator release in animals, 447
    subclasses in human respiratory secretions, 11
Immunoglobulin M
    in BALT, 43, 49
    cold-hemagglutinin with mycoplasma, 105
Immunoglobulins
    in human respiratory tract, 10

[Immunoglobulins]
quantitation IgA, IgG, IgE, 13
Immunoglobulin therapy, 193
Immunosuppression
effect on mycoplasma disease with
antilymphocyte serum,
118
Immunotherapy, 461
adverse effects, 475
for allergic rhinitis in adults,
466
with allergoids, 477
of bacterial allergy, 468
in children, 467
effect on IgE, 474
of house dust allergy, 467
long acting extract preparations,
476
Immunization of respiratory tract
with mycoplasma, 101
with sheep erythrocytes (SRBC),
74
with SRBC in dogs, 89
with SRBC in rabbits, 87
Influenza A virus, antigenic shift, 377,
384

K

Kinin system
in chemotaxis, 165

L

Lipopolysaccharide
chemotaxis, 165
from *Pseudomonas,* 145
Loeffler's pneumonia, 247
due to parasites, 290
Lung transplantation
bronchostenosis, 498
in humans, 503
immunosuppression, 501
lung preservation, 489, 509
reimplantation response, 490
rejection response, 492, 506, 509

[Lung transplantation]
technical considerations, 487
Lymphocytes
B and T cells in BALT, 40
human respiratory, 5, 9
Lymphoid tissue
BALT
in chicken, 31
in hamsters, 111
in rabbit, 31
bronchus-associated lymphoid
tissue (BALT), 30, 80, 111
Lymphomatoid granulomatosis, 249

M

Mast cells
IgE, 446
in lung tissue, 47
Mehotrexate-induced lung disease, 277
Methylxanthines, effect on cyclic
AMP, 450
Methysergide-induced lung fibrosis,
277
Migration-inhibition factor (MIF), 42
to *Pseudomonas* in rabbits, 151
Mycoplasma pneumoniae, 101, 184
pathogenesis, 121

N

Nitrofurantoin-induced pneumonitis,
269

O

Opsonic antibodies, 149

P

Periarteritis nodosa, 247, 294
Phagocytosis
associated processes, 202
by eosinophils, 297
Plasma transfusion, 335, 338, 343
adverse reactions to, 339

Prostaglandins, 452
Proteins in respiratory tract
    human, 10
    antibodies to mycoplasma, 106
    Pseudomonas antibodies in rabbits,
        146
Pseudomonas aeruginosa, 143
Pseudomonas vaccine to immunize
        rabbits, 145
Pulmonary eosinophilia, 290
    with asthma, 292
    due to drugs, 290
    due to parasites, 290
Pulmonary infections
    gamma globulin therapy in immuno-
        deficiencies, 340

R

Respiratory infection
    in immunodeficiency diseases, 192
Respiratory syncytial virus, 131
    immunity to, 136, 380
    pathogenesis, 140

S

Serum sickness, 247
Sinopulmonary infections related to
        IgA and IgE, 195
Slow-reacting substance of anaphylaxis,
    446, 448
Sputum, antibiotic levels, 364
Steroids
    in treatment of pulmonary hyper-
        sensitivity vasculitis, 254
Surfactant, 20

T

T-cells (dog lung), 83
    summary of functions, 60
Temperature sensitive virus mutants
    influenza vaccine, 390
    mycoplasma, 397
    respiratory syncytial virus, 396
Thermophilic actinomycetes
    in hypersensitivity pneumonitis,
        230
Thymus transplantation, 338
Tissue levels of antibiotic, factors which
        affect, 356
Transfer factor, 519, 528
    as chemotactic stimulus, 168
    in treatment of coccidioidomycosis,
        358
    in treatment of sarcoidosis, 526
    in treatment of tuberculosis, 536
Tuberculosis, 184, 410, 520

V

Vasculitis, 243
    in eosinophilic pneumonias, 291
Viral agents causing lower respiratory
        tract disease, 376
Viral-bacterial respiratory infection,
    184

W

Wegener's granulomatosis, 248